ADHD in Adults

ADHD
IN ADULTS

WHAT THE SCIENCE SAYS

Russell A. Barkley

Kevin R. Murphy

Mariellen Fischer

THE GUILFORD PRESS
New York   London

© 2008 The Guilford Press
A Division of Guilford Publications, Inc.
72 Spring Street, New York, NY 10012
www.guilford.com

Printed in the United States of America

This book is printed on acid-free paper.

Last digit is print number: 9 8 7 6 5 4 3

Library of Congress Cataloging-in-Publication Data
Barkley, Russell A., 1949–
   ADHD in adults : what the science says / Russell A. Barkley, Kevin R. Murphy,
Mariellen Fischer.
      p. ; cm.
   Includes bibliographical references and index.
   ISBN-10: 1-59385-586-9 ISBN-13: 978-1-59385-586-4 (cloth : alk. paper)
   1. Attention-deficit disorder in adults. I. Murphy, Kevin R. II. Fischer, Mariellen. III.
Title. IV. Title: Attention deficit hyperactivity disorder in adults.
   [DNLM: 1. Attention Deficit Disorder with Hyperactivity—psychology. 2. Adult.
3. Attention Deficit Disorder with Hyperactivity—diagnosis. 4. Data Interpretation,
Statistical. 5. Longitudinal Studies. WM 190 B256ab 2007]
   RC394.A85B37 2008
   616.85′89—dc22

                                                        2007028826

To our wives, Patricia Barkley and Bonnie Murphy,
in gratitude for their love, support,
and creation of a home and family life
within which we could achieve our dreams
—RUSSELL A. BARKLEY AND KEVIN R. MURPHY

With deep appreciation to the participants in our studies,
who generously and courageously opened their lives to us
so that we all might better understand
—MARIELLEN FISCHER

About the Authors

Russell A. Barkley, PhD, is Clinical Professor of Psychiatry at the Medical University of South Carolina in Charleston and Research Professor of Psychiatry at the State University of New York Upstate Medical University in Syracuse. He was previously Director of Psychology and Professor of Psychiatry and Neurology at the University of Massachusetts Medical School in Worcester (1985–2002), where a portion of the original research reported in this volume was conducted. A diplomate in three specialties (Clinical Neuropsychology, Clinical Psychology, and Clinical Child and Adolescent Psychology, ABCN, ABPP), he has published extensively on attention-deficit/hyperactivity disorder (ADHD) over his 30 years of conducting scientific research on the disorder and related topics. Dr. Barkley served as the principal investigator on the two large research projects reported in this volume (clinic-referred adults with ADHD and hyperactive children grown up) and has received numerous awards from professional associations for his scientific and clinical contributions and for the public dissemination of psychological science.

Kevin R. Murphy, PhD, is founder and Director of the Adult ADHD Clinic of Central Massachusetts in Northborough. He was previously Director of the Adult ADHD Clinic and an Associate Professor of Psychiatry at the University of Massachusetts Medical School in Worcester (1990–2002). He has published extensively on adults with ADHD, often with Dr. Barkley, and consults to numerous legal, educational, and commercial organizations on the clinical diagnosis and management of ADHD in adults. Dr. Murphy served as the coinvestigator on the research study of clinic-referred adults with ADHD reported in this volume and conducted the clinical evaluations of all of the adults in that project.

Mariellen Fischer, PhD, is a pediatric neuropsychologist and Professor in the Division of Neuropsychology, Department of Neurology, at the Medical College of Wisconsin in Milwaukee. A diplomate in Clinical Neuropsychology, ABPP/CN, Dr. Fischer has published numerous articles on ADHD, developmental psychopathology, and neuropsychology. She and Dr. Barkley have reported the earlier results of the Milwaukee longitudinal study of hyperactive children, the adult outcome of which is presented in this book. Dr. Fischer served as coinvestigator and the Milwaukee site principal investigator on the longitudinal study reported in this volume.

Acknowledgments

The research reported here was supported by two grants from the National Institute of Mental Health to Russell A. Barkley while he was at the University of Massachusetts Medical School. The opinions expressed here, however, do not necessarily represent those of the funding institute. We are exceptionally grateful to Tracie Bush for her assistance with the evaluation of the research participants in the study of clinic-referred adults with ADHD reported here and with their data entry. We also wish to thank Laura Montville for her administrative and data entry assistance on this same project. We are just as grateful to Lorri Bauer, Kelli Douville, and Cherie Horan for their assistance with the evaluation of the adult (mean age 27 years) research participants in the Milwaukee longitudinal study reported here; to physician assistants Hope Schrader and Kent Shiffert for their help with participant health evaluations; and to Peter Leo for assistance with data entry. We wish to thank Michael Gordon for his comments on the first three chapters of this book and, more generally, for challenging us to address clinically important controversies using the science-based results of these large research studies and the scientific literature. Last, but hardly least, is the encouragement and support we received from Kitty Moore and Seymour Weingarten at The Guilford Press for this book and for their agreement with the necessity of placing both research studies in the context of each other and the larger scientific literature relevant to both clinic-referred adults with ADHD and children growing up with ADHD.

Contents

Contents

CHAPTER 1

Introduction

Over the past 20 years, a relatively small but increasing body of scientific literature has begun to emerge on the nature of attention-deficit/hyperactivity disorder (ADHD) as it appears in adults who are self-referred to clinics (see Goldstein & Ellison, 2002; Spencer, 2004). While one might view this rather limited body of literature as being of little consequence, given the thousands of studies on ADHD in children in comparison, there is reason to suspect that adults with ADHD will not manifest identical problems to those seen in children having ADHD. The results of numerous longitudinal studies following ADHD (hyperactive) children to adulthood also suggest that they are not identical to self-referred adults diagnosed with ADHD. While it is clear that both groups experience the same disorder (O'Donnell, McCann, & Pluth, 2001; Wilens, Faraone, & Biederman, 2004), differences in comorbidity and other associated conditions and risks may differ significantly. That is one of the major topics of this book. It compares the results of an extensive evaluation of clinic-referred adults with ADHD, employing both a clinical and a community control group, to the results of the Milwaukee longitudinal study of hyperactive (ADHD combined type) children followed to adulthood (mean age 27 years), also involving a community control group, on many of the same measures. To our knowledge, this is the first and only such study or book to do so, giving a unique glimpse at the similarities and differences between these two populations of adults with ADHD.

Popular books on the subject of adults with ADHD abound, based largely on clinic-referred adults (Hallowell & Ratey, 1994; Kelly & Ramundo, 1992; Murphy & LeVert, 1995; Nadeau, 1995; Solden, 1995; L. Weiss, 1992), and a few clinical textbooks for professionals have also emerged (Gordon & McClure, 1996; Goldstein & Ellison, 2002; Nadeau, 1995; Wender, 1995; Weiss, Hechtman, & Weiss, 1999). But for all their good intentions, much of what is contained in most of these books is based solely on clinical experience

1

with self-referred adults, often seen in specialty practices and garnered without the benefit of scientific methods. Many of the assertions, especially those made in the popular trade books, about the nature of clinic-referred adults diagnosed with ADHD have not been put to the empirical test of controlled scientific research. For instance, some authors claim that adults with ADHD are more intelligent, more creative, more "lateral" in their thinking, more optimistic, more entrepreneurial, and better able to handle crises than those without the disorder. Similar advocates of adult ADHD have gone so far as to assert that the disorder conveys some positive benefit. To our knowledge, none of these claims have any scientific support at this time. Most, in fact, are refuted in this book. The information obtained from such clinical cases is also fraught with various confounding variables, not the least of which are referral bias and the effects of comorbid psychiatric disorders frequently associated with ADHD. Useful as clinical cases may be initially, when a vacuum exists in scientific information about a disorder, such case reports still remain, for better or worse, purely anecdotal. More scientifically oriented studies of samples of clinic-referred adults with ADHD have been published in the past 15 years, however. Also, many longitudinal studies of children with ADHD/hyperactivity have now followed them into adulthood, reporting their findings during this same period. The results of both types of research underscore both the legitimacy and the specificity of this diagnosis in adults while providing no support for the view that ADHD produces positive benefits in adults with the disorder (Spencer, 2004; Wilens et al., 2004). This is not to say that adults with ADHD do not have positive attributes; they certainly do. Rather, such attributes likely have nothing to do with their disorder. Nearly everyone possesses a profile of hundreds of psychological traits, including both numerous strengths and many weaknesses relative to the norm. Greater care must be taken in not attributing these strengths (or all weaknesses) to the presence of ADHD in an adult.

The overarching aim of this book is to report the results of two of the largest and most comprehensive studies of adults with ADHD conducted to date, juxtaposing the results for clinic-referred adults with the disorder against those for children with the disorder who have reached young adulthood. As noted above, one of these studies compared large samples of clinic-referred adults diagnosed with ADHD to both a large control group of adults having other disorders seen at the same clinic and to a large community control group. This project is referred to here as the UMASS Study, named for the University of Massachusetts Medical School where it was conducted. We here integrate those results with the small but growing literature on ADHD in adults and formulate what we believe are the clinical implications of those findings and the relevant literature for the diagnosis and management of adults with ADHD. The major purposes of that research project were to:

- Conduct a comprehensive study of the symptom presentation of ADHD in the adult stage of life as it occurs among clinic-referred adults so as to determine which symptoms were most likely to differentiate this population from clinic-referred adults without ADHD and community control adults.
- Examine the frequency of symptoms of ADHD from DSM-IV-TR (*Diagnostic and Statistical Manual of Mental Disorders*, 4th edition, text revision; American Psychiatric Association, 2000) across groups to determine the relative utility or predictive accuracy of these symptoms for adults with ADHD, since they were originally and exclusively developed in the study of children with the disorder (Lahey et al., 1994).
- Evaluate a large pool of new and potentially useful symptoms reflecting the adult stage of the disorder apart from those presented in the DSM-IV-TR.
- Reduce this pool of items to a limited set having the greatest utility for distinguishing adults with ADHD from a control group of other clinic-referred adults having other disorders (mostly anxiety and depression) and from a general community control group.
- Determine the necessity or diagnostic utility of specifying an age of onset of symptoms producing impairment by 7 years, as set forth in the DSM-IV-TR, and determining if another age of onset would be more useful for diagnosis.
- Better understand the other psychiatric disorders and psychological maladjustment most likely to be associated with ADHD in adults (comorbidity) as compared with these two control groups.
- Examine the specific impairments that ADHD is likely to produce across the major life activities characteristic of adult adaptive functioning, with specific attention to education, occupational and social functioning, marital adjustment, financial functioning, driving, criminal activity and drug use and abuse, and current health lifestyles.
- Assess the general cognitive and neuropsychological deficits that may be specifically associated with ADHD in adults relative to that functioning evident in the two control groups noted above, with specific attention given to the executive functions of sustained attention, behavioral inhibition, working memory, and problem solving.
- Analyze the extent to which women with ADHD may differ from men with the disorder apart from those more general sex differences that arise in the general adult population.
- Evaluate the risk of psychological maladjustment in the offspring of these adults with ADHD relative to that in the two control groups noted above.
- Formulate research and clinical recommendations from these findings that may serve to guide future studies of adults with ADHD as well as to improve their clinical assessment and management.

This book also reports the results of a second substantial study: the adult follow-up of one of the larger longitudinal studies of hyperactive (ADHD combined type) children followed into adulthood, known as the Milwaukee Study, so named for the city where it was conducted. The major purposes of that research project at this follow-up point were very similar to those of the UMASS Study described above. Specifically those purposes were:

- To conduct a comprehensive study of the symptom presentation of ADHD in the adult stage of life as it occurs among adults who, as children, were clinic-referred, rigorously diagnosed with the disorder, and thereafter followed; as above, the aim was to determine which symptoms were most likely to differentiate this population from community control adults. In doing so, we further subdivided these ADHD subjects into those who continued to meet criteria for the disorder as adults and those who no longer did so.
- To examine the frequency of symptoms of ADHD from DSM-IV-TR across the ADHD and control groups to determine the relative utility or predictive accuracy of these symptoms. The current DSM-IV-TR symptoms for ADHD were originally and exclusively developed on and for children with the disorder (Lahey et al., 1994); therefore, their utility for identifying adults with ADHD remains unproven.
- As in the UMASS Study, we evaluated the same large pool of new and potentially useful symptoms reflecting the adult stage of the disorder for their utility in identifying adults with ADHD—in this case, those who had grown up with the disorder diagnosed in childhood. Similarly, we reduced this pool of items to a limited set having the greatest utility for distinguishing adults with ADHD from our control groups in that study.
- Again, to determine the necessity or diagnostic utility of specifying an age of onset of symptoms producing impairment by 7 years, as set forth in the DSM-IV-TR, and whether another age of onset would be more useful for diagnosis. Given that all of the children with ADHD in the Milwaukee Study were required to have an onset of their symptoms prior to 6 years of age to enter the study, it is important to evaluate the accuracy of their own recall of symptom onset if the DSM-IV-TR age-of-onset criterion is to be extended to adult clinical diagnosis.
- To further understand the other psychiatric disorders and psychological maladjustments most likely to be associated with ADHD in children growing up with the disorder who continue to have it in adulthood as compared with the two control groups (children with ADHD who no longer qualify for the diagnosis as adults and community control children followed to adulthood).
- To examine, as above, the specific impairments that ADHD is likely to produce across the major life activities characteristic of adult adaptive functioning, with specific attention to education, occupational and social functioning,

marital adjustment, financial functioning, driving, criminal activity, drug use and abuse, and current health lifestyles. The Milwaukee Study, in fact, not only took a more detailed health history of its participants than did the UMASS Study but also conducted various blood and urine analyses to further document current health status, making it the first study of which we are aware to examine this topic in adults who grew up with ADHD. From these results, one can begin to obtain some idea of the future medical risks that may be associated with the disorder and take a first glimpse of the impact that ADHD may have on life expectancy.

• To assess the general cognitive and neuropsychological deficits that may be specifically associated with ADHD in adults who grew up with the disorder relative to the functioning evident in the two control groups noted above, with specific attention to the executive functions of sustained attention, behavioral inhibition, working memory, and problem solving.

• Last, as above, to formulate research and clinical recommendations from these findings that may serve to guide future studies of children growing up with ADHD as well as to improve their clinical assessment and management as adults.

Unlike the UMASS Study, the Milwaukee Study did not contain a sufficiently large sample of females in either the hyperactive ($n = 20$) or control group ($n = 5$) to permit reliable conclusions to be reached on sex differences that may be specific to the former group. Therefore, while some comparisons of males and females in this study are reported herein, specifically within the hyperactive groups who do and do not have ADHD at follow-up, we urge caution in placing much confidence in those findings until they can be replicated by much larger studies. We also did not examine the psychiatric status or psychological adjustment of the offspring of our hyperactive and control groups at this outcome. Only half (48%) of the hyperactive group had children, many of whom were too young to reliably document psychiatric status by current measures, while most of the control group (87%) had not yet had children. We hope to continue to track the existence and whereabouts of these offspring for evaluation in a later follow-up of these samples.

There are numerous reasons why clinic-referred adults with ADHD would differ from children growing up with the disorder, despite having the disorder in common. An obvious one is that not all of the children diagnosed in childhood with ADHD (then called hyperactivity or hyperactive child syndrome) would be expected to qualify for the clinical diagnosis as adults. As a group, then, one might expect the children with ADHD to be functioning better in various domains of major life activities than would the clinic-referred adults, all of whom currently have the disorder. For this reason, we will break out those hyperactive children in the Milwaukee Study who have ADHD at the adult follow-up from those who no longer qualify for the disorder so as to permit a more direct comparison of the former group to the clinic-referred adults with ADHD in the UMASS Study. Of course it is also possible that the children growing up with the disorder may have a worse condition or greater impairments, given that they likely had an earlier onset of their disorder or were brought into clinics for treatment much earlier than most clinic-referred adults. An earlier age of onset or earlier age of referral for a mental disorder may indicate greater severity. That is, it is possible that the children growing up with ADHD may have worse outcomes than clinic-referred adults being newly diagnosed with the disorder. Another reason this may be the case is that self-referred adults may, by this fact, be more concerned about their current adjustment and have greater psychological awareness of the condition and impairments that led them to seek treatment. As we shall see, most children growing up with ADHD are not seeking current treatment and may be less likely to recognize or accept that they even have a disorder once they leave their parents' home. It was, after all, their parents (and often teachers) who referred them for treatment as children, not themselves. For these and other reasons, it would seem to be extremely informative to contrast the nature of ADHD and its comorbid disorders and impairments as seen in clinic-referred adults with the same sort of information obtained from those who grew up with ADHD, having been diagnosed in childhood. This is why we have chosen to combine both of these large research projects into a single book, offering for the first time an opportunity to compare directly these two groups of adults.

We do not address the etiologies of ADHD in this book. These have been extensively researched in children with ADHD; that literature is reviewed elsewhere (Nigg, 2006). Genetic contributions are the most prominent domain of etiology in this disorder, followed in importance by acquired injuries or adverse developmental influences of varying sorts on the developing brain. We see little reason why these same etiologies would not apply to adults, with the possible exception that acquired injuries to the nervous system may account for an increasing number of cases of ADHD across development, thereby representing a somewhat greater proportion of the adult ADHD than the child ADHD population. This would result from the greater time frame over which such etiologies, such as accidental injuries or poisonings known to exist in child ADHD, have an opportunity to operate on adults. We also do not evaluate the standard available treatments for ADHD in adults, as these have been addressed elsewhere (Barkley, 2006). The medication treatments effective for child ADHD have been found to be just as applicable to the adult stage of the disorder. Counseling, workplace accommodations, cognitive-behavioral therapy, and other psychological therapies have some utility as well and are addressed in the text by Barkley (2006). What we do strive to address here are the clinical implications for diagnosis and management that arise from the numerous results of the two large projects reported here, some of which point to a need for additional treatment approaches in dealing with the various adaptive living impairments we have identified.

We are most grateful to the National Institute of Mental Health (NIMH) for its generous support of these two projects. The UMASS Study involved the better part of 4 years of research (2000–2003), while the Milwaukee Study has been going on since its inception in 1977–1980, with the most recent follow-up conducted from 1999 to 2003. Add to this the more than 2 years it has taken to enter and clean data and analyze all of the results of these two large projects—as well as to prepare this book—and you have some idea of the time and effort we have dedicated to it. We are most grateful for the NIMH and university support we have received along the way.

We could have chosen to present these findings in numerous smaller articles focused on highly specific topics or sections of our database published in various scientific journals. We elected not to do so for several reasons. Not the least of these is that such piecemeal publication, driven by space shortages in journals, would necessitate scattering these findings in small portions across as many as 20 different journals. That would make it very difficult for anyone, including our-selves, to appreciate the larger picture that these results paint for our scientific and clinical understanding of ADHD as it presents in adults. This is especially so for juxtaposing the results for clinic-referred adults against those of individuals who have grown up with the disorder. It would also have made it inconvenient for scientific and clinical colleagues as well as interested students to find those various articles so as to possess the totality of our results and gain this larger, multifaceted perspective. It would, moreover, have taken at least 5 more years to prepare, submit, revise, resubmit, and eventually publish the numerous papers that could have been derived from these two large projects, ensuring that our findings would grow progressively more dated (if not stale) over this period. This drawn-out process would surely have made our results of far less assistance to the field than this current comprehensive presentation of our findings. Finally, publication in journals would have been exceptionally limiting with regard to deriving the numerous clinical implications that arise from such a project; to appreciate them fully requires the perspective of the totality of the results of both projects and the relevant literature. For these and other reasons we have opted to publish these projects in book form. We are most grateful to The Guilford Press for allowing us to do so.

In bypassing the more traditional route of journal publications of our find-ings, however, we recognize that we have also bypassed a critical stage in the publication of scientific findings—the stage involving the peer review process. Clinical books written on ADHD adults do not need to undergo such peer review process, although one wishes at times that they would do so. But scien-tific studies, their methods, analyses, and findings demand such review to provide some assurance of their integrity. In an effort to at least partially address this issue, we will make the entire database from these two projects (in SPSS format) available to any practicing scientist who purchases this book in order to allow those interested to confirm our findings or to conduct further analyses of the data from these publicly funded projects. We extend this courtesy to fellow scientists only because of the necessary expertise required to understand these methods, procedures, analyses, results, and so on. To obtain the datasets, such currently practicing scientists should contact the first author at *russellbarkley@earthlink.net*, providing a cover letter explaining their scientific background, the purpose of the request, and the proposed plan for use of the databases. In making the data available, we recognize that others may wish to pursue additional analyses and even publications from those analyses beyond those we have presented here. If so, we require that permission to do so be obtained in writing in advance of such analyses and publication from the first author (*russellbarkley@earthlink.net*) and that the source of the databases (this textbook) be fully acknowledged in any such publications. For further information on making such requests, contact the first author (R. A. B.), who is the final arbiter for the release of these databases to others.

While we report the results of these original research projects, we strive to do so in a manner that is more easily read and digested than is typical of the format of most scientific journals. So that the flow of the text and the story we wish to tell is not unnecessarily impeded by methodology, measures, and statistics, we will follow a somewhat different format from that used in journal publication. Nearly all of the results are presented in tables and supplemented in some cases with figures, so that they may be readily visible and appreciated. For our scientific colleagues, we provide, beneath each table in a footnote format, the statistical methods used to derive those tabled results. This should allow the clinical or general readers to bypass such information ordinarily provided in the text in pursuing the more clinically informative story line we wish to retain in the text. For similar reasons, we provide descriptions of the measures that we collected in this project in gray-shaded sidebars, such that the scientific reader interested in those details about the particular measures under discussion may have that information available. We believe that this does not detract from the reasoning and general flow of the ideas we present for our clinical readers. We hope that this approach to formatting of this book and specifically our methods, findings, and conclusions will prove satisfactory to the diverse audiences we are striving to reach (scientists, clinicians, students, and the educated general audience).

CHAPTER 2

History and Prevalence
of ADHD in Adults

A Brief History of ADHD in Adults

The history of ADHD for the childhood stage of the disorder is extensive and is discussed in detail by Barkley (2006). Far less exists concerning the history of ADHD in adults, largely because, for most of the past century, ADHD was widely held to be strictly a disorder of childhood. While popular interest in the possibility that adults can have ADHD most likely originated with the bestseller *Driven to Distraction*, published in 1994 by psychiatrists Edward Hallowell and John Ratey, clinical and scientific papers acknowledging the existence of an adult version of this disorder date back at least 40 years and possibly even a century.

In his series of three published lectures to the Royal College of Physicians, George Still (1902) described 43 children in his clinical practice having serious problems with sustained attention and in the moral control of their behavior. By the latter symptom, Still meant the regulation of behavior relative to the moral good of all. He viewed the latter construct as a conscious comparative process in which one evaluates both the present and likely future consequences of one's actions both for oneself and others prior to choosing a course of action. Most of his patients were not only inattentive and lacking in forethought but also quite overactive. In addition, many were often aggressive, defiant, resistant to discipline, and excessively emotional or "passionate," showing little "inhibitory volition" over their behavior. A penchant for "lawlessness," spitefulness, cruelty, and dishonesty was also evident in a significant subset of his clinical sample, heralding the now well-established association of the ADHD triad of symptoms of inattention–hyperactivity–impulsivity with conduct disorder. He proposed that immediate gratification of the self was the "keynote" quality of these and other attributes of these children. And among all of them, passion (or heightened emotionality) was the most commonly observed attribute and the most noteworthy. Still noted further that a reduced sensitivity to punishment characterized many of these cases, for they would be punished, evenly physically, yet engage in the same infraction within a matter of hours. Still believed that the major "defect in moral control" so typical of these cases was relatively chronic. While it could arise from an acquired brain defect secondary to an acute brain disease and might remit on recovery from the disease, in most cases it was chronic. Here, then, likely arises the first mention that ADHD may persist into adulthood, thereby logically opening the door to the possibility, at least, that adults can possess this same pattern of symptoms dating back to their childhood.

Acknowledging that George Still may have first signaled the possibility that adults could have ADHD as an outcome of its chronic childhood course, the first papers on actual adults having ADHD seem to date to the late 1960s. At that time, the disorder was known as minimal brain damage or dysfunction (MBD), and its likely existence in adults arose from three sources. The first was the publication of several early follow-up studies demonstrating the persistence of symptoms of hyperactivity/MBD into adulthood in many cases (Mendelson, Johnson, & Stewart, 1971; Menkes, Rowe, & Menkes, 1967). The second source was the publication of research showing that the parents of hyperactive children were likely to have been hyperactive themselves and to suffer in adulthood from sociopathy, hysteria, and alcoholism (Cantwell, 1975; Morrison & Stewart, 1973). Later papers would further confirm this familial association of hyperactivity in which the biological parents of such children were also abnormal in their attention, impulse control, and activity levels (Alberts-Corush, Firestone, & Goodman, 1986). This early work began to suggest that children with ADHD symptoms were likely to have parents with ADHD symptoms logically implying that ADHD could therefore exist in adults.

The third source of evidence implying the existence of ADHD in adults was the publication of studies on samples of adult patients who were believed to have hyperactivity or MBD. The first of such papers appears to have been that of Harticollis (1968), who focused on the results of neuropsychological and psychiatric assessments of 15 adolescent and young adult patients (ages 15–25) seen at the Menninger Clinic. The neuropsychological performance of these patients suggested evidence of MBD or moderate brain damage. Their behavioral profile suggested many of the symptoms that Still initially identified in his own child cases, particularly impulsiveness, overactivity, concreteness, mood lability, and proneness to aggressive behavior and depression. Some of these individuals appeared to have demonstrated this behavior uniformly or consistently since childhood. Using psychoanalytic theory, Harticollis speculated that this condition arose from an early and possibly congenital defect in the ego apparatus in interaction with busy, action-oriented, successful parents. In short, an inborn error of cognition interacts with a particular pattern of child rearing by parents to result in the condition of MBD.

A year later, Quitkin and Klein (1969) described two behavioral syndromes in adults that may be related to MBD. The authors studied 105 patients at the Hillside Hospital in Glen Oaks, New York, for behavioral signs of "organicity" (brain damage). They searched for behavioral syndromes that might be considered soft neurological signs of central nervous system (CNS) impairment as well as the results of electroencephalographic (EEG) examination, psychological testing, and clinical presentation and history that might differentiate these patients' disorders from other types of adult psychopathology. They selected those cases having a childhood history suggesting CNS damage, including the early hyperactive and impulsive behavior which they believed might reflect the likelihood of such damage. These patients were further sorted into three groups based on current behavioral profiles: those having socially awkward and withdrawn behavior ($n = 12$), those having impulsive and destructive behavior ($n = 19$), and a "borderline" group that did not fit neatly into these other two groups ($n = 11$). The results indicated that nearly twice as many of these "organic" groups had EEG abnormalities and impairments on psychological testing, indicating organicity, as did the control group. Noteworthy for our purposes was their finding that an early history of hyperactive–impulsive–inattentive behavior was highly predictive of placement in the adult impulsive–destructive group, implying a persistent course of this behavioral pattern from childhood to adulthood. Of the 19 patients in the impulsive–destructive group, 17 had received a clinical diagnosis of character disorder (primarily emotionally unstable types) as compared to only 5 in the socially awkward group (which were of the schizoid and passive dependent types).

These results were in conflict with the widely held belief at the time that hyperactive–impulsive behavior tended to wane in adolescence. Instead, the authors argued that some of these children continued into young adulthood with this specific behavioral syndrome. Quitkin and Klein (1969) also took issue with Harticollis's psychoanalytic hypothesis that demanding and perfectionistic child rearing by parents was causal of or contributory to this syndrome, given that their impulsive–destructive patients did not uniformly experience such an upbringing. In keeping with Still's original position that family environment could not account for this syndrome, the authors hypothesized "that such parents would intensify the difficulty, but are not necessary to the formation of the impulsive–destructive syndrome" (p. 140) and that the "illness shaping role of the psychosocial environment may have been over-emphasized by other authors" (p. 141). Treatment with a well-structured set of demands and educational procedures as well as with phenothiazine medication was thought to be indicated.

The first paper to focus specifically on adult cases defined as MBD, as opposed to the earlier and more general concept of "organicity," may have

been that by Shelley and Reister (1972). These authors described 16 individuals seen at an Air Force training base psychiatric clinic (ages 18–23) because of
difficulties coping with their military basic training. These patients were
described as having marked difficulties concentrating, being emotionally labile,
fearing their loss of impulse control, and showing marked irritability as well as
anxiety and self-depreciation. Problems with poor motor skills and sluggish
reaction or response timing were noteworthy. While EEG and neurological
exams were normal for gross findings of hard neurological signs, all patients
showed "soft" signs of "neurointegrative disturbances" such as motor clumsiness, poor balance, confused laterality, and poor coordination. Psychological
testing also revealed evidence of perceptual-motor problems and motor inco-
ordination and timing. On history, 14 of the 16 patients reported difficulties
with temper tantrums and low frustration tolerance as children, with 12 (75%)
reporting behavior consistent with hyperkinetic behavior syndrome, among
other early behavioral symptoms. Over the ensuing 30 years, these problems
with motor development and coordination have been well documented in
children with ADHD (Barkley, 2006).

The following year, Anneliese Pontius (1973) summarized her clinical
observations of more than 100 adults with MBD. She proposed that many such
adults demonstrated hyperactive and impulsive behavior and that their disorder
likely arose from frontal lobe and caudate dysfunction. This would lead to "an
inability to construct plans of action ahead of the act, to sketch out a goal of
action, to keep it in mind for some time (as an overriding idea) and to follow it
through in actions under the constructive guidance of such planning" (p. 286).
Moreover, if adult MBD arises from dysfunction in this frontal-caudate network,
it should also be associated with an inability "to re-program an ongoing activity
and to shift within *principles* of action whenever necessary" (p. 286). She went on
to show that indeed adults with MBD demonstrated such deficits, indicative of
dysfunction in this brain network. Such observations would prove quite pro-
phetic. Two decades later, research demonstrated reduced size in the prefrontal–
caudate network in children with ADHD (Castellanos et al., 1996; Filipek et al.,
1997). And theories of ADHD argued that the neuropsychological deficits associated with it involved the executive functions, such as planning, the control of
behavior by mentally represented information (working memory), rule-governed
behavior, and response fluency and flexibility, among others (Barkley 1997a,
1997b).

Morrison and Minkoff (1975) would subsequently argue that adult patients
with explosive personality disorder or episodic dyscontrol syndrome may well
represent the adult outcome of the hyperactive child syndrome. By 1976, Mann
and Greenspan proposed that adults having MBD constituted a distinct diagnostic
entity (adult brain dysfunction), which they illustrated with two of their clinical

cases. They believed that MBD adults shared a basic impairment in attention and that they were also likely to manifest problems with hyperactivity, impulsiveness, depression, and anxiety. They recommended the use of Leon Eisenberg's (1973) behavior questionnaire for hyperactive child syndrome as part of the diagnostic workup, a rating scale actually developed by C. Keith Conners, who at the time was working with Eisenberg and whose rating scale would later become a mainstay of the evaluation of hyperactive children (Barkley, 1981). Mann and Greenspan also found that these symptoms were responsive to antidepressant medication (imipramine) or stimulants, echoing the same suggestion made earlier by Hans Huessy (1974). In a letter to the editor of a journal he suggested that both antidepressants and stimulants may be the most useful medications for the treatment of these hyperkinetic or MBD adults.

Around this time, the first truly scientific evaluation of the efficacy of stimulants with adults with MBD was conducted by Wood, Reimherr, Wender, and Johnson (1976). They used a double-blind, placebo-controlled method to assess response to methylphenidate in 11 of 15 adults with MBD followed by an open trial of pemoline (another stimulant) and the antidepressants imipramine and amitriptyline. The authors found that 8 of the 11 tested on methylphenidate had a favorable response, whereas 10 of the 15 tested in the open trial showed a positive response to either the stimulants or antidepressants. Others in this decade and into the next would also make the case for the existence of an adult equivalent of childhood hyperkinesis or MBD and the efficacy of using stimulants and antidepressants for its management (Gomez, Janowsky, Zetin, Huey, & Clopton, 1981; Mann & Greenspan, 1976; Packer, 1978; Pontius, 1973; Rybak, 1977; Shelley & Reister, 1972). Yet it would not be until the 1990s that both the lay public and the professional field of adult psychiatry would begin to seriously recognize the adult equivalent of childhood ADHD on a more widespread basis and to recommend stimulant or antidepressant treatment in these cases (Barkley, 1994, 1998; Spencer et al., 1995; Wender, 1995). Even then there remained skeptics concerning whether or not adults could have ADHD or should be treated for it (Shaffer, 1994).

Gomez and colleagues later published a study of 100 adult psychiatric patients, of whom 32% showed signs of childhood hyperactivity, attention deficits, and impulsivity compared to just 4% of a control group (Gomez et al., 1981). These investigators reported that 20% also had symptoms consistent with adult hyperkinetic syndrome, compared to none of their control group. The highest incidence of these symptoms was found in patients who traditionally would have been diagnosed as having a character disorder (47% had childhood and current signs of hyperkinetic syndrome). This study suggests that a sizable minority of adults evaluated at a psychiatric clinic were likely to have a childhood history of hyperkinetic syndrome and that perhaps one in five currently did so at clinical evaluation.

Another historical advance worth noting here is the initial development of diagnostic criteria for ADHD in adults. Besides initiating the first scientifically based study of medication treatment for ADHD noted earlier, Paul Wender was also the first to offer explicit criteria for the manner in which the diagnosis of ADHD in adults should be made. At the time this position was at odds with prevailing clinical opinion that children outgrew the disorder. Wender (1995) recognized that diagnostic criteria proposed for the syndrome of childhood hyperactivity (as in DSM-II; American Psychiatric Association, 1968) or the later attention-deficit disorder (as in DSM-III; American Psychiatric Association, 1980), were not developmentally appropriate for adult patients. While both recognized that ADHD might be a residual condition in some adults and that it could be diagnosed as such, the widespread existence of the full disorder in adults was not recognized at the time, nor were explicit criteria provided for doing so. Based on his empirical work, Wender developed an approach for the diagnosis of ADHD in adults (Wender, 1995) that was subsequently used in a number of research projects, especially medication trials. Patients and an additional informant, preferably a parent, are interviewed to assess retrospectively the childhood diagnosis of ADHD. Evidence is also obtained for continued impairment from hyperactive and inattentive symptoms. Seven symptoms were proposed to characterize the phenomenology of adult ADHD, namely (1) inattentiveness, (2) hyperactivity, (3) mood lability, (4) irritability and hot temper, (5) impaired stress tolerance, (6) disorganization, and (7) impulsivity. Known as the Utah criteria, these diagnostic guidelines required a retrospective childhood diagnosis, ongoing difficulties with inattentiveness *and* hyperactivity, and at least two of the remaining five symptoms. Wender also developed a rating scale, the Wender Utah Rating Scale (WURS), to aid in the retrospective diagnosis of childhood ADHD (Ward, Wender, & Reimherr, 1993). The WURS is a self-completed report of retrospective childhood behavioral symptoms. To its credit, the Utah approach to adult ADHD established the need for retrospective childhood diagnosis, careful elucidation of current symptoms, and the routine use of third-party informants of childhood and adult behavior. These stipulations have become standard practice for many clinicians and investigators, including ourselves.

Although it was clearly an advance in the diagnosis of ADHD in adults in view of their being no such guidelines prior to 1993 for doing so, Wender's approach would later be argued to be problematic for ongoing research and clinical work (McGough & Barkley, 2004). With subsequent editions of the DSM, the Utah criteria have diverged further and further from the current clinical conceptualizations of ADHD. It is difficult to apply knowledge derived from the study of child ADHD diagnosed by DSM to adults identified with alternative diagnostic schemes like the Utah criteria. By design, the Utah criteria include only individuals with lifelong inattention and hyperactivity and therefore exclude patients with the predominately inattentive ADHD subtype. Conversely, al-

though symptoms of irritability and hot temper were included in early concep-
tions of childhood ADHD, substantial research shows this dimension of behavior
to be semi-independent of ADHD symptoms, to have different associated
impairments, to be more closely associated with problems in the social environment, and to predict different developmental outcomes than do the symptoms of
ADHD (Hinshaw, 1987; Loeber, Burke, Lahey, Winters, & Zera, 2000). Permitting symptoms of irritability and hot temper to qualify a patient for the disorder creates an automatic confound of ADHD with oppositional defiant disorder,
conduct disorder, and possibly the mixed-mood dysphoric form of bipolar disorder. Likewise, the inclusion of symptoms of mood lability without additional
clarification may further confound the delineation of this disorder from other
mood disorders in adulthood. The Utah criteria exclude the diagnosis of ADHD
with coexisting major depression, psychosis, or severe personality disorder.
While these restrictions can be useful in research studies of medication response,
they will fail to diagnose significant numbers of patients who are clearly impaired
and would benefit from treatment. Studies indicate that a significant minority of
children and adults with ADHD are likely to have major depression or dysthymia
(20–27%) and personality disorders (11–24%) by adulthood (Barkley, 2006;
Fischer, Barkley, Smallish, & Fletcher, 2002; Murphy & Barkley, 1996). Likewise, adults who self-refer to clinics specializing in adult ADHD may have even
higher rates of anxiety disorders and depression than do children with ADHD
followed to adulthood (Murphy & Barkley, 1996a; Shekim, Asarnow, Hess,
Zauha, & Wheeler, 1990). A further problem with the criteria was the initial lack
of adequate norms for adults on the WURS in order to determine more precisely
an appropriate, empirically based cutoff score for developmental deviance of
symptoms as opposed to those proposed initially, which were based on the developers' clinical experience. For these reasons, the Utah criteria have declined in
use among investigators and clinicians in favor of the more current DSM-IV criteria (see Chapter 3). Later and better-constructed scales with adult norms, such
as those developed for adults by Conners, Erhardt, and Sparrow (1998) or those
more closely aligned with the DSM symptom lists, such as the scales offered by
Brown (1996) and ourselves (Barkley & Murphy, 1998, 2006), would offer
DSM-based criteria as alternatives to the WURS for clinical practice.

Also of historical significance was the first neuroimaging study of adults with
ADHD conducted by Zametkin and colleagues, published in 1990. These
researchers used positron emission tomography to study the cerebral glucose
metabolism of 25 adults who were currently hyperactive and had been so since
childhood in comparison to 50 normal control adults (Zametkin et al., 1990).
They found that the hyperactive adults manifested reduced metabolism globally
and particularly in the premotor cortex and superior prefrontal cortex, areas previously shown to be instrumental in the control of attention and motor activity.
As a consequence of this and other studies discussed later in this book, by the

early 1990s, ADHD (hyperactivity) was becoming recognized in clinical and scientific journals as a valid psychiatric disorder of adulthood distinct from other diagnostic conditions (Spencer, Biederman, Wilens, & Faraone, 1994).

A further watershed moment in the history of adults with ADHD was the development of a nonstimulant medication, atomoxetine (Strattera), by the Eli Lilly Company that would be studied in thousands of adults with ADHD in several randomized, placebo-controlled trials. Initially this drug was studied by the company as an antidepressant in approximately 1,200 adults. In this trial neither atomoxetine nor desipramine was significantly different from placebo, so atomoxetine was shelved as an antidepressant. But largely based upon the demonstrated efficacy of the tricyclic antidepressants in treating ADHD, mainly in children (see Spencer, 2006), a proof-of-concept study in adults with ADHD was encouraged by John Heiligenstein with the Eli Lilly Co. and subsequently initiated at Massachusetts General Hospital. In this study Spencer and colleagues, using a double-blind placebo-controlled design, demonstrated that atomoxetine was well tolerated and significantly more effective than placebo in reducing clinical symptoms of ADHD (Spencer et al., 1998). These initial positive findings led to the performance of two large multisite trials of atomoxetine in adult ADHD, evaluating more than 536 adults with ADHD. These trials likewise proved the drug to be efficacious for the management of ADHD in adults (Michelson et al., 2003). These studies were the largest ever done in evaluating a medication for adults with ADHD. More would follow. The drug would be the first new drug developed for the management of ADHD in more than 25 years and would be the first ever approved for treatment of ADHD in adults by the U.S. Food and Drug Administration. Later, the use of stimulants (methylphenidate, mixed amphetamine salts) would also be studied more thoroughly for adults with ADHD (Spencer et al., 2005; Spencer et al., 2001) and receive similar FDA approval for use in this age group. New delivery systems have also been recently developed that permit greater sustained therapeutic action across the day than did immediate-release preparations. These include osmotic pumps (Concerta), various timed-release pellets (Focalin XR, Metadate CD, Ritalin LA, Adderall XR, etc.), and skin patches (Daytrana) besides the earlier available but clinically disappointing wax-matrix sustained-release formulation of methylphenidate (Ritalin SR). As of this writing, a new nonabusable formulation of a mixed amphetamine compound has received FDA approval for use with ADHD (Vyvanse); here, the pills must be dissolved in stomach acid before the amphetamine compound can be activated and available for absorption through the gut.

Psychological treatments for adults with ADHD, though numerous in clinical practice, have to date not received much serious scientific scrutiny. This remains a glaring gap in the clinical scientific literature on the disorder in adults. Fortunately this may be changing. Safren and colleagues (Safren, Perlman,

Sprich, & Otto, 2005) have developed a group-delivered cognitive behavioral therapy program for adults with ADHD as a supplement to their medication treatment. Initial results from a small-scale study of this manualized therapy have been favorable in showing significant benefits beyond those achieved by medication alone (Safren, Otto, et al., 2005). More recently, Ramsay and Rothstein (2007) have also created a cognitive-behavioral program for adults with ADHD. More such research is to be encouraged, given that medication treatments are hardly likely to address all of the domains of impairment associated with ADHD, much less its frequent comorbid disorders such as anxiety, depression, and learning disabilities.

Given the growing acceptance of ADHD as a legitimate disorder in adults by the time of this writing, one can rightly ask just how prevalent ADHD is among adults. We address that issue next.

Prevalence of ADHD in Adults

Just how prevalent ADHD was in adults would remain controversial until 2005. One means of attempting to estimate adult prevalence is to determine, using longitudinal studies, the percentage of persistence of disorders in children followed into adulthood. Adult outcome studies of large samples of clinic-referred children with hyperactivity, or ADHD–combined type, are few in number. Only four follow-up studies have retained at least 50% or more of their original sample into adulthood. These are the Montreal study by Weiss and Hechtman (1993), the New York City study by Mannuzza and colleagues (see Mannuzza, Gittelman-Klein, Bessler, Malloy, & LaPadula, 1993), the Swedish study by Rasmussen and Gillberg (2001), and the Barkley and Fischer study from Milwaukee (Barkley, Fischer, Smallish, & Fletcher, 2002). The results regarding the persistence of disorder into young adulthood (middle 20s) are mixed. The Montreal study ($N = 103$) found that two-thirds of their original sample ($n = 64$; mean age of 25 years) claimed to be troubled as adults by at least one or more disabling core symptoms of their original disorder (restlessness, impulsivity, or inattention) and that 34% had at least moderate to severe levels of hyperactive, impulsive, and inattentive symptoms (Weiss & Hechtman, 1993, p. 73). In Sweden ($N = 50$), Rasmussen and Gillberg (2001) obtained similar results, with 49% of probands reporting marked symptoms of ADHD at age 22, compared to 9% of controls. Formal diagnostic criteria for ADHD, as in DSM-III or later editions, were not employed at any of the outcome points in either study, however. A follow-up study in China (Wenwei, 1996) found that nearly 70% of 197 children diagnosed 15 years earlier as having minimal brain dysfunction persisted in having symptoms of ADHD into young adulthood (ages 20–33, mean 25.5 years).

In contrast, the New York study has followed two separate cohorts of hyperactive children using DSM criteria to assess persistence of disorder. That study found that 31% of their initial cohort ($n = 101$) and 43% of their second cohort ($N = 94$) met DSM-III criteria for ADHD by ages 16 to 23 (mean age = 18.5 years) (Gittelman, Mannuzza, Shenker, & Bonagura, 1985; Mannuzza et al., 1991). Eight years later, (mean age 26), however, these figures fell to 8% and 4%, respectively (now using DSM-III-R criteria; American Psychiatric Association, 1987) (Mannuzza et al., 1993; Mannuzza, Klein, Bessler, Malloy, & LaPadula, 1998). Those results might imply that the vast majority of hyperactive children no longer qualify for the diagnosis of ADHD by adulthood.

The disparity in persistence to age 25 between the New York and the other two studies may have resulted in part from differences in their selection criteria. All studies began before systematic DSM criteria existed. The Montreal study accepted children who had received a clinical diagnosis of the hyperactive child syndrome based on significant levels of restlessness and poor concentration that were long-standing symptoms and caused problems both at home and at school. Nevertheless, explicit criteria for level of deviance in these symptoms, age of onset, pervasiveness, or other more exact criteria were not applied. The Swedish study selected children initially for having minimal brain dysfunction, a subset of whom had elevated teacher ratings of ADHD symptoms. Subsequently, 85% received a DSM-IV diagnosis of ADHD (American Psychiatric Association, 1994).

The New York studies, in contrast, required a clinical diagnosis of DSM-II hyperkinetic reaction of childhood (American Psychiatric Association, 1968), significantly elevated ratings of hyperactivity from parents, teachers, or clinical staff on the Conners rating scales, IQ of 85 or higher, and absence of gross neurological disorders or psychosis. Children with high levels of aggressive behavior or conduct problems were excluded from this study, however—a procedure not used in the Montreal or Swedish studies. This probably excluded many children with conduct disorder from participation (Mannuzza et al., 1993) and thus may have limited the severity of ADHD within the New York cohorts. More severe levels of ADHD are often associated with more severe levels of aggressiveness and conduct disorder (Achenbach, 1991; Hinshaw, 1987). For these reasons, it is possible that—while the New York study followed a more rigorously selected group of hyperactive children—their sample may also have comprised less severe disorder than the other studies.

The interpretation of the relatively low rate of persistence of ADHD into adulthood, particularly for the New York study, is clouded by at least two issues, apart from differences in selection criteria. One is that the source of information about the disorder changed in all of these studies from that used at the childhood and adolescent evaluations to that used at the adult outcome. At study entry and at adolescence, all studies used the reports of others (e.g., parents and teachers).

By midadolescence, all found that the majority of hyperactive participants (more than 70%) continued to manifest significant levels of the disorder (Klein & Mannuzza, 1991), findings consistent with other adolescent follow-up studies using DSM-III and DSM-III-R (70–86%; American Psychiatric Association, 1980, 1987) and parental reports (August & Stewart, 1983; Barkley, Fischer, Edelbrock, & Smallish, 1990; Claude & Firestone, 1995). In young adulthood (approximately at age 26 years) both the New York and Montreal studies switched to self-reports of the disorder.

The rather marked decline in persistence of ADHD from adolescence to adulthood could stem from this change in source of information. Indeed, the New York study found this to be likely when, at late adolescence (mean age 18–19 years), they interviewed both the teenagers and their parents about the psychiatric status of the teens (Mannuzza & Gittelman, 1986). There was a marked disparity between the reports of parents and teens concerning the presence of ADHD (11% vs. 27%; agreement 74%, kappa = .19). Other research also suggests that the relationship between older children's (age 11) self-reports of externalizing symptoms, such as those involved in ADHD, and those of parents and teachers is quite low (r = .16–.32; Henry, Moffitt, Caspi, Langley, & Silva, 1994). Thus, changing sources of reporting in longitudinal studies on behavioral disorders could be expected to lead to marked differences in estimates of persistence of those disorders.

The question obviously arises as to whose assessment of the proband is more accurate. This would depend on the purpose of the assessment, but the prediction of impairment in major life activities would seem to be an important one in research on psychiatric disorders. After all, the very definition of disorder may hinge on the demonstration of harm or impairment to the individual (Wakefield, 1999). The Milwaukee study by Barkley and Fischer (Barkley, Fischer, et al., 2002) examined this issue at the age 21 follow-up by interviewing both the participants and their parents about ADHD symptoms. It then examined the relationship of each source's reports to significant outcomes in major life activities (education, occupation, social, etc.) after controlling for the contribution made by the other source.

The Milwaukee Study addressed a second limitation in establishing persistence of ADHD into adulthood, and that is the contradiction inherent in the current conceptualization of it relative to the criteria actually used to diagnose it. ADHD has long been conceptualized as a developmental disability. This implies that it is a disorder because its symptoms occur to a degree that is *developmentally inappropriate* and thereby cause impairment in major life activities. All developmental disorders are diagnosed based on developmental relativity—age-inappropriateness in comparison to peers. That is because they reflect delays in the rate of development of a normal psychological attribute and not static pathological states or absolute deficits in or losses of formerly normal functioning.

From this perspective, the presence of ADHD at any stage in life must be partly determined by using age-relative thresholds for diagnostic symptom lists. However, such thresholds are not provided in the DSM. Despite requiring developmental inappropriateness, a fixed symptom threshold is imposed across all ages. Given that the frequency of ADHD symptoms declines substantially in normal populations with age (DuPaul, Power, Anastopoulos, & Reid, 1998; Hart, Lahey, Loeber, Applegate, & Frick, 1995), this application of a fixed threshold across a developmentally declining frequency curve means that the fixed threshold is becoming increasingly stricter or statistically rarer with age. Two predictable outcomes would flow from this circumstance. First, the diagnostic criteria will become less valid (sensitive to the disorder) with age—a situation noted in both the DSM-III-R and DSM-IV field trials (Applegate et al., 1997; Spitzer, Davies, & Barkley, 1990). And second, many of those having the disorder as children will appear to have outgrown it by adulthood when in fact they have only outgrown the criteria (Barkley, 2006).

To examine this issue, ADHD was determined in the Milwaukee Study (Barkley, Fischer et al., 2002), using not only the DSM-III-R threshold but also a developmentally referenced cutoff. The 98th percentile, or +2 standard deviations above the normal mean, was chosen for several reasons. First, it was the threshold used to select the probands into the study in childhood. Therefore we simply reapplied the entry criterion to the same sample at a later date using the control group to establish the 98th percentile. This threshold also is the one most commonly recommended in clinical practice for the interpretation of rating scale elevations as being clinically significant (Achenbach, 1991; DuPaul et al., 1998). And it is used as the demarcation on intelligence and adaptive behavior inventories for the diagnosis of another developmental disorder—mental retardation. So its extension to ADHD is in keeping with the practice used to define other developmental conditions.

We found a rate of only 3 to 5% of our hyperactive participants qualifying for a DSM-III-R diagnosis of ADHD when based on their self-report at young-adult follow-up (mean age approximately 20 years) (Barkley, Fischer, et al., 2002). However, when we subsequently interviewed their parents about the presence of disorder (using the recently released DSM-IV criteria), the rate rose to 42%. This clearly suggests that the source of information being used to judge persistence of disorder into adulthood is exceptionally important. If an empirical criterion for presence of disorder was employed with these same parent reports (e.g., 2+ standard deviations above the mean for the normal control group on DSM-IV symptom list at adult follow-up), 66% of the hyperactive group exceeded this cutoff score and could be said to have retained the disorder. This is a rather extreme developmental cutoff, reflecting the 98th percentile of the adult population. It was imposed because it was the same threshold employed to select the children as hyperactive (ADHD) at study entry in the late 1970s. It can therefore be said that at least 66% of the original hyperactive group continued to meet the entry criteria for the disorder at young adulthood. But clinicians are often counseled to use the 93rd percentile to judge the beginning of clinical deviance of symptom severity within a distribution, in which case the figure for the persistence of the disorder would have been markedly higher in this study.

All this means that the persistence of ADHD into adulthood is very much a matter of the source of information and the diagnostic criteria being employed, with parent reports yielding not only a far higher rate of persistence but also being more predictive of various impairments in major life activities (Barkley, Fischer, et al., 2002). If DSM criteria are applied to the person's own self-reports, low rates of persistence of ADHD are found in this study. But if parent reports of the subjects continue to be used, as they were in the prior follow-up assessments (and in other studies of ADHD into adolescence), persistence of disorder is 14 times greater. And if an empirical developmentally referenced criterion is established for disorder, rates are nearly 23 times greater.

This helps to explain the low rate of persistence of disorder predicted by Hill and Schoener (1996). They relied heavily on these earlier results to conjecture that, given a continuation of such trends, the disorder should occur in fewer than 2 in 1,000 adults by age 30 years or later. That review suffers from numerous other methodological and conceptual flaws, which undermine their conclusion (see Barkley, 1998, pp. 202–206). As the Milwaukee Study shows, the DSM criteria become increasingly less sensitive to the disorder with age. It also implies that subjects with ADHD may be prone to seriously underreporting their symptoms in early adulthood relative to what others may say about them—a problem noted in the Milwaukee Study at the earlier adolescent follow-up point as well (Fischer, Barkley, Fletcher, & Smallish, 1993a).

If one uses the Milwaukee Study follow-up to estimate the prevalence of ADHD in adults, it would lead to the following results. If 5 to 8% of children have ADHD (see Barkley, 2006) and 66% or more persist in maintaining the disorder into adulthood, one could extrapolate such findings to infer that 3.3 to 5.3% of adults are likely to have ADHD. Such a figure would not take into account any new cases of the disorder that could arise over time as a consequence of normal individuals experiencing neurological injuries which could give rise to the acquired form of the disorder as opposed to its more common familial-genetic form (Nigg, 2006).

We can now see whether such an inference actually squares with recent studies of prevalence using adult general population samples as opposed to the aforementioned approach, which attempts merely to infer prevalence from childhood longitudinal studies. An initial attempt at estimating prevalence was conducted by these authors in 1996, when we surveyed 720 adults (ages 17–84) in the central Massachusetts region who were renewing their driver's licenses (Murphy & Barkley, 1996b). At that time, all drivers had to renew their licenses in person, making this a fairly reasonable way of obtaining a representative sampling from the general adult population of this region or at least of its adult drivers. These adults completed two rating scales based on the DSM-IV symptom list for ADHD; one scale was for current functioning and the second for their recall of their own behavior as children, ages 5 to 12 years. When we required that adults meet the DSM symptom thresholds for clinical disorder (six of nine symptoms rated as often or more frequent) for both current and childhood functioning (a rather stringent criterion), the prevalence for ADHD (all types) was 4.7%.

This figure is well within the 3 to 5% estimate conjectured above from the follow-up studies of children. But it is certainly higher than those found in three previous studies of college students. Weyandt, Linterman, and Rice (1995) found a prevalence of 7% of 770 students reporting significant current symptoms of ADHD (+1.5 SD above the mean), while this figure fell to 2.5% if this threshold was imposed for both current and childhood functioning. DuPaul and colleagues found that 2.9% of men and 3.9% of women in their U.S. college sample ($N =$ 799) met symptom thresholds (six of nine) for current functioning (DuPaul et al., 2001). In a third study (Heiligenstein, Conyers, Berns, & Smith, 1998), a prevalence of 4% of 448 students was reported based on current symptoms, very similar to those of the DuPaul et al. study. No data were available, however, in the DuPaul and Heiligenstein studies concerning childhood ADHD symptoms. But it is likely, given the results of our own study and that of Weyandt and colleagues above, that their figures would be reduced by at least 50% if significant childhood symptoms also had been required for determining prevalence of disorder. This would likely reduce the prevalence figures for those two studies closer to 1.5 and 2%, again very similar to those of Weyandt et al. Studies of college students would likely result in underestimates of true adult ADHD prevalence given the significant adverse impact ADHD has on educational functioning and eventual attainment, such that the vast majority (approximately 80% or more) of children growing up with ADHD do not attend college (Barkley, 2006).

All of these prevalence figures may be an underestimate, however, given the problems discussed earlier, that they are based on the DSM symptom list and symptom thresholds that may be developmentally inappropriate and too severe, respectively, for use with adults. And the more symptoms of ADHD one may have, the more one may underestimate the occurrence and severity of those symptoms, as shown above, thus further limiting this estimate. But another problem with this research could render these figures as overestimates. That is because no imposition of a criterion for having evidence of impairment in major life activities was used in any of these studies, yet it is required as part of the DSM diagnostic criteria for this disorder. In studies of children, when such a criterion is imposed, it can result in a significant reduction in prevalence (see Barkley, 2006). Our own research is further limited by restricting its sample to central Massachusetts, while the sample at Weyandt et al. was chiefly Washington

state, and the samples of DuPaul et al. were also regionally limited to three locali-
ties, making it difficult to extrapolate these figures to other regions of the United
States. Indeed, it appears that a large part of the study sample ($N = 444$) of
Weyandt et al. may have been included in the study of DuPaul et al., which
may limit the status of the study of DuPaul et al. as a replication of that of
Weyandt et al.

The latter limitation has now been overcome as a consequence of a far
larger study of prevalence of ADHD in an adult general population sample
(Kessler et al., 2006). In that study, a screen for adult ADHD was included in a
probability subsample ($n = 3,199$) of 18- to 44-year-old respondents in the
National Comorbidity Survey Replication (NCS-R), a nationally representative
household survey that used a lay-administered diagnostic interview to assess a
wide range of DSM-IV disorders. Blinded clinical follow-up interviews of adults
with ADHD were carried out with 154 NCS-R respondents, oversampling
those with a positive screen. This study found an estimated prevalence of adult
ADHD to be 4.4%. Lifetime prevalence has been estimated by Kessler and colleagues to be 8.1% (Kessler, Berglund, Demler, Jin, & Walters, 2005). This figure
for current prevalence is highly similar to that found in the more regionally limited study by Murphy and Barkley (1996b) (4.7%) and falls well within the mid-
range of the prevalence estimate inferred above from childhood longitudinal
studies (3.3–5.3%). Most recently, a worldwide study of prevalence in adults estimated it to be 3.4%, being higher in higher-income countries (4.2%), and close
to the Kessler et al. estimate (Fayyad et al., 2007). The Kessler et al. study also
found that ADHD was significantly correlated with being male, being previously
married, being unemployed, and being of non-Hispanic white ancestry. ADHD
was also noted to be highly comorbid with many other DSM-IV disorders and
was associated with substantial role impairment. The majority of patients determined to have ADHD in this study had been untreated specifically for their
ADHD, although many had obtained treatment for other comorbid mental and
substance use disorders. Many of these issues of comorbidity, impairments, and
treatment history were also noted by Fayyad et al. (2007) and are recommended
later in this book in relation to our own results. For now, it is worth noting that
Kessler et al. (2006) concluded that efforts were needed to increase the detection
and treatment of ADHD in adults and that more research was required to determine whether effective treatment would reduce the onset, persistence, and severity of disorders that co-occur with adult ADHD—a call for more research with
which we heartily agree.

To summarize, it appears from both childhood follow-up studies and, more
directly, from studies of adult general population samples that the prevalence of
ADHD in adults in the United States is approximately 5%. The U.S. Census
Bureau (*www.census.gov*) estimates that in 2005, the U.S. population stood at
295,507,134, with 221,868,077 being 18 years of age or older. Based on this fig-

ure and the 5% estimated prevalence for ADHD in adults, it seems likely that at least 11,093,403 adults in the United States probably have ADHD. This is a sizable number, making it imperative that the mental health, medical, and educational professions as well as employers become more aware of the existence of this disorder and its treatments. It also makes it essential that we understand as much about the expression of this disorder in adulthood—along with its comorbid psychiatric disorders and impairments in major life activities—if we are to be able to better understand it and manage it and its consequences more effectively. These are major aims of this book.

We now turn our attention, in the next chapter, toward a description of the methods and procedures involved in our research projects. We also use this as an opportunity to acquaint the reader with some of the larger issues related to the clinical diagnosis of the disorder in adults, since those issues bear directly on how the adults in our projects were selected as having ADHD.

Conclusions and Clinical Implications

This chapter has provided a brief history of the clinical recognition and treatment of adults with ADHD as a background for the results of the two large-scale studies reported in this book. We have demonstrated that:

✓ History shows that the notion that ADHD can exist in adults is not new, having been intimated in papers on children with ADHD and its developmentally chronic nature as long ago as 1902 and certainly since systematic longitudinal studies began to appear in the 1970s.

✓ Studies appeared in the 1960s–1970s on small groups of clinical patients thought to have ADHD or its precursor diagnoses, thus beginning to establish the scientific legitimacy of the disorder as distinct from other adult conditions.

✓ The first systematic study of medication for adults with ADHD was published shortly thereafter, or 30 years ago, finding significant benefits for management of the condition.

✓ Despite such occasional research papers, clinical recognition of the disorder in adults did not become more widespread until the 1990s, spurring a marked increase in scientific research on the nature and management of the disorder in adults, including the studies presented here.

✓ The prevalence of ADHD in adults has been interpolated from longitudinal studies of ADHD children followed into adulthood to be approximately 3.3 to 5.3%. Actual studies of large general population samples have more recently placed the figure at nearly 5% of adults, representing more than 11 million adults in the United States alone. ADHD is therefore a relatively common mental disorder among adults, affecting at least 5% of the U.S. adult population.

✓ Clinicians should appreciate that ADHD is now a recognized and scientifically validated disorder in adults and has been so for at least 15 to 30 years, likely representing a sizable proportion of referrals to outpatient clinics.

✓ Stimulant and nonstimulant medications have proven effective in the management of the disorder in adults, similar to their efficacy in children with the disorder.

✓ With the increasing public awareness about ADHD in adults, clinicians should prepare themselves to properly recognize, diagnose, and manage these adults as they become an increasing percentage of the clinically referred outpatient population.

CHAPTER 3

Diagnostic Criteria
for ADHD in Adults

Before discussing the manner in which adults were selected into the UMASS and Milwaukee Studies as having ADHD or not, we wish to review some of the issues—some controversial—regarding the manner in which ADHD should be clinically diagnosed. This review helps to justify the decisions we made concerning the selection criteria employed in these two studies. We need to begin, then, with a quick review of the current diagnostic criteria for ADHD as set forth in the DSM-IV-TR (American Psychiatric Association, 2000), as shown in Table 3.1. Readers should understand that despite the criticisms and limitations we level at these criteria below, especially as they pertain to the diagnosis of adults, they are the most empirically based, rigorously tested, and logically coherent criteria of their time for the diagnosis of ADHD, especially in children. For more on the development of these criteria, see the paper by Lahey and colleagues (Lahey et al., 1994) and others (Applegate et al., 1997) and the earlier field trial for DSM-III-R (Spitzer et al., 1990).

A Critical Review
of the DSM-IV ADHD Criteria as Used for Adults

The discussion that follows is largely taken from Barkley's earlier paper on this same subject with James McGough (see McGough & Barkley, 2004). In contrast to the Wender Utah Criteria for diagnosing adults with ADHD discussed in Chapter 2 (see also Wender, 1995), which gained some popularity in the early

TABLE 3.1. DSM-IV-TR Criteria for ADHD

A. Either (1) or (2):

(1) six (or more) of the following symptoms of **inattention** have persisted for at least 6 months to a degree that is maladaptive and inconsistent with developmental level:

Inattention
(a) often fails to give close attention to details or makes careless mistakes in schoolwork, work, or other activities
(b) often has difficulty sustaining attention in tasks or play activities
(c) often does not seem to listen when spoken to directly
(d) often does not follow through on instructions and fails to finish schoolwork, chores, or duties in the workplace (not due to oppositional behavior or failure to understand instructions)
(e) often has difficulty organizing tasks and activities
(f) often avoids, dislikes, or is reluctant to engage in tasks that require sustained mental effort (such as school work or homework)
(g) often loses things necessary for tasks or activities (e.g., toys, school assignments, pencils, books, or tools)
(h) is often easily distracted by extraneous stimuli
(i) is often forgetful in daily activities

(2) six (or more) of the following symptoms of **hyperactivity–impulsivity** have persisted for at least 6 months to a degree that is maladaptive and inconsistent with developmental level:

Hyperactivity
(a) often fidgets with hands or feet or squirms in seat
(b) often leaves seat in classroom or in other situations in which remaining seated is expected
(c) often runs about or climbs excessively in situations in which it is inappropriate (in adolescents or adults, may be limited to subjective feelings of restlessness)
(d) often has difficulty playing or engaging in leisure activities quietly
(e) is often "on the go" or often acts as if "driven by a motor"
(f) often talks excessively

Impulsivity
(g) often blurts out answers before the questions have been completed
(h) often has difficulty awaiting turn
(i) often interrupts or intrudes on others (e.g., butts into conversations or games)

B. Some hyperactive–impulsive or inattentive symptoms that caused impairment were present before age 7 years.

C. Some impairment from the symptoms is present in two or more settings (e.g., at school [or work] and at home).

D. There must be clear evidence of clinically significant impairment in social, academic, or occupational functioning.

E. The symptoms do not occur exclusively during the course of a Pervasive Developmental Disorder, Schizophrenia, or other Psychotic Disorder, and are not better accounted for by another mental disorder (e.g., Mood Disorder, Anxiety Disorder, Dissociative Disorder, or a Personality Disorder).

(continued)

TABLE 3.1. *(continued)*

Code based on type:

    314.01 Attention-Deficit/Hyperactivity Disorder, Combined Type: if both criteria A1 and A2 are met for the past 6 months.

    314.00 Attention-Deficit/Hyperactivity Disorder, Predominantly Inattentive Type: if criterion A1 is met but criterion A2 is not met for the past 6 months

    314.01 Attention-Deficit/Hyperactivity Disorder, Predominantly Hyperactive–Impulsive Type: if criterion A2 is met but criterion A1 is not met for the past 6 months.

Coding note: For individuals (especially adolescents and adults) who currently have symptoms that no longer meet full criteria, "In Partial Remission" should be specified.

Note. From American Psychiatric Association (2000). Copyright 2000 by the American Psychiatric Association. Reprinted by permission.

1990s, Biederman and colleagues showed the utility of adhering to the DSM-based approach for the diagnosis of adults and demonstrated that those so identified had patterns of impairment, comorbidity, and neuropsychological functioning similar to those of children with ADHD (Biederman, Faraone, Knee, & Munir, 1990; Biederman et al., 1993). In their research, structured diagnostic interviews for adult psychopathology are supplemented with modules from child-diagnostic structured interviews, specifically the child module for ADHD. Patients report retrospectively on the occurrence and associated impairment of each of the ADHD symptoms from the DSM that occurred during their childhood. Where positive responses occur, further inquiries are made as to current DSM symptoms and related impairment. As with Wender's criteria, the diagnosis of adult ADHD based on this approach is contingent upon the retrospective recall of the patient, which is then used to infer a diagnosis of ADHD in childhood. In our clinical and research practices, we have followed a similar approach to assess childhood and current functioning (Barkley, Murphy, & Bush, 2001, Murphy & Barkley, 1996a; Murphy, Barkley, & Bush, 2001). But we developed our own structured interviews and rating scales for doing so (Barkley & Murphy, 1998, 2006) considering that none existed at the time specifically for the diagnosis of ADHD in adults and that the child-diagnostic structured interviews were not developed or intended for use with adults.

    DSM criteria have been employed in numerous studies of adult ADHD, comorbid conditions, and associated impairments, as discussed throughout this book, and in numerous clinical pharmaceutical studies. A number of findings support the validity of the DSM approach to diagnosing ADHD in adults. For instance, the children of adults diagnosed as having ADHD have also been found to be 7 to 10 times more likely to have ADHD than children of adults not so diagnosed (57% vs. the base rate of 5–7.7%) (Biederman et al., 1995). Our later chapter on the offspring of our adult ADHD sample in the UMASS Study corroborates this elevated risk for disorder. This clearly demonstrates a familial aggregation as well as a pattern of genetic inheritance of the disorder. Similarly, families ascertained through adult probands diagnosed by DSM criteria as having ADHD have demonstrated an association with a variant of the dopamine receptor gene (DRD4) that has also been associated with childhood ADHD (Faraone, Biederman, Weiffenbach, Keith, Chu, et al., 1999). A recent study by Barkley and colleagues (Barkley, Smith, Fischer, & Navia, 2006), using the Milwaukee Study findings up to age 21 years, has also shown a striking relationship between the DAT1 9/10 allele pairing and DSM symptoms of ADHD across a 13-year follow-up of children with ADHD into adulthood. Adults with DSM-based ADHD also show cognitive deficits typically seen in children with ADHD (Barkley, Murphy, et al., 2001; Murphy et al., 2001; Bekker et al., 2005a; Seidman et al., 2004) as well as substantial driving problems previously and frequently demonstrated in adolescents with ADHD (Barkley, 2004; Barkley & Cox, 2007). Further evidence of the validity of the DSM approach to diagnosing ADHD in adults comes from studies showing such adults to have increased striatal dopamine transporter density in SPECT (single photon emission computed tomography) imaging studies (Dougherty et al., 1999). These and numerous other findings to be discussed throughout this book attest to the validity of using the DSM criteria for diagnosing adults with ADHD.

Despite this successful adaptation of the DSM for the identification of adult patients with ADHD, significant limitations to this approach deserve notice. Indeed, the present research studies were designed to evaluate and recommend means of addressing several of these limitations. The DSM-IV-TR criteria are noted below *in italics* along with specific difficulties that arise from each criterion as it may be applied to the diagnosis of adults.

A. Either (1) or (2): (1) six (or more) of the following symptoms of **inattention** *have persisted for at least 6 months to a degree that is maladaptive and inconsistent with developmental level; (2) six (or more) of the following symptoms of* **hyperactivity–impulsivity** *have persisted for at least 6 months to a degree that is maladaptive and inconsistent with developmental level.* ADHD symptoms listed in DSM-IV-TR are based on symptoms from prior DSMs along with items chosen from empirically derived behavior rating scales that load on these same factors or dimensions, expert clinical opinion, and a field trial testing the psychometric properties and utility of the item pool (Lahey et al., 1994). Symptoms eventually selected for inclusion significantly correlated with parent and teacher ratings of impairment and differentiated clinically diagnosed ADHD from non-ADHD disorders in a sample of 380 clinically referred children ranging in age from 4 to 17 years. Field trial results further suggested that a threshold of six of nine hyperactive–impulsive symptoms or six of nine inattentive symptoms optimally predicted significant impairment and a clinically validated diagnosis of ADHD. It also produced the best interjudge reliability.

Despite the commendable empirical basis to the development of DSM-IV-TR, its shortcomings for use in diagnosing adults with ADHD are readily apparent. Symptoms were identified for application to children and by a workgroup concerned only with childhood disruptive disorders. Unlike Wender's Utah criteria, there was no attempt to test symptoms that were more developmentally representative of the adult stage of the disorder. Moreover, no adults were included in the DSM field trial. In fact, several DSM-IV-TR symptoms, such as "runs and climbs excessively" or "has difficulty playing . . . quietly" are clearly inappropriate and without face validity for use with adults. There is little evidence to suggest that current DSM symptoms designed for use with children best characterize adults with ADHD. This was one of the major purposes of the present UMASS Study and a secondary aim of the Milwaukee Study—to evaluate current DSM symptoms when used with adults as well as additional items that potentially may have greater applicability to and validity for detecting the adult stage of the disorder.

There is also a concern about whether the DSM symptom list represents the current conceptualization(s) of ADHD as accurately as it could or should. Since the late 1980s and early 1990s, ADHD has been conceptualized as involving a disorder of behavioral inhibition (Barkley, 1997; Nigg, 2001; Quay, 1988), and earlier conceptualizations certainly made it part of the trinity of symptom complexes (Douglas, 1972) even as far back as DSM-II (American Psychiatric Association, 1968). Yet if one examines the symptom lists in DSM-IV-TR, the greatest weight is given to inattention (nine symptoms) followed by hyperactivity (six symptoms), with the remaining three symptoms thought to reflect impulsiveness. Most of those impulsive items reflect principally verbal behavior. The words "impulsive" or "poorly inhibited" are not even mentioned in the symptom list despite being viewed currently as a core feature if not *the* core feature of this disorder. As our studies show, this has proved to be a glaring oversight, because the symptom of "makes decisions impulsively" and others related to it ("acts before thinking," "has difficulty waiting for things," etc.) are among the most useful symptoms for distinguishing ADHD from other psychiatric disorders as well as the general nondisordered population (Chapter 7). DSM-V will need to give greater balance to the triad of symptoms if it is to reasonably represent current conceptualizations of what is disordered in ADHD.

Similarly, there is no scientific basis for establishing nine symptoms as the best list length or six symptoms as the most appropriate threshold for adult diagnosis; it is a threshold based on and meant for children. As we noted in Chapter 2, we studied the prevalence of DSM-IV-TR symptoms in a sample of adults in Massachusetts (Murphy & Barkley, 1996a) and found that a threshold of six symptoms required for diagnosis of ADHD was 2 to 4 *SD*s above the normal adult mean for that sample, in essence representing the 98th to 99.9th percentiles of the adult population. The use of this threshold could therefore define adult ADHD almost out of existence or make it a statistical rarity at best. Likewise, this threshold was 3.5 *SD*s above the mean for the control group followed from childhood to adulthood in the Milwaukee Study of ADHD children at their age-21 follow-up (Barkley, Fischer, Smallish, & Fletcher, 2002). This study concluded that approximately one-third of individuals with severe symptoms (98th percentile) failed to meet the DSM criteria for clinical diagnosis. Our earlier study of a general population sample in Massachusetts (see Chapter 2) reported that cutoff scores of 4 for current symptoms of hyperactivity or inattention would be more commensurate with the 93rd percentile often recommended as being clinically significant in childhood diagnosis of ADHD. Others have recommended this same threshold to identify college students with sufficient difficulties to warrant treatment (Heilingenstein et al., 1998; Kooij et al., 2004). This suggests that DSM-IV-TR criteria are overly restrictive when extrapolated to adults and fail to identify a substantial minority of adults who suffer clinically meaningful levels of ADHD symptoms.

Clinicians should also take note of the fact that the majority of children who participated in the field trial were males (Lahey et al., 1994) by an average of at least 2:1. Many studies have found that males show higher frequencies of these symptoms than do females in general population samples (e.g., DuPaul et al., 1998). If symptom thresholds are based predominantly on males, as they were in the DSM-IV field trial, it is likely that those thresholds are more severe for females relative to the general female population than they would prove to be for males relative to the male population. This would make it more difficult for a female to obtain the diagnosis than a male despite equal levels of symptom deviance (developmental inappropriateness) relative to others of the same sex. Given that no adults were studied in the field trial, whether the symptom thresholds are equally valid (sensitive) at detecting females as males with ADHD in adulthood is open to question. The general population study by Murphy and Barkley (1996a) suggested that symptoms in adults were as frequent in females as in males but that this was not true for retrospective recall of childhood symptoms, in which the more typical pattern of greater male frequency of symptoms was evident.

B. Some hyperactive–impulsive or inattentive symptoms that caused impairment were present before age 7 years. DSM-IV-TR requires the onset of symptoms producing impairment prior to age 7 for diagnosis of ADHD, essentially at 6 years of age or earlier. ADHD has always been characterized as a disorder of early childhood, with the implication that ADHD-like symptoms arising later in life represent some other condition. But the use of a precise age of onset criterion was not introduced until DSM-III in 1980. Even then, it was not based on any sound scientific rationale or empirical basis. In its defense, it was commonplace at that time to include such a criterion in research studies of ADHD in children, but that was done mainly to ensure the presence of a developmental disorder (early onset of disorder) and to permit replication of the study by other researchers (Barkley & Biederman, 1997).

The age-of-onset criterion for symptoms and associated impairment poses particular difficulties for the diagnosis of adult patients. As we noted in Chapter 2, unlike assessment of children, the clinical evaluation of adults is highly dependent on patient self-report. Adults likely have a limited recall of the exact time course and nature of symptoms—a point we will prove to be the case later in Chapter 4, using the Milwaukee Study data. Adults are also likely to have a limited recall of the domains of childhood impairments related to those symptoms within the limited developmental time frame associated with so precise a childhood onset of age 7, as is required for diagnosis in DSM-IV-TR. Many adults who present for clinical care, moreover, are unable to provide independent evidence of the disorder, either through retrospective parental report or records of academic functioning. Adults do not typically come to clinical evaluations with their parents to provide the customary evidence for judging symptom onset, as is done in children. While it is implicit that the judgments of someone besides the patient (child) will provide this evidence in the use of the DSM-IV-TR criteria with children, it is not made explicit. Therefore it is typically not required when adults are being evaluated, even though that requirement is assumed to exist in child patients. A further problem here is the much greater time span over which these adults (or even their parents if interviewed) must retrospectively recall their childhood behavior relative to the time span upon which parents of children with ADHD must reflect. Add to this the likelihood that ADHD may create a positive illusory bias in adults concerning their possible impairment, as it does in children with ADHD (Knouse, Bagwell, Barkley, & Murphy, 2005), it is clear that this could possibly diminish self-awareness of symptoms and impairments. This is a further reason to question reliance upon the recall of adult patients for establishing the age of onset of their symptoms and associated impairments.

Given the lack of empirical evidence supporting the age-of-onset criterion as well as practical difficulties in demonstrating impairment prior to age 7 in older adolescents and adults, some have argued that the criterion should be abandoned or redefined to include the broader period of adolescence (ages 12–14) (Barkley & Biederman, 1997). The suggestion is not as radical as it may first appear. Consider that most mental disorders do not have a criterion requiring such an explicit age of onset for symptoms or impairment, if they have any at all. This state of affairs applies as well to other developmental disorders known commonly to arise in childhood, such as the specific developmental disorders (no age of onset), mental retardation (onset before 18 years), tic disorders and Tourette syndrome (onset before 18 years), and Asperger syndrome (none). Although such disorders are considered to be as much or even more "developmental" in nature as ADHD and that most cases have their onset in childhood, an age of onset is either not required for them or is quite broadly construed (before age 18). A case can now easily be made that ADHD is just as deserving of such liberal treatment concerning this diagnostic criterion as the other developmental disorders. A further point in favor of broadening or abandoning an age-of-onset requirement for ADHD rests on the fact that there was never a compelling rationale or empirical foundation for inserting this diagnostic criterion into the DSM. This criterion did not exist in DSM-II for the predecessor of this disorder (hyperkinetic reaction), and its insertion into DSM-III was based solely on committee consensus alone, without benefit of an empirical field trial. Its retention across DSM-III-R and IV appears to have been based more on a sense of tradition than on any empirical foundation for its diagnostic validity or utility.

But the greatest evidence against using so precise a criterion for age of onset as age 7 years is that the DSM-IV field trial not only failed to find evidence in support of this specific age as being diagnostically useful, it even found substantial evidence arguing against its retention (Applegate et al., 1997). This study found that using the onset of age 7 for this purpose reduced the classification accuracy of the remaining diagnostic criteria when compared to using older ages of onset (8, 9, or higher). It also reduced the interjudge reliability for the diagnosis significantly and failed to show any association with the types of impairments examined in that study. Unfortunately, DSM-IV had been published before these aspects of the field-trial analyses were completed and published, so the age-of-onset criterion was retained solely by default.

Last, to our knowledge, no evidence is available in the literature suggesting that onset of ADHD symptoms at or after age 7 years results in a qualitatively or even quantitatively different disorder than cases of ADHD having the earlier recommended symptom onset. The fact that some prior studies have reported a mean age of onset of initial ADHD symptoms as occurring between ages 3 and 4 years does not automatically argue for inclusion of a precise age-of-onset criterion into a diagnostic system for ADHD but only that ADHD, like retardation, appears to be "developmental," arising early in many cases. However, the range of symptom onsets around this mean is substantial, the reliability of parental identification of this precise onset is questionable, and the diagnostic or conceptual significance of a precise age of onset remains unexamined and unjustified (Barkley & Biederman, 1997). Furthermore, the early age of onset found in most studies of children with ADHD may be due in part to method artifact; it arises by virtue of studying clinic-referred children who, almost by definition if not by default, have developed their symptoms in childhood. And because they are children who do not self-refer to clinics on first appearance of their problem behavior, their symptom onset often occurs well before the decision to refer for mental health services is finally reached by the family, teachers, or primary care professionals. The DSM-IV field trial also demonstrated that a significant percentage of children meeting all other criteria for the disorder failed to demonstrate symptom onset prior to age 7, particularly those with the inattentive type (Applegate et al., 1997). Yet, in favor of broadening the criteria, that same field trial found that all patients with ADHD used in that study had developed their disorder by the more generous adolescent onset age of 14 years (Applegate et al., 1997). To continue to argue that the 7-year age-of-onset criterion must be applied to adults for a diagnosis of ADHD to be valid, just because the DSM-IV so stipulates, is an empirically indefensible justification smacking more of ritual or dogma than of supporting data. The issue is critical and deserving of study. All this supports another major purpose of the UMASS and Milwaukee Studies, and that was to explore the validity of the age of onset of 7 versus the more generous onset of symptoms by adolescence, approximately ages 14 to 16.

  C. Some impairment from the symptoms is present in two or more settings (e.g., at school [or work] and at home). Problematic here, obviously, is that adults are involved in far more numerous and important adaptive settings or domains of major life activities than this criterion stipulates. The settings specified here are not only too global to be of much good to the clinician evaluating domains of impairment (e.g., "home") but they ignore many more domains of major life activities that are not only more specific but also important domains of adult adaptive functioning. General functioning within the larger organized community, for instance, (e.g., participation in government or formally organized community groups, cooperation with others living in the same neighborhood, abiding by laws, driving), financial management (e.g., banking, credit, contracts, debt repayment), parenting and child rearing (e.g., protection, sustenance, financial and social support, appropriate education, discipline), marital functioning, and routine health maintenance activities are additional domains of major life activities in which symptoms may produce impairment that would not be evident in children. Current criteria fail to reflect these potential areas of impairment. This, too, represents another major aim of the present book—that is, to examine the major domains of important life activities in adulthood and the manner in which ADHD in adults affects them. The UMASS Study examines the degree to which each DSM symptom is associated with impairment in each of a number of domains of major life activities and also does so for a newly proposed set of symptoms to be recommended for consideration for inclusion in the DSM-V diagnostic criteria for adults with ADHD. Moreover, both the UMASS and Milwaukee Studies will also show how severity of ADHD pertains to severity of impairment both within and across multiple domains of major life functioning for adults.

D. There must be clear evidence of clinically significant impairment in social, academic, or occupational functioning. ADHD is conceptualized as a pervasive disorder of functioning, not as a reaction limited to a specific stressor or a specific circumscribed setting. It is expected that ADHD in childhood leads to some measurable impairment in multiple settings, most notably home, school, and with peers. DSM-IV briefly specifies substitution of "work" for "school" but fails to reference the full range of adult impairments noted above. Both children with ADHD followed to adulthood as well as clinic-referred adults with ADHD have demonstrated decreased educational achievement, poorer occupational functioning, a greater propensity for antisocial activities and drug use/abuse, greater divorce rates, poorer personal health choices, earlier parenthood, and increased driving risks compared with non-ADHD adults (Barkley, 2006; Barkley, Fischer, Smallish, & Fletcher, 2004, 2006; Biederman et al., 1993; Fischer & Barkley, 2006; Murphy & Barkley, 1996b). Although each of these domains is reviewed in detail, along with our results concerning them, in later chapters, the point here is that DSM-IV provides an insufficient array of major life activities for judging adult impairments. It also provides no guidance for differentiating among the various domains of functioning necessary to meet diagnostic criteria. Based on our results, our later chapters offer further recommendations as to the other domains that should be noted in DSM beyond just home, school, and work settings.

Conversely, many adults have adopted lifestyles that minimize self-reported dysfunction across multiple domains. For example, an adult with significant occupational impairment might live alone, no longer attend school, stay with less responsible part-time, unskilled, or entry-level work, become involved recreationally with the more liberal social mores of the performing arts, such as rock music or acting, be content with few or no friends or those with similar antisocial or drug abuse tendencies, and perhaps have minimal insight into the full range of his or her dysfunction. Therefore clinicians who adhere strictly to the requirement for multiple domains of impairment might fail to treat patients who would clearly benefit from treatment but who demonstrate impairment in only a single domain. These clinicians may fail to appreciate this form of adult niche-picking, which renders the patient's symptoms less impairing by virtue of the individual associating with these less culturally mainstream and more avant garde, asocial, or frankly antisocial arenas of life.

Because of an enormous increase in requests for special accommodations in employment and high-stakes academic testing under the Americans with Disabilities Act, controversy has arisen over the definition of impairment. Further specification of the meaning of impairment is necessary in DSM-V so as to avoid misunderstandings among clinicians and public agencies. Some clinicians assess impairment based on comparison of deficits relative to a person's intellectual level, much as had been done in the earlier history of defining learning disabilities as being significant discrepancies between IQ and some specific area of academic achievement, such as reading. Others believe that impairment is based on how well an individual, particularly if unusually intelligent or well educated, functions relative to his or her specialized peer group, such as fellow gifted individuals or colleagues in medical or law school. Still others have argued that impairment should mean serious dysfunction in the performance of the major life activities (family, marital, social, occupational functioning, etc.) required of society in general. More to the point, this view holds that impairment should be defined as being relative to the norm or average person, as required by the Americans with Disabilities Act (ADA), and not relative to some narrow, highly specialized and accomplished subset of adults or to an estimate of one's general cognitive ability, such as IQ (see Gordon & Keiser, 1998; Murphy & Gordon, 2006). We prefer the latter view of defining impairment because of a number of factors: its consistency with scientific views of valid mental disorders (harmful dysfunctions that are failures or severe deficiencies in mental adaptations; Wakefield, 1999); its consistency with the ADA, with associated court rulings, and with the legislative intent behind the ADA (granting protections and accommodations to subnormally functioning individuals); and simple fairness or justice—individuals should not be viewed as disordered and granted special protections, accommodations, disability financial benefits, or other societal privileges when they are not below the average of the population at large. It is inherently unfair to grant advantages to those who are not actually subnormal. And this latter view of impairment respects the fact that one's intelligence is not an indicator of functioning in all avenues of adult life, nor are disparities between IQ and some other measure of adaptive functioning. Future DSM committees should make the criterion for impairment clearer as to the domains it encompasses and the comparison group to be used for its determination.

E. *The symptoms are not better accounted for by another mental disorder.* Current DSM-IV-TR symptoms were selected in part for their ability to differentiate ADHD from other psychiatric disorders (Lahey et al., 1994). However, without adult studies, there is no evidence to suggest that childhood ADHD symptoms similarly differentiate ADHD adults from other adult psychiatric conditions. This, in fact, is another purpose of the present UMASS Study—to examine how well DSM-IV-TR symptoms distinguish adults with ADHD from other clinic-referred adults who do not have ADHD. Unlike the Utah criteria, which exclude significant comorbidities from the adult ADHD diagnosis (see Chapter 2), DSM-based studies report high rates of co-occurring psychopathology with adult ADHD—findings corroborated in both our projects later in this text. ADHD in adults is frequently described as having coexisting oppositional defiant disorder, conduct disorder, antisocial personality disorder, and psychoactive substance use disorders, as noted above. More controversial are increased rates of anxiety, depression, and possibly bipolar disorder (Faraone & Biederman, 1997; Faraone, Biederman, Mennin, Wozniak, & Spencer, 1997; Shekim et al., 1990). Several ADHD symptoms (i.e., concentration difficulties, restlessness, increased speech, acting "on the go") are also symptoms of other disorders, particularly anxiety, depression, and mania. It is unclear if these DSM symptoms adequately differentiate ADHD from other adult disorders or how other disorders might manifest when they co-occur with ADHD.

   F. DSM-IV subtypes. ADHD subtypes (i.e., inattentive, hyperactive–impulsive, and combined) are based on the DSM field trial suggesting that ADHD symptoms cluster around two partially distinct factors of inattentive and hyperactive–impulsive symptoms (Lahey et al., 1994). Subtyping based on any approaches using two lists would create three groups of entities not based on clinical or conceptual significance but by mere default. There is ongoing controversy as to whether ADHD subtypes so formed represent manifestations of the same or different conditions. Some researchers have found evidence that DSM subtypes breed true (Hudziak et al., 1998; Levy, Hay, McStephen, Wood, & Waldman, 1997), while other investigators report a lack of relationship in subtypes among family members (Faraone, Biederman, & Friedman, 2000; Smalley et al., 2000; Willcutt, Pennington, & DeFries, 2000). The question of subtypes is particularly vexing with adults. Evidence suggests that hyperactive–impulsive symptoms decrease significantly over development, earlier in development, and significantly more over development than do inattentive symptoms (Biederman, Mick, & Faraone, 2000; Hart et al., 1995; Mick, Faraone, & Biederman, 2004), at least as they are currently described in the DSM symptom list. Yet this could easily be the result of using symptom descriptions most applicable to early childhood that fail to capture the expression of the same construct at later developmental stages. Results from the field trial reveal that most children of the hyperactive–impulsive type develop the combined type during their early school years, while those of the inattentive type tend to remain in that category (Lahey et al., 1994). In many cases patients who might have been diagnosed with the combined type as youths will appear as inattentive types in adulthood simply by virtue of the aforementioned expected decline in their hyperactivity with age. That decline eventually may reach a point where fewer than six symptoms of hyperactivity–impulsivity exist, necessitating their reclassification from combined to inattentive type. The DSM provides no guidance as to whether an adult subtype should be assigned based on one's symptom presentation in childhood, adolescence, or adulthood. Once children have been diagnosed with combined type ADHD, should they always be considered combined type even if they no longer manifest a sufficient number of hyperactive–impulsive symptoms as adolescents or adults? Should the predominantly inattentive type be reserved only for "true" or "pure" inattentive types who have never had any developmentally inappropriate symptoms of hyperactivity or impulsivity? Or is it appropriate to assign the "inattentive type" label to those who met criteria for combined type as children and no longer have a sufficient number of HI symptoms as adults? These issues have relevance to investigations of potential biological differences between types and to practitioners who clinically diagnose patients. The current DSM subtype classification has, in fact, never been validated in adults with ADHD and has insufficient empirical evidence at present to justify its use after childhood, if even then.

G. *DSM residual categories*. In earlier versions of DSM the category ADHD residual type was reserved for adults who met criteria for ADHD in childhood and continued to have significant symptoms and impairment that fell below threshold for full diagnosis. This category has been replaced in DSM-IV-TR with ADHD in partial remission. The DSM-IV-TR category of ADHD not otherwise specified is employed when patients have impairment from symptoms of inattention or hyperactivity/impulsivity but fail to meet all criteria for ADHD. These diagnoses are default categories that are useful when clinicians are required to provide a diagnosis. Neither of these categories has defined or validated criteria, and their reliability is insufficient to support research efforts. Adult patients would be better served with developmentally appropriate and well-validated diagnostic criteria. Hence the justification for examining potentially new items for diagnosing ADHD in adults in the present book, along with evaluation of the symptom thresholds and age-of-onset criteria.

With this information on the background and limitations of diagnostic criteria for ADHD in adults, we discuss in the next chapter the criteria we employed for selecting adults with ADHD in the UMASS Study and for determining the presence of current ADHD in the Milwaukee Study of hyperactive (ADHD) children followed to adulthood.

Conclusions and Clinical Implications

In this chapter we have discussed the applicability of the DSM-IV-TR diagnostic criteria for ADHD when applied to adults being clinically evaluated for the disorder.

✓ Developed exclusively on and for children, the DSM-IV-TR criteria for ADHD as written could be expected to have some inherent difficulties when extended to use with adults.

✓ Not only the symptom items are developed and worded expressly for application to children (ages 4–16), but also the thresholds for the number of symptoms required to be met to establish the presence of sufficient inattention or hyperactive–impulsive behavior.

✓ Problems also exist in the restricted stipulation of the domains of impairment that must exist for a diagnosis (home, school, or work), which fall far short of the varied domains in which adults must be adaptively effective.

✓ The problems are compounded by an utter lack of guidelines for determining the meaning of and reference group for specifying impairment (intraindividual discrepancies, comparisons to similar peer groups, comparison to the normal population, etc.).

✓ Problematic as well is the imposition of an age of onset for symptoms that produce impairment (before 7 years), which is wholly unempirical in origin and imposes severe limitations on the use of this criterion with adults.

✓ Nor is it evident that the subtyping approach recommended for children has any merit for adults with ADHD, much less for the children themselves. This is particularly likely, since children may move from the hyperactive type into the combined type as they progress from early to middle childhood and from the combined to the inattentive type by adolescence or early adulthood by virtue of the differing developmental course of the two different lists of symptoms (the hyperactive symptoms declining earlier than the inattentive symptoms).

✓ Clinicians wishing to apply the DSM-IV-TR criteria to the diagnosis of adults need to be keenly aware of these limitations, adjusting the criteria as recommended above and supplementing them with other measures of developmental inappropriateness, such as behavior rating scales completed by both the patient and someone who knows him or her well.

✓ Clinicians need to exercise careful judgment in determining if symptoms reported by patients are in fact inappropriate and reflective of disorder rather than simply resulting from dissatisfaction with current performance in current activities or from a desire to obtain accommodations or performance-enhancing medications so as to be more competitive in high stakes examinations or circumstances.

✓ Consideration must be given to establishing that impairment is relative to the average or normal person and not to some high-functioning specialized peer group or index of general cognitive ability, such as IQ scores.

✓ Clinicians should consider utilizing several methods of establishing impairment, such as a combination of patient-reported history, corroboration through others who know the patient well, and archival records that may reflect such impairment, as in school, medical, mental health, employment, criminal, and driving records.

✓ It is certainly worth remembering the admonition in the DSM criteria that if the symptoms are better accounted for by the existence of another disorder, the diagnosis of ADHD may be inappropriate; this is particularly so for complaints of inattentiveness that may arise coincidentally with mood or affective disorders, especially of late-adolescent or adult onset.

CHAPTER 4

Defining ADHD in Adults
MAKING THE DIAGNOSIS
IN THE UMASS AND MILWAUKEE STUDIES

Chapter 3 raised the various issues involved in attempting to use the DSM-IV diagnostic criteria for ADHD with adults. In this chapter, we describe how we resolved these issues in creating the selection criteria for the groups in both the UMASS Study and the Milwaukee Study. As in the remaining chapters of this book, we first present the information for the UMASS Study of clinic-referred adults with ADHD, followed by that for the Milwaukee Study, an 18+-year prospective longitudinal study of hyperactive children followed to a mean age of 27 years. While these selection criteria may be of less interest to clinicians, they are crucial to scientists and students who wish to understand the formation of these groups and hence the very definition of the independent variable of interest in both of these projects, that being ADHD.

Diagnostic Criteria for ADHD Used in the UMASS Study

The UMASS Study recruited three groups of participants. The groups and sample sizes were 146 for the clinically diagnosed ADHD group, 97 for the clinic-referred non-ADHD control group, and 109 for the nonreferred community control group. Henceforth, these groups are referred to as the ADHD, Clinical control, and Community control groups respectively. As noted earlier, clinical control groups are very important in such studies because they help to control for referral biases that can result in differences between ADHD and normal groups

41

yet have little to do with ADHD. They can also help control for comorbid disorders, such as anxiety and depression, which may be present to an equivalent extent in both clinical groups yet would be a confounding factor in comparisons of ADHD with normal control groups. In short, what clinical control groups provide is the ability to examine evidence specific to the findings for ADHD and not just for being clinic-referred.

Recruitment

Both the ADHD and Clinical control adults were obtained from consecutive referrals to the Adult ADHD Clinic in the Department of Psychiatry at the University of Massachusetts Medical School. The Community control adults were obtained from advertisements posted throughout the medical school lobbies and from periodic newspaper ads in the regional newspaper. All participants signed statements of informed consent as approved by the medical school institutional review board and all were paid $100 for their participation. Significant others were paid $20 each for the forms we asked them to complete. After contacting the project, all participants were scheduled for their initial diagnostic interview with the second author and IQ screening test administered by a master's-level psychological assistant. These steps were done to determine eligibility for participation in any of the three groups.

To be eligible all subjects had to have an IQ of 80 or higher on the Shipley Institute of Living Scale (see sidebar). They also had to have no evidence of deafness, blindness, or other significant sensory impairment; significant and obvious brain damage or neurological injury or epilepsy; significant language disorders that would interfere with comprehension of verbal instructions in the protocol; a chronic and serious medical condition such as diabetes, thyroid disease, cancer, heart disease; or a childhood history of mental retardation, autism, or psychosis. To be placed in the ADHD group, clinic-referred participants had to meet the DSM-IV criteria for ADHD except for the age-of-onset criterion as judged by an experienced clinical psychologist (Murphy) using a structured interview for ADHD created by the authors (see sidebar). Participants in the Clinical control group were those evaluated at this same clinic but who did not receive a clinical diagnosis of ADHD.

As noted earlier, no precise age of onset of symptoms producing impairment was required for placement within the ADHD group so that we could examine the value of specifying various age ranges of onset for the diagnosis of ADHD in adults. Typically, we require corroboration of ADHD symptoms and impairment from someone else who knows the person well, such as parents, siblings, or spouses/partners, as part of a clinical diagnosis of ADHD. We did not do so here, although we did collect such information for most participants. This permitted us to specifically examine the degree of agreement between those sources and the

Shipley Institute of Living Scale (Shipley, 1946)

This short intelligence test served as a measure of IQ in the UMASS Study. It comprises a 40-item vocabulary test and 20 items assessing abstract thinking. The composite IQ score correlates well with other measures of intelligence (Zachary, 1988) and was employed here as a screening criterion for intellectual level as part of the study entry criteria.

Structured Clinical Interview for ADHD

A paper-and-pencil interview was created that consisted of the criteria from the DSM-IV for ADHD. This interview was employed by an experienced clinician during the initial interview with participants as part of the selection criteria used for identifying the groups as having ADHD or not. Symptoms of ADHD were reviewed twice, once for current functioning (past 6 months) and a second time for childhood between 5 and 12 years of age, with the requirement that the symptom be endorsed only if it occurs often or even more frequently. The onset of symptoms was also questioned in this interview. Six domains of impairment were also reviewed with participants, requiring them to indicate, as with the ADHD symptom list, whether or not these domains were impaired often or even more frequently. Also, participants indicated approximately at what age each domain became impaired. The domains were occupational, home, social, participation in community activities, education, and dating/marriage. The interview was used in both projects reported here.

Current Symptoms Scale and Childhood Symptoms Scale (Barkley & Murphy, 2006)

Besides interviewing the subjects about significant symptoms of ADHD, oppositional defiant disorder (ODD), and conduct disorder (CD), participants completed a rating scale containing these items from the DSM-IV. Each item can be reported on a 4-point scale (0–3) using the response format of not at all, sometimes, often, and very often. Participants completed the scale twice; once with reference to *current symptoms* and a second time with reference to retrospectively recalled *childhood symptoms* of ADHD/ODD (ages 5–12 years) and symptoms of CD (ages 5–18). A total score was calculated separately for each disorder, with the score for ADHD further subdivided into two scores, one for inattention and another for hyperactive-impulsive items. Participants also rated their current degree of impairment as a consequence of any ADHD symptoms in 10 different domains of current functioning and, for the childhood form, 8 different domains of childhood functioning. The 10 domains assessed for current functioning were work, social, community, education, dating/marriage, money, driving, leisure, and daily responsibilities. The 8 domains on the childhood ratings were family, social, community, school, sports, self-care, play, and chores. A separate impairment score was obtained for each scale by summing across these ratings. We also obtained the same two rating scales about

ADHD and impairment from their parents (or a sibling, should parents be deceased or unavailable to the study). Current spouses or cohabiting partners of the participants, if available, completed the current functioning version of this scale. Validity of the scale has been demonstrated through past findings of significant group differences between ADHD and control adults (Barkley et al., 2001; Murphy et al., 2001). An earlier DSM-III-R version of the current symptoms scale also correlated significantly with the same scale completed by a parent ($r = .75$) and by a spouse or intimate partner of the ADHD adult ($r = .64$) (Murphy & Barkley, 1996b). Correlations across these informants for the scales used in the present study are reported later in this book and are consistent with the results of these earlier studies supporting their validity. These scales were used in both the UMASS and Milwaukee Studies.

Vocabulary and Block Design Subtests from the Wechsler Adult Intelligence Scale, Third Edition (WAIS-III; Wechsler, 1997)

Two subtests were chosen from this standardized intelligence test to serve as a quick screening for level of verbal and nonverbal intelligence (Vocabulary and Block Designs) in the Milwaukee Study. They were chosen for having among the highest correlations with the Verbal and Nonverbal IQ scores, respectively, derived from the complete test administration. The scaled scores from both subtests were used here.

Peabody Picture Vocabulary Test (Dunn & Dunn, 1981)

This relatively simple assessment of receptive language was used at the childhood entry point in the Milwaukee Study as a measure of IQ. The test comprises a series of vocabulary words escalating in difficulty. When each word is spoken to the child, he or she is simultaneously shown four pictures on a single page and asked to report which picture represents the meaning of that word. Standard scores from this test were used in the Milwaukee Study.

Conners Parent and Teacher Rating Scales—Revised (CPRS-R, CTRS-R; Goyette, Conners, & Ulrich, 1978)

The parent version of this is a 48-item scale and is among the most widely used rating scales in the history of research on hyperactivity–ADHD in children (See Barkley, 1990, p. 288–289). Each item is rated on a 4-point Likert scale (0–3 for not at all, just a little, pretty much, and very much). The scale assesses five behavioral factors: conduct problems, learning problems, psychosomatic, complaints, impulsivity–hyperactivity, and anxiety. A 10-item Hyperactivity Index is also computed and was believed to represent the most frequently occurring items in children with hyperactivity. Scores are determined by summing the responses across all items for that factor and then dividing by the number of items to get the mean response. The Hyperactivity Index of this scale was used at the childhood study entry point to select subjects to be in the hyperactive group, as noted above.

The teacher version of the scale is shorter, containing 28 items that can be scored as three factors of conduct problems, hyperactivity, and inattention–passivity, along with the same 10-item Hyperactivity Index found on the parent scale. Both the parent and teacher scales have been used extensively in research in ADHD, including group identification as hyperactive, studies of medication effects, and studies of parent training outcomes (see Barkley, 1990, for a review). Norms for both scales were reported by Goyette et al. (1978) and are reprinted in Barkley (1981).

Home Situations Questionnaire (HSQ; Barkley, 1990)

This scale was developed to evaluate the situational pervasiveness of children's behavioral problems. Parents answer whether or not their child has a behavioral problem in 16 different home and public situations; if so, they rate that problem using a 0 to 9 Likert scale. Two scores are obtained from the scale, one reflecting the number of different problem settings and the other the mean severity rating for all settings claimed to be problematic. To be in the Milwaukee Study, the hyperactive children had to be posing problems in at least 6 of the 16 settings. Norms collected subsequent to the scale's use in this project indicate that this requirement approximates 1 SD above the normal mean on the scale (Barkley, 1990, p. 293).

Werry–Weiss–Peters Activity Rating Scale
(WWPARS; see Barkley, 1981, pp. 111–113; Barkley, 1990, pp. 660–662)

The original 31-item scale was developed to evaluate children's levels of hyperactive behavior in home and school situations (Werry & Sprague, 1970). It was subsequently modified to a 22-item scale for use with parents by Routh, Schroeder, and O'Tuama (1974) in which the school items were deleted. The modified scale was employed here at study entry to select the hyperactive children based on a threshold of +2 SD above the mean for a small sample of normal children ($N = 140$) studied by Routh, Schroeder, and O'Tuama (1974).

participants and the ecological validity of the reports of the participants as part of the aims of this study.

As for meeting DSM-IV diagnostic criteria by self-report, the clinician conducting the interview exercised his judgment as to whether the patient's reports on these matters could be considered to be realistic or to have some veracity. As a consequence, a few individuals were clinically diagnosed as having ADHD by the clinician despite their not meeting diagnostic criteria strictly by their own initial self-report. Others who did meet criteria based solely on their self-report may not have been granted the clinical diagnosis of ADHD. The latter would have been assigned to the Clinical control group instead. A moment's reflection will show several reasons for why this necessarily had to be the case; such reasons are informative for readers wishing to conduct clinical evaluations of adults for ADHD.

First, the self-reported ADHD-like symptoms may have been clinically judged to be better accounted for by the presence of another diagnosis (such as dysthymia, depression, anxiety, substance abuse, marital problem, a situational stressor). This is a requirement of the DSM criteria for ADHD that may often go overlooked in research studies that select their ADHD group merely by rating scales or solely on self-reported information. This criterion can be executed only via clinical judgment and knowledge of differential diagnosis; it cannot be incorporated into some mindless algorithm that relies exclusively on self-report.

Second, the symptoms patients endorsed and/or the associated impairment they alleged may not have risen to the level of being clinically significant or maladaptive in the clinician's judgment. DSM criteria require that symptoms be developmentally inappropriate and lead to impairment, both of which inherently involve clinical judgment. For example, patients may have endorsed 14 of the 18 symptoms, but the examples of their symptoms they gave were judged to be clinically trivial and the impact they had in producing clinically significant impairment was either minor or nonexistent. Likewise, they may have given evidence of having no real impairment other than an internal perception that they were somehow not working up to their potential or not being as successful or effective as they thought they should be. In other words, there was no other historical corroborative evidence in their reports that the behavior of which they complained was actually a symptom (abnormal) or that the impairment they claimed interfered with their functioning so severely that it resulted in their being well below the "average person" standard discussed above. For example, despite their reported symptoms, they may have suffered no problems in school, have received no prior psychological treatment, have received no accommodations for a disorder at school or at work, were happily married, and demonstrated no occupational impairment; or they may have failed to manifest convincing social or daily adaptive impairment that, in the clinician's judgment, was significant and a consequence of ADHD. In some cases, these were what one might call "ADHD wannabes" who were self-diagnosed before coming into the study, typically based on reading a popular trade book on ADHD in adults or hearing media accounts of the disorder and believing themselves to have it. The ease with which ADHD symptoms can be faked, either in interviews or on some tests, makes such efforts to seek consistency of current symptoms with the history and evidence for impairment critical to accurate diagnosis (Harrison, Edwards, & Parker, 2007). In short, to be eligible for the ADHD group, participants had to have a sufficient number of DSM-IV symptoms that, in the clinician's judgment, also produced clinically significant real-world functional impairment in major life activities.

Third, for the clinician to have rendered an ADHD diagnosis, he needed to see fairly compelling evidence of an onset of symptoms at some time during childhood or adolescence, a chronic (unremitting) and pervasive pattern of ADHD symptoms, and impairment that could be reasonably attributed to ADHD. The clinician did not simply record mere self-reported symptom counts or statements of impairment relying solely on a judgment-free algorithm. It was clear that some patients did not have a good perspective on what constitutes impairment. For example, they may have denied having any significant impairment, yet a closer look at their history and school records may have shown substantial struggles in school achievement and deportment, in conduct in the community (delinquency), in their job performance or social relationships, or in just managing daily major responsibilities. However, they might have simply chalked it up to "I just hated school" or their job, or their friend or partner, and so on, rather than viewing their difficulties as stemming from any sort of disorder.

Finally, there had to be convincing evidence that the symptoms had actually developed and produced impairment at some time during childhood or adolescence. Consistent with our criticisms—raised in the previous chapter—about the DSM criteria for ADHD, in many cases, when asked the question about onset, people had a hard time specifying an exact age. They used phrases such as "as long as I can remember," "always," "forever," and so on. Others evidenced a very poor memory of their childhood and could not remember when they first noticed problems, yet they may have given the clinician other information that helped attach an age to the onset of symptoms producing impairment (such as getting suspended or held back in first grade). In addition, some might have said their impairment began in high school, yet during the interview or from inspecting school records it became clear that the impairment had begun much earlier. Hence, differences could exist in self-reported perceptions of onset versus a clinician's determination of onset based on the totality of information received during the assessment.

The Clinical control group comprised all those patients referred to this same clinic who were not clinically diagnosed as having ADHD. The primary diagnoses given by the clinician to this group were varied but included the following: 43%, anxiety disorders; 15%, drug use disorders; 12%, mood disorders; 4%, learning disorders; 4%, partner relationship problems; 4%, adjustment disorders; 1%, personality disorders; 1%, oppositional defiant disorder; and 17%, no diagnosis.

The Community control group consisted of relatively normal adults drawn from the local central Massachusetts region via advertisements. To be eligible for this group, they must have met the criteria noted earlier for all participants. In addition, they had to have a score on the Adult ADHD Rating Scale (see sidebar) based on current symptoms (by self-report) *below* the 84th percentile (within +1

SD of mean) for their age (using norms reported in Barkley & Murphy, 1998, 2006). They also had to be free of any ongoing medication for treatment of a medical condition or psychiatric disorder that could be judged to interfere with the measures to be collected.

Determining the Diagnosis:
Patient Report versus Clinician Judgment

We can demonstrate what differences may exist in the pattern of diagnosis and assignment to groups in our study comparing the clinician judgment approach to group assignment versus an approach based only on patient report without intervening clinical judgment, since we recorded patient information about ADHD symptoms and other DSM criteria as it was reported during the interview. If we consider only current functioning while still using the relaxed age of onset of 14 years, we found that 13 (9%) of the 146 adults assigned to the ADHD group by clinical judgment did not meet the DSM criteria for current symptoms because seven did not have the requisite six symptoms on either list by their own report, two did not meet the more relaxed age of onset by 14, and five did not have two settings of impairment by their own report. The disagreement here between patient- and clinician-driven diagnosis seems to be minor and has little consequence for the composition of this group.

Now consider the non-ADHD Clinical control group, where a far different pattern emerged. Here we found that 45% of Clinical controls met these modified DSM criteria (*n* = 44) by their own report, which represents a sizable disagreement with clinical diagnosis. This disagreement is driven by all of the problems we noted above in relying exclusively on patient-driven information applied with only a DSM algorithm. This was especially so for criterion E, in which a judgment must be made as to whether the symptoms reported by the patient are not better understood as being due to another disorder. It is interesting to note that the majority of these cases of disagreement (64%, or *n* = 44) were in the inattentive subtype of ADHD based only on patient reports. This likely arises because symptoms of inattention are common in other clinical disorders besides ADHD—a circumstance that clinical diagnosis will weigh in reaching a diagnostic decision but that a patient-driven algorithm would not. As is shown below, it can also arise when this algorithm does not invoke a requirement for diagnostic levels of symptoms (six of nine) to be present in childhood, since it is based entirely on current functioning.

This situation improves considerably, however, if one imposes the requirement that patients must have met criteria for the disorder in childhood based on their retrospective recall in addition to meeting DSM criteria for current symptoms and functioning. Again, this would be based entirely on patient-driven information. If we now impose the additional requirement of having six or more patient-reported inattention or hyperactive symptoms in childhood by recall, then 82% of the clinician-diagnosed ADHD cases still meet all DSM criteria (27, or 18%, do not) which is a decline of just 9%—still a fairly respectable level of agreement between patient-driven and clinician-based diagnosis for that group. But now only 22% of those assigned to the Clinical control group would be considered to have ADHD based on a purely patient-driven algorithm. This is a reduction of 23%, or nearly half of the prior cases self-diagnosed as ADHD in this Clinical control group, and it yields a more acceptable level of disagreement between patient-driven and clinician-based diagnosis for assignment to this group. It is still possible that other clinicians might well have diagnosed some or all of this 22% of Clinical controls as having actual ADHD, given that disagreement can surely arise on whether or not the symptoms, especially those of inattention, can or cannot be better attributed to another disorder. Even if that were true, it would make our study a more conservative comparison of these two clinical groups (not an undesirable feature), since there would be some overlap in ADHD membership between these two groups that could attenuate any group differences that might exist on our measures. Given that our study is adequately powered to detect small to moderate effect sizes (group differences) on our measures, this is a conservative situation that we find acceptable. Therefore we continue to make up our study groups using a clinician-based diagnosis rather than a purely patient-driven algorithm.

ADHD Subtypes in the UMASS Study ADHD Group

Of the 146 adults assigned to the ADHD group, 30 were inattentive types (20%), 6 were residual (4%), and 110 were combined types (76%) by clinician diagnosis. But if we applied a mindless DSM algorithm that relied solely on patient self-reported information while also relaxing the age of onset to 14 years and considered only current symptoms and functioning (not childhood), then the subtyping breakdown would be 47% inattentive, 42% combined, 7% hyperactive, and 5% residual. It is evident here that far more ADHD patients would have been assigned to the inattentive type using a patient-driven algorithm approach to diagnosis than one relying on the application of clinical judgment to such patient information. This is most likely due to the fact that many combined type patients outgrow enough symptoms of hyperactivity to no longer qualify as that type by adulthood under DSM decision rules (as noted above). In our clinical practice, on the other hand, we typically consider that if an adult has ever previously met criteria for the combined type, including childhood, he or she remains in that category for clinical diagnostic purposes. Differences in the proportions of the other two types of ADHD are most likely to be a consequence of the aforementioned differences between patient perceptions of the occurrence of a developmentally inappropriate symptom versus that of an experienced clinician.

Demographic Characteristics of the UMASS Study Groups

The demographic characteristics of our three participant groups are shown in Table 4.1. The age of our ADHD group was significantly lower than that of the other two groups, by an average of 4 years from the Community control group and 5 years from the Clinical control group. This means that in all of the analyses of continuous measures to be conducted on these groups throughout this book, we must consider using age as a covariate. To do so, we first correlate age with the various measures and, where that correlation proves to be significant, we then include it as a covariate in the analysis of that measure. Throughout the tables of results in this book, we follow the convention of indicating that age was used as a covariate by placing a superscript A ([A]) next to that particular measure. We also examine our measures for any sex differences, and especially for the interaction of sex of participant with the grouping factor, as that would indicate that sex differences may be quite different within the various groups. The latter finding is important to note, as it could suggest that women with ADHD differ from men in various aspects of their disorder that are not merely the result of sex differences evident across all groups (main effects for sex). For instance, as Table 4.2 shows, the ADHD group had fewer years of education than either of the control groups, while the Clinical control group had more years of education than the Community control group. On average, however, the educational levels of our groups were several years beyond high school, indicating a relatively well-educated participant pool in this study. Yet here we also found a significant interaction of sex with group. We illustrate this relationship in Figure 4.1.

As Figure 4.1 appears to show, females in the ADHD group had more education than did males in this group, while the opposite was true in the Community control group. In the Clinical control group, however, there were no appar-

TABLE 4.1. Demographic Characteristics by Group for Dimensional Measures for the UMASS Study

Measure	ADHD		Clinical		Community		F	p	Pairwise contrasts
	Mean	SD	Mean	SD	Mean	SD			
Age (years)	32.4	10.9	37.8	13.2	36.4	12.0	6.78	.001	1 < 2,3
Education (years)[GxS]	14.2	2.2	16.3	2.8	15.4	2.7	15.05	< .001	1 < 3 < 2
IQ	106.6	8.8	109.6	8.8	108.3	7.9	2.79	NS	
Hollingshead[A]	38.2	26.8	54.1	31.3	42.3	26.7	64.93	< .001	1,3 < 2

Note. Sample sizes are ADHD = 146, Clinical control = 97, and Community control = 109. IQ is from the Shipley Institute of Living Scale. Hollingshead = Hollingshead Job Index from the Hollingshead Index of Social Position; SD = standard deviation; F = F-test results of the analysis of variance (or covariance); p = probability value for the F-test; NS = not significant, [S] = Significant main effect for sex (see text for details); [GxS] = significant group × sex interaction (see Figure 4.1 and text for details); [A] = age used as a covariate in this analysis.

Statistical analysis: Groups were initially compared using two-way (groups × sex) analysis of variance (or covariance as necessary). Where this analysis was significant (p < .05) for the main effect for group, pairwise comparisons of the groups were conducted the results of which are shown in the last column.

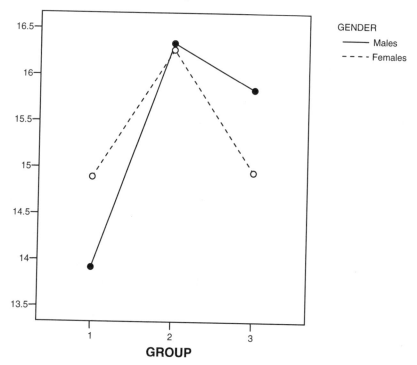

FIGURE 4.1. Graph showing the number of years of education for each sex within each group (the group × sex interaction was significant) for the UMASS Study. Group 1 = ADHD, 2 = Clinical control, 3 = Community control.

ent sex differences in education. This may suggest that ADHD has a significantly greater impact on educational attainment in males than in females with the disorder. Yet it could simply reflect differences in the recruitment of these samples—differences that are not characteristic of the general population of adults with ADHD. We return to these issues in a later chapter examining the various education-related outcomes for these groups.

We also found that the ADHD group ranked lower in their average Hollingshead Occupational Index than did the Clinical control group (Hollingshead, 1975) but did not differ from the Community control group, implying that the Clinical control adults held higher-ranked positions of employment than the other groups. Chapter 9 revisits this finding, along with others having to do with occupational functioning. For now, we have simply shown that adults with ADHD are significantly less educated than other adults and hold jobs of somewhat lower social status than do the Clinical control adults participating in this project. The groups are not different in their intellectual abilities, however.

Some of the demographic features of our groups were categorical in nature, such as sex; therefore these attributes are shown in Table 4.2. Slightly more than

TABLE 4.2. Demographic Characteristics by Group for Categorical Measures for the UMASS Study

Measure	ADHD		Clinical		Community		χ^2	p	Pairwise contrasts
	N	%	N	%	N	%			
Sex (males)	99	68	54	56	51	47	11.60	.003	1 > 3
Ethnic group (white)	138	94	91	94	103	94	6.06	NS	
Ever married	65	45	47	50	69	64	9.25	.01	1,2 < 3
Living with spouse	45	31	41	44	50	46	7.01	.03	1 < 2,3
Living alone	29	20	12	13	17	16	2.24	NS	
Living with parents	37	26	17	18	19	18	3.06	NS	
Currently employed	106	73	67	71	83	77	0.87	NS	

Note. N = sample sizes that fell into each categorical measure; % = the percentage of the entire group sample that fell into each categorical measure; χ^2 = results for the Pearson omnibus chi-square; p = probability value for the chi-square result. Pairwise contrasts = results for the paired comparisons of the groups with each other, if the omnibus chi-square was significant ($p < .05$).

two-thirds (68%) of our ADHD group were male, which differed from a nearly equal sex distribution (51%) in our Community control group but was not significantly different from that evident in the Clinical control group (56%). This finding is in keeping with many studies of children and adults with ADHD demonstrating a greater representation of the disorder in males than females (Barkley, 2006; Kessler et al., 2006). Typically, ADHD is approximately three times more common in males than in females, at least in childhood epidemiological (community-derived) samples, but this ratio may fall to 2:1 in adult epidemiological studies—a ratio similar to that found here. The vast majority of participants were white (94%) or of European-American ancestry; the groups did not differ in this respect. This finding therefore warrants caution in any efforts to extrapolate these results to adults with ADHD in ethnic groups other than that represented here.

In terms of marital status, both of our clinical groups were less likely to be married at the time of this evaluation than were the Community control adults. Yet even if married, significantly fewer of the adults with ADHD were likely to be currently living with their spouse, which was the consequence of a higher separation and divorce rate in the ADHD group. We examine this and other issues related to marital adjustment in a later chapter of this book; for now, there is some suggestion that adults with ADHD are less likely to marry. If they have married, they are more likely to be divorced—a finding that emerged in our earlier study of adults with ADHD (Murphy & Barkley, 1996b). The groups did not differ from each other in the likelihood that they were currently living alone or living with a parent. We also found that these groups were not different in the proportions that were currently employed, with over 70% of each group working at the time of their entry into our study.

These results give a quick snapshot of the demographic attributes of our samples and even begin to intimate some differences that distinguish the ADHD group from the others—differences that receive further attention in later chapters. But we can be confident going forward that any differences we may find among the groups are not the result of intellectual abilities or ethnic differences. However, a special effort will need to be made to examine and, if necessary, statistically control for any influence that age may have on our results, given the younger average age of our ADHD group.

Treatment History of the UMASS Groups

The history of psychological or psychiatric treatment received by our groups is shown in Table 4.3. As this table indicates, the majority (78% and 60%) of our two clinical groups had been previously evaluated by some type of mental health professional. Of interest, however, is that 34% of our Community control group had also been evaluated. A history of treatment from a mental health professional was not an exclusionary criterion for eligibility for this group, given that even otherwise normal individuals may seek mental health consultation for a variety of stressful or emotionally disturbing events in their lives yet not necessarily have a psychiatric disorder. This is evident in the subsequent rows in this table, where

TABLE 4.3. Evaluation and Treatment History by Group for the UMASS Study

Measure	ADHD N	ADHD %	Clinical N	Clinical %	Community N	Community %	χ^2	p	Pairwise contrasts
Ever evaluated	113	78	56	60	37	34	49.0	< .001	1 > 2 > 3
Prior Dx of ADHD[S]	49	34	15	16	0	0	48.2	< .001	1 > 2 > 3
Prior non-ADHD Dx	72	50	42	45	3	3	68.5	< .001	1,2 > 3
Psych treatment	116	80	76	81	43	40	55.9	< .001	1,2 > 3
Residential/halfway[S]	16	11	3	3	0	0	15.9	< .001	1 > 2,3
Hospitalized	17	12	5	5	0	0	14.5	.001	1,2 > 3
On psych meds now	39	17	29	30	0	0	37.9	< .001	1,2 > 3
Stimulants	12	8	6	6	0	0	9.0	.011	1,2 > 3
Antidepressants	21	14	20	20	0	0	22.8	< .001	1,2 > 3
Other meds	17	12	10	10	0	0	12.23	.001	1,2 > 3
Ever on psych meds	82	57	45	48	7	6	70.1	< .001	1,2 > 3

Note. Sample sizes are ADHD = 145, Clinical control = 94, and Community control = 108. N = sample sizes that fell into each categorical measure; % = the percentage of the entire group sample that fell into each categorical measure; χ^2 = results for the Pearson omnibus chi-square; p = probability value for the chi-square result; pairwise contrasts = results for the paired comparisons of the groups with each other, if the omnibus chi-square was significant (p < .05); [S]= significant main effect for sex; Dx = diagnosis; psych treatment = any prior psychological or psychiatric treatment; on psych meds now = on psychiatric medication at entry into the study; ever on psych meds = any treatment with psychiatric drugs; other meds = other psychiatric medications, predominantly antianxiety drugs.

none of the community controls had ever been diagnosed with ADHD and just 3% had received any other psychiatric diagnosis as a consequence of their contact with a mental health professional.

Significantly more adults in the ADHD group had been previously evaluated by a mental health professional compared to either the Clinical or Community control groups, perhaps implying that ADHD may be a more severe disorder that is more likely to lead to a mental health evaluation than are those disorders represented in the Clinical control group. Yet just one-third (34%) of our ADHD group had been previously diagnosed as having ADHD—a fact that serves to illustrate that ADHD in adults may not be widely recognized by mental health specialists working with adults. Nevertheless, this figure was significantly greater than the 16% found in our Clinical control group and in none of the Community controls. Yet nearly half of the adults in each of our clinical groups had received some other diagnosis than ADHD from a previously seen professional, with these two groups not differing in this respect. There was a significant main effect for sex on the measure of prior ADHD diagnosis, such that males were more likely than females to have been previously diagnosed as ADHD across all groups (22% vs. 14%, $p = .045$).

As for prior treatment, we found that at least 80% of our two clinical groups had received some form of prior psychiatric or psychological treatment and that approximately half of each of these groups had been previous treated with psychiatric medications; both groups certainly differed from the Community control group in these respects. The figures were significantly lower in the Community control group, where 40% had participated in some form of mental health treatment approach, while just 6% had taken a psychiatric medication. The figures were low for all groups in terms of prior hospitalization or residential treatment, although, as expected, the clinical groups were more likely than the Community control group to have experienced this form of treatment. Even so, the ADHD group was significantly more likely to have been previously treated in a residential or halfway house facility than either the Clinical or Community control groups. There was a sex difference that proved significant here, but it did not interact with the grouping factor and so characterized all the groups. We found that males were more likely than females to have participated in residential treatment (8% vs. 1%, $p = .004$).

Important to consider is the proportion of the groups that were currently receiving psychiatric medications, as these could have some potential biasing effect on the results of our various dependent measures, particularly those of impairment and the neuropsychological tests. We can see in Table 4.3 that 17% of the ADHD group was currently on some form of psychiatric medication, mostly antidepressants or antianxiety drugs (the principal class in the "other medication" category), while 30% of the Clinical control group were on medications at study entry—a figure that is not significantly different from that in the ADHD group. Again, the medication profile for this group was similar to that for the ADHD group, with the most frequent class of medications being antidepressants, followed by antianxiety drugs. To evaluate the potential effect that medication status may have had on our results, we compared those ADHD cases that were on medication to those not on medication in the following measures, reflecting severity of their disorder: the frequency of their ADHD symptoms from the interview, their age of onset, the number of domains of impairment from the interview, the number of childhood ADHD symptoms (interview), the total score for ADHD symptoms from self-ratings in adulthood and in childhood, self-rated impairment total scores on these same scales, the total score for ADHD symptoms from ratings provided by others for both current and childhood behavior, and the total impairment scores provided by others for both current and childhood functioning. None of these comparisons were significant. We conducted the same analyses for those patients in the Clinical control group who were and were not currently on medication. Again, none were significant. We therefore felt reasonably confident that the small proportion of patients in these two groups currently taking medication would not bias our results by significantly reducing the severity of their ADHD-related symptoms (the independent variable of interest to this project). If it were to do so, however, the bias would likely make the study a more conservative one by reducing differences between the two clinical groups and the Community control group. We therefore combined the medicated and unmedicated patients in each clinical group for all subsequent analyses reported in this book.

The Milwaukee Study Participant Selection Criteria

This study utilized a Hyperactive group, rigorously diagnosed as having been hyperactive in childhood ($N = 158$), and a matched Community control group ($N = 81$) that was followed concurrently. These two groups were originally evaluated in 1979–1980, when they were 4 to 12 years of age, to participate in studies of mother–child interactions in hyperactive and normal children so as to further evaluate the effects of age on these interaction patterns and, in a subset of these children, to examine stimulant drug effects on these interactions (see Barkley, Karlsson, Strzelecki, & Murphy, 1984; Barkley, Karlsson, & Pollard, 1985; Barkley, Karlsson, Pollard, & Murphy, 1985). The majority of these participants (hyperactive $n = 123$, or 78%; normal $n = 66$, or 81%) were evaluated again in 1987-88 when they were 12 to 20 years of age (see Barkley, Fischer, et al., 1990; Barkley, Fischer, et al., 1991; Fischer, Barkley, Edelbrock, & Smallish, 1990; Fischer, Barkley, Fletcher, & Smallish, 1993a, 1993b; Fletcher, Fischer, Barkley, & Smallish, 1996). The participants were reassessed in 1992–1996 when they were at least 19 years of age (ages 19–25 years of age; mean = 21 years) (see Barkley, Fischer, et al., 2002; Barkley et al., 2004; Barkley, Fischer, et al., 2006; Fischer et al., 2002; Fischer & Barkley, 2006; Fischer, Barkley, Smallish, & Fletcher, 2005, 2007). At that time, all of the participants in both groups were able to be located. The participation rate at that follow-up (completion of all measures) was 93% (147 of 158) for the Hyperactive group and 90% (73 of 81) for the Community control group. For this follow-up (at a mean age of 27), 135 (85%) of the original hyperactive participants agreed to participate, as did 75 (93%) of the original 81 control participants. One control subject died of a sudden cardiac arrest before the adolescent follow-up and another died prior to the age-21 follow-up in a car accident. One hyperactive participant died by suicide prior to this follow-up. Two of the hyperactive subjects had died since the previous evaluation (mean age 21 years), one from suicide and one from a drug overdose. Despite these tragic losses, we have an excellent retention and participation rate for a longitudinal study that has now followed its subjects for more than 18 years.

Recruitment at Childhood Entry

At childhood entry into the study, all participants were required to (1) have an IQ greater than 80 on the Peabody Picture Vocabulary Test (Dunn & Dunn, 1981), (2) be free of gross sensory or motor abnormalities, and (3) be the biological offspring of their current mothers or have been adopted by them shortly after birth. All parents signed statements of informed consent for their own and their child's participation in the study. The original gender composition was 91% male and 9% female. The racial composition was 94% white, 5% black, and 1% Hispanic.

The Hyperactive group was originally recruited from consecutive referrals to a child psychology service specializing in the treatment of hyperactive children at Milwaukee Children's Hospital. The Community control group was recruited using a "snowball" technique in which the parents of the hyperactive children were asked to provide the names of their friends who had children within the age range of interest to the study. These friends of the parents then were contacted about the study. Those volunteering were asked a series of questions over the telephone to ensure probable eligibility for the project. Those eligible were seen for the initial evaluation. At that time, they were asked about other friends of theirs who had children; these families then were contacted to participate, and so on.

For this follow-up, all participants were contacted by phone, given an explanation of the study, and urged to volunteer to be reevaluated. They were then scheduled for their evaluations over a 2-day period, at which time formal written consent was obtained. They were then given a battery of measures that assessed psychiatric disorders, history of mental health treatments, outcomes in major life activities (education, occupation, dating, sexual activity, driving, money management, etc.), antisocial activities and drug use, and medical history.

Some psychological tests and rating scales were also collected. Participants were asked to provide the name of another adult who could best describe their current functioning and to give permission for project staff to contact and interview this person about them. All interviews were conducted by an experienced psychological assistant under the supervision of a licensed, board-certified neuropsychologist (Fischer) after extensive training. This same assistant was not blind to original group membership. However, she was blind to the subgroup designation of whether or not a participant was classified here as having current disorder. Participants were paid a stipend for their time.

The breakdown for the relationship of the collateral providing information about the hyperactive participants was parent = 39%, sibling = 7%, spouse/partner = 42%, friends = 11%, and other relative = 1%. For the Community control group, this breakdown was parent = 27%, sibling = 4%, spouse/partner = 59%, friend = 11%, and other relative = 0%. The groups did not differ significantly in these sources of collateral information (χ^2 = 5.85, p = not significant).

Participant Selection Criteria at Childhood Entry

Formal and more empirically based diagnostic criteria were not available at the time these children were recruited. While the DSM-II (American Psychiatric Association, 1968) was available, it did not provide explicit criteria for the diagnosis of hyperkinetic reaction of childhood other than to say in a single sentence that *"The disorder is characterized by overactivity, restlessness, distractibility, and short attention span, especially in young children; the behavior usually diminishes by adolescence"* (p. 50). Based on research and conceptual statements in the field at the time, Barkley developed research criteria for identifying hyperactive children, and these were employed at the study entry (see Barkley, 1982).

To be considered hyperactive, the children had to (1) have scores on both the Hyperactivity Index of the Revised Conners Parent Rating Scale—Revised (CPRS-R; Goyette et al., 1978) and the Werry–Weiss–Peters Activity Rating Scale (WWPARS; see Barkley, 1981) that met or exceeded +2 *SD*s above the mean for severity for same-age, same-sex normal children; (2) have scores on the Home Situations Questionnaire (HSQ; Barkley, 1990) indicating significant behavioral problems in at least 6 or more of the 14 problem situations on this scale (a score exceeding +1 *SD*); (3) have elicited parent and/or teacher complaints (as reported by parent) of poor sustained attention, poor impulse control, and excessive activity level; (4) have developed their behavior problems prior to 6 years of age; (5) have had their behavioral problems for at least 12 months; and (6) show no indication of autism, psychosis, thought disorder, epilepsy, gross brain damage, or mental retardation.

The criteria listed in (1) above involving the CPRS-R Hyperactivity Index and WWPARS may appear very outdated and even laughable at this point in time. However, it is important to recognize that they represented not only the state of the art at the time that this longitudinal study began but also the first attempt to include *quantitatively based* diagnostic criteria in such a study of hyperactive (now ADHD) children.

Of critical importance to the purpose of this book (comparing children with ADHD grown up to adults with ADHD) is the degree to which these selection criteria for our hyperactive group are consistent with the current diagnostic criteria for ADHD in the DSM-IV. In view of these selection criteria and the close convergence of rating scale diagnoses with the clinical diagnosis of ADHD (Edelbrock & Costello, 1988), we believe it is likely that all participants would have met criteria for ADHD based on the earlier DSM-III-R had those been available. In fact, over 70% of them met those criteria for ADHD 8 to 10 years later, at the adolescent follow-up using parent-reported information (Barkley et al., 1990). At that follow-up, we also collected again the CPRS-R and HSQ rating scales that were used at study entry to select our groups. The correlations between these scales and the number of DSM-III-R symptoms at that time were (1) CPRS-R Hyperactive–Impulsive factor score, $r = .84$, $p < .001$; (2) CPRS-R Total Score, $r = .80$, $p < .001$; and (3) HSQ number of problem settings, $r = .70$, $p < .001$. Since the HSQ is a measure of problem pervasiveness and not strictly ADHD symptoms per se, it would not be expected to correlate as well with DSM-III-R symptom counts. Nevertheless, the correlations, especially between the CPRS-R scale and DSM-III-R symptoms, are impressive enough to suggest considerable consistency between our entry criteria and those of DSM-III-R, even when collected 8 to 10 years after study entry.

Although pervasiveness of symptoms across home and school settings was not required for this study, as it is in the DSM, the vast majority of children were experiencing problems in both settings as reported in the parent interview. This was also evident on the Conners Teacher Rating Scale—Revised (CTRS-R), which was available at that time, in 58% of the Hyperactive group and 37% of the Community control group. Where teacher ratings were available, the Hyperactive group differed substantially from the Community control group on the CTRS-R Hyperactivity Index (the teacher equivalent of the CPRS-R Index) (means = 19.1 vs. 4.3, SDs = 6.3 vs. 4.5, $F = 140.08$, $p < .001$), having an average more than four times that of our Control group. Teacher ratings on the inattention factor scale of the CTRS-R also were four times greater, on average, for the Hyperactive than the Community control group (means = 1.9 vs. 0.4, SDs = 0.8 vs. 0.5; $F = 52.18$, $p < .001$) and were more than 3 times greater on the hyperactive–impulsive factor scale (means = 1.5 vs. 0.4, SDs = 0.6 vs. 0.4; $F = 81.4$, $p < .001$). This makes it clear that, at least for the subsets on whom teacher ratings were available, our Hyperactive group manifested significant problems with inattentive, hyperactive, and impulsive behavior in the school setting, even if not formally required at study entry to be selected as hyperactive.

The DSM-III-R version of ADHD became ADHD combined type in DSM-IV. Consistent with both DSM-III-R and DSM-IV, our participants were initially required to demonstrate developmentally inappropriate levels (the 98th percentile in our study) on the same symptom constructs as in these DSMs (hyperactive, impulsive, and inattentive behavior) and to have developed these problems by 6 years of age (a year earlier than the age 7 requirement in the DSMs). The majority had problems at both home and school as reported in our parental interview and substantiated where teacher ratings were available, as above. That the impairment criterion was met would be obvious and inferred from the substantially deviant levels of symptoms required at study entry (98th percentile) based on parent ratings of behavior. These criteria would be consistent with current DSM requirements even if the DSM symptom items themselves were unavailable in 1979. Therefore it is our opinion—based on the selection criteria above, the evidence marshaled here, and the current requirements for ADHD combined type in DSM-IV—that these participants would easily have met DSM criteria for ADHD had they been available. We regard these participants as having had ADHD in childhood throughout this book.

Eligibility for the Community control group was based on (1) no history of referral to a mental health professional; (2) no current parental or teacher complaints of significant behavioral problems; (3) scores within 1.5 SDs of the mean for normal children on both the Hyperactivity Index of the CPRS-R and the WWPARS; and (4) no evidence of any other psychiatric disorder. Recruitment into the initial study did not begin until at least 6 months after the Hyperactive group to permit equating of the groups by age and school grade. As a consequence, at the teen and age-21 young-adult follow-up points, the Hyperactive group has been slightly older than the Community control group. This was not the case at the age-27 follow-up reported here, where groups no longer differed significantly in their ages (mean ages were 27 years for both groups, range was 22 to 31 years). This was achieved by calling participants in to be evaluated based on their birth dates as much as possible and evaluating the oldest participants first, irrespective of their group membership.

Determining Current ADHD in Adulthood

As noted above, we consider all of these children to have DSM-defined ADHD as they entered the study. Deciding who continues to be ADHD at this adult follow-up is not as straightforward as it may first appear. We could simply apply the DSM-IV criteria as written to these adults and be done with it, just as we did in the UMASS Study above. If we did so, then just 30% of the Hyperactive group would meet the threshold of having at least 6 of 9 symptoms on either symptom list by self-report (14% inattentive type, 12% hyperactive–impulsive type, and 4% Combined type). If we added the additional requirement—having impairment in at least one or more domains by self-report—the figure falls to 24%. The results for the control group would be 3% using symptoms only, all placing in the hyperactive–impulsive type, and 1% using symptoms and impairment. If the reports of others (the collaterals) are used instead to define ADHD, these figures would be 26% for having 6 of 9 symptoms and 25% for having those symptoms plus impairment for the Hyperactive group (1% for controls in either case).

However, as discussed in the previous chapter and above, there are good reasons to challenge this approach to diagnosing adults, especially in follow-up studies of children with ADHD. Not the least of those problems is that the DSM was designed for use with children, not adults. Given that ADHD symptoms decline significantly with age in both ADHD and normal populations (see previous chapter), symptom thresholds used with children may not be useful with adults, as they would prove to represent an increasing severity level with age. As noted earlier, the threshold of 6 symptoms has been found to be at or above the 99th percentile for the general population (and of our Community control group) on each list of symptoms. This would automatically limit the diagnosis in adults to just the top 1% of the population. Previous studies (Murphy & Barkley, 1996a) and results presented in Chapter 5 all suggest that a threshold of 4 symptoms on either list is sufficient to accurately classify ADHD in adults, representing as it does approximately the 93rd percentile or +1.5 SDs above the general population mean. In other words, people can outgrow the DSM criteria as they develop from childhood to adulthood while remaining highly symptomatic and without necessarily outgrowing the disorder (or at least the developmental inappropriateness of their symptoms). We demonstrated this at the age-21 follow-up, where we found that 46% of our Hyperactive group met criteria for DSM-III-R–defined ADHD based on parent report while 66% continued to be above the 98th percentile (+2 SDs) relative to our control group—that is, they remained developmentally inappropriate or excessive in their symptoms. Thus nearly one-third of cases that remain developmentally deviant in ADHD symptoms by age 21 do not meet the DSM criteria—a rather substantial rate of misclassification.

The DSM therefore offers a syndromal, or psychopathological, approach to diagnostic criteria for disorder as if the syndrome were detected by the same invariant set of symptoms and symptom thresholds at any age. But ADHD is conceptualized in the DSM as a developmental disorder that is supposed to be evident by having "developmentally inappropriate" symptom levels. If one holds true to that conceptualization, then the developmental or symptomatic definition of ADHD as defined relative to general population peers of the same age is the more accurate or valid definition of the disorder. The DSM approach wants to have it both ways, setting forth a fixed set of diagnostic criteria (symptoms and thresholds), as if ADHD were a psychopathology (syndrome), but then insisting it be defined by symptoms that are inappropriate for developmental stage or age group, which makes it a developmental disorder. The persistence of disorder over development is going to be quite different, as we have already shown, depending on which of these views of the disorder one adopts. There is far more persistence of the developmentally defined disorder of ADHD than of the syndromally defined psychopathological one.

We side with the developmentally defined view of ADHD, especially for longitudinal studies where children, at study entry, already meet criteria for the disorder. The criteria (both symptoms and thresholds) were designed for children; therefore children meeting them will meet *both* the syndromal and developmental definitions. But that is not true for these same cases followed to adulthood, where these same DSM criteria have no scientifically validated basis. Using a threshold of four symptoms from either list in the DSM would make more sense for the rediagnosis of our ADHD children as adults in our longitudinal study. That is because it continues to represent the same threshold of developmental deviance we used to select these cases as hyperactive (or ADHD) in childhood—that being +2 SDs above the mean or the 98th percentile. This is evident in Table 4.4, where we report the number of DSM-IV symptoms self-reported in the interview for current functioning and using rating scales of ADHD symptoms completed by participants and others who knew them well, again for current functioning. The interview and rating scales of ADHD employed here are the same as those used in the UMASS Study above and described in the sidebar. It is evident from this table that no matter which measure one uses for current functioning (interviews or rating scales) or which source (self or others), the hyperactive group remains significantly deviant from our control group at this follow-up in the average level of ADHD symptoms. Using the means and SDs for the Community control group and for the interview data shows that a threshold of four symptoms represents approximately the +2 SD threshold for our control group, or its 98th percentile. We use the interview data rather than the results for the rating scales because that method is how the DSM criteria are typically applied in practice. The threshold of four symptoms per list is also the threshold that best classified adults with ADHD in the UMASS Study and the threshold recommended for use with adults based on general population samples of adults (see Chapter 5; also Murphy & Barkley, 1996a). Applying this threshold results in 56% of the hyperactive group meeting this criterion for current ADHD (10% inattentive, 17% hyperactive-impulsive, and 29% combined types). Yet it also would result in 20% of the Control group meeting this threshold on either list (8% inattentive, 11% hyperactive–impulsive, and 1% combined types).

However, the DSM-IV criteria also require current impairment in major life activities (home, school, work, etc.). If we impose this additional requirement (self-reported as impaired in the interview), then the percentage of the Hyperactive group that could be considered to have current ADHD falls from 56% to

TABLE 4.4. Current ADHD Symptoms (DSM-IV) from Interviews and Self- and Other-Ratings by Group for the Milwaukee Study

Measure	Hyperactive		Control		F	p
	Mean	SD	Mean	SD		
Current self-report (interview)						
No. of inattention items	3.0	2.5	0.9	1.4	45.12	< .001
No. of hyperactivity–impulsivity items	3.3	2.2	1.3	1.6	45.22	< .001
Total no. of ADHD items	6.2	4.0	2.2	2.6	60.39	< .001
Current self-ratings						
Total ADHD score	12.9	10.0	7.4	7.2	16.91	< .001
No. of inattention items rated 2+	1.2	2.0	0.5	1.4	7.14	.008
No. of hyperactivity–impulsivity items rated 2+	1.8	2.2	0.7	1.4	13.57	< .001
Total No. of ADHD items rated 2+	3.0	3.9	1.3	2.6	12.05	.001
Current other-ratings						
Total ADHD score	19.3	12.3	6.9	5.9	66.72	< .001
No. of inattention items rated as 2+	2.5	2.7	0.5	1.0	35.18	< .001
No. of hyperactivity–impulsivity items rated as 2+	3.0	2.7	0.5	1.1	57.71	< .001
Total no. of ADHD items rated as 2+	5.5	5.0	1.1	1.7	51.03	< .001

Note. Sample sizes for self-reported interview information are Hyperactive = 135, Control = 75. For self-ratings they are 134 and 74. For other-ratings they are Hyperactive = 132, Control = 75.

Statistical analysis: Groups were compared using one-way (groups) analysis of variance. SD = standard deviation, F = F-test results of the analysis of variance; p = probability value for the F-test; NS = not significant.

44% ($n = 55$). Because an impairment requirement is part of the DSM criteria for ADHD and because we consider it to be an important feature in establishing the presence of any disorder (see Chapter 3), we use it here to determine who has current ADHD. To reiterate, to be considered as currently having ADHD in the Hyperactive group of the Milwaukee Study, we required that individuals report at least four or more symptoms on either the inattention or hyperactive–impulsive symptom list from the DSM-IV and self-report impairment in one or more domains of major life activity covered in the interview. Henceforth, we refer to this group as being H+ADHD, or hyperactive with current ADHD. The remaining 80 members of the Hyperactive group who did not meet these criteria are referred to as H–ADHD, or hyperactive without current ADHD.

A second problem in applying the diagnosis of ADHD to adults who were diagnosed as children in such longitudinal studies is deciding which source of information is the most valid means of determining presence of the disorder. At study entry in childhood, of course parent reports were used to make the diagnosis. At the adolescent follow-up, parent report was once again used to determine the presence of current ADHD. However, all previous longitudinal studies of hyperactive children shifted to using self-reports at their adult follow-up points to establish current ADHD (see Barkley, Fischer, et al., 2002). This makes some sense if one believes that young adults are the best informants of their ADHD symptoms. As in the other studies, when we used self-reported information at the age 21 follow-up, we found that just 5% of our Hyperactive group would still be considered to have ADHD by DSM criteria. However, when we used parent-reported information, this figure rose to 46%—a remarkable disparity. Moreover, only 10% of those receiving a parent-based diagnosis of ADHD also had the diagnosis based on self-report; owing of course to the very small percentage diagnosed as ADHD by self-report. The correlation between self- and parent-reported levels of ADHD symptoms was just .21. Parent-reported symptoms were found to have a far greater association with various measures of impairment at that age than were self-reported symptoms. For that reason, we chose to view the parent reports as providing a more accurate depiction of current ADHD in our hyperactive sample than self-reports at that follow-up.

But what is the situation for the current follow-up? Should self-reported information on ADHD and impairment now be relied upon to determine current ADHD rather than reverting to parent or other reported information? We believe there are many good reasons for us to now use self-reported information to determine ADHD at this later age.

1. Far fewer of the current hyperactive sample are now living with their parents (18%) than was the case at age 21 (52%). With increasing age and independence from parents, parents may no longer have the degree of contact or ongoing experiences with their hyperactive offspring, so that they are no longer the most useful informants about those offspring.

2. The decreasing access to parents as consented to by our samples. That is, when asked who they thought could provide the best information about their current functioning and thus whom they wished us to contact for an interview about them, only 39% of the hyperactive group and 27% of the control group nominated a parent to provide this information. In contrast, 42% of the hyperactive group and 59% of the control group nominated their spouse or the significant other with whom they were currently residing to obtain this information. Thus continuing to rely on parental information for determining current ADHD is becoming less practical or feasible and less acceptable to our samples.

3. The correlation between self- and parent-reported ADHD symptoms has increased substantially since the last follow-up. Previously these sources correlated just .21, as noted above, using the entire sample of the Hyperactive and Community control groups, and just .16 in the Hyperactive group. Now, the relationship has doubled to .50 using the entire sample and .41 using just the Hyperactive group—a considerable increase. While these levels of agreement are not ideal and remain below those found for the self-referred adults with ADHD

in the UMASS Study ($r = .70$, see Chapter 5), the doubling of the extent of these relationships may suggest an increasing accuracy or at least greater concordance with others' opinions now than 5 years ago. This increasing correspondence between self- and "other" reports was also evident in the agreement between those classified as ADHD now by self-report and the percentage of these cases that would have been so classified using other reported information (53%). In any event, there is a greater reason now to accept the self-reported information as probably more credible now than it had been previously.

4. Switching to other-reported information yields a similar breakdown in the proportion of the hyperactive participants who would currently be called ADHD as does using self-reported information. If we relied on our current criteria for diagnosis of ADHD (4+ symptoms on either symptom list and 1+ impairments) based on other reports, 40% of our hyperactive sample would be classified as currently having ADHD; the corresponding figure above was 44% for self-reported criteria. So there is no real change in sample sizes or gain in statistical power to be had by switching to other-reported information.

5. The basis for diagnosing ADHD in adults using current DSM criteria is self-report.

6. We wished to compare all subsequent results for the Milwaukee Study to those obtained in the UMASS Study, and the latter study used self-reported information to determine the presence of ADHD. It seemed wise therefore to stay with groups based on the same source of information for defining ADHD (self-reports) across these two projects than to do otherwise.

With this rationale as our basis, the present study elected to rely on self-reported information for determining the presence of current ADHD. This led to 44% of the Hyperactive group being classified as H+ADHD ($N = 55$) and the remaining 56% to be classified as H−ADHD ($N = 80$). These, then, are compared against each other and the Community control group ($N = 75$) for analyzing all dependent measures collected in this project.

The fact that 56% of our Hyperactive group is classified as not currently having ADHD (H−ADHD) should not lead readers to infer that they are all normal or no longer have any ADHD. Indeed, 32% of this group would have been classified as ADHD by our current criteria (4+ symptoms and 1+ impairments) had other reports been relied upon for this purpose. Additionally, as shown in subsequent chapters, while they were comparable to our Control group on some of our measures, they remained significantly different from this group on others, though often falling below the fully ADHD group in these instances.

All this being said, it may help the reader to visualize what is happening across development in terms of the percentage of the Hyperactive (child ADHD) group that is remaining ADHD by graphically illustrating the percentage of individuals at each follow-up point who are meeting these various definitions of

ADHD using parent/other reports. To do so, we define ADHD by three methods:

- *Syndromal*: Meets the DSM-recommended symptom threshold applied regardless of current age. This is a very conservative definition of disorder, as argued above. At childhood study entry, as noted above, we consider this to be 100% of the hyperactive group, even though no DSM criteria existed at that time. For age 15, we had available DSM-III-R symptoms so the threshold would be eight of 14 as recommended in that manual. At age 21, we had the same information available. At the current follow-up (age 27), we used DSM-IV criteria, in which case the threshold now would be having six of nine symptoms on either of the two symptom lists.

- *Symptomatic 2 SD*: Places at or above the threshold representing +2 *SDs* above the mean for the control group of the same age in this study on DSM symptom lists, approximating the 98th percentile. This is a developmental, not a syndromal, definition of disorder as stated above. We see it as more appropriate and in keeping with the view of ADHD as a developmental disorder defined by developmentally inappropriate symptoms. Note that DSM-III-R used a single symptom list of 14 items; therefore ages 15 and 21 are based on this list. The +2 *SDs* thresholds for those ages were 6 and 5, respectively, at these two follow-up points. At age 27, the DSM-IV is used, which has two symptom lists. Rather than compute symptom thresholds represented +2 *SDs* separately for each list, we chose the simpler course of using the threshold of +2 *SDs* based on the entire list of 18 symptoms so as to be consistent with the single-symptom list approach at the two earlier follow-ups. This threshold was five total ADHD symptoms for parent-reported information. Since +2 *SDs* (98th percentile) was the threshold used to select the hyperactive group in childhood on our hyperactivity/ADHD measures, we consider 100% of the hyperactive group to have met this criterion at study entry.

- *Symptomatic 1.5 SD*: This is also a developmental definition of disorder, though one less strict than that above. It defines disorder as placing at or above the threshold representing +1.5 *SDs* above the mean for the control group in this study on DSM symptom lists, approximating the 93rd percentile. Such a view is very consistent with standard clinical practice, in which individuals falling at or above this level in symptom severity are viewed as having clinically meaningful (i.e., nonnormal) levels of symptoms. Again, at ages 15 and 21, the single DSM-III-R symptom list is used and the thresholds were 5 and 4, respectively, for parent/other-reported information. At age 27, the entire list of 18 DSM-IV symptoms is used, as above, and the symptom threshold is a total of four for the entire list. Since all members of the hyperactive group had to be at the 98th percentile at study entry, then of course we can consider 100% of them to have met this criterion at that time as well.

The presence of impairment was not required for these definitions, as no explicit clinical interview questions in childhood or at adolescent follow-up dealt with the issue of impairment explicitly at home, school, and so on as part of the diagnostic criteria being applied. However, specific measures of various impairments were certainly being obtained then (such as educational functioning). So these three different definitions of ADHD reflect only meeting various symptom thresholds. Parent-reported information was used exclusively at the child, age-15, and age-21 follow-up points, while parent/other informants were used at the age-27 follow-up.

The graph illustrating the developmental changes in ADHD as defined by these three methods and using parent/other reports appears in Figure 4.2. As this diagram shows, there is a significant decline in the percentage of hyperactive patients meeting these definitions across development, with the steepest and greatest decline occurring using the DSM syndromal method (applying a fixed threshold regardless of age). Doing so results in just 26% of the Hyperactive group retaining the diagnosis of ADHD at age 27. This might suggest to some a remarkable recovery from ADHD, such as that voiced by Hill and Schoener (1996) using this syndromal perspective. But we believe this view would be quite mistaken, as noted in Chapter 3. Notice that a much larger percentage of cases at each follow-up remain remarkably symptomatic, whether defined as being the 93rd or 98th percentile (+1.5 and +2 SDs, respectively) relative to our Control group. By these definitions of disorder, 54% and 49% continue to have the developmentally defined disorder, respectively, at age-27 follow-up—that is, approximately double the level of disorder compared to the syndromal DSM approach to diagnosis.

We can create the same sort of graph based on self-reported information. However, such information was only collected at ages 21 and 27. The graph representing these developmental changes for each of the three methods defining ADHD above appears in Figure 4.3. The thresholds for the +1.5 and +2 SD thresholds at age 21 (DSM-III-R) were 5 and 6, respectively while at age 27 they were 6 and 7 (DSM-IV), respectively. When judged against the parent/other-reported information in Figure 4.2, a rather interesting pattern is apparent. The percentage of disorder by all three methods is *increasing* with age—the very opposite pattern for the parent/other-reported information. Examining the percentages at age 27 in particular shows that self-reported information is now converging on the same levels of disorder as were provided by parent/other-reported information. For full *syndromal* disorder, the figures rise from 5 to 30% between ages 21 and 27. For the *symptomatic 1.5* definition, the figure rises even more markedly, from 18 to 53% between these two follow-ups. And for *symptomatic 2.0*, the figures rise from 12 to 46%, an equally remarkable increase in disorder. It is our opinion that these changes in self-report reflect a growing self-awareness in our participants concerning their existence and inappropriateness of their symp-

Developmental Persistence and Normalization (parent/other reports)

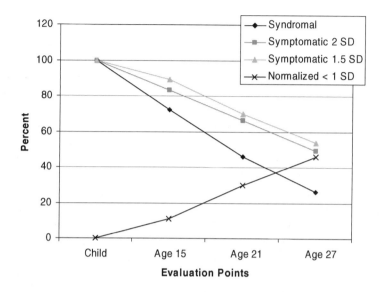

FIGURE 4.2. Developmental persistence of ADHD from the Milwaukee Study using parent information (at childhood, age-15, and age-21 follow-up points) and parent/other information (age 27 follow-up point) at each follow-up. ADHD is defined by full syndrome (DSM symptom thresholds), symptomatic at +1.5 *SDs* above the mean for the control group (93rd percentile), and symptomatic at +2 *SDs* above the mean for the control group (98th percentile). Normalization or recovery is defined as being within +1 *SD* (84th percentile) for the control group at these same follow-up points.

tomatic behavior across their 20s and early 30s—a change consistent with the continued maturity of various executive functions viewed as mediated by frontal-striatal brain circuitry during this time. Of course, this change could also be a consequence of the participants leaving home, engaging the larger society in which they live, and receiving feedback from others as they do so concerning the extent of their behavioral deviance. Whatever its source, this is the first study to document such a developmental increase in disorder in a longitudinal study based on self-reported information.

The reader may well wonder by now why we applied the DSM-based syndromal definition of the disorder in the UMASS Study of clinic-referred adults when we then adopted a developmental definition of the disorder for the Milwaukee Study (our preferred definition). One reason was stated above. The Milwaukee ADHD participants had already met the syndromal (and developmental) definition of the disorder at study entry by virtue of using criteria that

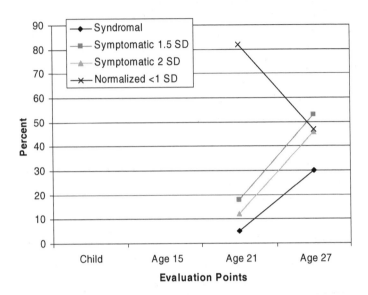

FIGURE 4.3. The same developmental changes as in Figure 4.2 but using self-reported information that began being obtained at age-21 and age-27 follow-up points for the Milwaukee Study. ADHD is defined by full syndrome (DSM symptom thresholds), symptomatic at +1.5 SDs above the mean for the control group (93rd percentile), and symptomatic at +2 SDs above the mean for the control group (98th percentile). Normalization means falling below the + 1 SD above the control mean or 84th percentile.

were developed with and most appropriate for children. The UMASS Study adults had not yet done so, as they were being evaluated in adulthood for ADHD, many for the first time. We felt it important to ensure that they met the syndromal DSM definition even though we knew it to be a more strict or developmentally severe one. Also, ADHD in adults is not yet a widely recognized or respected disorder in adult psychiatry, making it important (at least to us) that the clinic-referred adults defined as having ADHD in the UMASS Study have the syndromally defined disorder that is the preference or standard for disorder in adult psychiatry. The UMASS Study had as one of its aims to examine the validity of ADHD in adults as a full-fledged adult syndrome (disorder), so it was imperative that those adults meet the syndromal definition, and the stricter the better. Such a strict definition is often needed in trying to convince skeptical colleagues of the validity of an adult disorder. We did not wish that study, focused as it was on clinic-referred adults, to be criticized for employing some watered-down version of the DSM in defining the adult disorder (even though evidence above shows that such a "diluted" view still identifies highly symptomatic and developmentally inappropriate levels symptoms—a developmental disorder). Readers need to keep this difference between the studies in mind as we explore the numerous findings throughout the rest of this book. This is especially so when they (and we) try to compare the results for the clinic-referred and *syndromally* defined adults with ADHD in the UMASS Study to the childhood-selected and longitudinally followed H+ADHD cases who are *developmentally* defined as having ADHD at adult outcome (but defined as having both in childhood).

The above findings concerning the persistence of ADHD into adulthood in the Milwaukee Study lead to an equally interesting but opposite question: How many of the Hyperactive (child ADHD) group would be considered as having outgrown the disorder at adulthood? That is, what percentage is now falling within the largely normal range of functioning at adult follow-up?

Outgrowing ADHD by Adulthood

To address this question, one needs a definition of "normal" or at least of no longer having ADHD. We will consider someone as having become *symptomatically normalized* if their level of ADHD symptoms is in the normal range, which is considered to be falling at or below the 84th percentile (+1 *SD*) of the control group in symptoms. We first determined how many were within the normal range now in their number of self-reported symptoms. This figure came to five or fewer total ADHD symptoms. We considered a patient to be completely *recovered* if he or she met this threshold and was determined to be within the normal range in the number of impaired domains from the interview (falling within +1 *SD* of the control mean). That figure was 1 or fewer domains of the 6 reviewed in the interview. We then determined which participants met both conditions: 5 or fewer total ADHD symptoms and 1 or fewer impairments. *We found that 36% of the Hyperactive group met these two criteria and could be considered to be recovered or to have outgrown their disorder*—that is, placing within the normal range in both symptoms and impairments by self-reports. Using the more relaxed definition of being symptomatically normal, this figure would rise to 47%.

If we now examine the proportion of each of the two hyperactive groups (H+ADHD, H–ADHD) that met these criteria, we find that none of the H+ADHD group would meet these criteria for full recovery. This would not be surprising, given how we formed that group (4+ symptoms on either of the symptom lists and 1+ impairments). But it is reassuring for our subsequent analyses of our dependent measures to know this going forward. We found that 60% of the H–ADHD group would be considered to be recovered or to have outgrown their ADHD by this definition. This, too, is reassuring in the sense that a majority of these patients who had ADHD in childhood no longer have ADHD but are now normal. The comparable figure for the control group was 81%, which approximates and confirms our definition of "the normal range" above as being below the 84th percentile for our control group. These figures help to understand the numerous findings we report in this book in which the H–ADHD group did not differ from our Community control group on various dependent measures or, if they did, they still fell significantly below the H+ADHD group in most of these respects. To reiterate, by our definition of current adult ADHD based on self-reported information:

- Forty-four percent of the participants diagnosed as having ADHD (hyperactivity) in childhood would be considered to still have ADHD in adulthood (by mean age 27).
- Thirty-six percent would be considered to be recovered or to have outgrown their ADHD.
- Twenty percent would therefore be considered *subsyndromal* or symptomatic (as opposed to fully syndromal) but *not* within the normal range.

How does this compare to earlier follow-up points? We have self-reported information on ADHD symptoms only starting at age 21. Even then, we did not collect the same rating scale or interview information concerning domains of impairment as we did at this age-27 follow-up. Thus we can examine only the level of symptomatic normalization for the age-21 follow-up (as being within +1 SD of the control mean in self-reported symptoms, which is four or fewer symptoms in DSM-III-R). Using this more relaxed definition of symptomatic normalization rather than that of full recovery, 82% of the Hyperactive group would have been considered to be normal by their report at that earlier follow-up. When we compare this to the 47% figure computed above for current symptomatic normalization at the age-27 follow-up, we can see that it has declined markedly. That is hardly surprising, given that these participants are self-reporting more symptoms now than they did at age 21. We show these symptomatic normalization rates for the age-21 and age-27 follow-ups in Figure 4.3 as well.

Since these participants were originally selected as having ADHD based on someone else's (parental) reports, it is worth conducting the same analyses using other-reported information at follow-up. The distribution of scores for the number of symptoms rated 2 or higher (often or more) using the reports of others (mostly parents and spouses/partners) shows that 3 or fewer total symptoms represents the threshold of +1 SD above the control mean, which we accept as representing the normal range. Approximately 86% of control participants fell at or below this number. Again, we found that having 1 or no areas of impairment (out of 10 possible; each domain rated as "often" or more to be considered impaired) on the ADHD Rating Scale represented +1 SD above the control mean, again defining the normal range for impairments. Approximately 82% of that group fell at or below this threshold. We therefore considered any Hyperactive group member having 3 or fewer total symptoms and 1 or no areas of significant impairment on this scale to have completely outgrown their ADHD (to be within the normal range in symptoms and impairments). Using other reports, we obtained the following results:

- Forty-one percent of the participants diagnosed as having ADHD (hyperactivity) in childhood would still be considered to have ADHD in adulthood. (having 4+ symptoms and 1+ impairments).
- Thirty-five percent would be considered to be fully recovered or to have outgrown their ADHD and to fall within the normal (control) range for symptoms and impairments (having three or fewer symptoms and one or no impairments).
- The remaining 24% would be considered symptomatic or subsyndromal cases but not as falling within the normal range.

Such figures are comparable to the results obtained by self-reports. But are they the same people? We examined the overlap of these two definitions of who outgrew their disorder and found that just 45% of those outgrowing ADHD based on self-report were considered to have outgrown it based on other reports ($n = 19$). This represents 14% of the entire sample diagnosed as having ADHD (hyperactive) in childhood. The degree of agreement between sources was better for the category of who had not outgrown ADHD by self-report. We found that 70% of those considered not to have outgrown their ADHD by self-report were so classified by other reports. To conclude, if one wished to rely on other-reported information, 35% of our Hyperactive group had outgrown their ADHD. But if one wished to adhere to the strictest definition of "outgrowing ADHD," in which both self and other reports must fall within the normal range in symptoms and impairments, then just 14% had outgrown the disorder.

Given that we have parent-reported information at both the teen and age-21 follow-up points, we can compute a developmental course of normalization much as we did for persistence of disorder in Figure 4.2. Because we did not have a rating scale or interview component that assessed domains of impairment in the manner used at this (age 27) follow-up, as noted above, we do not use impairment as a criterion for defining what is normal. Instead, we simply use the same demarcation for being symptomatically normalized based on just the number of symptoms as we did above (below the +1 SD threshold above the normal mean, which was four or fewer symptoms at adolescent follow-up and three or fewer at age 21 using DSM-III-R symptom lists). Using this threshold, we found that 11% of the hyperactive group were symptomatically normalized at the teen follow-up (age 15) while 30% were symptomatically normalized by the age-21 follow-up. Using this somewhat more relaxed definition of being normal rather than that of full recovery above would have led to 46% of the hyperactive group being normalized by age 27 rather than the 35% cited above using an impairment criterion. This developmental course of symptomatic normalization is also shown in Figure 4.2.

Demographic Information for the Milwaukee Study Groups

Having defined our groups for the purpose of analyzing our numerous dependent measures, we can now examine the demographic characteristics of these groups (H+ADHD, H−ADHD, and Community controls). The categorical demographic information is shown in Table 4.5. This table shows that the groups did not differ in their sex composition (84–93% males). Therefore our findings largely reflect the outcomes of boys with ADHD grown up, which is true for all other longitudinal studies tracking participants to this age in adulthood. This means there were just 9 females in the H+ADHD group, 11 in the H−ADHD group, and 5 in the Control group, precluding us from examining our measures for any potential sex differences that could be considered reliable. Where we know sex to be an important factor in a measure, we conduct some preliminary analyses of such differences but urge caution in drawing any reliable conclusions from those results. The UMASS Study, above, is better powered to permit an

TABLE 4.5. Demographic Characteristics for Hyperactive Subgroup and Control Group for Categorical Measures for the Milwaukee Study

Measure	H+ADHD N	H+ADHD %	H−ADHD N	H−ADHD %	Control N	Control %	χ^2	p	Pairwise contrasts
Sex (males)	46	83.6	70	87.5	70	93.3	3.09	NS	
Ethnic group (white)	46	83.6	65	81.2	73	97.3	10.32	.006	1,2 < 3
Marital status							4.58	NS	
Single (not married)	37	67.3	52	65.0	41	54.7			
Married now	16	29.6	26	32.9	32	42.7			
Divorced/separated	2	3.8	2	2.6	2	2.7			
Living arrangements							18.85	NS	
Live alone	4	7.3	11	13.9	8	10.7			
Live with spouse	16	29.6	27	34.2	33	44.0			
Live with parents	9	16.7	15	19.0	8	10.7			
Live with others	26	48.1	27	33.7	26	34.7			
Currently employed	41	74.5	73	91.3	68	90.7	9.49	.009	1 < 2,3

Note. Sample sizes are H+ADHD = 55, H−ADHD = 80, and Controls = 75. N = sample sizes that fell into each categorical measure; % = the percentage of the entire group sample that fell into each categorical measure; χ^2 = results for the Pearson omnibus chi-square; p = probability value for the chi-square result; H+ADHD = Hyperactive group that currently has a diagnosis of ADHD at follow-up; H−ADHD = Hyperactive group that does not have a diagnosis of ADHD at follow-up.

Statistical analysis: Pearson chi-square.

examination of sex differences in adults with ADHD, and so more will be made of those findings on this matter than any results from the Milwaukee Study.

As we found at the childhood study entry point and all subsequent follow-ups, a slightly yet significantly lower percentage of the two hyperactive groups consisted of self-identified white or European American ethnic identity (81–84% white) in comparison to the control group (97% white). Despite such a difference, the small minority representation across these groups prevents us from examining specific ethnic groups within our data for any reliable or meaningful differences. For instance, just 7% of the hyperactive group identified themselves as black or African American, 4% as Hispanic or Latino, and 7% as "other," mostly Native American. There was no Asian representation in these samples. The comparable figures for the control group were 0%, 0%, and 3%, respectively. This problem also affected the UMASS Study samples, as noted earlier. We must leave it to other studies of larger minority samples and greater statistical power to examine possible ethnic differences in adults with ADHD to address that issue.

We observed no differences in the proportions of our groups who were currently single, married, or separated/divorced, with approximately 30 to 43% of our groups being currently married. This figure is somewhat lower than the 45 to 64% range observed in the UMASS Study but is understandable given the somewhat younger age of these groups (mean age = 27 years) relative to those in the UMASS Study (mean age = 32–37 years). Significantly fewer of the H+ADHD group were currently employed compared to the H–ADHD and Control groups. We have more to say about this finding in Chapter 9, on educational and occupational functioning. Yet the proportion of the H+ADHD group that was employed is comparable to that found in the UMASS Study (71–77% across groups, no group differences).

Other demographic characteristics were dimensional in nature and are displayed in Table 4.6. Despite resorting our original groups (Hyperactive and Control) into the revised sorting strategy based on being ADHD at follow-up (H+ADHD, H–ADHD, and Control), the ages of the groups remain comparable (age 27). Both of the H groups had significantly less education than our control group—a finding consistent with the age-21 follow-up results and with the UMASS Study of ADHD adults. Yet worth noting is that the ADHD adults in the UMASS Study had, on average, 2 more years of education than either the Milwaukee H+ADHD or H–ADHD groups in this study. As discussed later, children growing up with ADHD appear to be less educated as adults than are adults who self-refer to clinics and are then diagnosed as ADHD. As has been the case since the childhood entry point of this study, both of the H groups score significantly lower on the IQ tests at follow-up relative to our control group. And both H groups had a significantly lower Hollingshead Job Index and consequently lower Hollingshead (SES) ratings than the control group—a finding not unexpected in view of the lower educational level of the H groups.

TABLE 4.6. Demographic Characteristics by Group for Dimensional Measures for the Milwaukee Study

Measure	H+ADHD		H–ADHD		Control		F	p	Pairwise contrasts
	Mean	SD	Mean	SD	Mean	SD			
Age (years)	26.8	1.4	27.2	1.4	27.0	0.9	1.83	NS	
Education (years)	12.2	2.2	12.8	2.1	15.8	2.3	51.49	< .001	1,2 < 3
Verbal IQ (vocabulary)	10.5	3.4	10.6	3.3	14.1	2.6	29.55	< .001	1,2 < 3
Nonverbal IQ (blocks)	11.6	3.2	11.6	3.4	13.0	2.9	4.85	.009	1,2 < 3
Hollingshead	32.3	19.8	40.1	20.6	56.0	27.0	18.11	< .001	1,2 < 3
Hollingshead SES	28.4	11.2	33.2	12.7	45.4	15.1	28.80	< .001	1,2 < 3

Note. Sample sizes are H+ADHD = 55, H–ADHD = 80, Controls = 75 for age, education, and Hollingshead measure. For WAIS IQ subtests, they are H+ADHD = 52, H–ADHD, 79, and Controls = 73. Verbal IQ is from the WAIS-III Vocabulary subtest; Nonverbal IQ is from the Block Design subtest; SD = standard deviation; F = F-test results of the analysis of variance (or covariance); p = probability value for the F-test; NS = not significant; H+ADHD = hyperactive group that currently has a diagnosis of ADHD at follow-up; H–ADHD = hyperactive group that does not have a diagnosis of ADHD at follow-up; Hollingshead = Hollingshead Job Index; SES (socioeconomic status) = Hollingshead Index of Social Position.

Statistical analysis: Groups were initially compared using one-way (groups) analysis of variance. Where this analysis was significant ($p < .05$) for the main effect for group, pairwise comparisons (Student–Newman–Keuls tests) of the groups were conducted the results of which are shown in the last column.

Treatment History of the Milwaukee Study Groups

We inquired of our samples whether they had received any psychiatric or psychological evaluations or treatments in the interim since the age-21 follow-up. Those results appear in Table 4.7. At the time of the earlier follow-up, very few of them were in current treatment. Just 8% of the Hyperactive group and 1% of Community controls were taking psychiatric medication, and 22% of the Hyperactive group and 10% of Community controls were in some form of individual therapy or counseling. At this follow-up, we found that significantly more (nearly half) of the H+ADHD group had sought a psychiatric or psychological evaluation since the prior follow-up. While more (approximately one-third) of the H+ADHD group had received some form of outpatient treatment in the interim since the last follow-up, just 9% of the H+ADHD group and 4% of the H–ADHD group was currently in some type of psychological therapy—figures that are not different from those for the Community control group (8%). Likewise, only a small percentage of each group was currently taking a psychiatric medication (7–14%), and the groups did not differ in this respect. A small but significant minority of the H+ADHD group had ever been placed in residential treatment or had been psychiatrically hospitalized (18%), which differed only from the percentages for the Community control group (3–4%). As these figures suggest, the vast majority of individuals in the two Hyperactive groups are not currently receiving any form of treatment. We compared those hyperactive par-

TABLE 4.7. Psychiatric Evaluation and Treatment History Since Last Follow-Up (Age 21) by Group for the Milwaukee Study

Measure	H+ADHD		H−ADHD		Control		χ^2	p	Pairwise contrasts
	N	%	N	%	N	%			
Evaluated in interim	25	45.5	14	17.5	11	14.7	19.42	< .001	1 > 2,3
Dx of any psych disorder in interim	17	30.9	3	3.8	9	12.0	20.52	< .001	1 > 2,3
Outpatient treatment in interim	19	34.5	11	13.8	11	14.7	10.72	.005	1 > 2,3
Ever in residential treatment	10	18.2	10	12.5	3	4.0	6.86	.032	1 > 3
Ever psychiatrically hospitalized	10	18.2	6	7.5	2	2.7	9.94	.007	1 > 3
Ever treated with psych drugs	22	40.0	17	21.3	10	13.3	12.93	.002	1 > 2,3
Currently in therapy	5	9.1	3	3.8	6	8.2	1.88	NS	
Currently on meds	8	14.5	6	7.5	5	6.7	2.77	NS	

Note. Sample sizes are H+ADHD = 55, H−ADHD = 80, and Community = 73. N = sample sizes that fell into each categorical measure; % = the percentage of the entire group sample that fell into each categorical measure; χ^2 = results for the Pearson omnibus chi-square; p = probability value for the chi-square result; pairwise contrasts = results for the paired comparisons of the groups with each other, if the omnibus chi-square was significant ($p < .05$); H+ADHD = hyperactive group that currently has a diagnosis of ADHD at follow-up; H−ADHD = hyperactive group that does not have a diagnosis of ADHD at follow-up; Dx = diagnosis; psych = psychiatric; meds = psychiatric medication.
  Statistical analysis: Pearson chi-square.

ticipants currently receiving medication ($N = 14$) to those not on medication on current and childhood ADHD symptom and impairment totals and found no significant differences. This leads us to believe that current medication use is not likely to have influenced the impact of our independent variable in this study, that being level of ADHD. For this reason, and in view of the exceptionally small sample currently on medication, we do not examine current medication effects on our dependent variables any further in the Milwaukee Study.

These results are very similar to those found for adults with ADHD in the UMASS Study (see Table 4.4), where just 17% of those adults were currently taking psychiatric medication. Such findings are consistent with the recent report by Kessler et al. (2006) that fewer than 25% of the adults with ADHD identified in that epidemiological sample were receiving any form of psychiatric treatment and only 10% were receiving a form of treatment specifically for their adult ADHD. The vast majority of adults with ADHD—whether clinic-referred, children grown up, or epidemiologically identified—are not currently receiving treatment, particularly medications. Thus, stories in the popular media that portray an epidemic of overmedication of adults for ADHD have no scientific support.

Conclusions and Clinical Implications

✓ The UMASS and Milwaukee Studies were designed to address some of the issues and limitations concerning the diagnostic criteria for ADHD in adults currently in DSM-IV. Specifically they address the appropriateness of the DSM current item set for adults, the identification of additional symptoms that may better characterize the adult stage of the disorder, the significance or lack of it for specifying so precise an early an age of onset for impairing symptoms (age 7), and the domains of impairment most likely to be associated with the disorder as determined from a far larger array of those domains than is currently acknowledged by the DSM criteria.

✓ We have also used this opportunity to set forth the criteria adopted in the UMASS Study for determining the assignment of adults to our ADHD and other groups, illustrating the clinically important issues that arise in making the clinical diagnosis of ADHD. We have also explained the procedures used to determine current ADHD in the longitudinal Milwaukee Study. In both studies, self-reported information served as the basis for current diagnosis.

✓ Using the Milwaukee Study, we were able to demonstrate a developmental decline in rates of disorder with increasing age as defined by parent/other report, with this decrease being most obvious when full DSM symptom thresholds (from 100 to 26%) are considered. Somewhat less but still remarkable declines in disorder are evident from childhood to age 27 using definitions of disorder based on the 93rd percentile (from 100 to 54%) and the 98th percentile (from 100 to 49%) for the control group. Symptomatic normalization (falling below the 84th percentile) occurred in 46% of the patients, while full recovery (< 84th percentile and 1 or no impaired domains) was achieved by 35% of those deemed to be hyperactive.

✓ In contrast to these developmental changes using others' reports, when self-reported information is considered (at ages 21 and 27), a marked *increase* in disorder is documented by each of these definitions. Full disorder increases from 5 to 30%, being symptomatic at or above the 93rd percentile increases from 18 to 53%; being symptomatic at or above the 98th percentile increases from 12 to 46%, respectively. In contrast to other-reported information, rates of symptomatic normalization declined by half, from 82 to 47%, over this same period. The basis for these changes is uncertain but could reflect a growing self-awareness of symptoms and their inappropriateness as participants move through their 20s into their early 30s. Whatever its source, it begins to suggest some convergence between sources of information (self vs. others) as these participants grow up and develop a greater awareness of their symptoms and impairments. If a strict definition of full recovery is used, in which the person must be below the 84th percentile in symptoms and impairments using *both* self and others' reports, then just 14% of the hyperactive sample would be fully recovered.

✓ We presented the initial demographic attributes of the groups used in these two studies that already intimate that ADHD may result in less education, lower job status, and a lower socioeconomic status than is evident in control groups. For clinic-referred adults, the UMASS Study also found them to have a lower likelihood of being or remaining married than is typical of a non-ADHD clinical group; this was not the case for the children with ADHD by their adult follow-up, but that could be due largely if not entirely to their being somewhat younger (on average, 5 years) than the adults in the UMASS Study. These issues of the impact of ADHD on education, occupational, and marital functioning receive closer scrutiny in subsequent chapters.

✓ The prior treatment history of the groups in both studies was also described. Most members of the clinical groups, not unexpectedly, had prior evaluations by mental health professionals, and most had participated in some form of treatment. Small percentages of each clinical group were taking psychiatric medication at the time of their enrollment in our studies reported in this book. In the UMASS Study, subsequent analyses showed that those so treated did not differ from those who were not on medication in a variety of measures of current and child ADHD symptoms and impairments. This was also the case in the Milwaukee Study. This gave us reasonable assurance that drug treatment status was not likely to produce a significant bias in the results of these studies. Even so, should one have occurred, it would likely produce a conservative effect on the results, serving to reduce group differences in comparisons with the Community control group. These groups (treated and untreated) were therefore collapsed back together for all subsequent analyses in both studies presented in this book.

With these issues as a backdrop along with our participant selection criteria, we now proceed to address the major purposes of these large-scale studies. We begin in Chapter 5 by examining the ADHD symptoms (DSM-IV) across these groups and their utility in discriminating among them.

CHAPTER 5

DSM Symptom Utility
and the Issue of Age of Onset

This chapter first examines the frequency of the 18 symptoms of ADHD found in the DSM-IV-TR diagnostic criteria (American Psychiatric Association, 2000) among adults in the UMASS Study—those with ADHD, a Clinical control group, and a Community control group. It also determines the validity of these self-reported symptoms, both for current and childhood functioning, relative to the reports of others (parents, partners) who knew our study participants well. We also evaluate the extent to which each of these symptoms is likely to predict the presence of the full disorder as well as the best subset of symptoms that could be used to diagnose the disorder; that is, our intention is to be maximally accurate in predicting the presence of the disorder. We then examine these same issues using the Milwaukee Study of children with ADHD who have grown up.

This chapter also determines the validity of the age-of-onset criterion (onset by age 7) in the DSM-IV-TR when applied to the diagnosis of adults with ADHD. Using the UMASS Study, we address the question of whether this criterion distinguishes between qualitatively different patient groups among those who otherwise meet all other DSM criteria for the disorder. That is a very problematic issue with the DSM when used for diagnosing adults with ADHD, as discussed in the previous chapter. We also use evidence from the Milwaukee Study to examine this issue; its results are especially interesting given that all of the children with ADHD in that study had developed their symptoms by 6 years of age. How well can they or even their parents recall such an onset 18 or more years later? We shall see.

Chapter 7 examines the possibility that other symptoms, especially those reflecting executive functioning, that were not included in the DSM-IV-TR may be more representative of the adult stage of this disorder as it presents in clinical settings. Our intention is to show whether they may be better at predicting the presence of ADHD in adults than are those in the DSM-IV-TR that were developed exclusively on children (Lahey et al., 1994).

Symptoms and Their Predictive Accuracy

We are not the first to report on the frequency of the DSM-IV symptoms of ADHD in adults with and without the disorder. Most recently, Riccio and associates have done so with far smaller samples of ADHD ($N = 32$), clinical control ($N = 38$), and community control ($N = 30$) groups relative to our samples (Riccio et al., 2005). Earlier, O'Donnnell et al. (2001) presented information on both symptom frequencies and predictive utility of the DSM-IV-TR symptoms, but for even smaller samples of just 14 adults with ADHD and 28 control adults, all college students. Such small and demographically selective samples are likely to pose significant problems for validity of their findings or the extent to which they can be extrapolated to the larger population of adults with ADHD. In contrast, Milstein, Wilens, Biederman, and Spencer (1997) reported symptom frequencies for a much larger sample size similar to our own ($N = 147$) but only for an adult ADHD group and using the earlier DSM-III-R symptom list. Focusing only on an ADHD group makes it impossible to examine the utility of symptoms for the diagnosis of the disorder that requires comparisons to control groups. We had previously described the symptom occurrence of DSM-III-R symptoms in a sample of 172 adults with ADHD and 30 control adults seen in the same clinic who were not diagnosed with ADHD (Murphy & Barkley, 1996a). Many of those DSM-III-R symptoms were retained in the DSM-IV symptom lists, so those results have some relevance to the ones reported below. We refer to the results of these studies below so as to integrate our own results with the existing research.

DSM-IV-TR Symptom Severity

The UMASS Study Results

The number of inattentive, hyperactive–impulsive, and total symptoms self-reported by each group on both the interview and the rating scale formats (see Chapter 4 sidebar) for both current functioning and recall of childhood are shown in Table 5.1. As this table shows, the ADHD group reported significantly more symptoms during their interviews than did either the Clinical control or Community control groups. This finding is visually depicted in Figure 5.1. They did so not only for current functioning but also for their recall of childhood func-

TABLE 5.1. ADHD Symptoms (DSM-IV) from Interviews and Ratings by Group for the UMASS Study

Measure	ADHD Mean	SD	Clinical Mean	SD	Community Mean	SD	F	p	Pairwise contrasts
Current self-report									
No. of inattention items	7.3	1.5	5.8	2.1	0.3	0.8	642.7	< .001	1 > 2 > 3
No. of hyperactivity–impulsivity items	5.1	2.4	3.8	2.4	0.4	0.7	174.2	< .001	1 > 2 > 3
Total no. of ADHD items[S]	12.4	2.9	9.6	3.4	0.7	1.1	617.2	< .001	1 > 2 > 3
Childhood self-report									
No. of inattention items[A]	7.4	1.9	4.5	2.7	0.3	0.8	363.3	< .001	1 > 2 > 3
No. of hyperactivity–impulsivity items	5.5	2.9	3.6	2.8	0.6	1.2	110.1	< .001	1 > 2 > 3
Total no. of ADHD items[A]	12.9	3.9	8.1	4.8	0.9	1.6	297.1	< .001	1 > 2 > 3
Current self-ratings									
Total ADHD score [S,GxS]	32.1	10.1	28.5	11.0	5.1	4.7	309.6	< .001	1 > 2 > 3
Childhood self-ratings									
Total ADHD score[GxS]	34.3	12.1	25.7	13.2	5.4	5.8	205.8	< .001	1 > 2 > 3
Current other-ratings									
Total ADHD	28.9	11.9	23.9	12.4	3.7	5.4	146.8	< .001	1 > 2 > 3
Childhood other-ratings									
Total ADHD[A]	27.1	13.9	13.4	10.5	3.4	5.8	62.5	< .001	1 > 2 > 3
School ratings by others									
Total ADHD[A]	27.7	12.8	14.9	12.6	2.5	4.5	68.9	< .001	1 > 2 > 3
Employer ratings									
Total ADHD[GxS]	16.1	11.7	13.2	10.8	5.0	6.1	19.0	< .001	1,2 > 3

Note. Sample sizes for self-reported interview information are ADHD = 146, Clinical control = 97, and Community control = 109. For self-rated symptoms, 134, 91, and 105, respectively. For self-rated childhood ADHD, *N*s = 127, 81, and 105, respectively. For other ratings of current ADHD, *N*s = 108, 76, and 90, respectively. For other ratings of childhood ADHD, *N*s = 65, 25, and 65, respectively. For other ratings of school ADHD, *N*s = 82, 35, and 60, respectively. For employer ratings, they were 39, 25, and 50, respectively. *SD* = standard deviation; *F* = *F*-test results of the analysis of variance (or covariance); *p* = probability value for the *F* test; NS = not significant; [S] = significant main effect for sex (see text for details); [GxS] = significant group × sex interaction (see text for details); [A] = age used as a covariate in this analysis.

Statistical analysis: Groups were initially compared using two-way (group × sex) analysis of variance (or covariance as necessary). Where this analysis was significant (*p* < .05) for the main effect for group, pairwise comparisons of the groups were conducted the results of which are shown in the last column.

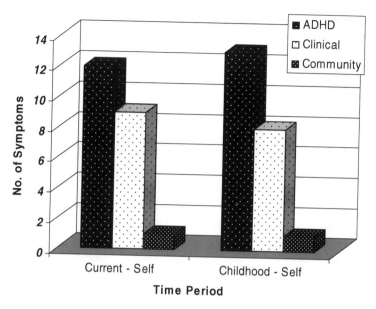

FIGURE 5.1. Number of ADHD symptoms currently and in childhood for each group based on self-reported interviews using DSM-IV-TR symptom lists in the UMASS Study.

tioning between the ages of 5 and 12 years. These results are not surprising given that these symptoms were used to make the diagnosis of ADHD and therefore to assign participants to the various groups. In essence, these results merely provide some reassurance that the group assignment procedure succeeded—the ADHD group was more symptomatic than the two non-ADHD groups on these ADHD symptom dimensions. Of some interest is that symptoms of inattention were endorsed more often than those of hyperactive and impulsive behavior. This likely reflects the fact that the latter symptoms emerge first in development, especially those related to hyperactivity, but decline more steeply with age than do symptoms of inattention, which arise somewhat later but decrease less with age (Hart et al., 1995; Loeber, Green, Lahey, Christ, & Frick, 1992). The impulsive items in the DSM are largely ones of verbal behavior and may remain especially problematic for adults more than for children, as becomes evident below. Across all participant groups, males reported more current symptoms of ADHD during the interview than did females. This was not the case for their recall of their childhood symptoms, where no gender differences emerged.

On the rating scales, a similar pattern of findings was evident for self-ratings, in which higher symptom ratings were found in the ADHD than in the two control groups, again, for current symptoms as well as recall of childhood symptoms. And once more, males on average reported higher current symptom ratings than did females across the groups (a main effect for sex). But we also noted a significant interaction of sex with group on these ratings and on those from childhood, suggesting that this was not the whole story—the groups may have differed among themselves in the pattern of sex differences. To study this further, we show the results for each sex within each group in Figures 5.2 (current symptoms ratings) and 5.3 (childhood recall ratings). Further analyses (pairwise comparisons) showed that for both current and childhood symptoms, men and women in the ADHD group did not differ from each other in their ratings. However, women in the Clinical control group reported significantly higher scores than men for both current and childhood ratings; in the Community control group, this pattern was reversed—men rated themselves as having somewhat more severe symptoms than women, both presently and in childhood. The message here for ADHD in clinic-referred adults seems to be that the typical or nor-

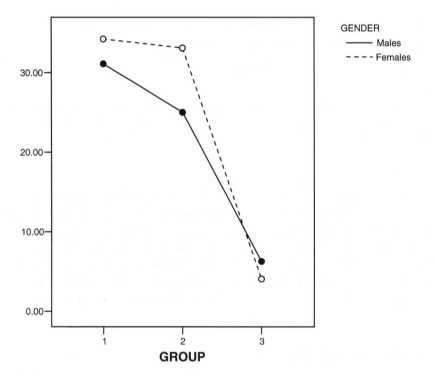

FIGURE 5.2. Results of the ADHD Rating Scale self-reported raw scores for current functioning showing each sex within each group (illustrating the significant group × sex interaction on this measure). Group 1 = ADHD, 2 = Clinical control, 3 = Community control.

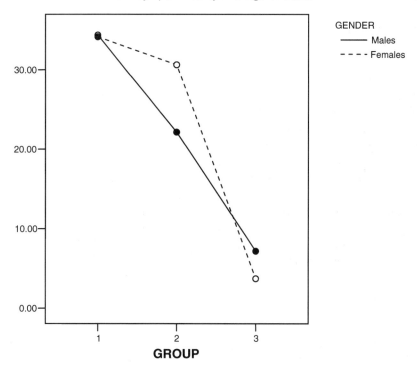

FIGURE 5.3. Results of the ADHD Rating Scale self-report raw scores for childhood functioning showing each sex within each group (illustrating the significant group × sex interaction on this measure). Group 1 = ADHD, 2 = Clinical control, 3 = Community control.

mal pattern of males reporting higher ADHD symptoms than females in the general population does not hold true for those with the disorder. Clinically referred women with ADHD rate themselves as having symptoms just as severe as those of men with the disorder when a rating scale is used to determine symptom severity, as might be done in a preevaluation screening process. But it is the non-ADHD clinical control group that actually defies the normal pattern here, with women reporting higher ratings than men at both developmental periods. Why this should be so is not obvious to us.

The Milwaukee Study Results

The same information was obtained in the Milwaukee Study from these ADHD patients as adults. These results appear in Table 5.2. As expected from the manner in which these groups were formed (see Chapter 4), the hyperactive group that currently has ADHD in adulthood (H+ADHD) reported significantly more symptoms of inattention as well as hyperactive-impulsive and total ADHD symptoms than did the hyperactive group no longer considered to have ADHD (H–ADHD) or control group. But the H–ADHD group also showed more such symptoms than the control group. Again, all this would be expected from the use of the DSM symptom lists to create these groups at adult outcome. More informative here is the fact that the hyperactive–impulsive symptoms were just as frequent as the inattention symptoms in adulthood for all groups, whereas in the UMASS Study above (Table 5.1), inattention appeared to be a more problematic

TABLE 5.2. ADHD (DSM-IV-TR) Symptom Totals from Interviews and Ratings for the Hyperactive and Community Control Groups from the Milwaukee Study

Measure	H+ADHD Mean	SD	H–ADHD Mean	SD	Community Mean	SD	F	p	Pairwise contrasts
Current self-report (interview):									
No. of inattention items	4.8	2.1	1.7	1.8	0.9	1.4	81.48	< .001	1 > 2 > 3
No. of hyperactivity–impulsivity items	4.8	1.8	2.1	1.6	1.3	1.6	73.52	< .001	1 > 2 > 3
Total no. of ADHD items	9.6	2.8	3.9	2.9	2.2	2.6	121.51	< .001	1 > 2 > 3
Childhood self-report (interview)									
No. of inattention items	7.2	1.9	5.7	2.7	1.8	2.6	86.1	< .001	1 > 2 > 3
No. of hyperactivity–impulsivity items	7.3	1.7	5.9	2.6	1.8	2.1	115.8	< .001	1 > 2 > 3
Total no. of ADHD items	14.5	2.9	11.6	4.8	3.6	4.2	126.1	< .001	1 > 2 > 3
Current self-ratings									
Total raw ADHD score	20.2	10.3	7.9	6.0	7.4	7.2	53.05	< .001	1 > 2,3
Childhood self-ratings									
Total raw ADHD score	34.9	11.2	23.7	13.5	10.1	10.2	70.25	< .001	1 > 2 > 3
Current other-ratings									
Total raw ADHD score	22.8	12.3	18.9	11.8	6.9	5.9	40.32	< .001	1 > 2 > 3
Childhood other-ratings	34.3	11.3	31.1	12.4	8.3	8.3	120.04	< .001	1,2 > 3
Total raw ADHD score									

Note. Sample sizes for self-reported interview information are H+ADHD = 55, H–ADHD = 80, and Community control = 75. For self-ratings scores, H+ADHD = 54, H–ADHD = 80, Community = 74. For self-rated childhood scores, H+ADHD = 54, H–ADHD = 80, Community = 74. For other ratings of current ADHD, H+ADHD = 54, H–ADHD = 78, Community = 75. For other ratings of childhood ADHD, H+ADHD = 54, H–ADHD = 77, Community = 74. SD = standard deviation; F = F-test results of the analysis of variance (or covariance); p = probability value for the F-test, NS = not significant; H+ADHD = Hyperactive group that currently has a diagnosis of ADHD at follow-up; H–ADHD = Hyperactive group that does not have a diagnosis of ADHD at follow-up.

Statistical analysis: Groups were initially compared using one-way (groups) analysis of variance. Where this analysis was significant (p < .05) for the main effect for group, pairwise comparisons of the groups were conducted, the results of which are shown in the last column.

domain of symptoms than hyperactive or impulsive behavior. This difference in findings undoubtedly owes itself to the fact that the Milwaukee ADHD sample was selected mainly on the basis of hyperactive symptoms at childhood study entry, which was not the case for the UMASS study adults, who were diagnosed in adulthood.

Another difference is evident between these two studies, and that is that the UMASS Study adults reported themselves to be more symptomatic in their current ADHD symptoms than did the H+ADHD adults in the Milwaukee Study. This was not the case for retrospective self-reports about childhood, where the groups appear to recall roughly equal levels of symptom severity. Such a difference between studies, however, may only reflect the fact that to be considered ADHD in the Milwaukee Study necessitated meeting a lower symptom threshold based on a developmental definition of ADHD (4+ symptoms on either symptom list, representing +2 SDs above the control mean). In contrast, ADHD in the UMASS Study was based on meeting the syndromal view of the disorder—that is, meeting full DSM-IV criteria (6+ symptoms on either list). We spelled out the reasons for this difference in Chapter 4.

The same pattern of findings was evident for the recall of these adult groups about their childhood behavior in the clinical interview. The H+ADHD group recalled having significantly more ADHD symptoms in their childhood than did either the H–ADHD or the control groups, who once more also differed from each other. Was this actually so in childhood? We know that both hyperactive groups had more such symptoms by their parents' reports at study entry than the control group, given the behavior rating scales used to form the groups. Yet when we examined the actual rating scale information collected at study entry from parents, we found that the H+ADHD and H–ADHD groups did not differ. We compared the parents ratings of these groups on the Conners Hyperactivity Index, the Hyperactive–Impulsive factor scores, the Werry–Weiss–Peters Activity Rating Scale, and the Home Situations Questionnaire (see Chapter 4 for details on these scales) and found no evident differences; their means and SDs were virtually the same (all Fs < 2.20, all ps = not significant). The same results were obtained when we examined parent reports of DSM-III-R symptoms at the adolescent (age 15) follow-up: the two hyperactive groups (+ vs. –ADHD) were not significantly different. In sum, those hyperactive children as adults who are no longer considered to have ADHD in adulthood (based on their self-reports) view themselves as having had fewer ADHD symptoms in childhood than do members of the H+ADHD group, even though their parents did not see things this way at the time they were children or when they were teenagers 8 to 10 years later. The parents saw members of both groups as being equally and substantially symptomatic. This lends some credence to our admonitions in Chapters 3 and 4 that clinicians need to corroborate the information provided to them by adults undergoing an evaluation for ADHD, particularly as concerns their childhood symptom severity, using either the reports of parents or archival information from school records. An adult's recall of his or her early childhood behavior does not necessarily accurately reflect the impression of others at the time.

The information obtained from the rating scales of ADHD symptoms were largely though not entirely the same as the results above for the interview method (see Table 5.2). Here, for current symptoms, the H+ADHD group differed from both groups, but the H–ADHD group did not differ from the Community control group, suggesting that the severity of their disorder as dimensionally rated on such a scale lies closer to that of the control group than of the group of adults with current ADHD. Yet in recall of childhood behavior, these self-ratings once again showed the H+ADHD group to be most symptomatic, followed by the H–ADHD group, who differed from the Community control group as well. Once more, the ratings of current symptoms for the H+ADHD group (mean = 20) appear to be below those reported in the UMASS Study by the those with ADHD (mean = 34). But the childhood self-ratings are much the same (both means = 34). Both ADHD-defined groups of adults see themselves as having been highly and comparably symptomatic in childhood but not currently. One reason for this may be that the adults in the UMASS Study were somewhat older. Recall from Chapter 4 that the hyperactive patients in the Milwaukee Study showed an increase with age in their self-reported ADHD symptoms (Figure 4.3), from the age-21 to the age-27 follow-up. It is possible that by the time they reach age 32, when they reach an average age similar to that of the adults in the UMASS Study, their reports of their current symptoms could rise still further and begin converging on the same level of symptom severity self-reported in the UMASS clinic-referred adults with ADHD.

What Is the Best Symptom Threshold for Diagnosing ADHD in Clinic-Referred Adults?

The DSM requires that an individual have at least 6 of 9 symptoms of inattention or 6 of 9 hyperactive-impulsive symptoms to qualify for the diagnosis of ADHD. But this threshold was based entirely on analyses of children (Lahey et al., 1994). Given that the symptoms of ADHD are far more common in child than adult populations, it is quite likely that a threshold for diagnosis based on children would not be the same as one that is best for discriminating ADHD from Community control adults. We examined that issue here by inspecting the distribution of total symptom endorsements in the ADHD and Community control groups in the UMASS Study. We found that 98% of the Community group endorsed three or fewer symptoms of inattention and 100% endorsed three or fewer of hyperactive impulsive behavior. In contrast, 100% of the ADHD group endorsed three or more inattention symptoms and 72% endorsed three or more hyperactive symptoms. In other words, a threshold of just four symptoms on the inattention or hyperactive-impulsive lists effectively rules out 100% of the Community control group (normal adults) and thus would appear to be a better diagnostic threshold than the now-recommended 6 symptoms. We made this same point in our earlier study of the prevalence of ADHD symptoms in a general population sample of adults (Murphy & Barkley, 1996b), where a threshold of four on either list would represent the 93rd percentile in that general population—a percentile often used in clinical practice to establish someone as clinically deviant or developmentally inappropriate in their symptoms. The threshold of four symptoms would accurately capture 96% of the ADHD group. And just three symptoms of hyperactive–impulsive behavior would accurately classify 72% of the ADHD group as ADHD. A total of seven current symptoms from the entire list of 18 in the DSM would effectively rule out 100% of our Community control group while accurately classifying more than 93% of our ADHD group. The same point can be made for childhood symptoms from our study. Using the threshold of four or more symptoms recalled from childhood on either symptom list would rule out 99% of the normal control group on the inattention list and more than 95% on the hyperactive list. A total of seven or more symptoms in childhood recall out of the 18 would effectively rule out 99% of our Community control group while ruling in 87% of the ADHD group.

We must therefore reiterate our earlier assertion that for DSM-V, a threshold for diagnosis for clinic-referred adults needs to be age-group referenced as opposed to relying on that threshold set for children. For now, we continue to advise clinicians based on these two studies that a threshold of four or more current symptoms on either list or a total of seven out of all 18 symptoms is more than enough to establish that a clinic-referred adult is abnormal or developmentally inappropriate in symptom frequency.

It is worth noting that 75% of the Clinical control group endorsed at least four or more inattention symptoms and 52% endorsed four or more hyperactive symptoms, with 70% endorsing seven or more total symptoms. Hence, a diagnostic threshold of four symptoms on either list may not differentiate ADHD from other clinical disorders as well as it does from the normal population. Nevertheless, the first step in clinical diagnosis is establishing that the patient's complaints constitute abnormality or developmental inappropriateness; for that purpose, these lower thresholds for adults function better than do current DSM guidelines. In conclusion, self-reporting of four or more symptoms of ADHD from either symptom list by clinic-referred adults is a good standard for discriminating patients with clinical disorders from the normal population but cannot be used to differentiate those with ADHD from those having other disorders that may affect attention or hyperactive behavior.

This issue was already examined in the Milwaukee Study and reported in Chapter 4, in discussing who retained ADHD into adulthood and who may have outgrown it. As in the UMASS Study, we found that having four symptoms on either DSM-IV symptom list or seven symptoms in total of all 18 items would represent the threshold of +2 SDs (or approximately the 98th percentile) for that Community control group. That was one of the reasons why we chose to define current ADHD at the age-27 outcome by this threshold. A second reason was based on the evidence given above—that this same threshold in the UMASS Study effectively ruled out all of the Community control group as having ADHD, while ruling in 87% of the ADHD group. Both studies show that such thresholds provide a clear delineation of symptom severity relative to these two adult control groups.

Symptom Ratings by Others

All of these results might be expected from the way in which these groups were initially formed (self-reported symptoms were used as part of the clinical diagnostic process, which led to these group assignments in both studies). As noted earlier, the results merely corroborate the method used to compose the groups. The external validity of these group compositions, however, can be found in the reports of others about the current and childhood ADHD symptoms of these adults. In both studies, we asked adults who knew the participants well to complete rating scales about the participants' current functioning.

The UMASS Study Results

In the UMASS Study, these reports were typically those of either the parents of these participants (ADHD = 67%, Clinical = 44%, Community = 53%) or their spouses/partners. A smaller percent were from siblings, with 3% or less of each group having friends complete the current symptom scale. As Table 5.1 shows, others rated the ADHD group as being significantly more symptomatic in their present functioning than was the case for the Clinical or Community control groups. Parents of the participants also completed the rating scale of childhood ADHD symptoms and, once again, rated the ADHD group as having significantly more severe symptoms in childhood than did the other two groups. We also had these parents rate the participants' ADHD symptoms specifically in the school environment during childhood, and the pattern of results was the same. We were also able to obtain ADHD ratings from employers for a small proportion of each group. These ratings showed that both the ADHD and Clinical control groups were rated as more symptomatic than the Community control group. Although the ratings were slightly higher for the ADHD group than for the Clinical group, they were not statistically significant. This may have resulted from the small sample sizes for employer ratings and the commensurate low statistical power to detect such differences as significant. Nevertheless, these ratings from others, both for current and childhood ADHD symptoms, serve to externally validate the group compositions in showing the ADHD group to indeed be more symptomatic than the control groups. The results largely agree with the findings of our earlier study of adults with ADHD using DSM-III-R symptoms (Murphy & Barkley, 1996a). We found that not only those with ADHD reported more ADHD symptoms in themselves for current and childhood time periods but so also did those who knew them well.

The only sex difference we detected on these various ratings was for those obtained from employers, where sex interacted with group membership. This result is depicted in Figure 5.4. Further analyses showed that employers did not rate men and women in the ADHD and Community groups as being significantly different from each other—a pattern found above for self-ratings in this group. But employers did rate males in the Clinical control group as manifesting more symptoms of ADHD at work than did females in that group—a pattern

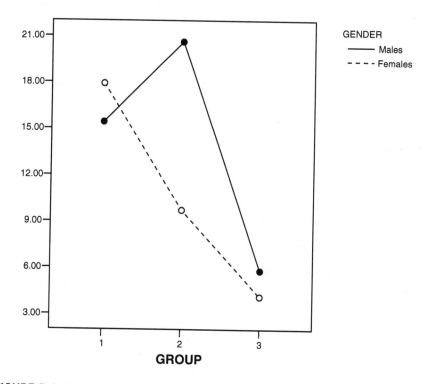

FIGURE 5.4. Results of the employer-completed ADHD ratings (raw scores) for workplace functioning showing each sex within each group (illustrating the significant group × sex interaction on this measure). Group 1 = ADHD, 2 = Clinical control, 3 = Community control.

opposite to that found for self-ratings in that group. Once more, it is the Clinical control group that is inconsistent with the pattern of sex differences found in the other groups; again, without apparent explanation.

The Milwaukee Study Results

Like those in the UMASS Study, the groups in the Milwaukee Study did not differ in the nature of the relationships found between the study participants and the collateral adult who provided information about them. Parents (27–41%) and spouses/partners (39–59%) were the majority of these informants, with friends (7–15%) and siblings (4–11%) representing a much smaller percentage of these informants. In this study, the ADHD ratings provided by others present a somewhat different picture than do the self-rated symptoms (see Table 5.3). While the H+ADHD group is still reported to be the most severely affected, the difference now is that the H–ADHD group is rated as more symptomatic than the control group, which was not the case for self-ratings. On average, then, others see this H–ADHD group as not being as close to normal or our Community control group as the group members see themselves. Note that the ratings for this group have a mean score more than double the mean for the self-ratings for this same group, a finding that is not evident for either the H+ADHD group or Community control group where others give ratings similar to the self-ratings of these groups. And in their ratings of the childhood behavior, others rate both the H+ADHD and H–ADHD groups as being highly symptomatic and as not being different from each other, though both clearly differ from the Community control group. These ratings from others compare favorably to those found in the UMASS Study, where total raw scores are relatively similar and the pattern of adults with ADHD having more symptom severity than the Community control groups is also evident. Just as in the UMASS Study, these ratings from others provide some corroboration of the manner in which the groups were formed as having ADHD on the basis of their self-reports.

When it comes to the retrospective childhood ratings provided by others, one could rightly wonder whether parents are the best informants here, providing a more accurate and more severe portrayal of these childhood and adolescent years of our participants than would nonparent informants. That may well be the case. But when we compared the current and childhood ratings for those participants whose parents provided this information to those participants who had a nonparent give that information, we found no significant differences. This is not the same as comparing the same participants on parent versus other-informant sources of the same information, which could tell us more specifically how these sources may differ in their views of the childhood and even current functioning of our participants. But it does indicate that the source of information did not contribute to any significant group differences in these ratings. It is possible that the nonparent informants may know enough about the childhood years of the participants to provide a "good enough" depiction of them, at least as far as detecting individual and group differences on our measures. Perhaps this judgment is achieved through conversations with the participants about their early years, conversations with their parents, other family members, and childhood friends, and possible access to some of the educational records of those participants.

Validation of Self-Reported Symptom Severity

To what extent do these various sources agree with each other on ADHD symptom severity? This question speaks to the validity of the self-reported symptoms provided by our participants. To examine this issue, we collapsed all three groups together in the UMASS Study. We then correlated the self-reported symptom severity on the rating scales with those provided by these other sources, using this entire sample. For ratings of current symptoms, the agreement (Pearson correlation, r) was a respectable .70 ($p < .001$; $N = 259$). This agrees with the results of our earlier study ($r = .76$, $N = 72$, $p < .001$) using just ADHD participants (Murphy, Barkley, & Bush, 2002) and with an even earlier paper (Murphy & Barkley, 1996a) using DSM-III-R symptom ratings with samples of ADHD and clinical control participants ($r = .75$). All three studies are consistent with a later paper by Murphy and Schachar (2000) ($r = .69$) based on adults whose children were undergoing an evaluation at a child psychiatry clinic compared to partner/ spouse ratings of those same adults. Most recently, Belendiuk and colleagues (Belendiuk, Clarke, Chronis, & Raggi, 2007) analyzed the degree of agreement between the self-reports of 69 mothers of children with ADHD and what others said about them using the K-SADS interview (ADHD module) adapted for adults. They found somewhat lower levels of agreement ($r = .54$ for inattention, $r = .29$ for hyperactive–impulsive symptoms). This disparity may be due to a difference in methods of assessing ADHD, given that all of the other studies used rating scales of DSM symptom lists while Belendiuk and associates used a structured interview—one originally intended for use with children. Rating scales permit a wider range of responses to each item than do interviews using a dichotomous (yes/no) response format, and that wider range could permit a greater distribution of scores and so a higher correlation between sources. Even so, the similarity of most research findings across studies is impressive and reassuring. It basically supports the important point that the reports of adult participants in the UMASS Study concerning their current symptoms are reasonably valid as judged against the reports of others who know them well.

Likewise, we found good agreement between the self-reports of the participants concerning their recall of their childhood ADHD behavior and the ratings provided by their parents concerning this same period of childhood ($r = .75$, $p <$ .001, $N = 143$). This is very important, given the concerns that have been raised by others on the accuracy of adult recall of childhood ADHD symptoms (Manuzza, Klein, Klein, Bessler, & Shrout, 2002; Shaffer, 1994). Our earlier study (Murphy, Barkley, & Bush, 2002) found virtually the same result ($r = .79$, $p < .001$) for an ADHD group, as did the much earlier paper using DSM-III-R symptoms ($r = .74$). Again, all three studies agree with that by Murphy and Schachar (2000) ($r = .79$). The degree of agreement here across studies is impressive and again provides some reassurance as to the validity of the childhood recall of the participant's about their own behavior, or specifically their ADHD symptoms.

Contrast these results with those from the Milwaukee Study of children with ADHD grown up. As we noted in Chapter 4, the degree of agreement between participants and their parents on current DSM-III-R symptoms at the previous age-21 follow-up was just .21 (Barkley, Fischer, et al., 2002). These findings are well below the correspondence documented above for clinic-referred adults. At this age-27 follow-up, we found that the correlations had doubled. For current symptom ratings (total rating scale scores), the degree of agreement was $r = .43$ ($N = 208$, $p < .001$) using the entire sample, and $r = .38$ using just the hyperactive group. For retrospectively recalled childhood ADHD symptom ratings, the degree of agreement was actually somewhat higher, being $r = .59$ ($N = 208$, $p < .001$) for the entire sample and $r = .31$ for the hyperactive group only. There is evidence of improvement between age 21 and 27 in the degree of agreement developing between the participants and others who know them well. Yet that agreement remains substantially below what is found in studies of the ratings of clinic-referred adults with ADHD, as we reported earlier, or in the parents of ADHD children about themselves as reported by Murphy and Schachar (2000).

The Milwaukee Study permits us another way of examining the validity of self-reported information about childhood ADHD-related behavior. Instead of just examining the degree of agreement between self and other reports of recall of childhood ADHD symptoms, we can actually examine the degree of agreement between self-rated childhood behavior and the actual parent reports from childhood. At the age-27 follow-up, we asked the participants to rate themselves on the precise scales that were used in childhood to determine if they were hyperactive (ADHD) or not. We then correlated these retrospectively recalled ratings with the actual parent ratings taken nearly 20 years ago. We found that the self-ratings on the Werry–Weiss–Peters Activity Rating Scale (see sidebar in Chapter 4) correlated .55 ($p < .001$) with the actual parent ratings on this scale collected at childhood entry using the entire sample. The correlation between self-ratings on the Conners Parent Rating Scale—Revised Hyperactivity Index (see sidebar in Chapter 4) and parent ratings on this same scale taken in childhood was .51, $p < .001$. These results are nearly the same as those obtained above between retrospectively recalled self-reports of childhood ADHD symptoms and others' retrospectively recalled results of those symptoms. We can therefore conclude that there is moderate agreement between retrospectively recalled self-reported information about childhood ADHD-related behavior and how parents actually rated that person in childhood. This agreement is actually higher than that between self-reports and other-reports for current ADHD behavior in this same sample.

Once more, it is worth remembering that the Milwaukee samples are at least 5 or more years younger than those in the UMASS Study. The trend here is for them to report increasing levels of ADHD with age since age 21; therefore one would expect increasing correspondence between self-reports and the reports of others over that same time frame. Such a trend could continue into the 30s or later years of the Milwaukee participants and thus begin to correspond to what is seen in older samples of studies using clinic-referred adults with ADHD.

These findings are of considerable importance to the clinical diagnostic process concerning ADHD in adults. They address the issue of how good or trustworthy the reports of clinic-referred adults are concerning their childhood behavior (ages 5–12 here) and not just their current functioning. The answer would seem to be good enough for clinical purposes. Shaffer (1994) previously raised a valid point that the recall of patients about their childhood may not have much veracity to use for clinical diagnosis. The evidence presented here addresses this issue. It provides some confidence in the reports of these patients as compared to the reports given by others if the participants are at least in their early 30s or older. It suggests great caution if the participants are in their early 20s, yet a somewhat better though still cautious acceptance of the reports of participants in their late 20s. This pattern implies that the older participants or patients are when they provide ratings of themselves about ADHD, particularly after their early 30s, the more likely are those reports to agree with the ratings provided by others.

This does not mean that there are no absolute differences between the level of symptom severity reported by our participants and that reported by others. It shows only that as self-reports increase in severity, so do the reports of others. Inspection of the means, for instance, between the self-ratings of current symptoms and other-rated current symptoms in the UMASS Study shows that self-ratings tend to be somewhat higher in all three groups relative to the ratings provided by others. This difference is also apparent in comparing self-rated childhood symptoms with those provided by parents for this same period of time. The differences are not striking with one exception. Noteworthy is the rather larger disparity between self and parent ratings in the Clinical control group for childhood functioning—a disparity far greater than that seen in the other two groups. Apparently, Clinical control adults recall their childhood ADHD behavior to be substantially greater than do their parents. Remember, these are patients who thought they had ADHD, came to an adult ADHD clinic, but were eventually not diagnosed with the condition. Perhaps their belief that they had ADHD served to distort their recollections of childhood ADHD symptoms relative to what their parents had to say about them as children. Regardless, an important point here is that the corroboration of patient reports through the reports of others, particularly concerning the childhood functioning of the patients, is an essential part of differential diagnosis of ADHD from other disorders and is to be encouraged whenever possible.

The differences between the self-rated symptoms and those provided by employers are even greater than between the self- and other-ratings for current functioning. Again, adults self-report more symptoms than what their employers say about them. For the two clinical groups at least, employers reported approximately 50% less symptom severity than did the participants' own self-ratings. While there was much closer agreement between these sources in the Community control group, this could easily have been the result of a "floor effect," given such low symptom ratings in this group. This disparity in the two clinical groups can be at least partially attributed to the fact that employers do not witness the behavior of these participants across as wide a range of situations as do others who know the participants well. And we must mention again the possibility that the far smaller sample sizes for the employer ratings may make them less representative of the actual workplace behavior of these population groups at large.

All of this is to say that while there is sufficient correspondence between the severity of ADHD symptoms reported by adults with what others are likely to say about them, the correspondence is far from perfect and is inexact with regard to absolute levels of severity. In general, there is a tendency for self-ratings to be somewhat higher than ratings provided by others and especially those provided by employers. None of these findings can speak to whose reports are the more accurate or valid, in which case information gleaned from several sources should be an essential part of the clinical diagnosis of ADHD in adults, as discussed in Chapter 2.

Percentage Endorsing Specific Symptoms

We now turn our attention to the percentage of each group that endorsed each specific symptom of ADHD from the DSM-IV. Such results may seem rather tedious to many readers, but they are important for other researchers studying the specific symptoms of adults with ADHD and for committees deliberating on changes to the DSM diagnostic criteria. The percentages are derived from the symptoms reported during the interview. We present only the results for the UMASS Study, as these have the greatest bearing on the utility of current

ADHD symptoms for diagnosis in this self-referred clinical population. For current functioning of the groups in the UMASS Study, the results are shown in Table 5.3, while for childhood functioning they appear in Table 5.4. For current functioning—with three exceptions—we found that adults with ADHD were more likely to endorse every particular symptom than were the Clinical control adults, who endorsed symptoms significantly more often than did the Community control adults. The exceptions were for the symptoms of difficulty organizing tasks under the inattention symptom list and having difficulty staying seated and refraining from talking excessively under the hyperactive–impulsive symptom list. For these three symptoms, we found that the ADHD and Clinical control groups did not differ from each other, but more members of both groups were likely to endorse these items than were the Community control adults.

Our results for the current inattention symptoms are generally similar if not somewhat higher than those reported for much smaller samples by Riccio et al.

TABLE 5.3. Frequency of Each Current DSM-IV-TR ADHD Symptom from Interview by Group for the UMASS Study

Measure	ADHD		Clinical		Community		χ^2	p	Pairwise contrasts
	N	%	N	%	N	%			
Inattention symptoms									
Is inattentive to details	108	74	46	47	3	3	128.5	< .001	1 > 2 > 3
Can't sustain attention	142	97	80	82	3	3	261.6	< .001	1 > 2 > 3
Fails to listen	106	73	54	56	2	2	130.8	< .001	1 > 2 > 3
Fails to follow instructions	110	75	48	50	1	1	140.6	< .001	1 > 2 > 3
Has difficulty organizing tasks	118	81	72	74	5	5	166.0	< .001	1,2 > 3
Avoids sustained mental effort	118	81	62	64	2	2	163.9	< .001	1 > 2 > 3
Loses necessary things	110	75	58	60	11	11	110.6	< .001	1 > 2 > 3
Is easily distracted	142	97	84	87	2	2	277.0	< .001	1 > 2 > 3
Is forgetful in daily activities	114	78	56	58	4	4	141.9	< .001	1 > 2 > 3
Hyperactivity–impulsivity symptoms									
Fidgets or squirms	115	79	54	56	4	4	143.1	< .001	1 > 2 > 3
Leaves seat	44	30	31	32	2	2	37.2	< .001	1,2 > 3
Feels restless	112	77	60	62	3	3	144.4	< .001	1 > 2 > 3
Can't do things quietly	56	38	15	15	3	3	50.1	< .001	1 > 2 > 3
Have to be "on the go"	91	62	43	44	13	12	65.5	< .001	1 > 2 > 3
Talks excessively	65	44	36	37	4	4	53.1	< .001	1,2 > 3
Blurts out answers	83	57	39	41	8	7	66.3	< .001	1,2 > 3
Has difficulty awaiting turn	98	67	52	54	3	3	110.8	< .001	1 > 2 > 3
Interrupts others	84	57	37	38	3	3	82.6	< .001	1 > 2 > 3

Note. N = sample size endorsing this item; % = percent of group endorsing this item; χ^2 = results of the omnibus chi-square test; p = probability value for the chi-square test; pairwise contrasts = results of the chi-square tests involving pairwise comparisons of the three groups.

TABLE 5.4. Frequency of Each Childhood DSM-IV-TR ADHD Symptom from Interview by Group for the UMASS Study

Measure	ADHD N	ADHD %	Clinical N	Clinical %	Community N	Community %	χ^2	p	Pairwise contrasts
Inattention symptoms									
Is inattentive to details	118	86	42	45	6	6	155.9	< .001	1 > 2 > 3
Can't sustain attention	132	94	57	61	6	6	194.1	< .001	1 > 2 > 3
Fails to listen	116	82	45	47	3	3	153.2	< .001	1 > 2 > 3
Fails to follow instructions	115	82	40	42	2	2	159.0	< .001	1 > 2 > 3
Has difficulty organizing tasks	114	80	52	54	5	5	141.6	< .001	1 > 2 > 3
Avoids sustained mental effort	120	84	45	47	5	5	156.9	< .001	1 > 2 > 3
Loses necessary things	92	66	43	45	3	3	101.7	< .001	1 > 2 > 3
Is easily distracted	132	94	66	70	6	6	203.0	< .001	1 > 2 > 3
Is forgetful in daily activities	105	74	35	36	1	1	137.9	< .001	1 > 2 > 3
Hyperactivity–impulsivity symptoms									
Fidgets or squirms	108	76	56	59	9	8	115.6	< .001	1 > 2 > 3
Leaves seat	71	50	24	25	8	7	55.4	< .001	1 > 2 > 3
Feels restless	104	74	58	61	5	5	126.4	< .001	1 > 2 > 3
Can't do things quietly	68	48	23	24	1	1	70.0	< .001	1 > 2 > 3
Has to be "on the go"	89	63	42	44	9	8	76.7	< .001	1 > 2 > 3
Talks excessively	77	55	33	34	9	8	58.0	< .001	1 > 2 > 3
Blurts out answers	89	63	40	42	12	11	67.6	< .001	1 > 2 > 3
Has difficulty awaiting turn	87	61	45	46	6	6	81.9	< .001	1 > 2 > 3
Interrupts others	84	57	34	35	2	2	89.8	< .001	1 > 2 > 3

Note. N = sample size endorsing this item; % = percent of group endorsing this item; χ^2 = results of the omnibus chi-square test; p = probability value for the chi-square test; pairwise contrasts = results of the chi-square tests involving pairwise comparisons of the three groups.

(2005), both for their ADHD and clinical control groups. They also found these two groups to differ significantly on all but one of the inattention items, that item being does not seem to listen to instructions. In contrast, a smaller percentage of our ADHD group endorsed the various symptoms of hyperactive–impulsive behavior relative to the ADHD group in the Riccio et al. study, most likely due to their limiting that analysis to just those adults who had the Combined type of ADHD, in which such symptoms would be higher than in the Inattentive type, whereas our analysis collapsed the types together. Only the item of fidgeting failed to discriminate among their ADHD and control groups, whereas it did so in our study.

Again, such findings would be expected, given the procedures used to create the ADHD and control groups (reliance on the DSM symptoms) in the UMASS Study. More informative, however, is the pattern of symptom endorsement. It is clear that difficulties sustaining attention to tasks and distractibility are the two most common symptoms of inattention in the ADHD group, being endorsed by 97% of the adults with ADHD. Yet these two symptoms are also the most commonly endorsed items in the Clinical control group, though not to the same extent (82–87%). Note that symptoms of inattention are quite rarely endorsed by the Community control group except for losing things necessary for tasks, yet even here it was endorsed in only 11% of these participants. Likewise, the two hyperactive symptoms most often endorsed in the ADHD group were (1) fidgeting with hand or feet or squirming in seat and (2) feeling restless, both of which were endorsed by more than 70% of members of the ADHD group. While they were endorsed somewhat less often in the Clinical control group, these two items were still the most frequently endorsed in that group as well relative to the other hyperactive items. Except for being on the go (11%), these symptoms of hyperactivity were quite rare in the Community control group.

What all this seems to show is that inattention and hyperactive–impulsive symptoms are relatively common in clinical samples, whether representing ADHD or not, while being relatively rare in community samples. Such findings conflict with the general notion among laypeople and probably some professionals that symptoms of ADHD are commonplace in the normal population in their current functioning—a finding we refuted in an earlier paper using a general population sample of 720 adults in central Massachusetts (Murphy & Barkley, 1996b). While symptom endorsements were somewhat higher in that sample, it is most likely because we did not screen out ADHD or other clinical disorders from that sample, as was done here to create the Community control group. Nevertheless, symptoms of inattention were endorsed by 5 to 19% of that sample and of hyperactive–impulsive behavior between 6 and 22%. The one exception was the finding that over 39% of the general population sample in that study endorsed feeling "on the go," a symptom that could have as much to do with the busyness of modern life than of just reflecting hyperactivity. On average, adults in that study endorsed between one and three symptoms of either inattention or hyperactivity—well below the threshold of six required in the DSM for clinical diagnosis. Similar results were reported by Riccio et al. (2005) and earlier by O'Donnell et al. (2001) for their ADHD and control groups. Thus, symptoms of ADHD are nowhere near as common among community or general population samples of adults as they are among adults with ADHD.

Table 5.3 shows the same information for recall of childhood symptoms. In this instance, the adults with ADHD were more likely to endorse each of the 18 symptoms than were members of the Clinical control group, which did so more often than did those in the Community control group. Again, difficulties with sustaining attention and with distractibility were the most common inattention symptoms in the ADHD group, being endorsed by 94% of this group. They were also the most common symptoms endorsed in the Clinical control group (61 and 70% respectively) while being rare in the Community control group

(6%). And once more, fidgeting and feeling restless were the two most commonly recalled symptoms of hyperactivity in childhood in the ADHD group (74–76%) as well as in the Clinical group (56–58%), while occurring in less than 8% of the Community control group. In our prior general population study, these various symptoms were endorsed by just 13 to 34% of adults recalling their childhood behavior. Such findings make the point, once again, that symptoms of ADHD are not recalled as occurring very often by a majority of a general population sample and far less in more carefully screened Community control samples (< 10%). When symptoms of ADHD are endorsed as occurring often or more frequently by adult clinical patients, they should therefore be taken seriously as likely reflecting the presence of a psychiatric disorder; this is especially so when at least four or more such symptoms are endorsed (as shown earlier).

Identifying the Best
Current DSM-IV ADHD Symptoms for Classifying Adults

Another issue we wished to study in this project dealt with identifying which among the 18 symptoms in DSM-IV was best at accurately discriminating those with ADHD from normal individuals (Community controls) and clinic-referred adults not having ADHD (Clinical controls). Simply stated, does one really need 18 symptoms to diagnose this condition or might a smaller set of these items be just as useful in the clinical evaluation of adults for ADHD? A smaller set of symptoms is conceivable, given that many items on the same list are highly intercorrelated and thus provide redundant information about inattentiveness or hyperactive–impulsive behavior. We addressed the issue using both of our studies. We employed binary logistic regression, a form of multiple regression for dealing with dichotomous variables (categorical) like the symptoms of ADHD endorsed in our clinical interview. They were recorded as positive (endorsed as occurring often or more) or negative (not occurring to this degree).

The UMASS Study Results

We first examined which of the 18 symptoms best differentiated (classified) the ADHD group from the Community control group. Those results appear in Table 5.5. We studied the nine inattention and nine hyperactive–impulsive symptom sets separately and then combined.

Incredibly, *just a single inattention symptom emerged from the analysis for accurately identifying an adult as being a control (normal) or not, that symptom being "Often easily distracted by extraneous stimuli,"* or symptom *1h* in the DSM-IV symptom list. This single item of distractibility accurately classified 97% of the ADHD cases

TABLE 5.5. ADHD Symptoms (Interview) That Best Discriminate the ADHD Group from Community Clinical and Control Groups (Both Current and Childhood Self-Reports) in the UMASS Study

Symptom	Beta	SE	Wald	p	Odds ratio	95% CI
From Community control group						
Inattention symptoms (current)						
Is easily distracted	7.54	.87	74.63	< .001	1899.24	341.51–10562.2
Hyperactivity–impulsivity symptoms (current)						
Fidgets with hands/feet or squirms	3.03	.68	19.70	< .001	20.69	5.43–78.82
Feels restless	3.50	.74	22.17	< .001	33.23	7.73–142.86
Blurts out answers	1.77	.66	7.22	.007	5.88	1.61–21.42
Has difficulty awaiting turn	3.22	.77	17.42	< .001	24.96	5.51–113.05
All current symptoms analyzed together						
Is easily distracted	7.54	.87	74.63	< .001	1899.24	341.51–10562.2
All childhood symptoms analyzed together						
Has difficulty sustaining attention	2.64	1.36	2.79	.095	9.62	0.67–137.09
Has difficulty listening when spoken to directly	4.13	1.81	5.23	.022	62.18	1.80–2142.77
Has difficulty organizing tasks and activities	7.21	2.40	9.04	.003	1358.26	12.31–149809.0
Has to be "on the go" or acts as if "driven by a motor"	8.00	2.85	7.89	.005	2976.28	11.23–789066.0
Loses things necessary for tasks or activities	4.71	1.77	7.05	.008	110.92	3.43–3585.86
Is easily distracted	4.42	1.72	6.64	.01	83.35	2.88–2408.86
From Clinical control group						
Inattention symptoms (current)						
Fails to give close attention to details	.91	.29	9.23	.002	2.48	1.38–4.47
Has difficulty sustaining attention to tasks	1.77	.59	8.84	.003	5.84	1.82–18.72
Fails to follow through on instructions	.74	.30	5.85	.016	2.09	1.15–3.80
Hyperactivity–impulsivity symptoms (current)						
Fidgets with hands/feet or squirms in seat	1.02	.32	10.27	.001	2.78	1.49–5.20
Leaves seat in settings requiring sitting	−.69	.33	4.43	.035	.50	0.26–0.95
Has difficulty engaging in leisure quietly	1.01	.35	8.22	.004	2.74	1.38–5.47
Interrupts or intrudes on others	.60	.29	4.35	.037	1.82	1.04–3.19
All current symptoms analyzed together						
Fails to give close attention to details	.83	.31	7.36	.007	2.30	1.26–4.22
Has difficulty sustaining attention to tasks	1.47	.60	5.88	.015	4.34	1.32–14.20
Fails to follow through on instructions	.93	.32	8.33	.004	2.55	1.35–4.80
Has difficulty engaging in leisure quietly	1.26	.36	12.16	< .001	3.51	1.73–7.12

(continued)

TABLE 5.5. (continued)

Symptom	Beta	SE	Wald	p	Odds ratio	95% CI
All childhood symptoms analyzed together						
Fails to give close attention to detail	0.84	.39	4.68	.03	2.31	1.08–4.94
Has difficulty sustaining attention	1.09	.49	5.07	.024	2.99	1.15–7.75
Avoids, dislikes, or is reluctant to engage in working requiring sustained mental effort	0.86	.38	5.26	.022	2.37	1.13–4.96
Is forgetful in daily activities	1.10	.33	11.07	.001	3.01	1.57–5.76
Interrupts or intrudes on others	0.65	.33	3.82	.051	1.91	1.00–3.64

Note. SE = standard error for beta; odds ratio = Exp(B); 95% CI = 95% confidence interval for the odds ratio. *Statistical analysis:* Logistic regression using forward conditional entry method.

and 98% of the Community controls. Adding the symptoms of poor sustained attention, being poorly organized, and being forgetful would bump this classification accuracy up to 99% for each group, but they are hardly necessary. If the set of nine hyperactive–impulsive items is considered alone, then four symptoms appeared to make a significant contribution to accurately classifying participants as being normal or ADHD in the UMASS Study, these being:

- Fidgets with hands/feet or squirms.
- Feels restless.
- Blurts out answers.
- Has difficulty awaiting turn.

These four symptoms accurately classified 91% of the Community control cases and 94% of the ADHD cases. It is interesting to note that just the single symptom of "Often fidgets with hands or feet or squirms in seat" was enough to accurately classify 96% of the Community control group and 78% of the ADHD group. Adding the additional items simply serves to classify more accurately the ADHD group while slightly diminishing the accuracy for classifying the Community controls. Again, if you wish to know whether someone is normal, then the single item of often fidgeting with hands or feet or squirming in his or her seat would suffice.

When all 18 items were studied simultaneously, *once again being easily distracted was the only symptom required for accurately classifying participants as a Community control or ADHD.* This single item of distractibility once more accurately classified 97% of the ADHD cases and 98% of the Community controls. We do not believe this to be a fluke, "one-off," or chance event. Milich, Widiger, and Landau (1987) found precisely this same result in studying the positive and negative predictive power of the ADHD item set from the earlier DSM-III-R. Being easily distracted was the best and only symptom necessary in their study for determining if a child was normal or not. We have therefore replicated this same finding and extended it upward to adults. This means that you really do not need 18 symptoms to tell if someone you are evaluating is normal or not—just this one symptom of being easily distracted will suffice.

In the next analysis, we evaluated the equally important issue of which items were best at discriminating those with ADHD from those adults in the Clinical control group. This issue speaks more directly to the ability of DSM-IV symptoms to aid in the differential diagnosis of ADHD from other clinical disorders. The results appear in Table 5.5 as well. Again, we studied the inattention items separately from the hyperactive–impulsive items before studying them jointly for their ability to classify these two groups accurately. In this case, the following three symptoms of inattention worked best:

- Fails to give close attention to details.
- Has difficulty sustaining attention to tasks.
- Fails to follow through on instructions.

Taken together, these items correctly classified 87% of the ADHD group correctly but just 44% of the Clinical control group. All of this suggests that while those with ADHD are highly likely to have these particular inattention symptoms, so are a significant portion of adults with other disorders.

Studying just the nine hyperactive–impulsive symptoms, we found these four items to be the most useful for classifying ADHD cases against Clinical control cases:

- Fidgets with hands/feet or squirms in seat.
- Leaves seat in settings requiring sitting.
- Has difficulty engaging in leisure quietly.
- Interrupts or intrudes on others.

These four hyperactive symptoms accurately classified 76% of ADHD cases and 49% of clinical control cases. Of note here was the finding that the item involving leaving one's seat in settings requiring sitting still was reverse weighted in the regression equation, meaning that it was more likely to have been endorsed by the Clinical control cases than the ADHD cases and so served to classify the former cases somewhat better than the ADHD cases.

When all of the 18 symptoms are considered together, the same inattention items appear once more to be the best at classifying these cases while a single item from the hyperactive–impulsive list now joins them to further assist in this purpose, that item being difficulty engaging in leisure activities quietly. In considering all symptoms together, these four ADHD symptoms accurately classify 86%

of ADHD cases but just 47% of Clinical control cases. Again, a point to be made here is the same as that made above for inattention symptoms—adults with ADHD are more likely to have this set of symptoms than adults with other disorders, yet a significant number of the latter adults may demonstrate them as well. This means that any individual item or set of items poses some difficulty in assisting with differential diagnosis of ADHD from other disorders with great accuracy. Yet another point of importance from these results is that 18 symptoms are hardly needed to distinguish ADHD from Community control adults or even from Clinical control adults. A much smaller, more cost-efficient item set for adults is feasible. Given the results above, this item set should at least include those items that were found to be useful in both of these sets of analyses. For inattention, they would be the DSM symptoms corresponding to the abbreviated ones below:

- Is easily distracted by extraneous information.
- Fails to give close attention to details.
- Has difficulty sustaining attention to tasks.
- Fails to follow through on instructions.

For hyperactive–impulsive, they would be the DSM symptoms corresponding to:

- Feels restless.
- Blurts out answers.
- Has difficulty awaiting turn.
- Leaves seat in settings requiring sitting.
- Interrupts or intrudes on others.
- Has difficulty engaging in leisure activities quietly.

This shows that only 10 items provide real discriminating ability for identifying adults with ADHD, not the 18 developed on and for children in the DSM-IV. But a single symptom list is really all that is needed for adults, as there is some redundancy across these two lists in contributing information that helps to distinguish ADHD. That list would involve five total items: the four inattention symptoms above and just the last symptom on the hyperactive–impulsive list (Has difficulty engaging in leisure activities quietly).

The Milwaukee Study Results

We repeated the same analyses as above using the Milwaukee Study samples. The results appear in Table 5.6. The following items from the inattention list were the most useful at discriminating the H+ADHD group from the community control group:

- Is easily distracted by extraneous information
- Has difficulty sustaining attention to tasks
- Is forgetful in daily activities

The first two of these are the same as those found in the UMASS Study. Once again, the single symptom of being easily distractible is, by itself, a very good symptom that could accurately classify 85% of the cases (ADHD = 88%, Controls = 81%). The classification accuracy for the entire list of three symptoms was 84% (ADHD = 89%, Controls = 79%).

The following items were the best from the hyperactive-impulsive symptom list, again several of which appeared to be the best in the UMASS Study (the second and fourth below):

- Fidgets with hands/feet or squirms.
- Feels restless.
- Talks excessively.
- Has difficulty awaiting turn.

The single symptom of feels restless resulted in a classification accuracy of 83% (ADHD = 81%, Control = 85%) with the additional items adding just 2% more overall accuracy. But once again, if the entire list of 18 symptoms is evaluated together, the following shorter list proved to be the best:

- Is easily distracted.
- Has difficulty sustaining attention to tasks.
- Is forgetful in daily activities.
- Feels restless.
- Blurts out answers.

Here, being easily distracted remains the best single symptom, with an overall accuracy of 85% and the remaining symptoms providing only slight improvement over this one.

Now what symptoms are best in discriminating the H+ADHD group from the H–ADHD group? The results are also found in Table 5.6. For inattention symptoms, they were:

- Has difficulty sustaining attention to tasks.
- Fails to listen when spoken to directly.

TABLE 5.6. Current ADHD Symptoms That Best Discriminate Hyperactive Children Having ADHD at Adult Follow-Up from the Community Control Group (Interview) and the Hyperactive Group without ADHD in the Milwaukee Study

Symptom	Beta	SE	Wald	p	Odds ratio	95% CI
From Community control group						
Inattention symptoms						
Has difficulty sustaining attention to tasks	1.36	.643	4.44	.035	3.88	1.10–13.69
Is easily distracted	2.77	.507	29.85	< .001	15.96	5.91–43.11
Is forgetful in daily activities	1.52	.497	9.42	.002	4.59	1.73–12.15
Hyperactive–impulsive symptoms						
Fidgets with hands/feet or squirms	1.02	.500	4.15	.042	2.77	1.04–7.39
Feels restless	2.19	.497	19.34	< .001	8.90	3.36–23.60
Talks excessively	1.00	.507	3.89	.048	2.71	1.01–7.33
Has difficulty awaiting turn	1.69	.625	7.30	.007	5.41	1.59–18.44
All symptoms analyzed together						
Has difficulty sustaining attention to tasks	1.92	.809	5.62	.018	6.81	1.39–33.26
Feels restless	2.70	.634	18.14	< .001	14.87	4.29–51.50
Blurts out answers	1.25	.629	3.98	.046	3.50	1.02–12.02
Is easily distracted	2.45	.620	15.56	< .001	11.56	3.43–39.00
Is forgetful in daily activities	1.47	.622	5.95	.018	4.35	1.29–14.74
All childhood symptoms together						
Has difficulty sustaining attention to tasks	2.62	.984	7.08	.008	13.71	1.99–94.33
Leaves seat when required to sit	2.37	.993	5.67	.017	10.65	1.52–74.65
Fails to listen when spoken to directly	2.03	1.01	4.03	.045	7.60	1.05–55.08
Feels restless	4.97	1.66	8.94	.003	144.37	5.55–3754.47
Has difficulty engaging in leisure quietly	2.49	1.09	5.18	.023	12.11	1.41–103.65
Talks excessively	2.87	1.09	6.94	.008	17.63	2.08–149.09
From H–ADHD group						
Inattention symptoms						
Has difficulty sustaining attention to tasks	1.13	.513	4.85	.028	3.09	1.13–8.46
Fails to listen when spoken to directly	2.03	.555	13.38	< .001	7.61	2.56–22.55
Avoids work requiring sustained mental effort	1.36	.515	6.93	.008	3.88	1.41–10.66
Loses things necessary for tasks	1.19	.510	5.47	.019	3.30	1.23–8.97
Hyperactive–impulsive symptoms						
Fidgets with hands/feet or squirms	1.38	.517	7.14	.008	3.98	1.44–10.97
Feels restless	1.61	.521	9.55	.002	5.00	1.80–13.89
Has difficulty awaiting turn	1.35	.588	5.25	.022	3.85	1.21–12.20
Interrupts or intrudes on others	1.59	.604	6.88	.009	4.88	1.49–15.97

(continued)

TABLE 5.6. (continued)

Symptom	Beta	SE	Wald	p	Odds ratio	95% CI
All symptoms analyzed together						
Fidgets with hands/feet or squirms	2.04	.660	9.51	.002	7.66	2.10–27.96
Fails to listen when spoken to directly	1.21	.694	3.05	.081	3.36	0.86–13.11
Feels restless	1.60	.578	7.70	.006	4.97	1.60–15.40
Avoids work requiring sustained mental effort	1.94	.660	8.60	.003	6.93	1.90–25.26
Loses things necessary for tasks	1.84	.616	8.98	.003	6.39	1.89–21.16
Interrupts or intrudes on others	1.37	.684	4.00	.046	3.92	1.03–14.98
All childhood symptoms together						
Feels restless	2.46	.773	10.13	.001	11.71	2.57–53.27
Loses things necessary for tasks	1.26	.392	10.35	.001	3.52	1.63–7.59

Note. SE = standard error for beta; odds ratio = Exp(B); 95% CI = 95% confidence interval for the odds ratio; H–ADHD = Hyperactive group that does not have a diagnosis of ADHD at follow-up.
Statistical analysis: Binary logistic regression using forward conditional entry method.

- Avoids work requiring sustained mental effort.
- Loses things necessary for tasks.

These symptoms had an overall classification accuracy of 84%. And only one of them (the first) is found on the list above, which worked best for discriminating the H+ADHD from the control group. The best hyperactive–impulsive symptoms turned out to be:

- Fidgets with hands/feet or squirms.
- Feels restless.
- Has difficulty awaiting turn.
- Interrupts or intrudes on others.

The first three of these four were also useful in discriminating the H+ADHD from the control group. The overall accuracy of this list was 83%. When all symptoms were analyzed together, the best symptoms were the following six (three of which come from each symptom list above):

- Fidgets with hands/feet or squirms.
- Fails to listen when spoken to directly.
- Feels restless.
- Avoids work requiring sustained mental effort.
- Loses things necessary for tasks.
- Interrupts or intrudes on others.

In comparison to the results of the UMASS Study, the Milwaukee study found that several more hyperactive–impulsive symptoms might be useful for group discrimination. But we feel compelled to admit that in developing diagnostic criteria for clinic-referred adults with ADHD, the UMASS Study results should carry greater weight, because such adults were the focus of that study, whereas most of the hyperactive group in the Milwaukee Study were not self-referred to clinics for evaluation or treatment. Still, there are points of overlap between these two studies that could provide further corroboration of the symptoms identified as being the best in that UMASS Study.

Identifying the Best Childhood DSM-IV ADHD Symptoms for Classifying Adults

The diagnosis of ADHD in adults, unlike the process in children, requires not only that symptoms of the disorder be present currently but that a significant number of symptoms should have been present in childhood as well. That is, the symptoms must have had their onset sometime during childhood (DSM-IV recommends by age 7 years, but see "Age of Onset," below). It is often recommended with adults that the DSM-IV symptoms be reviewed with a patient not just for current functioning, but also for recall of childhood behavior (Barkley, 2006; McGough & Barkley, 2004). This naturally raises the question of which of the 18 symptoms of ADHD when recollected from their childhood years serves to best differentiate the groups. The self-reports of ADHD symptoms experienced in childhood were included as part of the structured interview used with participants in both studies.

The UMASS Study Results

We analyzed these childhood symptoms initially for their ability to discriminate the ADHD from the Community control group and these results also appear in Table 5.7 (center). Six of the 18 symptoms served to discriminate these groups with an overall accuracy of 98% (97% for Community and 99% for ADHD cases). These were:

- Has difficulty sustaining attention.
- Has difficulty listening when spoken to directly.
- Has difficulty organizing tasks and activities.
- Has to be "on the go" or acts as if "driven by a motor."
- Loses things necessary for tasks or activities.
- Is easily distracted.

TABLE 5.7. Factor Structure and Item Loading of the DSM-IV ADHD Symptom List for Adult Self-Reports (Interview Results) in the UMASS Study

Item	Factor		
	I. Inattention	II. Hyperactivity	III. Impulsivity
Inattention symptoms			
Is inattentive to details	**.688**	.086	.263
Can't sustain attention	**.757**	.368	.229
Fails to listen	**.634**	.166	.316
Fails to follow instructions	**.770**	.108	.088
Has difficulty organizing tasks	**.768**	.053	.124
Avoids sustained mental effort	**.699**	.263	.131
Loses necessary things	**.630**	.210	.121
Is easily distracted	**.751**	.386	.210
Is forgetful in daily activities	**.728**	.135	.199
Hyperactivity symptoms			
Fidgets or squirms	.455	**.592**	.235
Leaves seat	.090	**.701**	.060
Feels restless	.396	**.656**	.226
Can't do things quietly	.038	**.513**	.427
Has to be "on the go"	.164	**.739**	.128
Has difficulty awaiting turn	.329	**.475**	.407
Impulsivity symptoms			
Blurts out answers	.249	.149	**.764**
Talks excessively	.150	.298	**.627**
Interrupts others	.301	.102	**.788**

Statistical analysis: Factor analysis using Varimax rotation. Loadings in **bold** represent the highest loading of the item.

Five of these represent inattention symptoms and just one comes from the hyperactivity list, suggesting that symptoms of inattention recalled from childhood may be more useful in the diagnosis of adult ADHD than hyperactive or impulsive symptoms. Of interest is that the single symptom of difficulty sustaining attention did a reasonable job of discriminating these groups, correctly identifying 94% of each group. Where being easily distracted was the best single symptom for discerning these two groups in current functioning, having difficulties sustaining attention achieves nearly the same degree of accuracy from childhood recollections of symptoms.

We repeated this same analysis of childhood symptoms for discrimination of the ADHD from the Clinical control group. Those results appear in Table 5.7 (bottom). Five symptoms proved useful in this discrimination, with an overall accuracy of 77% (60% for Clinical control and 89% for ADHD cases):

- Fails to give close attention to detail.
- Has difficulty sustaining attention.
- Avoids, dislikes, or is reluctant to engage in working requiring sustained mental effort.
- Is forgetful in daily activities.
- Interrupts or intrudes on others.

Only one of these symptoms (difficulty sustaining attention) appears on the earlier list for discriminating ADHD patients from Community controls. Yet once again, the domain of inattention seems more useful than that of hyperactivity or impulsivity. No hyperactive symptoms proved useful in this respect, while one of the impulsive symptoms did so (interrupts or intrudes on others). It would seem that the nature of the inattention symptoms recalled from childhood that work best to distinguish ADHD from Community controls are not necessarily those that discriminate ADHD from Clinical cases. This implies that a review of all nine inattention symptoms in the DSM may be important when evaluating childhood recall of symptoms.

The Milwaukee Study Results

We conducted the same analyses on the item set from the Milwaukee Study for recall of childhood ADHD symptoms. When all 18 symptoms were considered, these six were the best at discriminating the H+ADHD group from the Community control group, having an impressive overall classification accuracy of 94%:

- Has difficulty sustaining attention to tasks.
- Leaves seat when required to sit.
- Fails to listen when spoken to directly.
- Feels restless.
- Has difficulty engaging in leisure quietly.
- Talks excessively.

In comparing the H+ADHD group to the H−ADHD group, only two symptoms were significant, having an overall classification accuracy of just 69%. This is hardly surprising, given that both of these groups were selected as being hyperactive (ADHD) in childhood; thus finding symptoms that may differentiate their childhood recall of themselves would prove difficult. The two symptoms were:

- Feels restless.
- Loses things necessary for tasks or activities.

The absence of the first of these symptoms identified the H–ADHD group with 100% accuracy, suggesting that it is the symptom best recalled from childhood for separating these two formerly hyperactive groups. The second symptom was more likely to identify the H+ADHD group with some accuracy—only 64%. As noted above, in differentiating clinic-referred adults with ADHD, the UMASS Study results have a greater bearing on trying to identify symptoms of ADHD recalled from childhood than do the results of the Milwaukee study.

Identifying a Diagnostic Threshold for Current Symptoms

Would the situation be any different if we just used the number of these "best" symptoms endorsed by an adult rather than employing them individually? After all, if severity of symptoms is the better indicator of ADHD relative to other clinical disorders, rather than symptom presence or absence, a numerical symptom count might work better for classification purposes. To answer this question, we took the three best inattention and three best hyperactive–impulsive symptoms (ignoring the reverse-weighted item dealing with leaving one's seat when required to sit) from the UMASS Study results above and created a total symptom score for each participant. This in essence is what DSM-IV recommends when it advises using six of nine symptoms from either list to establish the diagnosis, except that in this case you really do not need all nine symptoms. But those lists were based on studies of children—just three from each list seems to be necessary in dealing with adults. Based on this scoring system (0 to 6), we found that 100% of community controls endorsed three or fewer, 99% endorsed two or fewer, and 98% endorsed one or fewer (87% endorsed none). Put another way, just 2% of the Community group endorsed two or more items as occurring often or very often. This is just another way of proving the point made earlier, that one needs only one symptom of ADHD to determine if someone is a Community control (or normal adult): being easily distracted. For the patients with ADHD, 99% endorsed two or more, 91% endorsed three or more, 72% endorsed four or more. For the Clinical controls, 78% endorsed two or more, 62% endorsed three or more, 33% endorsed four or more. Therefore requiring just two symptoms would easily discriminate ADHD from Community controls while four symptoms would be needed to discriminate ADHD from Clinical controls. Using these six best symptoms, logistic regression shows 86% classification of ADHD cases and 55% of Clinical control cases. Even then, this score would be far from perfect at doing so, yielding a 45% false-positive rate for ADHD among the Clinical controls and a 14% false-negative rate in the ADHD group (classifying ADHD adults erroneously as Clinical controls). The mean symptom scores from

this 6-item list were ADHD group: mean = 4.2 (SD = 1.2); Clinical control
group: 2.9 (1.4); and Community control group: 0.1 (0.4) (F = 415.17, df = 2/
349, p < .001).

The use of a total symptom score seems to be somewhat better at differentiating ADHD from Clinical control cases than is the use of the individual symptom endorsement approach used earlier. But clinical judgment is still going to be
needed beyond this actuarial approach to further distinguish ADHD from other
adult disorders. That judgment certainly needs to include the age of onset of
symptoms, which significantly distinguished the ADHD and Clinical groups, as
shown earlier. And, as a later chapter shows, the number of domains of impairment and the specific nature of those impairments may provide further means of
distinguishing between these two groups. All of this also raises the interesting
issue of whether or not the DSM-IV symptom list comprises the best possible
symptoms for identifying ADHD in adults, given that they were originally developed for use in identifying children with the disorder. Would other symptoms
not on this list but thought to characterize the adult stage of the disorder prove
better at classifying cases of ADHD? We consider this issue in detail in a later
chapter.

Factor Structure of DSM-IV Symptoms in Adults

Several previous studies have examined the factor structure of the 18 DSM-IV
items to see if the two-factor structure (two symptom lists) set forth in the DSM-
IV, and based on children, is the same when adult self-reports are evaluated. All
of these studies of adults found that a three factor solution fit the symptom structure, rather than the two presented in DSM-IV (Conners, Erhardt, Epstein,
Parker, & Sitarenios, 2006; Span, Earleywine, & Strybel, 2002). We also found a
similar factor structure when we analyzed the results of a general population survey of these symptoms in adults, although the results of that factor analysis were
not published in that paper (Murphy & Barkley, 1996b). The factors found across
all studies show the same factor of inattention symptoms as presented in DSM-
IV. But instead of the hyperactive and impulsive symptoms forming a single
dimension, as presented in DSM-IV, three items largely assessing verbal impulsiveness form their own separate factor from the remaining symptoms of hyperactivity and the one symptom of behavioral impulsiveness—difficulty waiting
one's turn. Volk, Henderson, Neuman, and Todd (2006) also found a talkative
impulsive cluster in their cluster analysis of ADHD symptoms from the Child
Behavior Checklist. Use of latent class analysis with a large sample of twins identified nearly 7% as falling into a cluster best identified as being talkative–
impulsive. Although not based on factor analysis, like the other studies above,
this study also implies that this pattern of behavior may represent a semi-

independent dimension of ADHD symptoms in children provided that large enough samples are evaluated.

All of these prior studies were based on rating scales of ADHD symptoms, which provide a range of responses to each symptom, typically 0 to 3 ("not at all" to "very often"). Such scaling can lead to somewhat different factors being derived than if interview results are used, in which items are coded dichotomously (yes or no) as being present or not to a degree that is at least often or more in frequency. It will be the results of interviews using dichotomous scaling that can best inform the construction of DSM-V, given that the symptoms presented in the DSM are considered to be binary in nature (present or absent) and are not presented to patients as a rating scale with four or more possible responses to each symptom. We factor-analyzed the self-reports of our entire samples for both studies (separately) using the results from the clinical interview.

The UMASS Study Results

We found a three-factor solution, as presented in Table 5.7, identical to that found in the three prior studies noted above, which used rating scales to assess these symptoms. The three factors were inattention, hyperactivity, and impulsivity representing 29%, 16%, and 13% of the variance, respectively. This suggests that the dimensions representing adult self-reports of ADHD symptoms are not quite the same as those seen in children, in which the two-factor structure presented in DSM-IV is frequently found (DuPaul et al., 1998; Lahey et al., 1994). Also noteworthy in Table 5.7 is that the item reflecting "difficulty awaiting one's turn" loads as much on the hyperactivity dimension as on the impulsivity dimension, suggesting that it does not exclusively reflect difficulties with poor impulse control. Interestingly, excessive talking, which DSM-IV implies represents hyperactivity more than impulsivity, loads as much or more on the latter factor (impulsivity) than on the former, again suggesting a more complex symptom than DSM-IV reflects. And all three items loading on the impulsivity factor found here could be construed to represent verbal impulsiveness (talks excessively, blurts out answers, interrupts others). This could suggest that verbal impulsiveness is a separate and more distinct problem for adults than it is for children with ADHD. It may also arise from a steeper or more rapid developmental decline in symptoms of motor activity relative to those of impulsive (largely verbal) behavior.

The Milwaukee Study Results

For the sake of completeness here, we present the same factor analysis of the Milwaukee sample, collapsing all participant groups together as was done above. Yet we continue to believe that, in terms of informing the development of diagnostic criteria for adults with ADHD, the UMASS Study may have greater relevance, as it is based on clinic-referred adults for whom any DSM would be intended for use. The results for the factor analysis of the Milwaukee samples are shown in Table 5.8. The findings essentially replicated the three-factor structure found in the UMASS Study. An inattention factor accounted for 29% of the variance, while the hyperactive factor explained 9% and the impulsive factor (largely verbal) accounted for 7%. The only difference was that a small fourth factor, barely reaching an Eigenvalue of 1.00 (1.065), emerged that was based on a single symptom: Often has difficulty engaging in leisure activities or doing fun things quietly. It explained 6% of the variance. "Avoids sustained mental effort" also had a moderate loading on this last factor, besides loading on the inattention one to a somewhat greater degree. Underlying both may be the fact that "doing things quietly" may also require sustained mental effort, such as reading for pleasure. Nevertheless, this fourth factor is not likely a reliable one, given that it comprises largely a single symptom and was not replicated in the

TABLE 5.8. Factor Structure and Item Loading of the DSM-IV-TR ADHD Symptom List for Adult Self-Reports (Interview Results) in the Milwaukee Study

Item	Factor			
	I. Inattention	II. Hyperactivity	III. Impulsivity	IV. Noisy
Inattention symptoms				
Is inattentive to details	**.746**	.066	−.142	.101
Can't sustain attention	**.608**	.203	.074	.295
Fails to listen	**.501**	.286	.291	−.028
Fails to follow instructions	**.625**	.141	.023	−.051
Has difficulty organizing tasks	**.645**	−.017	.130	−.010
Avoids sustained mental effort	**.440**	.182	.093	.396
Loses necessary things	**.489**	.128	.233	.282
Is easily distracted	**.536**	.297	.418	.029
Is forgetful in daily activities	**.552**	.086	.353	.021
Hyperactivity symptoms				
Fidgets or squirms	.251	**.494**	.379	−.274
Leaves seat	.277	**.697**	−.224	.025
Feels restless	.252	**.548**	.414	.139
Can't do leisure things quietly	.038	.028	.029	**.857**
Has to be "on the go"	−.064	**.649**	.170	.025
Has difficulty awaiting turn	.171	**.588**	.268	.273
Impulsive symptoms				
Blurts out answers	.098	.116	**.694**	.287
Talks excessively	.048	.079	**.726**	−.124
Interrupts others	.219	.329	**.432**	.274

Statistical analysis: Factor analysis using Varimax rotation. Loadings in **bold** represent the highest loading of the item.

UMASS Study results. The remaining three-factor structure seems to be far more reliable.

These findings support the point made earlier, in Chapter 3, that the DSM-IV may not accurately weight or balance the concepts thought to be involved in ADHD as fairly or accurately as it should. Problems with inhibition or impulsiveness are thought to represent a core feature, if not *the* core feature, of this disorder. Yet they are represented in just three of the 18 symptoms, and these are principally problems with verbal impulsiveness. It is quite likely that had more symptoms of behavioral inhibition problems (makes decisions impulsively, is impatient or has difficulty waiting for things, acts without considering the consequences, cannot delay gratification, etc.) been represented in the DSM, this third factor may well have emerged in the studies of children and might well have been a stronger factor (accounting for more variance) than was found in these studies of adults with ADHD. As we noted earlier, the next DSM needs to do a better job of representing the constructs of the disorder in a more balanced fashion, and particularly this core one of poor inhibition.

Screening Adults for ADHD with a DSM-IV Based Scale

As noted above, the results derived from interviews will not necessarily be the same as those derived from rating scales when one examines the best symptoms for identifying adults who may have ADHD. Adults in the present studies completed a rating scale of their DSM-IV symptoms, both for current functioning and for recall of childhood behavior (see sidebar in Chapter 4). We first analyzed these ratings from the UMASS Study to see which symptoms best discriminated the ADHD group from the Community control group. Our results appear in Table 5.9 and, not unexpectedly, are somewhat different from those identified above for the dichotomous interview format using these same symptoms.

Considering just the inattention symptom list, we found the following four symptoms to provide the best discrimination between these two groups, having 97% overall accuracy at doing so (95% for Community control and 98% for ADHD cases):

- Fails to give close attention to details.
- Has difficulty organizing tasks.
- Loses things necessary for tasks.
- Is easily distracted.

Notice that, once again, the symptom of being easily distracted has considerable predictive power among the inattention symptoms and has the highest odds ratio

TABLE 5.9. ADHD Rating Scale Items That Best Discriminate ADHD from Community Control Group (Both Current and Childhood Self-Ratings)

Symptom	Beta	SE	Wald	p	Odds ratio	95% CI
Inattention symptoms (current)						
Fails to give close attention to details	1.31	.69	3.61	.057	3.72	0.96–14.41
Has difficulty organizing tasks	1.92	.55	12.21	< .001	6.81	2.32–19.98
Loses things necessary for tasks	1.40	.64	4.78	.029	4.05	1.15–14.18
Is easily distracted	2.53	.63	16.24	< .001	12.56	3.67–42.98
Hyperactivity–impulsivity symptoms (current)						
Feels restless	1.46	.33	19.90	< .001	4.33	2.27–8.23
Has difficulty engaging in leisure quietly	1.17	.40	8.52	.004	3.23	1.47–7.11
Talks excessively	.75	.33	5.21	.022	2.13	1.11–4.07
Has difficulty awaiting turn	1.58	.39	16.65	< .001	4.83	2.27–10.30
All current symptoms analyzed together						
Fails to give close attention to details	1.51	.74	4.19	.041	4.54	1.07–19.30
Has difficulty organizing tasks	1.69	.57	8.70	.003	5.41	1.76–16.62
Loses things necessary for tasks	1.47	.65	5.16	.023	4.36	1.22–15.54
Is easily distracted	2.58	.65	15.66	< .001	13.22	3.68–47.46
All childhood symptoms together						
Has difficulty organizing tasks	2.07	.63	10.74	.001	7.83	2.29–26.81
Loses things necessary for tasks	1.77	.54	10.86	.001	5.85	2.05–16.74
Is easily distracted	1.87	.41	19.85	< .001	6.46	2.84–14.68

Note. SE = standard error for beta; odds ratio = Exp(B); 95% CI = 95% confidence interval for the odds ratio. *Statistical analysis:* Logistic regression using forward conditional entry method.

of identifying ADHD from Community control cases, as it did when presented in the interview. By itself, this symptom accurately classified 93% of cases overall (96% of Community control and 90% of ADHD cases). As is discussed in a later chapter, these four items likely reflect more than just problems with inattention but seem more indicative of executive deficits, especially in working memory and its protective function from distractibility, known as interference control (Barkley, 1997).

For the hyperactive symptom list, the best rating scale items for discriminating the ADHD from the Community control group, doing so with 90% accuracy (89% for Community and 91% for ADHD cases), were:

- Feels restless.
- Has difficulty engaging in leisure quietly.
- Talks excessively.
- Has difficulty awaiting turn.

Such items are indicative not just of hyperactivity but also of behavioral inhibition (impulse control) and possibly the larger domain of metacognitive functioning of self-monitoring (Knouse et al., 2005).

But if all 18 DSM-IV symptoms are evaluated together for their discriminative ability, then just the four symptoms of inattention noted above appear to be all that are necessary for usefully separating the ADHD from Community control adults, again with 97% accuracy overall (95% for Community control and 98% for ADHD cases). And once more, the single item of being easily distractible accounts for a sizable proportion of this accuracy.

Noteworthy here is that these are not entirely the same symptoms that proved useful in this regard from the interview format presented earlier. There, a single symptom sufficed to separate these two groups with surprisingly high accuracy, and that, as already noted was the symptom of being easily distractible. Using ratings, however, results in several other items adding significantly (though not impressively) to the ability to differentiate ADHD from Community control adults. This should serve as a note of caution to both clinicians and investigators who would extrapolate from studies of the predictive power of ADHD symptoms based on one format (interviews with dichotomous answers) to the other (rating scales dimensional scaling, typically a 4-point Likert scale). In sum, if a screening scale were to be developed for adult self-ratings to assist in identifying adults who may likely have ADHD, then the above four items should be used to do so. If one felt it was important to present both inattention and hyperactive–impulsive items on such a scale, then the earlier item sets above, containing four symptoms from each list, would serve this purpose—keeping in mind, of course, that there is some redundancy of predictive power across those eight items, and those assessing hyperactivity are not necessary to achieve the best group discrimination.

Just as important to evaluate is the extent to which the DSM items presented in a rating-scale format can accurately distinguish between those with ADHD and the Clinical control group in the UMASS Study. Again, this is the issue of differential diagnosis. We conducted the same three analyses of the 18 current symptoms as above, using these two groups and logistic regression. Our results found that no symptoms of hyperactive–impulsive behavior contributed significantly to this discrimination. Just one item of inattention was significant in separating these two groups, that being "Avoids sustained mental effort," but it was rather mediocre at doing so. While it identified 89% of those with ADHD correctly, it did so for just 12% of the Clinical controls, thereby yielding an overall classification accuracy of just 58%, or little better than tossing a coin. And when all 18 symptoms were considered together, again just this single inattention symptom proved significant, yielding essentially the same rather poor classification accuracy. This indicates that while most ADHD patients rate themselves as having this type of attention problem, so do many of those in the clinical group who do not receive a diagnosis of ADHD.

In examining the self-ratings of childhood symptoms for discriminating the ADHD from the Community control group, we considered them all together in doing so, rather than analyzing the inattention and hyperactive–impulsive items separately. The results are also shown in Table 5.9. Three symptoms appeared to be useful in doing so, all of which were from the inattention list: Has difficulty organizing tasks, Loses things necessary for tasks, and Is easily distracted. Once again, they did so with good overall accuracy of 94% (97% for Community controls and 91% for the ADHD group). And once again, the single item of being easily distracted accounted for much of this accuracy (92% overall; 95% Community controls and 90% ADHD group). Just as with the current ratings of symptoms and much less with the interview format of presenting symptoms, this single symptom possesses surprisingly good power for accurately distinguishing those with ADHD from Community controls (or, more accurately, for ruling out the latter). In comparing the ADHD and Clinical control groups, we found just two inattention symptoms that significantly contributed to classifying these groups. They did so with a somewhat better overall accuracy of 78% (56% of Clinical controls and 82% of the ADHD group) than did the current ratings. These symptoms were those of (1) not following through on instructions or failing to finish work (odds ratio = 1.93) and (2) being easily distracted (odds ratio = 1.64).

All of these results serve to show that while a screening scale using DSM-IV symptoms (either current or recalled from childhood) could be used effectively to rule out those who may be normal (Community controls here) from those having a clinical disorder, such screening scales would not be of as much help in differential diagnosis, where the clinical interview using the DSM symptoms may be of somewhat greater help. Even then, as noted above, the added advantage of the interview comes not just from a more careful review of dichotomously classified symptoms and more careful probing for examples but also its coverage of additional issues of diagnostic importance, the age of onset of symptoms, the nature of the impairments they produce, and especially the ruling out of other clinical disorders that seem to better account for the patient's complaints.

We chose not to analyze the results of the Milwaukee Study for this purpose, given our belief that the UMASS Study has a greater bearing on developing diagnostic criteria and screening scales for identifying clinic-referred adults who may have ADHD. Our belief is further buttressed by the fact that we required those adults to meet full DSM-IV criteria as adults, whereas in the Milwaukee study we did not do so, employing instead a more developmentally referenced definition of disorder at adult outcome.

The Issue of Age of Onset

The DSM-IV requires that symptoms producing impairment must have developed before 7 years of age. As noted in Chapter 2, this is not based on any scientific research and is in conflict with the findings from the DSM field trial (Applegate et al., 1997) that found this criterion to reduce the reliability of diagnosis between clinician judges and to miss as many as 35% of otherwise legitimate patients with ADHD, particularly those having the inattentive type. It also poses considerable problems for diagnosing adults due to this very early and narrow window of recall of childhood, which is likely to have limited reliability or validity (Barkley & Biederman, 1997). It moreover asserts that ADHD has a clear demarcation in nature for its onset, contrary to nearly all other diagnoses listed in the DSM. For these reasons, we sought to evaluate the legitimacy of this criterion in these two large studies. As noted in earlier chapters, we allowed adults in the UMASS Study to be clinically diagnosed with ADHD for group assignment purposes regardless of their age of onset as long as it was before adulthood (age 21). This would permit us to evaluate the actual utility of imposing this age of onset on our ADHD sample.

The Validity (Utility) of the DSM-IV Onset by Age 7 Years in the UMASS Study

In Table 5.10 are shown the ages of onset of initial ADHD symptoms for the two clinical groups from the UMASS Study (ADHD patients and Clinical controls).

TABLE 5.10. Age of Onset (Years) of ADHD Symptoms and Impairments from Interview for ADHD and Clinical Control Groups for the UMASS Study

Measure	ADHD			Clinical			F	p
	Mean	SD	N	Mean	SD	N		
Global onset[A]	7.3	3.5	146	12.1	8.3	96	32.6	< .001
School impairment	8.2	3.3	143	12.3	7.8	89	27.5	< .001
Social impairment[A]	10.3	6.5	117	12.6	7.5	52	2.4	NS
Home impairment[A,GxS]	9.4	6.3	131	16.0	11.6	69	20.2	< .001
Community impairment[A]	13.2	8.2	65	14.7	6.8	31	0.5	NS
Occupational impairment[A,S]	19.1	6.6	129	22.1	7.7	65	1.7	NS
Dating or marriage impairment[A]	20.1	7.3	118	23.8	8.5	70	3.0	NS

Note. SD = standard deviation; *F* = *F*-test results of the analysis of variance (or covariance); *p* = probability value for the *F*-test; NS = not significant, [S] = significant main effect for sex (see text for details); [GxS] = significant group × sex interaction (see text for details); [A] = age used as a covariate in this analysis.

Statistical analysis: Groups were initially compared using two-way (group × sex) analysis of variance (or covariance as necessary).

This information was not obtained on the Community control group as we did not expect them to have many symptoms or to lead to any impairment in most cases, and this proved to be the case. As this table shows, despite relaxing the DSM-IV age-of-onset criterion generously to age 21 from age 7, the mean age of onset of symptoms was 7 years of age for the ADHD group but a considerably later onset of 12 years for the non-ADHD Clinical control group. The distributions for the age of onset for these groups are shown in Figures 5.5 (ADHD group) and 5.6 (Clinical control group). The distribution for the ADHD group is largely unimodal, with its peak centered around 7 years of age, though a smaller peak may be evident in the early adolescent years. The distribution for the Clinical control group is bimodal, with an initial narrow peak at 4 to 8 years of age and a second broader peak spanning 12 to 16 years of age. Such a multimodal distribution would be expected, given the mixture of various disorders that comprise this clinical control group, where each of these disorders may be associated with somewhat different mean ages of onset. The later average age of onset for this group (12–13 years) is consistent, however, with findings that mood disorders such as anxiety and depression, which generally characterize this clinical

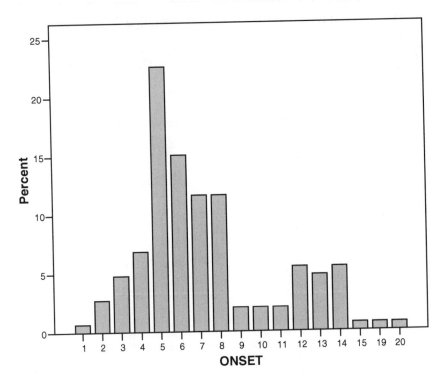

FIGURE 5.5. Distribution for age of onset for the ADHD group in the UMASS Study.

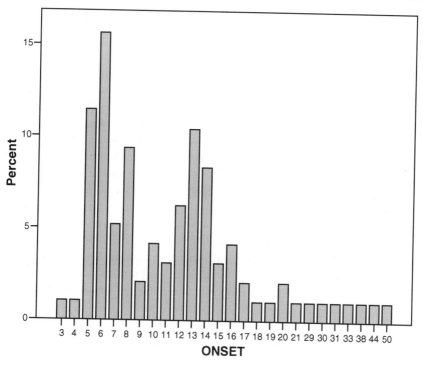

FIGURE 5.6. Age-of-onset distribution for the Clinical control group in the UMASS Study.

control group, often have their onset in the late-childhood to early-adolescent years. In contrast, ADHD in our adults had a mean onset, as shown above, of 7 years in adults, and has been found in studies to be 3 to 5 years in clinic-referred children with the combined type and somewhat later in those with the inattentive type (Applegate et al., 1997; Biederman & Barkley, 1997).

We compared males and females in the ADHD group on DSM-recommended onset before (6 or less) or after 7 years (7 or more). We found that 47% of males and 64% of females had onset before age 7 ($\chi^2 = 3.42$, $p = .064$)—a sex difference that was marginally significant. For the clinical controls, it was 24% males and 36% females (NS). Overall, 53% of the ADHD group and just 29% of clinical controls had an onset before age 7 years ($\chi^2 = 12.90$, $p < .001$). While this is noteworthy in demonstrating once again that many individuals with ADHD have an onset to their disorder below the threshold recommended by DSM-IV, nearly half of the clinic referred adults who otherwise meet criteria for the diagnosis do not. If clinicians were to impose the age-of-onset criterion religiously, nearly half of this sample would not have received a diagnosis of ADHD, although they meet all other criteria, underscoring a serious problem with this particular DSM criterion. A similar finding also emerged from the recent study of prevalence of adult ADHD by Kessler and colleagues (Kessler et al., 2005), who found that only 10% of ADHD adults self-reported an onset by age 6, while 99% had an onset by age 16 years. Again, this general population study supports our contention that many adults who otherwise meet criteria for ADHD would not be granted the diagnosis if the age-of-onset criterion were scrupulously applied. It is likely that the reason more of our cases had an earlier onset than in the study of Kessler et al. is that our study focuses on clinic-referred adults who likely have more severe disorder, whereas Kessler et al. studied a general population sampling. This implies that clinic-referred adults are somewhat more likely to have an earlier onset of their disorder than do those who are not clinic-referred.

If the DSM age-of-onset threshold were raised to 14 years, as recommended previously by Barkley and Biederman (1997), 98% of the ADHD group would have met this revised threshold (just 2% did not) compared to 78% of Clinical controls ($N = 21$) ($\chi^2 = 25.47$, $p < .001$). There was no significant sex difference within either group in the percent meeting this revised criterion. For the ADHD group, it was 99% of males and 96% of females (NS). For Clinical controls, it was 76% versus 81% (NS). These data support the recommendation by Barkley and Biederman (1997) that raising the threshold for age of onset would aid greatly in capturing those adults who otherwise meet all other DSM criteria except this one and who should receive a clinical diagnosis of ADHD.

There is another way of making the case that the age of onset of 7 years has no merit in the diagnosis of ADHD and should be jettisoned in DSM-V. The specification of so precise an age of onset implies that there ought to be either large quantitative differences or even qualitative ones between those having an onset at age 6 or below compared to those with an onset at 7 or above in various measures of symptoms severity, comorbidity, and impairments in major life activities, not to mention etiologies. We examined this issue by taking our UMASS ADHD group and subdividing it using this age of onset (6 and younger vs. 7 and older). We then compared these two groups on important measures of symptom severity, comorbidity, and impairment in the various major life activities reported later in this book. When we compared these groups on severity of ADHD symptoms from the interview, both currently and in childhood, we found that the early-onset group had an average of one more ADHD symptom currently (13 vs. 11.8) and an average of two more in childhood (mean = 13.8 vs. 11.8) than did the later-onset group. The groups did not differ in the number of domains in which they reported being impaired in the interview. They also did not differ in the proportion reporting impairment in any single domain among the six covered in the interview. They also did not differ in age, education, Hollingshead occupational index, intelligence estimate, or any of the achievement tests discussed in later chapters. And they did not differ in any scales of psychological adjustment from the Symptom Checklist 90—Revised, in the proportion having any of the other clinical diagnoses in the Structured Clinical Interview for DSM Disorders (SCID), or in the proportion having clinical risks (or concerns) on any scale assessing health and lifestyle on the Skinner Lifestyle Assessment (all described in later chapters). In sum, apart from having slightly more symptoms of ADHD, the early-onset group had no positive predictive value and was not different in any other important respects from the late-onset group of ADHD participants in this study. The same was found by Faraone et al. (2006).

The Validity of the DSM Age of Onset in the Milwaukee Study

Another way of examining this issue of the validity or utility of the age of onset by 7 years is to evaluate just how well adults can recall the onset of their symptoms. The Milwaukee study data can speak directly to this issue because all children with ADHD (hyperactivity) in that study had to have an onset of their symptoms by age 6 by parent report in order to enter the study. The participants ranged in age from 3 to 12 with the average being 7 years, which was not significantly different across our groups. The average age of onset in this study as reported by parents at study entry for all hyperactive children was 3 to 4 years. At the teen follow-up 8 to 10 years later, parents were asked again about the age of onset of their children's ADHD symptoms as part of the diagnostic criteria for DSM-III-R used at that follow-up. The average age was 3.8 years, being almost identical to that actually reported at study entry.

Now let us examine the age of onset reported by the children themselves when they were age 27, the current follow-up, and then by the parents' own recall at this follow-up. Like the adults in the UMASS Study, these young adults in the hyperactive group reported an average onset of their symptoms at 8.0 years of age (SD = 4.7), this being 7.1 for the H+ADHD group and 8.8 years of age (SD = 5.5) for the H–ADHD group (difference not significant, F = 3.73). The distribution of the ages of onset they reported is shown in Figure 5.7 and is very similar to that reported by the UMASS ADHD adult group (Figure 5.5). Note that both ADHD groups in these two studies report a typical peak onset at 5 to 6 years of age and that the average age of 7 for the hyperactive cases classified as currently having ADHD at follow-up is nearly identical to that of the adults with ADHD in the UMASS Study. Seventeen members of the hyperactive group (most in the H–ADHD group) did not provide an age of onset, believing that they did not have significant symptoms and so had no onset to recall. We found that 90% of the hyperactive group who reported an onset had an onset of symptoms by age 14, while just 52% had an onset by age 6 (before 7) as required by DSM criteria. As in the UMASS Study, we found that 96% of those who currently had ADHD claimed to have had an onset by age 14. Only 55% of those

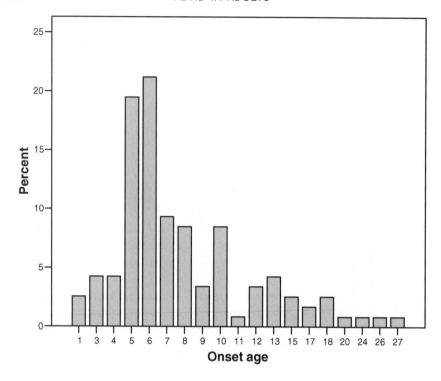

FIGURE 5.7. Distribution of age of onset of ADHD symptoms as retrospectively recalled by participants in the interview for all hyperactive participants who reported having significant ADHD symptoms at age-27 follow-up in the Milwaukee Study (percent of group at each age, $N = 118$).

with current ADHD had an onset by age 6 (before age 7), virtually matching the 52% for the clinic-referred adults in the UMASS Study.

The point here is this: Children with ADHD who were documented as having an onset of disorder by 6 years of age in childhood (mean onset of 3.8 years) recalled that onset as being, on average, approximately 4 years later than reported by their parents. Nearly half reported it as being after the age of 7 years, as required by the DSM-IV, even though ADHD was clearly there before then.

We had collected information about the ADHD symptoms of participants from others who knew them well at this age-27 follow-up. We asked them at what age those symptoms developed. For present purposes, we examined only the reports provided by parents and only for the hyperactive group ($N = 49$). The distribution of responses is shown in Figure 5.8. The average age of onset was 7.8 ($SD = 8.3$), with a range of 8 to 28 years of age. Remember, all of these parents reported an onset of ADHD before 6 years in these participants. Like the participants themselves, the parents are now off by an average of 4 years from the

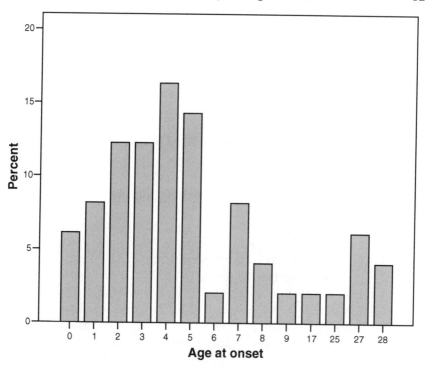

FIGURE 5.8. Distribution of age of onset of ADHD symptoms as retrospectively recalled by parents of the hyperactive participants at age-27 follow-up in the Milwaukee Study (percent of group at each age, *N* = 49). All parents had reported in childhood at study entry that their children had developed symptoms by 6 years of age.

mean age of onset they actually reported for these participants at childhood study entry. Forty-six percent of the parents reported an onset of 7 years of age or later. In summary, even the recall of parents about what they told us when the participants were children is biased toward a later age of onset than was actually the case. The findings above for self-report and parent report of symptom onset should give considerable pause to anyone wishing to retain this age-of-onset criterion in future DSMs as if it could be ascertained with any degree of validity in adult self-reports of childhood behavior.

We also compared those in the hyperactive group who reported an age of onset before 7 years to those reporting after 7 years, as we had done above for the UMASS Study. After all the issue here, using the DSM criteria, is technically not when their disorder started in some objective sense but their recall of when their disorder started. We compared them on severity of ADHD symptoms currently and in childhood both self- and other-reported, number of current impairments both self- and other-reported, number of childhood impairments self- and other-reported, and severity of ODD and CD self- and other-reported. The groups did not differ on any of these important parameters of the disorder, indicating that they have essentially the same disorder. This replicates what was found in the UMASS Study above.

All of the foregoing evidence leads us to conclude that:

The age of onset before 7 recommended in the DSM-IV therefore has no clinical or scientific value in the diagnosis of ADHD in adults. It is unreliable and substantially inaccurate when applied to adult recall of actual childhood behavior. It identifies no important qualitative or quantitative distinctions within the group otherwise having the disorder. It therefore should either be abandoned entirely in DSM-V or raised to encompass all of childhood and adolescence (14–16 years of age) if keeping the concept of childhood onset of ADHD remains important to defining this disorder.

More than 25 years ago, the first author argued for the imposition of an age of onset by 6 years of age for research criteria for studying hyperactivity/ADHD in children (Barkley, 1982). That recommendation, however, was largely intended for studies of children, to ensure an early onset to what was then considered a developmental disorder arising in early childhood and to permit replication of research methods across laboratories. The latter was important to consider at the time, given that just four of 210 studies of hyperactive children reviewed at that time had required any sort of age of onset to the disorder. That situation could easily lead to failures to replicate findings across labs. This recommendation was not intended to be applied to adults with ADHD, a group not considered to exist 25 years ago. It is obvious now that this recommendation for so early an age of onset, well intentioned as it was at the time, is without merit and especially when applied to the diagnosis of ADHD in adults. There are no data of which we are aware that would support its retention in DSM-V for ADHD in adults as well as for children. And as we show here, there is much evidence against it.

The Age of Onset of Impairment in Specific Major Life Activities

We asked participants in both studies about their recollection of the onset of specific domains of impairment in major life activities stemming from their ADHD symptoms.

The UMASS Study Results

Table 5.10 shows the self-reported ages of onset for experiencing impairment in six domains of major life activities discussed in the clinical interview with the ADHD and Clinical Control adults in this study. The ADHD group had a significantly earlier average age of onset of their impairment in both the home and school settings than did those in the Clinical control group, differing by at least 4 years from each other, on average. The age of onset of impairment in the other domains of social, community, occupation, dating, or marriage did not differ between the groups. We did find a significant interaction of group × sex on two of these specific domains of impairment, those being home and occupational impairment. Further analysis revealed that men and women in the ADHD group did not differ in their onset of impairment in home functioning, nor did men and women in the Clinical control group differ from each other. The significant effect is due to the fact that men in the ADHD group have an earlier onset of impairment in home functioning than do men in the Clinical control group. The same pattern of results was evident for the onset of occupational impairment.

The Milwaukee Study Results

Table 5.11 reports the same information for the two hyperactive groups in the Milwaukee Study. They did not differ in their onset of impairment in any specific domains. Thus growing up as hyperactive/ADHD is associated with the onsets of these various impairments regardless of current ADHD status in adulthood.

Also apparent in both of these tables is that as those with ADHD matured and entered into domains of major life activity outside of home, they experienced impairment in those newly available major life activities. Viewed another way, with advancing age, the number of domains available to the individual in

TABLE 5.11. Age of Onset (Years) of ADHD Symptoms and Impairments from Interview for Hyperactives Currently Having ADHD Compared to Hyperactives Not Currently Having ADHD in the Milwaukee Study

Measure	H+ADHD			H−ADHD			F	p
	Mean	SD	N	Mean	SD	N		
Global onset	7.1	3.5	54	8.8	5.5	64	3.73	NS
School impairment	8.1	3.4	51	8.4	3.6	56	0.21	NS
Home impairment	8.1	5.0	44	7.8	3.9	38	0.14	NS
Community impairment	9.1	2.6	22	9.1	3.2	11	0.01	NS
Occupational impairment	17.3	2.8	36	17.2	3.5	17	0.02	NS
Dating or marriage impairment	18.2	4.1	38	18.0	4.9	9	0.01	NS

Note. SD = standard deviation; F = F-test results of the analysis of variance (or covariance); p = probability value for the F-test; NS = not significant; H+ADHD = hyperactive group that currently has a diagnosis of ADHD at follow-up; H−ADHD = hyperactive group that does not have a diagnosis of ADHD at follow-up.

Statistical analysis: Groups were compared using one-way (groups) analysis of variance.

which they can be impaired increases. As it does so, the opportunity for the individual with ADHD to now experience such impairment in those domains increases as well, creating a virtual layering effect of these impaired domains with development, one atop another and each atop those that came beforehand.

This, too, poses problems for the DSM-IV–recommended onset of age 7. It shows that the onset of symptoms producing impairment is largely determined by the specific domains of major life activity previously available to the individual to be impaired. It will all depend on which of these more specific domains the clinician may choose to focus in the clinical evaluation of the age of onset to be reported. All impairment does not have the same age of onset.

Conclusions and Clinical Implications

This chapter evaluated the DSM-IV-TR symptoms of ADHD in detail for their prevalence among ADHD, Clinical control, and Community control adults in the UMASS Study and their utility for discriminating among these groups. It also conducted similar analyses of these same symptoms as they exist in children with ADHD as adults. The issue of symptom specificity for the DSM symptom list for ADHD in adults is exceptionally important in view of the fact that the symptom list was developed specifically on and for children (4–16 years of age, specifically). In the absence of data concerning their prevalence and especially their ability to differentiate those with ADHD from normal adults or from persons with other clinical disorders, the increasing clinical use of this set of symptoms to identify adults with ADHD is open to considerable challenge.

✓ Our UMASS Study results demonstrated that adults with ADHD display most of the DSM-IV symptoms to a degree that is significantly greater than do either the Clinical or Community control groups. Indeed, these individual symptoms are rather uncommon among the Community control adults. Similar findings were evident in the Milwaukee study of ADHD children grown up. While these results are not surprising given the use of the DSM-IV criteria to create our groups, the low rate of symptoms in the Community groups certainly suggests that the concern among the general public that such symptoms are commonplace in normal individuals and may lead to misdiagnosis or overdiagnosis of ADHD in the normal population is unwarranted.

✓ When we evaluated the number of symptoms from each of the DSM lists that might best serve to accurately identify the ADHD from the Community control group in the UMASS Study, we found that just four symptoms on either list would effectively rule out 100% of the normal or Community control adults and would capture 100% of the ADHD group. If DSM-V is to retain these same 18 items for the diagnosis of ADHD, then our results indicate that a threshold of four symptoms for either list (or seven overall) works well at identifying ADHD adults from normal or Community control adults. This is the case for both current symptoms and for recall of childhood symptoms using a clinical interview.

✓ This same set of thresholds is not as useful, however, at distinguishing ADHD from other clinical disorders that may present to a clinic for adult ADHD. As the UMASS Study found, those disorders may also be associated with elevated levels of inattentive or hyperactive–impulsive symptoms, albeit to a lesser degree. In such instances, differential diagnosis (knowledge of what constitutes other disorders) will be required to further differentiate the legitimate cases of ADHD from those cases best conceptualized as due to another mental disorder.

✓ We also found satisfactory agreement between the symptom ratings of adults in the UMASS Study in comparison to others who knew them well (all *r*s .70–.80), both for current symptoms of ADHD and for their recall of childhood symptoms. This agreement was much lower for those who had grown up with ADHD and were 21 years of age at the time of the Milwaukee Study ($r = .21$). But it nearly doubled by age 27 ($r = .43$), though still falling well below that seen in clinic-referred adults with the disorder. Nevertheless, the combined results of these studies suggest that agreement between self-reported information and that given by others about ADHD may increase with age and be of acceptable levels especially by the early 30s. Such information should not be trusted as reliable (agreeing with others), however, in those with ADHD in their teens and early 20s.

✓ The adults with ADHD in both studies received significantly higher ratings of ADHD symptoms from significant others than did adults in the other two groups. Such findings corroborate the group selection procedures employed (Chapter 4) with these groups in showing that adults who self-identify as having high levels of ADHD symptoms are likely to be so described by others who know them well.

✓ We also found that the participants in the UMASS Study tended to report more symptoms in themselves than were reported by others about them. Clinicians can therefore place reasonable confidence in the severity of symptoms reported by adults, yet they should still seek to corroborate the severity of those reports through others who know the patients well. Understand, however, that in dealing with clinic-referred adults, such reports of others may prove to be somewhat lower than the severity reported by the adult patient.

✓ This chapter also presented considerable information showing that a list of 18 symptoms is not required to accurately identify adults with ADHD from either Community or Clinical control adults. In fact, just one symptom in the UMASS Study ruled out the normal adult sample with over 97% accuracy, and that is the item of "often being easily distracted by extraneous stimuli." If, therefore, determining whether someone is normal (nondisordered) or not is the issue, this single item works very well at doing so.

✓ We also found that a small set of three attention items and three hyperactive–impulsive items best distinguished the ADHD from the Clinical control group, though not with the same degree of accuracy as was shown in the ADHD versus Community control comparisons in the UMASS Study. Still we found that a set of six rather than 18 items (three from each list) was sufficient for classification purposes, with the remaining items adding nothing further to the accuracy of this process. Having four of these "best" six items appeared to be a reasonable threshold as one of the diagnostic criteria for screening for ADHD in adults.

✓ The two-factor (dimensional) structure of symptoms represented in DSM-IV and based on children does not accurately represent the factor structure of these same symptoms in adults. There, a three-factor solution emerges, representing inattention, hyperactivity, and impulsiveness (especially verbal). This factor structure was also found in the Milwaukee Study and agrees with the results of three other studies of adults. This separation of impulsivity from hyperactivity in adults compared to children suggests that it is becoming a relatively distinct domain of symptomatic behavior apart from excessive motor activity. This could be due to the relatively more rapid developmental decline in symptoms of hyperactivity than those of inattention and impulsivity, or possibly to the fact that impulsiveness (mostly verbal in the DSM items) causes greater problems in adults than in children.

✓ We also examined the important issue of whether the DSM-IV requirement of an age of onset of symptoms producing impairment by age 7 years is valid or useful in diagnosing ADHD in adults. We found that the ADHD group in the UMASS Study had an earlier age of onset (7 years) of symptoms than did the Clinical control group (12 years) by an average of nearly 5 years, in keeping with the view that ADHD is a disorder of largely childhood onset. Yet the results of various analyses using both studies showed that this diagnostic criterion of age 7 years has no scientific or clinical merit and misses nearly half of all adults who otherwise meet all other DSM criteria for this clinical diagnosis. The Milwaukee Study, in fact, showed that a sample of children documented in childhood to have an onset of symptoms before age 6 (mean age 3.8 years) and followed to age 27 years could not accurately recall the age of onset of their disorder. Their recall demonstrated at least a 4-year disparity (on average) from that documented in childhood, recalling a later onset than was actually the case. Their recollected onset, in fact, resembled that of the ADHD adults in the UMASS Study. Our results support the earlier recommendation of Barkley and Biederman (1997) that either the age-of-onset criterion be abandoned in DSM-V for adults or be raised to at least 14 to 16 years of age, in which case it will capture 98% of adults meeting the other clinical criteria for this diagnosis.

✓ This chapter provides substantial evidence that the construction of the next version of DSM criteria for ADHD in adults must establish separate criteria for them, rather than automatically assuming that criteria developed on children apply equally well to the diagnosis of adults presenting with this disorder.

✓ DSM-V can also reduce the symptom list to a more manageable number given that just one symptom was needed to determine if a patient was normal or not (often easily distracted) and a six-symptom list worked well to maximize the classification accuracy of the ADHD adults from the other groups. Clinicians should also ignore the currently recommended age of onset of before 7 years, instead requiring that symptoms have developed and produced impairment at some time in childhood or early adolescence prior to 16 years of age.

CHAPTER 6

Impairment in Major Life Activities

Anecdotal accounts of adults with ADHD have repeatedly noted their difficulties in a variety of domains of major life activities, including workplace behavior and occupational functioning, educational settings, social functioning, dating or marital relations, and behavior in community activities (Adler, 2006; Hallowell & Ratey, 1994; Wender, 1995). Clinicians, likewise, have noted these areas of impairment as well as complaints by these adults of problems in managing their money, driving, obeying laws (antisocial behavior), excessive substance use or outright dependence and abuse, child-rearing and behavior management, running a household, maintaining their health, and even sexual functioning (Goldstein & Ellison, 2002; Triolo, 1999; Weiss et al., 1999). Despite such clinical wisdom, more rigorous, quantitative, and scientific examinations of these and other domains of impairment have been few in number. Most studies focused largely on self-reports of global impairment generally or about specific domains (e.g., work) but did not seek to validate these reports against others who know the adult ADHD patients well. Nor did these studies rely on well-developed measures to assess specific domains of impairment. Past research does show that many of these domains are, indeed, self-reported as more impaired in adults with ADHD than in normal control groups (De Quiros & Kinsbourne, 2001; Murphy & Barkley, 1996; Murphy et al., 2002; Roy-Byrne et al., 1997).

One area that has received in-depth evaluation in adults with ADHD is driving, or the operation of motor vehicles. This body of research comprises a variety of measures, including self-reports, others' ratings, official archives, behind-the-wheel road tests, driving simulators, video-based testing of driving knowledge, and tests of basic cognitive abilities required for driving. The totality of findings in this area of research (see Chapter 12) has established this domain of major life activities as being often impaired by ADHD in adults (see Barkley, 2004; Barkley & Cox, 2007 for reviews). Most other domains, however, have been studied largely at the level of patient self-reports about them.

In this chapter we explore the number of different domains that are self-reported as being generally impaired by adults with ADHD in comparison to our two control groups. We examine each domain in more detail in later chapters. Comparisons to a clinical control group is crucial in order to establish what, if any, domains of impairment are relatively specific to ADHD compared to other disorders. We also obtained similar information on these general domains from others who knew the participants well—something rarely done in past research on impairment. Such reports are essential to corroborating the findings based on self-reported information. We also wished to explore the degree to which the overall relationship of ADHD severity relates to the severity of impairment in each domain and to the pervasiveness (number of domains) of impairments. Just as important, we examined each of the various symptoms of ADHD for its predictive value for each of the different domains of impairment studied here.

The DSM-IV-TR (American Psychiatric Association, 2000) makes establishing the presence of impairment in two or more domains a separate criterion for the clinical diagnosis of ADHD besides just establishing the presence of symptoms that are developmentally inappropriate and have an onset in childhood. Yet no guidance is given in the DSM-IV-TR as to how to evaluate impairment under this criterion. And only three domains are suggested for review with patients (home and school for children and occupation for adults), even though other domains of functioning are also important in adulthood, as suggested above. We therefore sought to evaluate impairment by several means, largely developing our own measures to do so (see sidebar). In the UMASS Study, we started by using interviews with participants in which we questioned them about the presence of significant impairment in six different domains (occupational, home, social, participation in community activities, education, and dating/marriage). Next, we used rating scales of both current and childhood functioning to obtain more dimensional, quantitative judgments of these six domains and up to four others thought to be important (money, driving, leisure, and daily responsibilities). We also obtained the same ratings from others who knew the participants well. Third, we collected ratings from both the participants and these other informants about childhood impairments, retrospectively recalled. The eight domains on the childhood ratings were family, social, community, school, sports, self-care, play, and chores. Fourth, we obtained employer ratings of workplace symptoms and impairment. Finally, we used a clinician rating of the extent of social, educational, and occupational functioning; the Social and Occupational Functioning Assessment Scale (SOFAS) developed by Patterson and Lee (1995). In the Milwaukee Study, we collected the same interview and rating scale infor-

Structured Clinical Interview of ADHD in Adults

As reported in prior chapters, we created a structured interview for this project in order to review the presence of DSM symptoms and symptoms of executive functioning deficits with study participants (see Chapters 3 and 4). This interview also reviewed information on each of the following major life activities as to whether or not the participants believed themselves to be impaired in them: occupation or job; life at home; social life; participation in clubs, sports, or other community organizations; educational activities; and dating or marital relationships. Participants were asked whether their symptoms had led them to be impaired in each of these major life activities. The score derived from the interview was the number of domains reported as impaired. The participants were also asked about the age of onset of impairment in each of these domains of daily life activity, as discussed in Chapter 3.

Impairment Rating Scales (Barkley & Murphy, 2006)

As noted in previous chapters, we also created rating scales of ADHD and executive functioning symptoms to be completed by the adult participants about their current functioning and again about their childhood functioning. We also obtained these scales from others who knew them well and from their employers, with the participants' permission. And we had someone who knew the participant well complete a scale concerning ADHD in school settings with regard to the childhood and adolescent years of these participants. Embedded within these symptom rating scales were questions about major life activities and whether they were impaired by the ADHD symptoms. The 10 domains of major life activities listed in the current functioning rating scale were work, social, community, education, dating/marriage, money, driving, leisure, and daily responsibilities. The eight domains on the childhood ratings were: family, social, community, school, sports, self-care, play, and chores. In the school ratings completed by others, the domains were classwork, homework, classroom behavior, on the bus, in sports, clubs, or other organizations, with classmates, at recess, at lunch, in time management. On the employer ratings, the 10 domains were relations with coworkers, relations with supervisors, relations with clients or customers, completing assigned work, educational activities, punctuality, meeting deadlines, operating equipment, operating vehicles, managing daily responsibilities. All ratings were done using a Likert scale of 0 to 3 (rare to very often impaired). This permitted us to obtain three different types of scores: A total rated impairment score reflecting a simple summation of the answers given across all items, a pervasiveness score reflecting the number of different domains rated as "often" or more impaired, and a score for each specific domain that was rated.

Social and Occupational Functioning Assessment Scale (SOFAS; Patterson & Lee, 1995)

Much like the clinician global assessment of functioning scale, the SOFAS is offered as an alternative for more specifically evaluating social, occupational, and educational functioning. Clinicians provide a rating on a scale from 1 (grossly impaired) to 100 (superior or excellent functioning) and are instructed to base this rating specifically on the individual's social, occupational, and educational functioning. Impairment must be a direct consequence of the mental and physical health problems of the individual and not due to lack of opportunity or other environmental limitations. Descriptors are provided at each 10-point marker on the scale to guide clinicians in making this rating. For instance, a score of 10 is indicated if the patient has "Persistent inability to maintain minimal personal hygiene, or unable to function without harming self or others or without considerable external support (e.g., nursing care and supervision)." In contrast, a score of 70 would be given if there is "Some difficulty in social, occupational, or school functioning but generally functioning well, has some meaningful interpersonal relations."

Adolescent Life Events Scale

For the teen follow-up in the Milwaukee Study, we created a scale of 65 items having yes/no answers that comprised potentially stressful life events. The score was the total number of stressful life events endorsed by the teen (see Barkley, Fischer, et al., 1991).

mation, but we did not collect employer ratings at this follow-up (although we had done so at age 21), nor did we collect the clinician SOFAS rating.

Before proceeding to our results for these measures, we wish to make clear the difference between symptoms and impairments. To us, *the symptoms of ADHD are the behavioral expressions associated with this disorder*—they are the actions demonstrated by those having the disorder that are believed to reflect that disorder (e.g., inattention, distractibility, impulsive responding, hyperactivity, poor executive functioning). In contrast, *impairments are the consequences that ensue for the individual as a result of these cognitive-behavioral expressions*. In short, symptoms are actions of an individual (cognition/behavior) and impairments are the consequences of those actions (outcomes or social costs). For instance, distractibility while performing school work is a symptom because it represents a behavior of the individual. Getting a low grade-point average, being retained in grade, not completing high school, getting less education more generally, and even losing friends may be consequences of such perennial distractibility in school. They represent the types of educational impairment that may ensue from that distractibility. The terms are easily confused and often are so in discussions of ADHD. Even within the symptom list in the DSM, some symptoms may overlap with impairment, such as avoiding tasks that require sustained mental effort (one symptom) could be a consequence of another (being distractible). Yet both are behavior and by the definitions offered here, both would be treated as symptoms for our purposes.

We also wish to make it clear that the term "impairment" refers to deficits that are relative to the functioning of the normal population or "average person" and not to an intrapersonal disparity. The latter is often seen in efforts to define learning disabilities as a significant discrepancy between one's intelligence or general cognitive ability and performance in a specific area of academic achievement. Some have extended this discrepancy concept to defining impairments in adults with ADHD. That is, if they are found to be functioning in any cognitive-behavioral trait significantly below their level of intelligence, they are impaired. We disagree for many reasons, not the least of which is that one's intelligence is not a guidepost or harbinger of how well one should perform in all other psychological abilities. It was originally developed as a predictor of likely academic success, not of all human endeavors. We also do not define impairment as being performance that is substandard for a local, high-functioning peer group such as other college or graduate students, professionals, etc. From our perspective, the fact that one may not do as well in an Ivy League university or a highly specialized profession does not necessarily mean one is impaired. Our definition coincides with that used in many rulings based on the Americans with Disabilities Act (Gordon & Keiser, 1998; Gordon et al., 2006) which have stipulated that impairment should be defined relative to the norm or average population and represents functioning significantly below that average.

The Extent of Impairment in Adults with ADHD

The methods we used to obtain the information on the various domains of major life activities are shown in the side bar. They are the same methods used in previous chapters to assess ADHD symptoms and those reflecting impaired executive functioning (Chapters 5 and 7). These measures also included questions concerning functioning in specific domains of major life activities, both currently and in childhood.

The UMASS Study Results

The total number of domains endorsed as impaired on the different interviews and rating scales completed by various sources are shown in Table 6.1. From the interview results, we can see that adults with ADHD reported themselves to be impaired in more domains of major life activity than either the Community or the Clinical control group. Not surprisingly, the latter group was also impaired in more domains than the Community group but not as much as were the adults with ADHD. The same pattern of results emerged on each of the various rating scales. It did so not only for self-reports but also for the reports from others, and

TABLE 6.1. Impairment Scores from Interviews and Ratings by Group for the UMASS Study

Measure	ADHD		Clinical		Community		F	p	Pairwise contrasts
	Mean	SD	Mean	SD	Mean	SD			
Current (interview)									
No. of domains impaired	4.8	1.2	3.8	1.5	0.2	0.5	543.8	< .001	1 > 2 > 3
Current (self-ratings)									
Total impairment[S]	18.7	5.8	15.8	6.0	2.0	3.7	243.8	< .001	1 > 2 > 3
No. of domains often impaired	6.5	2.6	5.2	2.6	0.2	1.1	184.2	< .001	1 > 2 > 3
Childhood (self-ratings)									
Total impairment	13.6	5.3	9.1	6.0	1.9	3.2	134.9	< .001	1 > 2 > 3
No. of domains often impaired	4.5	2.5	2.5	2.7	0.2	1.0	89.4	< .001	1 > 2 > 3
Current (other-ratings)									
Total impairment[A]	18.1	6.1	13.8	6.6	2.2	3.8	134.1	< .001	1 > 2 > 3
No. of domains often impaired[A]	6.1	2.9	4.4	2.9	0.2	1.2	90.8	< .001	1 > 2 > 3
Childhood (other-ratings)									
Total impairment[A]	11.6	6.1	6.4	6.1	1.8	2.6	45.4	< .001	1 > 2 > 3
No. of domains often impaired[A]	3.7	2.7	1.7	2.4	0.1	0.3	36.6	< .001	1 > 2 > 3
School ratings (others)									
Total impairment[A]	9.1	5.8	4.1	4.5	1.0	1.9	38.8	< .001	1 > 2 > 3
No. of domains often impaired[A]	3.3	2.7	1.4	1.8	0.1	0.4	30.6	< .001	1 > 2 > 3
Employer ratings									
Total impairment[S, GxS]	6.8	6.6	4.3	5.6	2.5	4.4	6.1	.003	1 > 3
No. of domains often impaired	0.4	1.2	0.2	0.7	0.2	0.9	101	NS	

Note. Sample sizes for self-reported interview information are ADHD = 146, Clinical control = 97, and Community control = 109. For self-rated impairment ratings, ADHD = 123, Clinical = 83, Community = 81. For self-rated childhood impairment, ADHD = 128, Clinical = 83, Community = 86. For other ratings of current impairment, ADHD = 97, Clinical = 53, Community = 64. For other ratings of childhood impairment, ADHD = 86, Clinical = 39, Community = 54. For other ratings of school impairment, ADHD = 75, Clinical = 38, and Community = 61. SD = standard deviation; F = F-test results of the analysis of variance (or covariance); p = probability value for the F-test; NS = not significant, [S] = significant main effect for sex (see text for details); [GxS] = significant group × sex interaction (see text for details); [A] = age used as a covariate in this analysis.

Statistical analysis: Groups were initially compared using two-way (group × sex) analysis of variance (or covariance as necessary). Where this analysis was significant (p < .05) for the main effect for group, pairwise comparisons of the groups were conducted, the results of which are shown in the last column.

it did so not only for current but also for recollected childhood functioning. In nearly all measures, the ADHD group was rated as having a higher impairment total score and as having more domains impaired than either of the two control groups. The Clinical control group was also significantly different from the Community control group in these respects but the former were always less impaired and had fewer domains of impairment than the ADHD group. These results are depicted graphically in Figure 6.1, where we show the percentage of the total possible domains on each measure that were rated as being impaired. To reiterate: *ADHD in clinic-referred adults is a more impairing disorder than are other common disorders likely to be seen in outpatient clinics, such as anxiety disorders, dysthymia, and even some cases of major depression.*

Only on the employer rating scale did this pattern differ. There the ADHD group was rated as having a higher total impairment score than that of the Community control group only but not that of the Clinical controls. And the groups did not differ among themselves in the number of different domains rated as impaired on this scale. But there was a significant interaction here on the total impairment score between the groups and the sex of participant. This interaction is shown graphically in Figure 6.2. We found that men and women in the

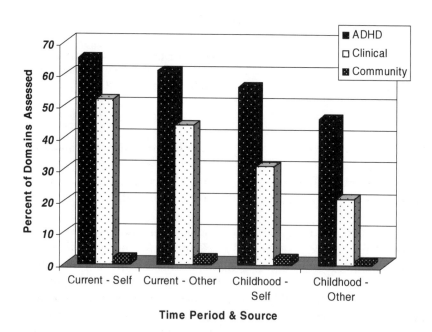

FIGURE 6.1. Percentage of domains of major life activities rated as often or very often impaired for each group currently (out of 10 possible domains) and in childhood (out of eight possible domains) for the UMASS Study.

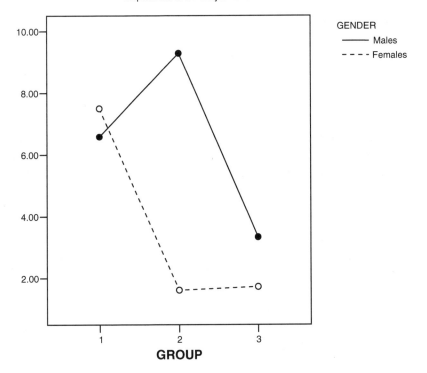

FIGURE 6.2. Results of the employer-completed ratings (raw scores) for workplace impairment showing each sex within each group (illustrating the significant group × sex interaction on this measure) for the UMASS Study. Group 1 = ADHD, 2 = Clinical control, 3 = Community control.

ADHD and Community control group were not very different in this measure of total impairment. In contrast, males in the Clinical control group were rated as being significantly more impaired in workplace functioning than were females in that group, who were rated as no more impaired than females in the Community control group.

   Thus, whether using interviews or rating scales, self-reports, reports of significant others, or ratings of current or childhood functioning, the adults with ADHD were more severely impaired and found more domains of life activities to be impaired than did the other groups. If nothing else, these results provide support for the notion that ADHD in adults is not a benign disorder. Nor are adults with ADHD simply part of the general population who have occasional difficulties from time to time with attention and who are perceived as exaggerating the extent to which their symptoms may be producing impairment in major life activities—a point sometimes asserted in the popular media and by critics of ADHD.

TABLE 6.3. Impaired Major Life Activities by Group (from Interview) from the UMASS Study

Measure	ADHD		Clinical		Community		χ^2	p	Pairwise contrasts
	N	%	N	%	N	%			
Occupation	130	89	63	65	4	4	188.9	< .001	1 > 2 > 3
Home responsibilities	131	90	76	78	3	3	215.5	< .001	1 > 2 > 3
Social activities	112	77	49	50	1	1	145.2	< .001	1 > 2 > 3
Community activities	68	47	33	34	0	0	68.0	< .001	1 > 2 > 3
Educational activities	143	98	81	83	3	3	268.1	< .001	1 > 2 > 3
Dating or marriage	120	82	71	73	7	6	161.2	< .001	1,2 > 3
Any domain	145	100	96	99	12	11	289.4	< .001	1,2 > 3

Note. N = sample size endorsing this item; % = percent of group endorsing this item; χ^2 = results of the omnibus chi-square test; p = probability value for the chi-square test; pairwise contrasts = results of the chi-square tests involving pairwise comparisons of the three groups.

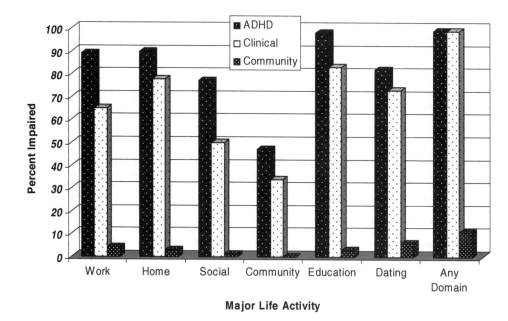

FIGURE 6.3. Percentage of each group reporting impairment in various domains of major life activities (by interview) for the UMASS Study.

more of these six domains, compared to 11% of the Community control group. This finding is not surprising, given that impairment in a major life activity is a requirement for a clinical diagnosis of any disorder, including ADHD. More informative are the specific areas of impairment. With the exception of dating or marriage, the ADHD group showed a significantly greater percentage as being impaired in each of these domains than was the case for either of the control groups. Again, a higher percentage of the Clinical control group was also impaired in each domain relative to the Community control group, but not as many as in the ADHD group. The rank ordering of the domains from most to least impairment for the ADHD group was as follows:

1. Education
2. Home responsibilities
3. Occupation
4. Dating or marriage
5. Social activities
6. Community activities

The vast majority of adults with ADHD reported being impaired in the first three of these major life activities, with the greatest percentage of ADHD cases being impaired in educational activities. If clinicians are most interested in identifying impairment in ADHD cases, they should focus chiefly on these three domains (education, home, and occupation) where the majority of ADHD cases are likely to be impaired and more so than are Clinical control cases. Community activities, in contrast, were impaired in only a minority of ADHD cases.

We had also assessed a larger variety of major life activities on the rating scales beyond the six evaluated in the interview, including money management, driving, and leisure activities as well as general daily responsibilities. The results of those ratings of impairment are displayed in Table 6.4, which shows the percentage of each group that was rated as being "often" or more impaired in each domain. Education, daily responsibilities, work, money management, and dating or marriage were the principal domains in which a considerable majority (more than 70%) of adults with ADHD rate themselves as being often impaired. In all domains, more of the ADHD group than the Community adults are rated as impaired. Of these, education, money management, daily responsibilities, and community activities are the domains that significantly distinguish the ADHD group from the Clinical control group. This is also true for the ratings provided by significant others except that here, work and social activities are also identified as areas more likely to distinguish the ADHD adults from those in the Clinical control group. Without a doubt, ADHD in adults has a relatively severe impact on many domains of major life activities.

TABLE 6.4. Domains of Major Life Activities Rated as Often Impaired by Group (from Rating Scales) from the UMASS Study

Measure	ADHD		Clinical		Community		χ^2	p	Pairwise contrasts
	N	%	N	%	N	%			
Current self-ratings									
Home life	97	69	54	59	2	2	96.2	< .001	1,2 > 3
Work or occupation	105	75	62	67	2	2	117.4	< .001	1,2 > 3
Social interactions	80	56	41	44	1	1	67.1	< .001	1,2 > 3
Community activities	60	44	27	30	1	1	45.7	< .001	1 > 2 > 3
Educational activities	127	89	62	70	1	1	172.5	< .001	1 > 2 > 3
Dating or marital activities	100	73	61	66	1	1	116.5	< .001	1,2 > 3
Money management	104	73	43	46	1	1	107.4	< .001	1 > 2 > 3
Driving	54	38	29	31	2	2	34.7	< .001	1,2 > 3
Leisure activities	65	46	35	38	1	1	49.2	< .001	1,2 > 3
Daily responsibilities	122	86	59	63	2	2	150.8	< .001	1 > 2 > 3
Childhood self-ratings									
Home life	79	58	27	30	3	3	70.8	< .001	1 > 2 > 3
Social interactions	80	58	35	38	2	2	72.6	< .001	1 > 2 > 3
Community activities	54	41	16	18	2	2	44.3	< .001	1 > 2 > 3
School	126	91	48	53	5	6	159.8	< .001	1 > 2 > 3
Sports, clubs, organizations	68	51	25	29	3	3	55.3	< .001	1 > 2 > 3
Self-care	55	41	25	28	3	3	38.6	< .001	1 > 2 > 3
Daily chores/responsibilities	101	75	37	42	1	1	118.0	< .001	1 > 2 > 3
Current other-ratings									
Home life	87	70	54	67	2	3	86.8	< .001	1,2 > 3
Work or occupation	87	73	38	52	1	1	87.5	< .001	1 > 2 > 3
Social interactions	71	57	29	36	1	1	56.0	< .001	1 > 2 > 3
Community activities	53	46	16	22	1	1	42.1	< .001	1 > 2 > 3
Educational activities	87	63	40	56	2	3	84.8	< .001	1 > 2 > 3
Dating or marital activities	76	66	42	57	3	4	67.3	< .001	1,2 > 3
Money management	80	64	35	43	3	4	63.0	< .001	1 > 2 > 3
Driving	43	34	23	28	1	1	26.0	< .001	1,2 > 3
Leisure activities	53	43	24	30	0	0	38.7	< .001	1,2 > 3
Daily responsibilities	96	77	51	64	2	3	98.5	< .001	1 > 2 > 3
Childhood other-ratings									
Home life	45	49	8	20	1	2	39.8	< .001	1 > 2 > 3
Social interactions	42	46	7	17	0	0	39.7	< .001	1 > 2 > 3
Community activities	26	29	3	8	0	0	24.2	< .001	1 > 2 > 3
School	59	66	15	37	1	2	57.7	< .001	1 > 2 > 3
Sports, clubs, organizations	35	39	7	17	0	0	30.7	< .001	1 > 2 > 3
Self-care	31	34	7	17	0	0	25.1	< .001	1 > 2 > 3
Play and leisure	32	35	6	15	1	2	24.1	< .001	1 > 2 > 3
Daily chores/responsibilities	56	61	14	35	2	4	48.0	< .001	1 > 2 > 3

(continued)

TABLE 6.4. (continued)

Measure	ADHD		Clinical		Community		χ^2	p	Pairwise contrasts
	N	%	N	%	N	%			
School ratings (others)									
Classwork	57	64	13	30	1	2	63.1	< .001	1 > 2 > 3
Homework	59	66	19	44	2	3	61.0	< .001	1 > 2 > 3
Classroom behavior	33	37	6	14	0	0	33.2	< .001	1 > 2 > 3
School bus behavior	12	15	2	5	0	0	11.3	.004	1 > 3
Interactions with classmates	31	35	2	5	0	0	37.9	< .001	1 > 3
Recess activities	23	27	3	7	0	0	24.0	< .001	1 > 2 > 3
Lunchroom activities	16	19	0	0	0	0	22.3	< .001	1 > 2,3
Time management	57	65	16	37	1	2	62.1	< .001	1 > 2 > 3

Note. N = sample size endorsing this item; % = percent of group endorsing this item; χ^2 = results of the omnibus chi-square test; p = probability value for the chi-square test; pairwise contrasts = results of the chi-square tests involving pairwise comparisons of the three groups.

In the self-ratings of childhood, a significantly greater proportion of the ADHD group than of the Clinical control or Community control groups rated themselves as being often impaired in all eight of these domains. Those results are illustrated in Figure 6.4. Among these domains, education or the school setting was far and away the domain most likely to be adversely impacted by ADHD (over 90%), followed by daily chores and responsibilities (75%). The same was true for the ratings provided by significant others about the childhood impairments in these groups. While a smaller proportion of each group was rated as being impaired in the reports of others compared to self-reports, once more, a higher proportion of the ADHD group was rated as impaired in each of the eight domains than was the case for either control group. And again, the educational setting was the domain in which more of the ADHD group had been affected relative to the other domains surveyed.

We also surveyed significant others for their views of the specific school settings in childhood that were impaired in the school histories of these participants. The adults with ADHD had a greater proportion rated as impaired in six of the eight domains relative to the Clinical control group, with only the school bus setting and peer interactions being the exceptions. More of the ADHD group was rated as impaired in all eight domains compared to the Community control group. Classwork, homework, and time management were the domains in which the largest percentage of adults with ADHD were reported to be often impaired.

One way to evaluate the veracity of these reports is to examine the correlation across sources for each developmental period being rated. Self-ratings of the number of domains of current impairment correlated moderately with other ratings of the same domains ($r = .68$, $p < .001$, $N = 184$), sharing nearly 50% of the

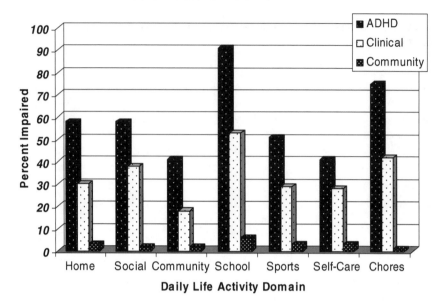

FIGURE 6.4. Percentage of each group rated as impaired in various domains of daily life activities in childhood (retrospectively recalled) in the UMASS Study.

variance. The correlation for ratings of impaired domains in childhood between self-reports and other reports was lower but still satisfactory considering the span of time over which such ratings had to be recollected (since childhood) (r = .55, p < .001, N = 160). A moderate degree of confidence can be placed in the reports of adults about their current and childhood impairments when considered relative to the reports of others who know them well.

Taken in their entirety, these findings clearly demonstrate that clinic-referred adults with ADHD experience more severe impairment and in more numerous domains of major life activities than do other clinic-referred adults without ADHD or members of a Community control group of adults. Also, more of the adults with ADHD are impaired in most of the domains assessed here than is the case for the control groups, whether in current or childhood functioning or whether by their own reports or the reports of others.

The Milwaukee Study Results

We collected the same sorts of information via the same methods in the Milwaukee Study as we did in the UMASS Study above except for employer ratings and specific ratings of school functioning. The results for the six domains of impairment reviewed in the interview are shown in Table 6.5, which can

TABLE 6.5. Impaired Major Life Activities by Group (from Interview) from the Milwaukee Study

Measure	H+ADHD		H–ADHD		Community		χ^2	p	Pairwise contrasts
	N	%	N	%	N	%			
Occupation	32	58.2	5	6.3	5	6.7	67.90	< .001	1 > 2,3
Home responsibilities	38	69.1	11	13.8	7	9.3	68.97	< .001	1 > 2,3
Social activities	29	52.7	6	7.5	6	8.0	52.29	< .001	1 > 2,3
Community activities	10	18.2	2	2.5	3	4.0	13.82	.001	1 > 2,3
Educational activities	18	32.7	6	7.5	5	6.7	22.43	< .001	1 > 2,3
Dating or marriage	34	61.8	10	12.5	5	6.7	62.43	< .001	1 > 2,3
Any domain	55	100.0	22	27.5	17	22.7	92.32	< .001	1 > 2,3

Note. N = sample size endorsing this item; % = percent of group endorsing this item; χ^2 = results of the omnibus chi-square test; p = probability value for the chi-square test; pairwise contrasts = results of the chi-square tests involving pairwise comparisons of the three groups; H+ADHD = hyperactive group that currently has a diagnosis of ADHD at follow-up; H–ADHD = hyperactive group that does not have a diagnosis of ADHD at follow-up.

Statistical analysis: Pearson chi-square.

be directly compared to those in Table 6.3 for the UMASS Study adults with ADHD. These results also appear in Figure 6.5, which can be compared to Figure 6.3 for the UMASS adults. Once more, one should not be surprised to see that 100% of the H+ADHD group is impaired in at least one of these domains, as this was a requirement for classifying them as currently ADHD (see Chapter 4). Noteworthy, though, is that just 27% of the H–ADHD group thought of themselves as currently impaired in at least one domain, a figure very near to the 23% reported in the control group. More informative are the specific domains in which impairment was reported. Like the clinic-referred adults, a majority of the H+ADHD group reported being impaired in home responsibilities and occupational functioning, though the percentages are lower than in the UMASS study of adults with ADHD. In the UMASS Study, educational activities were also reported by most adults (98%) with ADHD as being impaired, while here, in the H+ADHD group, just 33% reported this domain as being impaired. Instead, these ADHD children grown up reported that dating or marriage was their third domain of greatest impairment (62%). While that domain was also impaired in a sizable majority of clinic-referred adults with ADHD (82%), it ranked lower than occupation, home, and educational functioning, but not by much. Nevertheless, the overall pattern of results for the Milwaukee Study is quite similar to the pattern found in the UMASS clinic-referred adults with ADHD in that the H+ADHD group rated themselves as being more likely to be impaired in every one of the six domains of major life activities than was the case for the H–ADHD and control groups, who did not differ from each other in these self-reports.

impaired in six of the 10 domains assessed on the rating scale. In short, others perceive more of these hyperactive individuals to be impaired in adulthood than do the hyperactive persons themselves, and they view the groups as equivalently so in most domains. Only in home, social, dating/marital, and daily responsibilities were the H+ADHD group seen as having more cases impaired than in the H−ADHD group, yet here too the H−ADHD group was so rated more often than was the Community control group.

An interesting pattern emerges in the other reports of childhood impairments when contrasted with the self-reports for this time period. Whereas the H+ADHD group had more members self-reporting impairment than the H−ADHD group in most domains of childhood functioning, others did not see it that way. They viewed both hyperactive groups as being more likely to be impaired in seven of the eight domains (play being the exception) than the control group and to be equivalently so. School, home life, and daily responsibilities were rated as having been impaired in the majority of patients of both hyperactive groups. As we concluded above for current functioning, in childhood we find that others perceive more of these hyperactive individuals to have been impaired than is the case in self-perceptions, and in most domains they perceive the two hyperactive groups to be relatively equivalent in risk for impairment. There seems to be more risk of impairment as judged by others than is evident in self-reports, particularly for the H−ADHD group.

Some clinicians and advocates for the adult ADHD community have claimed that ADHD has a good side, and that it brings with it positive traits or special gifts individuals would not otherwise possess. "People with ADD have special gifts, even if they are hidden. The most common include originality, creativity, charisma, energy, liveliness, and unusual sense of humor, areas of intellectual brilliance, and spunk" (Hallowell & Ratey, 2005, p. 6). Others have claimed likewise (Hartmann, 1993; Sarkis, 2005). We wish we could say there is evidence in these two large projects supporting such a romantic view of this disorder. But none was found above. Nor is any found in the remaining chapters of this book, at least not at the group level of analysis. In not a single instance on hundreds of measures did we find that ADHD conferred some advantage over our various control groups. Admittedly we did not examine any specific and positive affinity ADHD may have with hunting or military combat ability, but neither did those who have asserted such special adaptive capacities as being associated with ADHD. Certainly there is nothing here that would suggest such special talents as likely to exist within those domains of life activities. Yet if this ideal were true, we should see it at the group level, not just in a few individual and exceptional cases cited by advocates. The exceptions are just that—exceptions. They likely represent unique individual positive traits in those cases, which have no relationship to ADHD and would have been present anyway, whether the disorder had been present or not. Clinicians should, by all means, help patients identify and celebrate their individual strengths and use them where feasible to compensate for their disorder. But let us not portray those individual talents as somehow resulting directly from the presence of this disorder. It is not only false to claim so but—given the prevailing scientific evidence mustered here—also misleading.

The Most Discriminating Domains for ADHD in Adults

It is reasonable to ask which of the numerous domains evaluated here are most effective in identifying adults with ADHD versus the control groups. The results we report are based on the rating scales.

The UMASS Study Results

The results for the UMASS Study appear in Table 6.7. As this table suggests, three domains were most effective in distinguishing adults with ADHD from the Community control group: *occupational functioning, educational activities, and money management*. The highest predictive power (odds ratio) was found for functioning in educational activities. In comparison to the Clinical controls, again, educational activities and money management are the most effective in identifying the adults with ADHD. Occupational functioning, however, was not a domain that distinguished these two clinical samples from each other, most likely because a high proportion of both groups reported impairment in that domain. Even though the Clinical controls were also shown to be more likely to experience impairment in both the education and money management domains, adults with ADHD were even more likely to have such impairments. This suggests that clinicians ought to explore these two domains more thoroughly in diagnosing adults with ADHD so as to distinguish them from other psychiatric patients (such as our non–ADHD clinical patients).

In childhood, the impairments most salient in discriminating between the ADHD group and Community controls were in *their home life, school, and performance of daily chores and other responsibilities*. Among these three domains, educational activities (school) once again proved to be the domain having the highest predictive value in identifying the ADHD group members. In contrast, it was only school functioning that significantly distinguished the ADHD and Clinical control groups. This suggests that it is important to pursue retrospective reports of adults with ADHD about the educational domain in helping clinicians to distinguish ADHD from other psychiatric disorders, such as our non–ADHD clinical patients. In fact, of all the domains for current and childhood functioning, one could say that educational functioning is routinely the most important domain to explore in identifying adults with ADHD. This is not to say that clinicians should not review all of these domains with all clinical cases but that in

TABLE 6.7. Current and Childhood Domains of Impairment That Best Discriminate between the Groups (from Rating Scales) in the UMASS Study

Symptom	Beta	SE	Wald	p	Odds ratio	95% CI
ADHD vs. Community—current						
Work or occupation	0.90	.412	4.74	.029	2.45	1.09–5.51
Educational activities	1.85	.391	22.49	< .001	6.39	2.97–13.74
Management of money	1.37	.440	9.74	.002	3.95	1.67–9.35
ADHD vs. Clinical—current						
Educational activities	0.64	.157	16.70	< .001	1.90	1.40–2.58
Management of money	0.40	.130	9.71	.002	1.50	1.16–1.93
Clinical vs. Community—current						
Work or occupation	0.86	.372	5.35	.021	2.36	1.14–4.90
Educational activities	1.48	.391	14.23	< .001	4.37	2.03–9.42
Dating or marriage	1.08	.406	7.08	.008	2.94	1.33–6.52
Management of money	0.77	.406	3.62	.057	2.16	0.98–4.80
ADHD vs. Community—childhood						
Home life with immediate family	0.90	.477	3.58	.058	2.46	0.97–6.28
School	1.74	.449	14.72	< .001	5.61	2.32–13.52
Daily chores and other Responsibilities	1.31	.534	6.01	.014	3.70	1.30–10.54
ADHD vs. Clinical—childhood						
School	1.08	.183	35.01	< .001	2.96	2.06–4.24
Clinical vs. Community—childhood						
School	0.57	.285	3.98	.046	1.76	1.01–3.09
Sports, clubs, or other organizations	0.73	.326	5.03	.025	2.08	1.10–3.93
Daily chores and other responsibilities	1.39	.378	13.55	< .001	4.03	1.92–8.46

Note. SE = standard error for beta; odds ratio = Exp(B); 95% CI = 95% confidence interval for the odds ratio. *Statistical analysis:* Logistic regression using forward conditional entry method.

reaching diagnostic decisions, the greatest predictive or distinguishing value will be reports of impairment in educational activities, followed by occupational functioning and money management.

The Milwaukee Study Results

We conducted the same analysis for the self-reported domains of current impairment in the Milwaukee Study, the results for which appear in Table 6.8. The domains that best discriminated the H+ADHD group from the Community control group were the domains of home, work, money management, and daily responsibilities. But note here that the domain of work was reverse-weighted in the regression results, indicating that the higher the impairment rating, the more likely the individual was to be in the Community control group. This suggests that controls were more inclined to rate themselves as having some degree of impairment at work than were the H+ADHD cases. For the other domains, the more impairment that was rated, the more likely the person was to be in the H+ADHD group. These findings differ from those for ADHD patients in the UMASS study only in that education was also a significantly predictive domain for having ADHD in that study, whereas it was not so here. Here, home life appeared to be a more useful domain of impairment for predicting current ADHD than was education. Otherwise, the results are similar in showing the importance of work and money management as useful domains for predicting current ADHD.

TABLE 6.8. Current Self-Rated Domains That Best Discriminate between the Groups in the Milwaukee Study

Symptom	Beta	SE	Wald	p	Odds ratio	95% CI
H+ADHD vs. Community—current						
Home life	1.42	.460	9.60	.002	4.16	1.69–10.24
Work or occupation	−2.31	.754	9.42	.002	.099	0.23–0.43
Money management	2.02	.516	15.30	< .001	7.52	2.74–20.67
Daily responsibilities	1.93	.664	8.49	.004	6.92	1.88–25.44
H+ADHD vs. H–ADHD—current						
Social activities	1.18	.383	9.47	.002	3.25	1.53–6.90
Dating and marital activities	.91	.304	9.00	.003	2.49	1.37–4.52
Daily responsibilities	.753	.310	5.92	.015	2.12	1.16–3.90
H–ADHD vs. Community—current						
Work or occupation	−.641	.288	4.95	.026	0.53	0.30–0.93
Money management	1.14	.299	14.49	< .001	3.12	1.74–5.62
H+ADHD vs. Community—childhood						
Social activities	1.16	.315	13.72	< .001	3.21	1.73–5.94
Sports, clubs, etc.	−.695	.312	4.96	.026	0.50	0.27–0.92
H+ADHD vs. H–ADHD—childhood						
Social activities	1.05	.231	20.71	< .001	2.87	1.82–4.51
H–ADHD vs. Community—childhood						
None						

Note. SE = standard error for beta; odds ratio = Exp(B); 95% CI = 95% confidence interval for the odds ratio; H+ADHD = hyperactive group that currently has a diagnosis of ADHD at follow-up; H–ADHD = hyperactive group that does not have a diagnosis of ADHD at follow-up.

Statistical analysis: Binary logistic regression using forward conditional entry method with the self-ratings of impairment for each of 10 self-rated domains, each domain rated 0–3.

In distinguishing the H–ADHD group from the control group, two of the same domains were again useful: work and money management. Here again the work domain was reverse-weighted; these hyperactive patients were less inclined to see themselves as being impaired in work than were members of the Community control group, just as we saw in the H+ADHD group. The domains found to contribute most to discriminating the two hyperactive groups from each other were social activities, dating and marital activities, and daily responsibilities, where higher impairment scores were associated with being in the group currently having ADHD.

When we examined the ratings of childhood impairments, we found that just two domains significantly discriminated the H+ADHD group from the control group: (1) social activities and (2) sports, clubs, and other organizations. Again, as with work functioning above, the domain of sports was reverse-weighted, suggesting that controls were more inclined to rate themselves as impaired in that childhood domain than were those hyperactives with current ADHD. The H–ADHD group could not be discriminated from the community control group on any domain of self-rated childhood impairments. The two hyperactive groups were best discriminated by just a single domain, that again being social activities. The H+ADHD group was more likely to be associated with impairment in this domain than was the H–ADHD group. Relative to the UMASS Study results, we find that school and home life and daily responsibilities were more discerning of ADHD as domains of impairment in childhood compared to controls, whereas here it was social activities.

Relationship of ADHD
Symptom Measures to Impairment Measures

The severity of an individual's ADHD symptoms does not automatically guarantee that impairment will ensue as a consequence of those symptoms. The DSM-IV makes establishing the presence of impairment in two or more domains a separate criterion (criterion D; see Chapter 3, Table 3.1) for the clinical diagnosis of ADHD besides just establishing the presence of symptoms that are developmentally inappropriate and have an onset in childhood. Yet no guidance is given in the DSM-IV as to how to evaluate impairment under this criterion and only three domains are suggested for review with patients (home and school for children, occupation added for adults). Yet other domains of functioning are also important in adulthood, such as dating or marital functioning, social functioning, participation in community activities, money management, driving, and so on. As noted above, these too should be assessed by clinicians.

Little information exists on the extent to which ADHD symptoms are related to measures of impairment. We and our colleagues have previously shown that severity of ADHD in children may be only modestly related to the degree of impairment in any single domain or on any specific measure of functioning in that domain (Gordon et al., 2006).

Here we explore this issue more thoroughly by examining correlations between various measures of ADHD severity using the interview and rating scales and the reports of self, other, employer, and clinician. We examined relationships not only within each source of information but also across sources, thus providing further evidence for the validity of each source's reports.

The UMASS Study Results

Our findings appear in Table 6.9 and are based on the entire sample (all groups collapsed together). Self-reports of ADHD symptoms on the interview, regardless of whether they were inattentive or hyperactive–impulsive symptoms, were highly correlated with the number of self-reported domains of impairment in this interview (rs = .70–.84), reflecting pervasiveness of impairment. Symptoms of inattention were more highly related to pervasive impairment than were those of hyperactive-impulsive behavior, but both showed very acceptable levels of association with impairment. Overall, the number of ADHD symptoms (severity of disorder) shared 70% of the variance with the number of self-reported domains that were impaired. Likewise and also impressive, we found relatively high correlations between self-reported symptoms on the interview and clinician ratings of severity of impairment on the SOFAS scale (rs = −.67 to −.80) (see sidebar).

The information collected on the rating scales provided both a larger number of domains of major life activities to be rated and a finer dimensional rating for each (0–3) than was the case in the interview, where symptoms and impairments were reported in a binary or dichotomous format (yes or no). This finer scaling for both symptoms and impairments resulted in even higher correlations being found between self-rated ADHD symptoms and self-rated impairments (rs = .78–.88). ADHD symptom severity was found to share as much as 77% of the variance with severity of impairment, whether using the total impairment score (severity) or the number of different domains rated as "often" or more impaired (pervasiveness). Essentially the same results emerged for the ratings provided by others concerning the current functioning of these participants (rs = .72–.88). Virtually the same pattern of results emerged for self-ratings of childhood symptoms in relation to childhood impairment scores as well as for other-rated childhood symptoms and impairment scores, whether concerning multiple domains or childhood school functioning specifically. Ratings provided by employers were also found to be only slightly lower in their relationships to employer-rated impairments in the workplace than were found in the other sources (self, others). Such findings indicate that the reports of adults about themselves or those provided by others who know them well

concerning ADHD symptoms are likely to be impressively correlated with reports within each of these sources about the degree and pervasiveness of impairment. These relationships are strong, whether they pertain to current functioning or to recall of childhood functioning.

Of course, the relationships described above are based upon using the same source of information for symptoms of ADHD and for impairments from those symptoms. This common source effect could inflate the correlation to some degree. An indicator of validity in these relationships would be to examine the relationship of self-reported symptoms with other reports of impairment and vice versa. That information is also provided in the lower half of Table 6.9. Here we find that self-rated symptoms on the rating scales, although lower, were still reasonably well correlated with degree of impairment as rated by others. The only exception was between self-rated symptoms and employer-rated impairments, which was quite low (r = .21). This could be due to the fact, reported in earlier tables, that most participants, especially in the Community and Clinical control groups, had very little employer-rated impairment. When we reversed the source of information concerning symptoms and impairment, equally moderate relationships were evident (rs = .55–.65). And this same level of agreement was found for information concerning childhood when sources of information were crossed.

These results show that self-ratings of either symptoms or impairment share 29 to 46% of their variance with the ratings of either symptoms or impairment provided by others, whether about current or childhood functioning. While crossing sources of information concerning symptoms vs. impairment does lower the degree of relationships to some degree from that found in same-source information, the relationships are still significant, are of moderate degree, and share a considerable degree of variance with each other. In one of the few other studies to do so, Kooij and colleagues (Kooij et al., 2005) also found significant relationships between ratings of ADHD symptoms in a general population sample of 1,813 adults and various measures of impairment. All of this information suggests that the severity of ADHD is related to both severity of impairment (total impairment across domains) and pervasiveness of impairment (number of different domains often impaired).

Another way of demonstrating this relationship of symptoms to impairment is shown in Figure 6.6. It shows the percentage of domains of major life activity self-reported often or very often as impaired for both current and childhood functioning juxtaposed against the percentage of self-reported ADHD symptoms. To make the comparison clearer, each measure is expressed as a percentage of the maximum possible score. This figure graphically shows that the higher the percentage of possible ADHD symptoms found across the groups, the greater the percentage of domains rated as impaired. Clearly, severity of ADHD links up with severity of impairment.

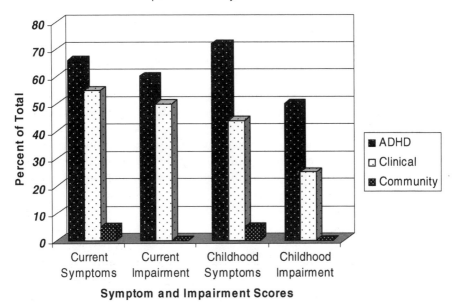

FIGURE 6.6. Percentage of possible ADHD symptoms (out of 18 in DSM-IV-TR) and percentage of possible impaired domains (out of 10 for current and eight for childhood) for each group for current and childhood functioning for the UMASS Study. Graph visually illustrates the relationship of symptoms to impairments. Groups are ADHD adults, Clinical control adults, and Community control adults.

Prior research has indicated that four or more symptoms of ADHD in adults reflects significant deviancy in the population (93rd percentile) and could serve as a clinical cutoff score instead of the six symptoms recommended in the DSM (see Murphy & Barkley, 1996). We also found this to be the case in Chapters 4 and 5, where four symptoms from the DSM-IV were more than enough to accurately classify the ADHD cases versus the Community control cases. We therefore examined the probability of being impaired if one had at least this many symptoms of ADHD. While four symptoms may sound like a very low threshold, it handily identified risk of impairment. In using this threshold, we found that 100% of those reporting four or more ADHD symptoms on the interview reported being impaired in at least one domain of major life activity. This is yet another way of showing that ADHD symptom severity is related to likelihood of impairment.

The Milwaukee Study Results

We then examined the same relationships using the Milwaukee sample. As in the UMASS Study, we collapsed all participants together for examination of these relationships. The results appear in Table 6.10. While the degree of relationship between symptoms and impairments is somewhat lower, it is still impressive in magnitude, especially for the rating scale results, where a wider range of quantitative scoring of impairment was available. Once again, relationships were stronger when both symptoms and impairments were measured using the same source than when sources were crossed, such as self-rated symptoms with other-rated impairment. But even here relationships were of a moderate degree. All of this again makes the point that the severity of ADHD, variously measured, is significantly related to the severity of impairment, variously measured, whether using ratings of current functioning or retrospectively recalled functioning in childhood.

TABLE 6.10. Relationship of ADHD Symptom Measures to Impairment Measures in the Milwaukee Study

Correlated measures	r	p	N
Interview			
No. of inattention symptoms with # of domains impaired	.60	< .001	210
No. of hyperactive symptoms with # of domains impaired	.48	< .001	210
Total no. of ADHD symptoms with # domains of impairment	.61	< .001	210
Self-ratings of current functioning			
Total ADHD symptom scores with impairment scores	.75	< .001	201
Other-ratings of current functioning			
Total ADHD symptom scores with impairment scores	.87	< .001	200
Self-ratings of childhood functioning			
Total ADHD symptom scores with impairment scores	.89	< .001	205
Other-ratings of childhood functioning			
Total ADHD symptom scores with impairment scores	.87	< .001	200
Self-rated current symptoms with other-rated impairment			
Total ADHD symptom scores with impairment scores	.37	< .001	199
Other-rated current symptoms with self-rated impairment			
Total ADHD symptom scores with impairment scores	.45	< .001	198
Self-rated childhood symptoms with other-rated impairment			
Total ADHD symptom scores with impairment scores	.53	< .001	199
Other-rated childhood symptoms with self-rated impairment			
Total ADHD symptom scores with impairment scores	.49	< .001	200

Note. r = Pearson correlation; p = probability value of the correlation; N = sample size.

The Milwaukee Study offers an additional means of exploring the predictive value of ADHD symptoms for determining severity of impairment. In this case, it can address the extent to which severity of childhood ADHD–related behavior is predictive of adult severity of impairment. Table 6.11 shows the results of linear regression analyses in which we explored the extent to which 13 measures collected earlier in development predicted current severity of ADHD and of impairment. The latter was determined using both self and other ratings and represented the total raw impairment rating across the 10 domains on the scale. Five predictors came from the childhood entry point, these being the scales used to select the cases as hyperactive (WWPARS, CPRS-R Hyperactivity Index, and HSQ number of problem settings scores) as well as the childhood IQ measure (PPVT) and the CPRS-R conduct problem scale (see sidebar in Chapter 4 for these measures). This set examines whether childhood IQ or our measure of oppositional behavior and conduct problems in childhood (CPRS-R) might be related to adult symptoms and impairment. Four more predictors came from the teen follow-up, these being parent reports of the number of ADHD, ODD, and CD symptoms (from a DSM-III-R–based interview) as well as the Teen Life Events Scale (see sidebar). This scale measures the number of disruptive or stressful life events a teen reports ever having experienced, such as home relocations, parental separations or divorces, and so on. From the age-21 follow-up, we selected four measures self-reported ADHD, ODD, and CD symptoms (DSM-III-R) and parent reports of ADHD symptoms.

As Table 6.11 shows, the number of current self-reported symptoms of ADHD at age 27 was significantly predicted chiefly by two of the subject selection scales at childhood entry into the study: the WWPARS and HSQ scales. The number of ADHD symptoms self-reported at age 21 also made an additional contribution to predicting current ADHD severity. In combination, these findings suggest that both severity of ADHD, especially hyperactivity, at study entry and persistence of ADHD to age 21 (by self-report) are predictive of severity of ADHD at age 27. A surprise was that the number of teen-reported stressful life events at the adolescent follow-up made an additional significant though small contribution to the degree of ADHD severity at adult outcome. It is possible that such events reflect indirectly the degree of ADHD severity in the parents, which may have contributed to both these greater stressful life events and to the severity of teen disorder through shared genetics. Or it could also obviously indicate a contribution of childhood and teen life stress to severity of disorder in adulthood. Our study is unable to tease apart such a genetic versus social environmental effect or its interaction. These four predictors accounted for nearly 28% of the variance in severity of ADHD symptoms (self-reported) at age 27. None of the other nine predictors significantly predicted current ADHD severity.

More to the point of this discussion, we used this same set of predictors to evaluate what may have contributed to severity of current impairment, both self-

TABLE 6.11. Predicting ADHD and Impairment Severity from Childhood, Teen, and Young Adult Follow-Up Measures in the Milwaukee Study

Outcome/predictors (step entered)	Beta	R	R^2	$R^2\Delta$	F	p
No. of current ADHD symptoms						
Childhood hyperactivity (WWPARS)	.266	.422	.178	.178	50.56	< .001
Childhood HSQ no. of problem settings	.152	.440	.184	.016	4.72	.031
Teen Life Events Scale (adversities)	.107	.457	.209	.015	4.43	.036
Age-21 no. of ADHD symptoms (self-reported)	.264	.527	.278	.068	21.88	< .001
NS: Childhood IQ (PPVT) and CPRS hyperactivity index and conduct problems; adolescent ADHD, ODD, and CD symptoms (parent); age-21 ADHD symptoms (parent), ODD and CD symptoms (self)						
Total impairment score (self-rated)						
Childhood hyperactivity (WWPARS)	.221	.325	.105	.105	27.57	< .001
No. of ODD symptoms at age 21 (self)	.234	.414	.172	.066	18.63	< .001
No. of ADHD symptoms at age 21 (parent)	.154	.434	.188	.016	4.66	.032
NS: Childhood IQ (PPVT), HSQ no. of problem settings, and CPRS hyperactivity index and conduct problems; teen ADHD, ODD, and CD symptoms (parent) and teen Life Events Scale; age-21 ADHD, and CD symptoms (self)						
Total impairment score (other-rated)						
Childhood hyperactivity (WWPARS)	.207	.410	.168	.168	47.18	< .001
Teen no. of ADHD symptoms (parent)	.017	.443	.196	.029	8.31	.004
Age-21 no. of ADHD symptoms (parent)	.361	.516	.266	.069	21.95	< .001
NS: Childhood IQ (PPVT) and CPRS hyperactivity index and conduct problems; teen ODD and CD symptoms (parent) and teen Life Events Scale; age-21 ADHD, ODD, and CD symptoms (self)						

Note. Beta = standardized beta coefficient; R = regression coefficient; R^2 = percent of explained variance accounted for by all variables at this step; $R^2\Delta$ = percent of explained variance accounted for by this variable added at this step; F = results of F test for the equation at this step; p = probability value for the F-test; NS = not significant; WWPARS = Werry–Weiss–Peters Activity Rating Scale; HSQ = Home Situations Questionnaire; PPVT = Peabody Picture Vocabulary Test; CPRS = Conners Parent Rating Scale; ODD = oppositional defiant disorder; CD = conduct disorder. Adolescent ADHD, ODD, and CD symptoms are from DSM-III-R. Age-21 self-reported symptoms of ADHD are from DSM-III-R. Age-21 parent-reported ADHD symptoms are from DSM-IV.

Statistical analysis: Multiple linear regression using stepwise conditional entry method and three steps (childhood, teen, and age-21 measures) with the entire sample (N = 208) and substituting the mean for any missing data.

rated and as rated by others. Table 6.11 shows that self-rated current impairment at age 27 was again predicted by severity of childhood hyperactivity (WWPARS). It was also, once again, predicted in part by persistence of ADHD at age 21 (this time from parent- rather than self-reported). But severity of ODD symptoms self-reported at age 21 made an additional contribution to current impairment, implying that current impairment is not being driven solely by severity of earlier ADHD or its persistence over time. These three predictors accounted for approximately 19% of the variance in current self-rated severity of impairment. Again, none of the other 10 predictors contributed to severity of current self-rated impairment.

Severity of current impairment as rated by others was predicted entirely by earlier levels of ADHD—at childhood (WWPARS), at adolescence (parent-reported DSM-III-R symptoms), and at age 21 (parent-reported ADHD symptoms). These predictors accounted for nearly 27% of the variance in impairment ratings at age 27. The higher the childhood symptom severity and the greater it remained at adolescence and early adulthood, the more severely impaired were these participants at age 27 as perceived by others. Such findings show that impairment is not simply associated with current ADHD but with severity of the disorder at earlier developmental periods.

Conclusions about Symptom–Impairment Relations

As shown above, using the same source (e.g., self, others) and the same method (interview, rating scale, clinician judgment) can result in higher relationships being found than if different sources and methods are used for one (symptoms) than the other (impairment) side of this relationship. Crossing sources and methods does lower the observed relationship more than when same sources are used. The resulting relationships, however, are still statistically significant and of a moderate magnitude. Neither approach to addressing this issue of symptoms versus impairment is a "gold standard," as each suffers from its own set of limitations. Individuals having just rated their symptoms highly may, on the same scale, inflate their ratings of impairment accordingly. That sword may cut both ways, however. Research suggests that children and adults with ADHD show a positive illusory bias in self-ratings of their competence and task performance, often rating themselves as functioning significantly better than they actually do when that domain of performance is tested (see Barkley, 2006; Knouse et al., 2005). Such findings would imply that self-ratings of impairment are likely to be an underestimate of actual functioning in that major life activity. We found this to be particularly so in the Milwaukee Study results, discussed above, when we compared the self-ratings of impairment in each of a number of domains of major life activities to others ratings of impairment in those same domains. Other ratings yield a higher percentage of cases being impaired in the hyperactive groups as adults than did self-reports.

Using a different source to obtain the impairment rating than the symptom rating is equally problematic. Those other sources may not have as complete a knowledge of the daily activities of the person they are rating as does the person being rated. Participants in both studies were mainly living away from home rather than with their parents. Thus parents or others are unlikely to be aware of the full range of social, occupational, driving, financial, and other domains of major life activities of these participants and hence of any impairment within them.

One should not be surprised that we found such a strong relationship between severity of ADHD and likelihood of impairment in major life activities. After all, many of the thousands of studies comparing ADHD and control groups, though mostly on children, have used various measures of social, educational, adaptive, occupational, and other areas of life functioning and found substantial differences between those groups (see *www.russellbarkley.org* for more than 2,500 such references). More recently, studies have controlled for comorbid disorders and have still found links between having ADHD and being impaired in particular life activities. All of these studies provided a different means of addressing the same issue raised here: the relationship of symptoms to impairment. After all, the groups having ADHD were selected for having more severe symptoms of ADHD than the control groups, which resulted in subsequent differences being found in major life activities. Those numerous studies provided just as much evidence that ADHD is linked to likelihood of impairment in a variety of major life activities as has the largely correlational approach taken here. More informative now would be studies that examine what factors like ADHD and other characteristics are likely to predict impairment in various major life activities in study samples (especially epidemiologically derived ones) using multivariate approaches such as regression, as has been done in several recent studies (Barkley, Fischer, et al., 2006; Deutscher & Fewell, 2005; Kooij et al., 2005).

Despite showing relatively strong relationships between symptoms (both current and from childhood) and impairment, clinicians should still evaluate both symptoms *and* domains of impairment separately as part of their clinical diagnostic assessment and not automatically assume that assessing the former is sufficient. All evidence points to this need to respect criterion D in the DSM-IV diagnostic criteria for ADHD (impairment) and to assess it specifically apart from just evaluating symptoms. In clinical practice, there will always be a small subset of patients who for a variety of reasons may endorse large numbers of ADHD symptoms on a rating scale or during an interview. But they do not evidence any significant objective impairment beyond a self-perception that they are not doing as well in life as they believe they should, as noted previously (Gordon et al., 2006).

There is also no doubt that better methods of assessing impairment, especially in adults, are in need of development, validation, and normative data if they are to provide clinicians with more efficient ways of evaluating impairment in their patients. The impairment scales used here for current, childhood, workplace, and school functioning along with the SOFAS scale seem to be a positive step in that direction. Our interviews and scales can be found in our clinical manual (Barkley & Murphy, 2006). In the future, other approaches, such as factor analysis or structural equation modeling, may also yield some useful composite approaches to evaluating impairment in various domains of major life activities with adults.

That said, the present findings provide some assurance that the severity of ADHD symptoms is not merely a meaningless expression of normal variation in the adult population devoid of or decoupled from risks for impairment in major life activities. Such severity, especially at clinically elevated levels, is highly likely to be associated with risk of impairment in one or more major life activities. If disorders are conceptualized as deficiencies in, or failures of, human psychological and behavioral adaptations that result in harm (impairment) to those individuals (Wakefield, 1992), then it is clear that ADHD in adults is just such a disorder with a high risk for associated impairment.

How Well Does Each DSM Symptom Predict Impairment in Each Domain?

A related issue to those raised above is the degree to which each symptom of ADHD is predictive of the likelihood of impairment in each domain of major life activity. The issue is important for constructing diagnostic criteria for ADHD in adults, as it helps to identify the best (most useful) symptoms for this purpose, where best is here defined as most likely to predict impairment. Table 6.12 shows this information based on the interview information we obtained in the UMASS Study. We report only the results for the UMASS Study, as they have the most direct bearing on constructing diagnostic criteria for use with clinically referred adults (the participants in that study). Note that the base rate for being impaired in any specific domain is shown across the top of the table. For a symptom to have much positive predictive value, the probability of impairment in each domain associated with that single symptom should exceed the base rate shown at the top of the column for each specific domain. Keep in mind that the base rates are so high because two of the three groups that were collapsed together for these analyses are clinic-referred patients, who would be expected, on that basis alone, to have some impairment in some settings. Table 6.13 shows the corresponding odds ratios for the same data shown in Table 6.12. In interpreting these tables, one should understand that positive predictive power (PPP) refers to the probability of being impaired in that domain, given that the symptom was endorsed as occurring often. Negative predictive power (NPP) is also

TABLE 6.12. The Positive (and Negative) Predictive Power of Each ADHD Symptom for Each Impaired Domain of Major Life Activities (from Interview) for the UMASS Study

		Work	Family and home	Social	Community	School and education	Dating/ marriage	Any impairment
				Impaired major life activities				
Symptom	Base rate:	56%	60%	46%	29%	64%	56%	72%
Inattention								
Is inattentive to details		83 (66)	85 (61)	66 (70)	44 (84)	92 (57)	78 (61)	99 (50)
Can't sustain attention		80 (87)	86 (87)	67 (91)	43 (96)	92 (84)	80 (85)	99 (76)
Fails to listen		83 (67)	88 (64)	72 (76)	41 (82)	94 (60)	83 (66)	98 (50)
Fails to follow instructions		82 (66)	89 (64)	70 (74)	43 (83)	92 (58)	83 (66)	99 (51)
Has difficulty organizing		80 (74)	87 (74)	66 (78)	41 (87)	89 (66)	78 (71)	98 (60)
Avoids sustained effort		81 (71)	87 (70)	69 (78)	43 (86)	94 (68)	78 (67)	99 (58)
Loses necessary things		80 (69)	84 (65)	66 (75)	41 (84)	87 (59)	78 (66)	96 (53)
Is easily distracted		80 (88)	86 (89)	67 (93)	42 (95)	92 (85)	79 (85)	99 (78)
Is forgetful		83 (70)	88 (68)	71 (78)	44 (86)	92 (62)	78 (65)	98 (54)
Hyperactivity–impulsivity								
Fidgets, squirms in seat		82 (69)	84 (64)	68 (75)	42 (84)	92 (63)	80 (66)	97 (52)
Leaves seat		78 (50)	84 (47)	70 (61)	38 (74)	91 (43)	80 (50)	96 (35)
Feels restless		83 (71)	87 (67)	71 (78)	43 (85)	93 (64)	82 (69)	98 (54)
Can't do things quietly		74 (49)	86 (47)	68 (60)	34 (73)	88 (42)	84 (51)	97 (35)
Is on the go		77 (59)	82 (57)	66 (68)	36 (77)	86 (51)	81 (61)	92 (42)
Talks excessively		81 (55)	85 (51)	72 (65)	36 (74)	88 (45)	85 (56)	96 (38)
Blurts out answers		77 (57)	87 (56)	72 (69)	41 (79)	88 (49)	82 (59)	95 (42)
Has difficulty waiting turn		82 (64)	87 (61)	74 (75)	42 (81)	92 (57)	81 (63)	98 (48)
Interrupts or intrudes		83 (59)	87 (55)	77 (71)	48 (82)	91 (50)	83 (58)	96 (41)

Note. PPP = positive predictive power, or the percentage of people endorsing the symptom who reported being impaired in that specific domain of major life activity; NPP = negative predictive power, or the percentage of people who did not endorse that symptom and who did not report being impaired in that specific major life activity. Symptoms in **bold** type are the five symptoms from DSM-IV-TR discovered earlier (Chapter 3) to be the best at discriminating ADHD from both the clinical and community groups. Base rate refers to the percentage of the entire sample (*N* = 352) endorsing impairment in each domain.

shown in parentheses in Table 6.12 and refers to the likelihood of *not* being impaired in that domain, given that the symptom was *not* endorsed. Ideally, one would like to see both PPP and NPP be as high as possible.

In Table 6.12, notice that even though the overall base rates for impairment in any domain are not trivial, each of the ADHD symptoms can be seen to elevate the risk above the base rate. Put another way, each symptom when endorsed affirmatively does predict an increase in risk of impairment in each domain. If it did not, its choice for being in the DSM-IV diagnostic criteria would be questionable. The DSM-IV symptoms are best at predicting impairment in educational, family, and work settings (from the interview), consistent with those being the major domains found to most likely be impaired in the ADHD group, as discussed above. All symptoms predicted risk of impairment quite well in terms of having any impairment in at least one domain (last column).

In most cases, the absence of the symptom was not necessarily predictive of the absence of any impairment, although being easily distracted and being unable to sustain attention were good at this, having NPPs of 78 and 76%. This made them the two best of any symptoms for predicting being impaired or not. But ADHD symptoms were not very good at predicting impairment in participation in community activities (clubs, sports, organizations, etc.), suggesting that in this domain people are least affected by symptoms of ADHD. Here, if you did not have the symptom, NPP was good, meaning that you were unlikely to be impaired. But having the symptom produced low PPP, meaning that you were not especially likely to be impaired in community activities even if you endorsed the symptom.

Table 6.13, for the odds ratios, makes it far easier to appreciate the relative predictive power of each ADHD symptom for each domain of major life activ-

TABLE 6.13. The Odds Ratios for Each ADHD Symptom in Predicting Each Impaired Domain of Major Life Activities (from Interview) for the UMASS Study

				Impaired major life activities			
Symptom	Work	Family and home	Social	Community	School and education	Dating/ marriage	Any impairment
Inattention							
Is inattentive to details	9.84	9.12	4.40	3.99	14.97	5.79	76.71
Can't sustain attention	25.88	39.03	21.52	18.16	61.52	22.12	360.52
Fails to listen	10.32	12.74	7.89	3.24	23.31	9.42	39.50
Fails to follow instructions	9.00	14.08	6.81	3.86	17.30	9.41	162.99
Has difficulty organizing	12.08	18.39	6.91	4.87	16.26	8.53	73.16
Avoids sustained effort	10.08	16.13	7.88	4.79	35.96	7.23	246.36
Loses necessary things	8.75	9.74	6.00	3.81	9.74	7.12	27.91
Is easily distracted	28.75	48.12	26.07	14.05	64.78	22.08	405.96
Is forgetful	11.32	16.77	8.60	4.75	18.93	6.32	66.73
Hyperactivity–impulsivity							
Fidgets, squirms in seat	10.33	9.72	6.58	3.94	20.57	7.82	37.16
Leaves seat	3.55	4.86	3.63	1.70	7.52	4.22	13.23
Feels restless	11.62	13.56	8.89	4.36	23.98	10.58	67.95
Can't do things quietly	2.77	5.79	3.09	1.36	5.17	5.39	19.29
Is on the go	4.79	6.07	4.18	1.84	6.18	6.78	8.29
Talks excessively	5.12	5.79	4.91	1.66	5.87	7.04	15.78
Blurts out answers	4.34	8.50	5.87	2.70	6.93	6.77	12.53
Has difficulty waiting turn	7.87	10.54	8.65	3.15	15.44	7.22	46.60
Interrupts or intrudes	6.99	8.34	7.87	4.02	10.27	6.87	16.70

Note. Symptoms in **bold** are the five symptoms from DSM-IV-TR discovered earlier (Chapter 3) to be the best at discriminating ADHD from both the clinical and community groups. Odds ratios are from the Mantel–Haenszel common odds ratio estimate as computed using chi-square analyses. All odds ratios were statistically significant at $p < .001$.

with a somewhat lower likelihood of being impaired in any particular domain, relative to levels seen in the UMASS study. Home and occupational domains were the most likely to be impaired, as were money management and daily responsibilities. Unlike the findings of the UMASS Study, the educational domain was not as likely to be self-reported as impaired in those hyperactive children retaining ADHD at follow-up.

✓ When rating scales of impairment were used so as to provide finer-grained dimensional judgments of impairment, the following were the principal domains in which a considerable majority (more than 70%) of adults with ADHD in the UMASS Study rated themselves as being often impaired: education, daily responsibilities, work, money management, and dating or marriage. With the exception of education, these domains were also those most likely to be affected by current ADHD at the age-27 follow-up in the Milwaukee Study.

✓ We also collected information from retrospective reports on the childhood domains most likely to be impaired. For the ADHD group in the UMASS Study, education or the school setting was far and away the domain most likely to be adversely impacted by ADHD (over 90%), followed by daily chores and responsibilities (75%). The same was true for the ratings provided by significant others about the childhood impairments in these groups. While a smaller proportion of each group was rated as being impaired in the reports of others compared to self-reports, a higher proportion of the ADHD group was rated as impaired in each of the eight domains from childhood than was the case for either control group. And again, the educational setting was the domain in which more of the ADHD group had been affected relative to the other domains surveyed. The Milwaukee Study found that the domain of social (peer) interactions was the one most likely to be associated with the ADHD group in childhood.

✓ These findings clearly demonstrate that adults with ADHD are more likely to experience impairment in numerous domains of major life activities and to experience more such impaired domains than are the control groups studied here.

✓ We then evaluated the relationship between the severity of ADHD and the likelihood of being impaired and the number of domains in which one was impaired. Our findings in the UMASS Study indicated that the reports of adults about themselves or those provided by others who know them well concerning ADHD symptoms are likely to be impressively correlated with reports within each of these sources about degree of impairment ($rs = .70–.80$). These relationships are strong whether they pertain to current functioning or to recall of childhood functioning. Such severity, especially at clinically elevated levels (four or more symptoms), is highly likely to be associated with risk of impairment in one or more major life activities (100% are impaired).

✓ Although finding somewhat lower levels of association between symptoms and impairments, the Milwaukee Study essentially replicated the pattern of results in the UMASS Study and found moderate to strong levels of such associations, depending on the method of measurement (interviews versus scales). The Milwaukee Study was also able to show that severity of ADHD-related symptoms at the childhood study entry point (mainly hyperactivity) and its pervasiveness across home settings, as well as the persistence of more severe ADHD symptoms to age 21, was associated with current severity of ADHD at age 27. That study also found that childhood, teen, and young adult ADHD severity were all predictive of greater impairment at age 27, implying that initial childhood ADHD severity as well as its persistence across development are also related to impairment at adult outcome.

✓ Finally, we analyzed the degree to which each specific symptom of ADHD in the DSM-IV was predictive of the likelihood of being impaired in each of six specific major life activities from our interviews in the UMASS Study. Among the hyperactive symptoms, feeling restless and having difficulties awaiting one's turn were the best for predicting impairments across all domains. Among the inattention symptoms, being easily distracted and being unable to sustain attention to tasks were the two best across these various domains.

✓ We found that those domains most likely to be impaired by the various ADHD symptoms were educational activities, followed by family responsibilities and then occupational functioning.

✓ The results of this chapter show that ADHD in adults is not a benign condition. It is associated with a high risk of impairment in one or more major life activities and more numerous such impaired activities than was the case for non-ADHD adults and certainly for Community control adults. The symptoms of ADHD, when they occur often or more frequently, are not trivial and produce an adverse impact on the ability of these adults to function satisfactorily in the vast majority of major life activities important to adult adjustment.

✓ These results also provided no evidence to support the contention of some advocates and clinicians working in this field that ADHD conveys special gifts, benefits, or other positive attributes to adults with the disorder. Indeed, it refutes such assertions by showing that virtually every domain of major life activities studied here is adversely affected to some extent by this disorder.

CHAPTER 7

Identifying New Symptoms of ADHD in Adulthood

Chapter 6 dealt with the utility of the current symptom list for ADHD in the DSM-IV-TR (American Psychiatric Association, 2000) to identify cases of ADHD relative to Community control adults and adults with other clinical disorders than ADHD. But is this the best symptom list for use with adults? As noted there, the current DSM-IV-TR symptoms were developed on children and were field tested using only children (Lahey, Applegate, McBurnett, Biederman, Greenhill et al., 1994; Spitzer, Barkley, & Davies, 1989). The utility of extending them to adults with ADHD is therefore an open question and should not be automatically assumed. As the previous chapter demonstrated, the nature of these symptoms, their underlying factor structure, their prevalence in both ADHD and non-ADHD clinical samples, their age of onset, and those symptoms most likely to distinguish the individuals with ADHD are not identical to what may be found in children with the disorder. This chapter addresses a separate but related issue, and that is whether or not better symptoms could be identified for the adult stage of this disorder than those 18 symptoms currently represented in the DSM-IV-TR.

To initially address this important issue, we began by making a list of the most common complaints made by adults presenting at the Adult ADHD Clinic at the University of Massachusetts Medical Center, where more than 100 adults were evaluated each year. This chart review included more than 200 patients who had eventually been diagnosed with ADHD. We also used items that represented the forms of adaptive behavioral difficulties they had reported, such as difficulties with workplace organization and time management, money management, and driving, among others. Furthermore, we used the theory of executive functioning (EF) developed by Barkley (1997) and its extension to understanding ADHD in order to generate potential symptoms that deal with each of the five executive components of his model. To understand those items better, a brief review of that model is now provided.

Inhibition, EF, and Self-Regulation

Barkley (1997) reviewed several previous models of the functions of the executive or prefrontal lobe developed by others in neuropsychology, noted their points of overlap and distinction, argued for their combination into a hybrid model, and discussed evidence from both neuropsychology and developmental psychology for the existence of behavioral inhibition and four separable executive functions. Research consistently shows these functions to be mediated by the prefrontal regions of the brain and to be disrupted by damage or injury to these various regions. The hybrid model is also a developmental neuropsychological model of human self-regulation. This theory specifies that behavioral inhibition, representing the first and foundation component in the model, is critical to the development, privatization, and proficient performance of the four EFs. "Privatization" refers to the fact that the model views each EF as a form of behavior or action done to oneself, where these actions are initially publicly observable but become internalized or "cognitive" over development. Behavioral inhibition permits this to occur, creates their internalization, and protects them from interference, just as it does for the generation and execution of the cross-temporal goal-directed behavior developed from these EFs. The four EFs are nonverbal working memory, internalization of speech (verbal working memory), self-regulation of affect/motivation/arousal, and reconstitution (planning and generativity). These EFs can shift behavior from control by the immediate environment to control by internally represented forms of information by their influence over the last component of the model, motor control.

"Behavioral inhibition" refers to three interrelated processes that, while distinguishable from each other, are treated here, for simplicity of explication, as a single construct: (1) inhibiting the initial prepotent response to an event; (2) stopping an ongoing response or response pattern, thereby permitting a delay in the decision to respond or continue responding; and (3) protecting this period of delay and the self-directed responses that occur within it from disruption by competing events and responses (interference control). The prepotent response is defined as that response for which immediate reinforcement (positive or negative) is available or has been previously associated with that response. The initiation of self-regulation must begin with inhibiting the prepotent response from occurring or with the interruption of an ongoing response pattern that is proving ineffective. This inhibition or interruption creates a delay in responding during

---

Structured Clinical Interview of EF

No clinical interview exists to our knowledge that provides an extensive review of symptoms of poor executive functioning (EF); therefore one was created for this project. This occurred at the end of the structured interview of ADHD symptoms and other DSM-IV-TR criteria for ADHD noted in Chapter 3. This interview instructed the participant to consider his or her behavior during the previous 6 months and to indicate whether or not each symptom had occurred as often or more so than would be typical of someone of the interviewee's age group. After every 20 items, the instruction was repeated that the participant was to respond affirmatively to an item only if it occurred as often or more so relative to peers in order to help the participant keep this important DSM-IV-TR item descriptor in mind in replying to this lengthy list of items. The 91 items shown in Table 7.1 are those taken verbatim from this interview.

---

which the EFs can occur. Thus those EFs are dependent on inhibition for their effective execution and for their regulation over the motor programming and execution component of the model (motor control). Preventing a prepotent response from occurring is critical to self-control. The individual cannot engage in self-control to maximize later outcomes related to a particular event if he or she has already acted to maximize the immediate ones related to that event or context. In essence, this situation reflects a conflict between the external now and the internally represented hypothetical future—the present self versus the future self, if you will. That future stands no chance of affecting current behavior if the individual cannot inhibit responding to the moment in order to give our sense of time and the future a chance to influence that behavior.

The third inhibitory process is interference control, often thought of as resistance to distraction. Interference control is as important to self-regulation as are the other inhibitory processes, especially during the delay in responding when the other EFs are at work. This is a time that is particularly vulnerable to both external and internal sources of interference or distraction. Task-irrelevant events playing out around the individual may be disruptive to those EFs taking place during the delay, as may be irrelevant internal thoughts of the individual; the more similar those distracting events are to the information being generated by these EFs (private behaviors), the more difficult it is to protect those functions from disruption, distortion, or perversion. Though represented here as a form of inhibition, interference control may be an inherent part of the EF of working or representational memory. The second form of inhibition (ceasing ongoing responses) may arise as an interaction of two functions. The working memory function retains information about outcomes of immediately past performance that feed forward to planning the next response. Coupled with the ability to inhibit prepotent responses, the combination thereby creates a sensitivity to errors—a capacity to track errors and use them to rapidly inhibit and shift behavior to other potentially more effective strategies. Research reviewed elsewhere (Barkley, 1997, 2006) suggests that all three inhibitory activities are impaired in ADHD, yet it is becoming increasingly evident that the inhibition of prepotent responses, termed "executive inhibition" by Nigg (2001), may be the most impaired in ADHD.

Barkley's model is one of human self-regulation. Self-regulation contains six key ingredients, implicit in its definition (Barkley, 1997):

1. Self-regulation means behavior by an individual that is directed at the individual rather than at the environmental event that may have initiated the self-regulation. It is self-directed action.

2. Such self-regulatory actions are designed to alter the probability of a subsequent response by the individual—they serve to change subsequent behavior from what it otherwise might have been had the person acted on impulse.

3. Behavior that is classified as self-regulatory serves to change the likelihood of a later rather than an immediate outcome for the greater long-term benefit of the individual. It is future directed. This process achieves a net maximization of beneficial consequences across both short- and long-term outcomes of a response for the individual, particularly when there is a discrepancy between the valences (negative vs. positive) of the short- and long-term outcomes. The individual is striving to create a net maximization of the immediate *and* the delayed consequences.

4. For self-control to occur or to even be desired by the individual, he or she must have developed a preference for the often larger long-term over the usually smaller short-term outcomes of behavior.

5. Self-regulatory actions by an individual have as an inherent property the bridging of time delays among the elements comprising behavioral contingencies. As long as there is little or no time between these elements (events, responses, and their outcomes), there is less or even no need for self-regulation. However, when time delays are introduced between these elements, self-directed actions must be undertaken to bridge them successfully—that is, to bind them together into a contingency despite the delays in time—so as to maximize the longer-term outcomes. Thus, a capacity for the cross-temporal organization of behavioral contingencies is implicit in the definition of self-regulation.

6. For self-control to occur, some neuropsychological or mental faculty must exist that permits this capacity to bind the parts of the contingency together despite large gaps in time between them. It requires a sense of time and the ability to conjecture the future and to put them to use in the organization and execution of behavior. To conjecture the future, the past must be capable of recall and analysis in order to detect patterns among chains of events and their behav-

ioral contingencies. It is from the recall of the past that such hypothetical futures can be constructed. This mental faculty is believed by Barkley to be working memory.

As noted previously, behavioral inhibition delays the decision to respond to an event. This gives self-control time to occur. The self-directed actions occurring during the delay in the response constitute, we believe, the EFs. They are often not publicly observable in older children and adults, although it is likely that in early development many of them are so. Over development, they become progressively more private or covert (cognitive) in form. The development of internalized, self-directed speech seems to exemplify this process. Although eventually "internalized," or better yet, privatized, these self-directed actions remain essentially self-directed forms of behavior despite the fact that they have become less or even not observable to others. Therefore, the term "executive function" refers here to a specific class of self-directed actions by the individual that are being used to self-regulate toward the future.

Barkley (1997) argues that there are four such classes of self-directed actions, or four EFs. Despite having distinct labels, these four executive abilities are believed to share a common purpose: to internalize or privatize behavior to anticipate change and to guide behavior toward that anticipated future. All this is done, as already noted, to maximize the net long-term outcomes or benefits for the individual. Barkley believes that these four EFs share a common characteristic: all represent private, covert forms of behavior that at one time in early child development and in human evolution were entirely public behavior and directed at managing others and the world around us. They have become turned back on the self (self-directed) as a means to control one's own behavior and have become increasingly covert, privatized, or "internalized" in form over human evolution and over a child's maturation. The four are often called by neuropsychologists (1) nonverbal working memory, (2) verbal working memory, (3) emotional self-regulation, and (4) planning or generativity. Such terms obscure the public behavioral origins of each function, however. Nonverbal working memory is, Barkley believes, the privatization of sensory-motor activities (resensing to or behaving toward the self). Verbal working memory is self-directed, private speech—the internalization of speech as Vygotsky conceived it. The third EF (emotional self-regulation) is the self-regulation of affect, motivation, and arousal. It occurs in large part, Barkley asserts, as a consequence of the first two EFs (self-directed sensory–motor behavior and speech) as well as the privatization of emotional behavior and its associated motivational features. Finally, planning and generativity, or reconstitution (analysis and synthesis), represent the internalization of human play.

The EFs represent the privatization or internalization of self-directed behavior to anticipate change in the environment (the future), where change represents essentially the concept of time. Thus, what the internalization of behavior achieves is the internalization of a conscious sense of time that is then used for the organization of behavior in anticipation of likely changes in the environment—events that probably lie ahead in time. Such behavior is therefore future-oriented and the individual who employs it can be said to be goal-directed, purposive, and intentional—or self-disciplined—in his or her actions. These EFs are interactive and coreliant in their naturally occurring state. It is the action of these functions in concert that permits and produces normal human self-regulation, especially by adulthood. Deficits in any particular EF will produce a relatively distinct impairment in self-regulation, different from that impairment in self-control produced by deficits in the other functions. Barkley argues that ADHD disrupts the EFs (private behavior) largely through its adverse impact on behavioral inhibition, the foundation of his model. By failing to inhibit prepotent responses to immediate events, those with ADHD are less able to activate and effectively utilize their system of self-directed actions (the executive system) so as to anticipate the probable future and to maximize the larger future consequences over the immediate and smaller ones. They cannot delay gratification and organize cross-temporal behavioral sequences so as to more effectively deal with the likely future as well as others of their age and intelligence.

A New Item Pool
of Potential Symptoms for ADHD in Adults

With this theory in mind and combined with the other sources of item generation noted earlier, we created the potential symptom lists for adults with ADHD. We developed a list of 91 new items that might have some potential for being associated with and predictive of ADHD at the adult stage of its development. These items are displayed in Table 7.1. We included items that further elaborated on the problems with behavioral and cognitive inhibition that are thought to be a core feature of ADHD (Barkley, 1997; Douglas, 1972; Nigg, 2001; Quay, 1988) yet which are represented by only three items in the current DSM-IV-TR list, most of which may reflect verbal impulsiveness. We therefore added items dealing with impulsive decision making, making impulsive comments to others, poor delay of gratification, doing things without considering their consequences, inability to wait (impatience) and so forth, that better reflect this construct. Other items dealt with working memory (holding information in mind that is guiding behavior), the sense and use of time (organization and time management), emotional self-regulation, and planning and forethought, all of which are derived from Barkley's theory. Other items of a less theoretical nature were included because they were often voiced by adults with ADHD as being problematic or

TABLE 7.1. EF Items from Interview by Group

Measure	ADHD %	Clinical %	Community %	χ^2	p	Pairwise contrasts
1. Finds it difficult to tolerate waiting; is impatient	75	63	5	139.9	< .001	1,2 > 3
2. Makes decisions impulsively	79	49	3	143.9	< .001	1 > 2 > 3
3. Is unable to inhibit reactions or responses to events or others	61	35	2	95.3	< .001	1 > 2 > 3
4. Has difficulty stopping activities or behavior when necessary	72	38	2	128.0	< .001	1 > 2 > 3
5. Has difficulty changing behavior when given feedback about mistakes	68	56	4	111.0	< .001	1 > 2 > 3
6. Is easily distracted by irrelevant thoughts when he or she must concentrate on something	96	84	3	255.9	< .001	1 > 2 > 3
7. Is prone to daydreaming when he or she should be concentrating on something	89	78	8	187.8	< .001	1 > 2 > 3
8. Procrastinates or puts off doing things until the last minute	94	88	27	152.7	< .001	1,2 > 3
9. Makes impulsive comments to others	56	31	3	80.9	< .001	1 > 2 > 3
10. Is likely to take shortcuts in work and not do all that he or she is supposed to do	65	36	6	91.0	< .001	1 > 2 > 3
11. Is likely to skip out on work early if it is boring or unpleasant to do	58	34	5	77.1	< .001	1 > 2 > 3
12. Can't seem to defer gratification or to put off doing things that are rewarding now so as to work for a later goal	69	49	2	116.5	< .001	1 > 2 > 3
13. Is likely to do things without considering the consequences for doing them	60	36	1	94.5	< .001	1 > 2 > 3
14. Changes plans at the last minute on a whim or last minute impulse	72	51	9	98.6	< .001	1 > 2 > 3
15. Starts a project or task without reading or listening to directions carefully	89	64	11	157.5	< .001	1 > 2 > 3
16. Has poor sense of time	63	57	3	103.8	< .001	1,2 > 3
17. Wastes or mismanages time	86	83	5	201.1	< .001	1,2 > 3
18. Fails to consider past relevant events or past personal experiences before responding to situations	44	34	1	60.4	< .001	1,2 > 3
19. Does not think about the future as much as others of his or her age seem to do	47	34	8	43.9	< .001	1,2 > 3
20. Is not prepared for work or assigned tasks	58	41	1	89.2	< .001	1 > 2 > 3
21. Fails to meet deadlines for assignments	65	43	1	109.0	< .001	1 > 2 > 3
22. Has trouble planning ahead or preparing for upcoming events	81	61	6	144.1	< .001	1 > 2 > 3
23. Forgets to do things he or she is supposed to do	82	64	5	152.7	< .001	1 > 2 > 3
24. Has difficulties with mental arithmetic	55	45	14	45.8	< .001	1,2 > 3
25. Is not able to comprehend what he or she reads as well as he or she should be able to do; has to reread material to get its meaning	81	58	12	119.3	< .001	1 > 2 > 3
26. Can't seem to remember what he or she previously heard or read about	77	53	12	106.3	< .001	1 > 2 > 3

(continued)

TABLE 7.1. (continued)

Measure	ADHD %	Clinical %	Community %	χ^2	p	Pairwise contrasts
27. Can't seem to accomplish the goals he or she set for him- or herself	84	62	7	68.6	< .001	**1 > 2 > 3**
28. Is late for work or scheduled appointments	55	44	5	68.6	< .001	1,2 > 3
29. **Has trouble organizing his or her thoughts or thinking clearly**	75	57	2	138.7	< .001	**1 > 2 > 3**
30. Is not aware of things he or she says or does	39	23	1	50.7	< .001	**1 > 2 > 3**
31. **Can't seem to hold in mind things he or she needs to remember to do**	83	69	7	153.4	< .001	**1 > 2 > 3**
32. Has difficulty being objective about things that affect him or her	64	51	5	91.5	< .001	1,2 > 3
33. Finds it hard to take other people's perspectives about a problem or situation	48	33	6	50.1	< .001	**1 > 2 > 3**
34. Has difficulty keeping in mind the purpose or goals of activities	51	34	1	74.5	< .001	**1 > 2 > 3**
35. **Forgets the point he or she was trying to make when talking to others**	75	51	2	133.9	< .001	**1 > 2 > 3**
36. When shown something complicated to do, cannot keep the information in mind so as to imitate or do it correctly	53	47	1	82.6	< .001	1,2 > 3
37. Gives poor attention to details in work	60	34	1	92.8	< .001	**1 > 2 > 3**
38. **Finds it difficult to keep track of several activities at once**	68	56	8	90.7	< .001	1,2 > 3
39. **Can't seem to get things done unless there is an immediate deadline**	89	82	6	195.3	< .001	1,2 > 3
40. Dislikes work or school activities where one must think more than usual	60	39	2	88.6	< .001	**1 > 2 > 3**
41. **Has difficulty judging how much time it will take to do something or get somewhere**	72	68	6	119.4	< .001	1,2 > 3
42. **Has trouble motivating self to start work**	80	72	6	147.4	< .001	1,2 > 3
43. Quick to get angry or become upset	63	46	7	77.6	< .001	**1 > 2 > 3**
44. **Easily frustrated**	86	70	8	156.6	< .001	**1 > 2 > 3**
45. **Overreact emotionally**	68	49	6	97.0	< .001	**1 > 2 > 3**
46. **Has difficulty motivating self to stick with work and get it done**	84	70	4	167.8	< .001	**1 > 2 > 3**
47. **Can't seem to persist at things he or she does not find interesting**	96	86	13	203.0	< .001	**1 > 2 > 3**
48. Does not put as much effort into my work as he or she should or that others are able to do	60	43	4	81.9	< .001	**1 > 2 > 3**
49. **Has trouble staying alert or awake in boring situations**	86	70	11	145.8	< .001	**1 > 2 > 3**
50. **Easily excited by activities going on nearby**	70	48	15	72.7	< .001	**1 > 2 > 3**
51. **Not motivated to prepare in advance for things that must be done**	80	62	4	147.2	< .001	**1 > 2 > 3**

(continued)

had been identified as problematic in previous studies, such as excessive speeding while driving, poor management of money, motor clumsiness, poor handwriting, and a proneness to accidents (see Barkley, 2006). Because most of these symptoms originated in Barkley's theory of EF, we consider this list to largely reflect that model and its component constructs.

These 91 items were collected in a structured interview with the participants in both studies, with each item requiring a dichotomous response format (yes/no). The participant was to indicate "yes" to an item if it was occurring "often" or more frequently, than that, as in the DSM-IV-TR. These items would have the greatest bearing on any effort to develop new symptoms to be listed in DSM-V for ADHD in adults because they would be of the same binary or dichotomous nature as those in the current DSM-IV-TR symptom list. We also collected them with reference to the same time period stipulated in the DSM-IV-TR, that being the previous 6 months as reported by participants. And we used the same descriptor of symptom frequency as in DSM-IV, that being the word "often."

We focus first and most heavily on the results for these items from the UMASS Study. We believe these results have the greatest bearing on developing new items for later DSM diagnostic criteria because this study utilized clinic-referred adults being evaluated for ADHD and that is the intended target of any such DSM criteria. Moreover, the adults with ADHD in that study had to meet the full syndromal definition for the disorder except for age of onset and so make a more convincing test for developing new diagnostic items. If, after having been defined as ADHD by the DSM items and other criteria, new symptoms can be found that do a better job at identifying (classifying) these same adults with ADHD, then the item(s) pass a more stringent and convincing test than if a non-DSM or modified DSM set of criteria were used to form the ADHD group, which was the case in the Milwaukee Study. A further concern here was the problem shown in the Milwaukee Study with relying on self-reported symptoms to capture the disorder when these cases of children with ADHD are in their early to mid-20s. As that study found, young adults growing up with ADHD are likely to significantly underreport symptoms of ADHD at age 21 and so are unlikely to meet diagnostic criteria for it at that age relative to what others report about them and their symptoms. While this situation appeared to be improving by the time these patients reached their late 20s (mean age 27) with regard to the agreement of their reports with those of others and an increase in their reported symptoms over time, the interjudge reliability of their self-reports is still lower than that of adults in their 30s and older (on average). The self-reports of the older and clinic-referred adults in the UMASS study are more reliable or valid when judged against those from others and so form a better basis for developing clinical diagnostic criteria for ADHD in adults.

Identifying New ADHD Symptoms for Adults: The UMASS Study

Obviously, as Table 7.1 shows, the symptom list served its purpose very well. *All* items occurred significantly more often in the ADHD than in the Community control group. In that sense, all 91 symptoms were problematic for the ADHD group, supporting the developmental inappropriateness of their severity, and thus had the potential to be used further in a diagnostic item set. Yet all but one of these items occurred in more of the Clinical control adults than in the Community controls as well, the exception being item No. 91. To reduce this item set down to those likely to have the greatest promise for characterizing ADHD in adults, we imposed two additional criteria. First, the item had to occur in at least 65% (roughly two-thirds) of the ADHD group (considered to be a symptom of the majority). Second, it had to occur in significantly more of the ADHD group than in the Clinical control group. There were 42 such items. However, 4 of these overlapped significantly with the DSM-IV-TR item list, so that they were not considered further for examination (Nos. 6, 23, 52, and 57 in Table 7.1). This left 38 items for further analysis.

These 38 items constituted the pool of those symptoms offering the greatest potential for characterizing ADHD in adults. They were analyzed further for their ability to accurately discriminate among the groups using logistic regression. The results of those analyses appear in Table 7.2. The items that best discriminated the ADHD patients from those in the Community control group were:

- Makes decisions impulsively.
- Has difficulty stopping activities or behavior when he or she should do so.
- Is prone to daydreaming when he or she should be concentrating.
- Have trouble planning ahead or preparing for upcoming events
- Can't persist at things not interesting to him or her.

These five items had an impressive overall classification accuracy of 99% (99% for the Community control group and 99% for the ADHD group). But just as important, a test of any new EF items for adult ADHD would be identifying those that differentiated the ADHD group from the Clinical control group. Six items did so and they were:

- Makes decisions impulsively.
- Has difficulty stopping activities or behavior when he or she should do so.
- Starts projects or tasks without reading or listening to directions carefully.
- Shows poor follow-through on promises.
- Has trouble doing things in their proper order.
- Drives with excessive speed.

TABLE 7.2. EF Deficits (Interview) That Best Discriminate ADHD from Both Control Groups

EF deficit	Beta	SE	Wald	p	Odds ratio	95%CI
From Community control group						
Makes decisions impulsively	4.57	1.30	12.40	< .001	96.79	7.6–1233.8
Has difficulty stopping activities or behavior when he or she should do so	2.70	1.20	5.12	.024	14.94	1.4–155.6
Is prone to daydreaming when you should be concentrating	2.54	1.02	6.15	.013	12.48	1.7–91.8
Have trouble planning ahead or preparing for upcoming events	3.51	1.11	10.06	.002	33.45	3.8–292.7
Can't persist at things not interesting to me	2.96	1.17	6.38	.012	19.33	1.9–192.4
From Clinical control group						
Make decisions impulsively	0.87	0.36	5.76	.016	2.40	1.2–4.9
Difficulty stopping activities or behavior when I should do so	0.62	0.35	3.08	.079	1.86	0.9–3.7
Start projects or tasks without reading or listening to directions carefully	1.22	0.43	8.14	.004	3.37	1.5–7.8
Shows poor follow-through on promises	1.06	0.34	9.50	.002	2.88	1.5–5.6
Trouble doing things in proper order	0.97	0.35	7.72	.005	2.64	1.3–5.2
Drive with excessive speed	1.35	0.34	15.47	< .001	3.84	2.0–7.5

Note. SE = standard error for beta; odds ratio = Exp(B); 95% CI = 95% confidence interval for the odds ratio. Statistical analysis: Logistic regression using forward conditional entry method.

These six items had an overall classification accuracy of 77% (65% for Clinical control group and 85% for ADHD group). This overall classification accuracy is superior to that of the interview items discussed in Chapter 4 from the DSM-IV-TR symptom list. The first two of these new EF items are the same items that proved so effective at discriminating the ADHD and Community control groups above. Readers also should not be surprised at the last symptom here (speeding), given that past studies of driving performance in adults and teens with ADHD have repeatedly identified excessive speeding with a motor vehicle as a significant problem (see Barkley, 2004; Barkley & Cox, 2007).

In view of these findings, we should consider the following nine symptoms that largely reflect EF as a potential item set for ADHD in adulthood:

- Makes decisions impulsively.
- Has difficulty stopping my activities or behavior when he or she should do so.
- Starts a project or task without reading or listening to directions carefully.
- Shows poor follow-through on promises or commitments he or she may make to others.

- Has trouble doing things in their proper order or sequence.
- Is more likely to drive a motor vehicle much faster than others (excessive speeding).
- Is prone to daydreaming when he or she should be concentrating on something.
- Has trouble planning ahead or preparing for upcoming events.
- Can't seem to persist at things he or she does not find interesting.

Factor Structure of New EF Symptoms and Old DSM-IV-TR Symptoms

Do these new items reflecting EF represent a different dimension of symptoms than those already identified as characterizing the DSM-IV-TR symptom list? Or do they more likely reflect an upward extension of the same symptom constructs used in defining child ADHD to defining adult ADHD? In Chapter 5, we showed that the DSM-IV-TR symptom list may best be characterized as involving three dimensions or factors in adults rather than the two presented in DSM-IV-TR and based on children. These three factors were inattention, hyperactivity, and impulsivity (largely verbal). To find out how these new EF symptoms related to the existing 18 symptoms from DSM-IV-TR, we conducted a factor analysis involving all 27 symptoms. The results appear in Table 7.3.

As this table clearly shows, the new EF symptoms do not constitute new constructs separate from those dimensions already thought to conceptualize ADHD in the DSM-IV-TR. This is important, because a major goal of discovering new items is to try to extend the same dimensions involved in ADHD in children up to its adult stage. Instead, these new items map quite nicely on to the three dimensions we found in Chapter 5 that comprise the DSM-IV-TR item set in adults. Factor I is largely a sustained attention–working memory–distractibility dimension and explains 44% of the variance. It is identical to that found in DSM-IV-TR for children yet clearly extends the construct of attention (sustained attention, distractibility) to include problems with working memory and organization in adults. Factor II is one of hyperactive–impulsive behavior and accounts for 7% of the variance. Noteworthy is that it also contains some item overlap with EF symptoms reflecting impulsive decision making and perseverative behavior. Finally, factor III is the same verbal impulsiveness factor noted in Chapter 5 and explains 4% of the variance. Therefore the new symptoms achieve our purpose, and that is to extend the constructs involved in ADHD from their childhood representation in DSM-IV-TR to their representation in adults with the disorder. It is no different than adding items to a vocabulary test designed for children so that it can be extended upward as a measure of vocabulary in adults.

Looking Ahead to DSM-V: A New List of Adult ADHD Symptoms

Rather than add nine new EF symptoms to the 18 symptoms already in the DSM-IV-TR, is it possible to reduce this pool of 27 items down to a more manageable size for use in the clinical diagnosis of adults? We tried to do so by using logistic regression with the entire 27-item set. We first examined those symptoms that might best distinguish the ADHD group from the Community control group. The results are shown in Table 7.4. As we saw in Chapter 5, just one item was required to achieve an overall classification accuracy of 97% for both groups—the DSM-IV-TR item of being easily distracted proved an excellent discriminator from normal cases. Three other items were able to add another 3% to this classification accuracy, and these were: difficulty sustaining attention (DSM), difficulty organizing tasks and activities (DSM), and the new EF item of poor follow through on promises or commitments I may make to others. But the latter are not really necessary for clinical purposes, as the single item of being easily distracted worked the best of all items.

Where the new EF items had greater value was in helping to distinguish the ADHD from the Clinical control group. Our analysis found seven symptoms

TABLE 7.4. DSM-IV-TR Symptoms and New EF Symptoms (from Interview) That Best Discriminate ADHD from Both Control Groups

EF deficit (origin)	Beta	SE	Wald	p	Odds ratio	95% CI
From Community control group						
Is easily distracted by extraneous stimuli (DSM)	7.43	.88	71.95	< .001	1686.62	302.96–9389.76
From Clinical control group						
Has difficulty remaining seated (DSM)	−.92	.37	6.25	.012	0.40	0.19–0.82
Makes decisions impulsively (EF)	1.04	.37	7.95	.005	2.84	1.37–5.87
Has difficulty stopping activities or behavior when he or she should do so (EF)	.70	.35	3.84	.05	2.02	1.00–4.08
Starts projects or tasks without reading or listening to directions carefully (EF)	1.29	.43	8.80	.003	3.64	1.55–8.56
Shows poor follow-through on promises (EF)	.96	.34	7.71	.005	2.61	1.33–5.13
Has trouble doing things in proper order (EF)	1.10	.36	9.44	.002	3.00	1.49–6.04
Drives with excessive speed (EF)	1.34	.35	14.89	< .001	3.84	1.94–7.60

Note. SE = standard error for beta; odds ratio = Exp(B); 95% CI = 95% confidence interval for the Odds Ratio; DSM = item is from DSM-IV-TR; EF = item is from executive function list.

Statistical analysis: Logistic regression using forward conditional entry method were needed to maximize group discrimination, with just one being from the DSM list and the remaining six from the new list of EF symptoms. These are listed in abbreviated form below and each began with the word often:

- Often leaves seat in classroom or in other situations in which remaining seated is expected (DSM). *Noteworthy here was that this item was reverse-weighted, meaning that it was significantly related to being in the Clinical control group rather than in the ADHD group.*
- Makes decisions impulsively (EF).
- Has difficulty stopping activities or behavior when he or she should do so (EF).
- Starts projects or tasks without reading or listening to directions carefully (EF).
- Shows poor follow-through on promises (EF).
- Has trouble doing things in their proper order (EF).
- Drives with excessive speed (EF).

The overall classification accuracy for these seven symptoms was 77% (88% for the ADHD cases and 64% for the Clinical control group). The one DSM hyperactive symptom making it into this classification analysis (Often leaves seat . . .) actually characterized the Clinical control group better than the ADHD group and served to rule out ADHD rather than rule it in. It should therefore not be considered a symptom of adult ADHD as it is an indication of likely not having the disorder but having some other disorder instead.

One symptom identified on this list may prove problematic in certain countries, geographic locations, or subcultures, and that is the one related to often driving a motor vehicle with excessive speed. While this proved to be a highly useful symptom for identifying our ADHD group from the Clinical control group, there will be situations in which an adult has had no experience or opportunity to drive a motor vehicle. To identify an alternate symptom that could be used in such circumstances in place of the one for driving, we reanalyzed the DSM-IV-TR symptoms and best EF symptoms as above but left out the item related to driving. The results for comparing the ADHD and Clinical control groups showed that a seven-item solution was best, with six of these items being the same as those found above. The new symptom that entered in place of speeding while driving was that of often having difficulty engaging in leisure activities or doing fun things quietly. The overall classification accuracy for this item set was 78%, virtually the same as that for the previous seven-item set found above, but the classification accuracy for the ADHD group was slightly lower, being 85% instead of 88%, while that for the Clinical control group rose slightly, from 64% to 66%. Given that the goal of this list is to try to identify the maximum percentage of ADHD cases, we recommend retaining the item pertaining to driving with excessive speed whenever patients undergoing evaluation for ADHD have experience with driving. Where they do not, the symptom related to being unable to engage in leisure activities quietly could be substituted, with only a very slight decline in ADHD classification accuracy.

We can combine the one DSM-IV item that best differentiated adults with ADHD from the Community control group with the six new EF items that served to best differentiate adults with ADHD from the Clinical control group (ignoring the reverse-weighted symptom related to staying seated when required to do so). This gives us a list of the seven best symptoms for identifying cases of ADHD. If desired, the additional two DSM items that made a nominal increase in classification accuracy between the ADHD and Community group could also be added to lengthen the list to nine symptoms. *These would be the nine items to be recommended to the DSM-V committee in considering the adoption of a specific item set for the diagnosis of ADHD in adults*:

- Is often easily distracted by extraneous stimuli (DSM-IV-TR) or irrelevant thoughts (EF).
- Often makes decisions impulsively (EF).
- Often has difficulty stopping his or her activities or behavior when he or she should do so (EF).
- Often starts a project or task without reading or listening to directions carefully (EF).
- Often shows poor follow-through on promises or commitments he or she may make to others (EF).
- Often has trouble doing things in their proper order or sequence (EF).
- Often more likely to drive a motor vehicle much faster than others (excessive speeding) (EF).
  - Substitute item for adults without driving experience: Often has difficulty engaging in leisure activities or doing fun things quietly.
- Often has difficulty sustaining attention in tasks or play activities (DSM—optional).
- Often has difficulty organizing tasks and activities (DSM—optional).

We fully realize that such a list does not incorporate symptoms of motor hyperactivity, perhaps violating the very conceptualization of ADHD or at least how it is currently subtyped in DSM-IV-TR (inattentive type, hyperactive–impulsive type, and combined type). The substitute symptom of having difficulty engaging in leisure activities quietly could be thought of as assessing this aspect of behavior, but we believe it has as much to do with impulsivity and not being able to sustain attention to more quiet activities, such as reading for pleasure, than with motor hyperactivity per se. As we noted above and in Chapter 3, ADHD is currently thought of more as a disorder of inhibition and not merely one of hyperactivity. Furthermore, if empirical grounds are the main basis for constructing a symptom list, then our analyses show that symptoms of hyperactivity do not contribute significantly to identifying adults with ADHD when evaluated in the context of the entire set of DSM-IV-TR symptoms along with the best EF items. Such a single set of symptoms, loading as it does largely on a single factor or dimension of inattention-EF symptoms, would certainly preclude using the current DSM subtyping approach to ADHD, as it would eliminate the hyperactive–impulsive subtype. But two symptoms of inhibitory problems are evident on this list, those items being makes impulsive decisions and excessive speeding (or its alternate, of not engaging in leisure activities quietly), along with several inattention items that load heavily on that dimension as well (distractibility, starting projects without reading or listening carefully to directions, failing to stop activities when one should do so). There is clearly an inhibitory problem dimension here embedded in or overlapping with the inattention one but there is no evidence here for one of motor hyperactivity that is useful for diagnosing ADHD in adults.

That is not such a bad thing however considering that the hyperactive–impulsive type is not a very common subtype diagnosed in adults with ADHD, as discussed in earlier chapters. It also has not been shown to differ in any qualitative way from the combined type of the disorder and declines markedly in prevalence with age, with most such children placed in this category ultimately moving on to the combined type within a few years (see Barkley, 2006). But if the DSM-V committee felt strongly about retaining some symptoms of hyperactivity in the official diagnostic symptom list, then the ones we identified in Chapter 3 that best distinguished the ADHD from the Community control group could be added to the symptom list as well. These were:

- Fidgets with hands/feet or squirms.
- Feels restless.
- Blurts out answers.
- Has difficulty awaiting turn.

We are not supportive of this idea, as these items lost all of their discriminatory value between ADHD and the Community control groups once a single attention–impulsivity item (being easily distracted) was entered in the regression equation. This item dwarfed all other DSM-IV-TR items in its predictive value for discerning this control group from patients with ADHD. Likewise, these symptoms of hyperactivity were of no predictive value in discriminating adults with ADHD from the Clinical control adults when inattention symptoms were entered with them in our regression analyses. In short, it is not hyperactivity that distinguishes adults with ADHD from normal adults or those having other disorders but distractibility, impulsive decision making, and poor EF (inattention). So why mislead clinicians and the public otherwise by keeping symptoms of hyperactivity in any adult symptom list? We see little merit to the idea, either for clinical diagnosis or for subtyping ADHD in adults.

As noted above, if all one wants to do in clinical diagnosis is determine if someone is normal (Community control) or not, than a single symptom (being easily distracted) does that quite well. But most adults coming to clinics for assistance are not normal and usually have some disorder. Given this circumstance, it appears from our work here that the inclusion of new EF symptoms increases the ability of this symptom set to accurately distinguish ADHD from non-ADHD clinical patients beyond that shown for the DSM items alone (see Chapter 5). While it would be nice if these symptoms could classify subjects into these two groups as well as the new symptom set has done between ADHD and normal (Community) patients (97–100%), this is asking too much. Considering that other clinical disorders are likely to have some effects on attention, executive functioning, and inhibition, this makes it more difficult for symptom presence alone to result in perfect differential diagnosis of ADHD from other disorders. Here again it will be the inclusion of additional diagnostic criteria (onset, chronic and pervasive symptoms, impairment, etc.) and clinical training concerning the core nature of other non-ADHD disorders that facilitate this differential diagnostic process. Still, the new items we have found here are not a bad start in this process of differential diagnosis.

A New Symptom Threshold for Adult ADHD for DSM-V

If the new symptom list generated above for diagnosing ADHD in adults were to be adopted in DSM-V, it would require a new threshold for the number of symptoms needed for diagnosis. Recall that the current DSM-IV recommends a threshold of six out of the nine symptoms on either the inattention list or the hyperactive–impulsive list. To examine this issue, we created a symptom summary score for both the "seven-best" symptom list and the somewhat longer "nine-best" symptom list above. We then examined the distributions of these scores for each of the three groups of participants. If the shorter list of the best seven symptoms above were to be used for diagnosis, inspection of the distribution shows that a cutoff score of four or more would work very well. We found that 99% of the Community control group fell below this threshold, so it would have a false-positive rate of just 1% for that group. And this same threshold would accurately classify or capture 94% of the ADHD group, yielding a false-negative rate of just 6%. These are very acceptable error rates for a diagnostic threshold. However, 56% of the Clinical control group would also exceed this threshold (false-positive rate), although nearly half of them would not (44% true negatives).

If the longer list of nine best symptoms from above were to be adopted, then our results show that a threshold of six symptoms would work reasonably well. Again, only 1% of the Community control group would meet or exceed that threshold, while 92% of the ADHD group would do so. But nearly half of the Clinical control group would do so as well (47%). Dropping the threshold to five symptoms would falsely identify no more Community cases than the previous 1% and would capture an additional 4% of ADHD cases (96% true positives) but would also raise the false-positive rate in the Clinical group by 18% to 65% meeting this threshold. We do not recommend doing so. Our preference would be to adopt the list of nine symptoms and to apply the threshold of six out of nine symptoms in view of the above findings. Of course, our results should be cross-validated against another sample of clinic-referred ADHD and control adults before they should be considered to be reliable, but our study does provide a starting point—it is an initial DSM-V field trial for guiding subsequent efforts at criteria development.

When we compared our three groups on their total score for the 9-best symptom list, we found that the ADHD group had significantly more such symptoms ($M = 7.3$; $SD = 1.3$) than the Clinical group ($M = 5.2$, $SD = 2.0$), which had more such symptoms than the Community control group ($M = 0.4$, $SD = 0.9$). We also found a significant interaction of group × sex on this score. Further analyses showed that males and females within the ADHD group did not differ on their average total symptom score. This was also true for the Clinical control group. But males in the Community control group had significantly higher scores than did females ($Ms = 0.7$ vs. 0.2, respectively). These results suggest that a separate threshold is not required for either males or females with ADHD in these diagnostic criteria, as they show an equivalent severity on this best symptom list. This was not the case for the DSM-IV-TR symptom totals (see Chapter 5), where we found that males in general reported more such symptoms than females across groups. This implied that a gender-based threshold on the DSM-IV-TR symptom list might be required for clinical diagnosis so as not to bias the DSM criteria against females with the disorder.

After reviewing this list of symptoms with clinical patients, clinicians might also review the list of the best symptoms of ADHD recalled from childhood (ages 5–12 years) that discriminated these groups (see Chapter 5). This serves to establish the presence of clinically significant levels of symptoms in childhood. Those symptoms were mainly ones of inattention, though one symptom of hyperactivity (always on the go or driven by a motor) and one of impulsivity (interrupts or intrudes on others) also proved useful. Added to this procedure should be establishing the onset of symptoms producing impairment by the more generous age of 14 to 16 years of age, as also recommended in Chapters 3 and 5. This would serve as an additional recommendation for the DSM-V committee to consider. Impairment would be defined relative to the average or normal population and could focus on those domains we found to be most likely to discriminate the ADHD group from the others (education, occupation, home functioning,

TABLE 7.5. Proposed DSM-V Criteria for ADHD in Adults

A. Has six (or more) of the following symptoms that have persisted for at least 6 months to a degree that is maladaptive and developmentally inappropriate:
   1. Often is easily distracted by extraneous stimuli or irrelevant thoughts
   2. Often makes decisions impulsively
   3. Often has difficulty stopping activities or behavior when he or she should do so
   4. Often starts a project or task without reading or listening to directions carefully
   5. Often shows poor follow-through on promises or commitments he or she may make to others
   6. Often has trouble doing things in their proper order or sequence
   7. Often is more likely to drive a motor vehicle much faster than others (excessive speeding) [Alternate symptom for those adults with no driving experience: Often has difficulty engaging in leisure activities or doing fun things quietly]
   8. Often has difficulty sustaining attention in tasks or play activities
   9. Often has difficulty organizing tasks and activities

B. Some symptoms that caused impairment were present in childhood to adolescence (before age 16 years).

C. Some impairment from the symptoms is present in two or more settings (e.g., work, educational activities, home life, community functioning, social relationships).

D. There must be clear evidence of clinically significant impairment in social, educational, domestic (dating, marriage or cohabiting, financial, driving, child-rearing, etc.), occupational, or community functioning.

E. The symptoms do not occur exclusively during the course of a Pervasive Developmental Disorder, Schizophrenia, or other Psychotic Disorder, and are not better accounted for by another mental disorder (e.g., Mood Disorder, Anxiety Disorder, Dissociative Disorder, or a Personality Disorder).

Coding note: For individuals who currently have symptoms that no longer meet full criteria, "in partial remission" should be specified.

Note. Copyright 2007 by Russell A. Barkley. Reprinted by permission.

money management), although other domains such as social, marital/dating, driving, should be considered for listing as well. Hypothetically, then, the DSM-V criteria for adult ADHD might resemble something like those set forth in Table 7.5.

Identifying New Symptoms for ADHD in Children Grown Up: The Milwaukee Study

We now examine some of these same issues using the groups in the Milwaukee Study of children with ADHD at adult follow-up (mean age 27). In Table 7.6 we show the results for the group comparisons for the proportion endorsing each of the nine best symptoms identified in the UMASS Study above. More of the

H+ADHD group manifested nearly all of these nine symptoms than was found in the H–ADHD, the only exception being driving at excessive speeds, where both hyperactive (H) groups were more likely to have done so than the Community control groups. The H+ADHD group also had a higher percentage of its members endorsing each of the nine symptoms than did the Community control group. On five of the nine symptoms, the H–ADHD and Community groups did not differ. The most commonly endorsed symptoms in the H+ADHD group (a majority) in decreasing order were being easily distracted, making decisions impulsively, starting projects without reading or listening carefully to directions, difficulty stopping activities when they should do so, driving at excessive speeds, difficulty sustaining attention, and poor follow through on promises. Eight of the nine symptoms appeared to work well in discriminating those children with ADHD retaining ADHD in adulthood from the other two groups. Yet the symptoms were also endorsed by a somewhat lower percentage of these cases than was found in the UMASS Study for its adults with ADHD. This was also true for the DSM-IV-TR symptoms (see Chapter 5), however, and so should

TABLE 7.6. Proportion of Each Group Experiencing the Nine Best EF Symptoms Found in the UMASS Study in the Milwaukee Study Participants

Measure	H+ADHD		H–ADHD		Community		χ^2	p	Pairwise contrasts
	N	%	N	%	N	%			
Has 6+ of 9 best EF items	28	51	7	9	4	5	51.83	< .001	1 > 2,3
Has 4+ of 9 best EF items	48	87	17	21	8	11	92.51	< .001	1 > 2,3
Has difficulty sustaining attention	28	51	11	14	4	5	44.07	< .001	1 > 2,3
Has difficulty organizing tasks	25	45	17	21	9	12	19.96	< .001	1 > 2,3
Is easily distracted	49	89	38	47	14	19	63.06	< .001	1 > 2 > 3
Makes decisions impulsively	45	82	34	42	15	20	49.31	< .001	1 > 2 > 3
Has difficulty stopping activities	32	58	12	15	7	9	47.24	< .001	1 > 2,3
Starts projects without reading or listening to directions	42	76	29	36	24	32	29.42	< .001	1 > 2,3
Shows poor follow-through on promises or commitments	28	51	13	16	6	8	36.43	< .001	1 > 2,3
Has trouble doing things in proper order or sequence	24	44	5	6	0	0	56.97	< .001	1 > 2 > 3
Drives at excessive speeds	30	54	38	47	24	32	7.27	.026	1,2 > 3

Note. Sample sizes are H+ADHD = 55, H–ADHD = 80, Community = 75. N = sample size endorsing this item; % = percent of group endorsing this item; χ^2 = results of the omnibus chi-square test; p = probability value for the chi-square test; pairwise contrasts = results of the chi-square tests involving pairwise comparisons of the three groups. H+ADHD = hyperactive group that currently has a diagnosis of ADHD at follow-up; H–ADHD = hyperactive group that does not have a diagnosis of ADHD at follow-up.

Statistical analysis: Pearson chi-square.

not be viewed as a limitation of this nine-item set of symptoms. As noted above, there are good reasons for this, including the greater propensity of these young adults to underreport their symptoms and the lower level of agreement between their own reports and those of others concerning their ADHD symptoms when compared to the clinic-referred adults in the UMASS Study.

For this reason, it is not surprising to see that only 51% of the H+ADHD participants in the Milwaukee Study endorsed enough symptoms on this list to surpass the threshold of six symptoms recommended for diagnosis above and in Table 7.5. This was, however, substantially higher than the adults in the H– ADHD (9%) and the Community control (5%) groups, providing some support for the validity of this item set. In this study, a threshold of just four symptoms would place at the +1.5 SD level above the control group mean, or approximately the 93rd percentile. As noted in earlier chapters (see, e.g., Chapters 3 and 5), this threshold is often used to define cases that are clinically significant or symptomatic. If this threshold is applied to the Milwaukee groups, we can see that the vast majority of H+ADHD adults (87%) fall above this clinical threshold. The figure is just 21% of the H–ADHD. Again, this provides some support for the validity of this nine-item set in identifying those with ADHD, even in follow-up studies of children with ADHD into adulthood. The mean number of symptoms for each group also differed significantly, with the H+ADHD group having more such symptoms (mean = 5.5, SD = 1.9) than the H–ADHD group (mean = 2.5, SD = 2.0) or than the Community control group (mean = 1.5, SD = 1.8)(F = 72.68, df = 2/207, p < .001). The latter two groups did not differ in this respect.

In Table 7.7, we show the results for all 91 of the EF symptoms studied above, this time for the Milwaukee Study groups. All symptoms were found in significantly more of the H+ADHD group than the Community control group, so this comparison is not shown in that table. Instead, the table shows just the comparison between those hyperactive children still retaining ADHD at adult follow-up and those not doing so. This is an indicator of which symptoms might prove most useful at distinguishing these groups. The items shown in boldface type are those that occurred in a majority (65% or more) of the H+ADHD group—one of the criteria used in the UMASS Study to reduce this list to those items occurring in a majority of cases of ADHD. Just 17 of these items met this requirement, compared to the 42 that did so in the UMASS Study.

We then subjected this list of 17 items to the same type of statistical analysis used in the UMASS Study (binary logistic regression) to identify the best among them at discriminating the H+ADHD group from the other two groups. Those results are shown in Table 7.8. The results identified six symptoms that worked well at differentiating the H+ADHD from the Community control group, these being:

TABLE 7.7. EF Items (from Interview) That Differed Significantly between the H+ADHD and H–ADHD Groups in the Milwaukee Study

Measure	H+ADHD %	H–ADHD %	Community %	χ^2	p	Pairwise contrasts
1. **Find it difficult to tolerate waiting; impatient**	73	39	29	25.82	< .001	1 > 2
2. **Make decisions impulsively**	82	42	20	49.31	< .001	1 > 2
3. Unable to inhibit my reactions or responses to events or others	44	15	4	34.05	< .001	1 > 2
4. Have difficulty stopping my activities or behavior when I should do so	58	15	9	47.24	< .001	1 > 2
5. Have difficulty changing my behavior when I am given feedback about my mistakes	54	14	11	40.79	< .001	1 > 2
6. **Easily distracted by irrelevant thoughts when I must concentrate on something**	84	37	19	56.21	< .001	1 > 2
7. Prone to daydreaming when I should be concentrating on something	64	40	25	19.30	< .001	1 > 2
8. **Procrastinate or put off doing things until the last minute**	87	61	71	10.85	.004	1 > 2
9. Make impulsive comments to others	56	25	15	27.78	< .001	1 > 2
10. Likely to take shortcuts in my work and not do all that I am supposed to do	51	17	13	27.71	< .001	1 > 2
11. Likely to skip out on work early if its boring or unpleasant to do	45	20	19	14.34	< .001	1 > 2
12. Can't seem to defer gratification or to put off doing things that are rewarding now so as to work for a later goal	42	20	11	18.15	< .001	1 > 2
13. Likely to do things without considering the consequences for doing them	56	26	15	27.14	< .001	1 > 2
14. **Change my plans at the last minute on a whim or last minute impulse**	69	45	17	35.71	< .001	1 > 2
15. **Start a project or task without reading or listening to directions carefully**	76	36	32	29.42	< .001	1 > 2
16. Poor sense of time	45	9	9	35.62	< .001	1 > 2
17. Waste or mismanage my time	62	27	17	30.14	< .001	1 > 2
18. Fail to consider past relevant events or past personal experiences before responding to situations	47	25	7	28.49	< .001	1 > 2
19. Do not think about the future as much as others of my age seem to do	31	17	4	18.78	< .001	1,2
20. Not prepared for work or assigned tasks	14	5	4	6.21	.045	1,2

(continued)

TABLE 7.7. (continued)

Measure	H+ADHD %	H−ADHD %	Community %	χ^2	p	Pairwise contrasts
63. Unable to work as well as others without supervision or frequent instruction	25	5	7	16.18	< .001	1 > 2
64. Have trouble doing what I tell myself to do	36	9	5	27.99	< .001	1 > 2
65. Poor follow through on promises or commitments I may make to others	51	16	8	36.43	< .001	1 > 2
66. Lack self-discipline	51	21	13	24.81	< .001	1 > 2
67. Have difficulty using sound judgement in problem situations or when under stress	40	7	7	33.20	< .001	1 > 2
68. Trouble following the rules in a situation	49	10	7	43.89	< .001	1 > 2
69. Not very flexible in my behavior or approach to a situation; overly rigid in how I like things done	51	32	15	19.65	< .001	1 > 2
70. Have trouble organizing my thoughts	53	14	5	47.08	< .001	1 > 2
71. **Have difficulties saying what I want to say**	66	31	12	41.05	< .001	1 > 2
72. Unable to come up with or invent as many solutions to problems as others seem to do	36	12	7	21.76	< .001	1 > 2
73. Am often at a loss for words when I want to explain something to others	44	34	15	13.91	.001	1,2
74. Have trouble putting my thoughts down in writing as well or as quickly as others	47	32	17	13.45	.001	1,2
75. Feel I am not as creative or inventive as others of my level of intelligence	25	16	5	10.44	.005	1,2
76. In trying to accomplish goals or assignments, find I am not able to think of as many ways of doing things as others	36	5	5	34.21	< .001	1 > 2
77. Have trouble learning new or complex activities as well as others	29	7	3	23.86	< .001	1 > 2
78. Have difficulty explaining things in their proper order or sequence	47	12	8	113.7	< .001	1 > 2
79. **Can't seem to get to the point of my explanations as quickly as others**	71	34	20	35.98	< .001	1 > 2
80. Have trouble doing things in their proper order or sequence	44	6	0	56.97	< .001	1 > 2
81. Unable to "think on my feet" or respond as effectively as others to unexpected events	36	10	5	26.40	< .001	1 > 2

(continued)

TABLE 7.7. (continued)

Measure	H+ADHD %	H–ADHD %	Community %	χ^2	p	Pairwise contrasts
82. Am clumsy; not as coordinated in my movements as others	31	11	7	16.09	< .001	1 > 2
83. Poor or sloppy handwriting	69	41	33	17.39	< .001	1 > 2
84. Have difficulty arranging or doing my work by its priority or importance; can't "prioritize" well	36	11	7	22.95	< .001	1 > 2
85. Am slower to react to unexpected events	31	11	4	20.01	< .001	1 > 2
86. Get silly, clown around, or act foolishly when I should be serious	58	44	20	20.64	< .001	1,2
87. Can't seem to remember things I have done or places I have been as well as others seem to do	44	19	19	13.36	.001	1 > 2
88. Accident prone	25	11	9	7.71	.021	1 > 2
89. More likely to drive a motor vehicle much faster than others (excessive speeding)	54	47	32	7.27	.026	1,2
90. Have difficulties managing my money or credit cards	71	42	19	35.75	< .001	1 > 2
91. I am less able to recall events from my childhood compared to others	66	36	19	29.70	< .001	1 > 2

Note. Sample sizes are H+ADHD = 55, H–ADHD = 80, Community control = 75. % = percent of group endorsing this item; χ^2 = results of the omnibus chi-square test; p = probability value for the chi-square test; pairwise contrasts = results of the chi-square tests involving pairwise comparisons of the three groups (in view of the large number of analyses conducted here, significance was set a $p < .001$ for all omnibus chi-square initial tests and a $p < .01$ for all pairwise comparisons); H+ADHD = hyperactive group that currently has a diagnosis of ADHD at follow-up; H–ADHD = hyperactive group that does not have a diagnosis of ADHD at follow-up. Items in **bold** type were those endorsed by at least 65% of the ADHD group.
Statistical analysis: Pearson chi-square.

- Finds it difficult to tolerate waiting; is impatient.
- Makes decisions impulsively.
- Is easily distracted by irrelevant thoughts.
- Can't seem to hold in mind things he or she needs to remember to do.
- Has trouble staying alert or awake in boring situations.
- Is less able to recall events from his or her childhood compared to others.

The first four of these are very similar to those items found in the UMASS Study to be of some utility in diagnosing ADHD in adults. The latter two are new and obviously have more pertinence to children with ADHD as adults who have retained their disorder. Again, being easily distracted was the best symptom for distinguishing these two groups, alone producing an accuracy of classification of 82%. The remaining five items added just 11% more accuracy to this discrimination. Again, this illustrates how useful this symptom is at ruling out individuals who are essentially normal (or at least qualify for a control group). A more stringent test is to see which items significantly distinguished the two hyperactive groups from each other. These results are shown in Table 7.8 as well, and the five surviving symptoms are listed below:

- Makes decisions impulsively.
- Is easily distracted by irrelevant thoughts.
- Starts projects or tasks without reading or listening to directions carefully.
- Can't seem to hold in mind things he or she needs to remember to do.
- Can't seem to sustain his or her concentration on reading, paperwork, lectures, or work.

All of these are either identical or highly similar to the symptoms that emerged as the best in the UMASS Study, and several overlap with those found just above to differentiate the H+ADHD from the Community control group. Combining them, then, would give the best list of symptoms from the Milwaukee Study for identifying ADHD in those who, now grown up, had the disorder as children. That combined list of eight symptoms is shown below:

TABLE 7.8. EF Deficits (from Interview) That Best Discriminate H+ADHD from H–ADHD and Community Control Groups in the Milwaukee Study

EF deficit	Beta	SE	Wald	p	Odds ratio
From Community control group					
Find it difficult to tolerate waiting; impatient	1.69	.753	4.84	.028	5.25
Make decisions impulsively	2.84	.998	8.10	.004	17.10
Easily distracted by irrelevant thoughts	1.34	.772	3.00	.083	3.81
Can't seem to hold in mind things I need to remember to do	2.96	.864	11.74	.001	19.33
Have trouble staying alert or awake in boring situations	1.81	.879	4.26	.039	6.13
I am less able to recall events from my childhood compared to others	3.47	1.07	10.55	.001	32.00
From H–ADHD group					
Make decisions impulsively	1.22	.510	5.69	.017	3.38
Easily distracted by irrelevant thoughts	1.27	.509	6.21	.013	3.56
Start projects or tasks without reading or listening to directions carefully	1.03	.489	4.40	.036	2.79
Can't seem to hold in mind things I need to remember to do	1.65	.481	11.71	.001	5.19
Can't seem to sustain my concentration on reading, paperwork, lectures, or work	1.25	.478	6.81	.009	3.48

Note. SE = standard error for beta; odds ratio = Exp(B); H+ADHD = hyperactive group classified as having ADHD at adult follow-up; H–ADHD = hyperactive group not classified as having ADHD at adult follow-up.
Statistical analysis: Logistic regression using forward conditional entry method.

- Makes decisions impulsively.
- Is easily distracted by irrelevant thoughts.
- Starts projects or tasks without reading or listening to directions carefully.
- Can't seem to hold in mind things he or she needs to remember to do.
- Can't seem to sustain his or her concentration on reading, paperwork, lectures, or work.
- Finds it difficult to tolerate waiting; is impatient.
- Has trouble staying alert or awake in boring situations.
- Is less able to recall events from childhood compared to others.

If we combine these 8 items with the 18 in the DSM-IV-TR, we can determine whether any of the new items might work better than the DSM-IV-TR items at identifying ADHD in adulthood in children growing up with the disorder, much as we did above for the UMASS Study. Those analyses appear in Table 7.9. The results of those analyses show that the following are the best eight symptoms for achieving significant discrimination of the H+ADHD group from

TABLE 7.9. Best EF Deficits and DSM-IV-TR Symptoms (from Interview) That Best Discriminate H+ADHD from H–ADHD and Community Control Group in the Milwaukee Study

EF deficit	Beta	SE	Wald	p	Odds ratio
From Community control group					
Feel restless (DSM)	2.93	1.07	7.28	.007	18.72
Easily distracted by extraneous events (DSM)	3.11	1.02	9.32	.002	22.53
Difficulty awaiting my turn (DSM)	2.47	1.12	4.88	.027	11.88
Make impulsive decisions (EF)	2.68	1.30	4.17	.041	14.12
Can't seem to hold in mind things I need to remember to do (EF)	3.17	1.08	8.60	.003	23.95
I am less able to recall events from my childhood compared to others (EF)	4.01	1.39	8.46	.004	55.00
From H–ADHD group					
Fail to listen when spoken to directly (DSM)	1.82	0.70	6.67	.010	6.20
Feel restless (DSM)	1.05	0.59	3.13	.077	2.86
Fail to follow through on instructions (DSM)	1.43	0.73	3.88	.049	4.19
Difficulty awaiting my turn (DSM)	1.90	0.68	7.72	.005	6.60
Easily distracted by irrelevant thoughts (EF)	1.27	0.62	4.23	.040	3.57
Can't seem to hold in mind things I need to remember to do (EF)	1.44	0.58	6.30	.012	4.24
Can't seem to sustain my concentration on reading, paperwork, lectures, or work (EF)	1.67	0.60	7.67	.006	5.30

Note. SE = standard error for beta; odds ratio = Exp(B).
Statistical analysis: Logistic regression using forward conditional entry method.

the other two groups. The origin of the symptom is shown in parentheses as either coming from the DSM list of the new pool of EF items:

- Feels restless (DSM).
- Is easily distracted by extraneous events or irrelevant thoughts (DSM/EF).
- Has difficulty awaiting his or her turn (DSM).
- Makes decisions impulsively (EF).
- Can't seem to hold in mind things he or she needs to remember to do (EF).
- Is less able to recall events from his or her childhood compared to others (EF).
- Can't seem to sustain his or her concentration on reading, paperwork, lectures, or work (EF).
- Fails to listen when spoken to directly (DSM)

While these are not entirely the same as the best symptoms found in the UMASS Study for clinic-referred adults with ADHD, some are identical and others are conceptually very similar. Problems with making impulsive decisions, being easily distracted, difficulty waiting for things, problems with concentration and listening, and working memory (hold information in mind) clearly overlap with the same constructs found to be useful in developing the best symptom list in the UMASS Study. In that sense, these results serve to replicate, further validate, and extend those earlier results giving some confidence in their utility for identifying ADHD in adults.

We found that a score of 4 or more of these 8 symptoms would do very well at distinguishing the H+ADHD group from the Community control group (92% H+ADHD and 94% for Community controls). Though not as good, this threshold would do a pretty fair job at distinguishing the H+ADHD from the H–ADHD group, where 24% of the latter group would place above this threshold. Yet we feel it necessary to reiterate the point here that the results from the UMASS Study seem to us to have greater utility for developing diagnostic criteria for use in adults with ADHD given that the focus of that study was clinic-referred adults, the very target population to which the DSM-IV-TR diagnostic criteria would be intended.

Conclusions and Clinical Implications

This chapter addressed a very important question of whether or not the symptoms as currently presented in DSM-IV-TR, and developed solely on children, are the best that can be developed for the evaluation of ADHD in adults. Here we attempted to identify potentially better symptoms for doing so from a pool of 91 new items for comparison with the 18 DSM-IV symptoms.

✓ We analyzed of a large item pool originally of 91 symptoms in the UMASS Study that mainly comprised difficulties with EF. While results indicated that more adults with ADHD were likely to have problems with all of these largely executive symptoms than were Community control adults, we were able to reduce this pool down to 38 symptoms that were present in at least 65% of ADHD cases while also being significantly more likely to be present in those cases than in the Clinical control group.

✓ Regression analyses were used to reduce this item pool down to the nine best EF symptoms for discriminating among these groups. These nine symptoms appeared to load on the same dimensions (factors) of inattention and hyperactive–impulsive behavior as was found to exist for the DSM symptom list in Chapter 5.

✓ This suggests that these two symptom dimensions actually assess a broader domain of cognitive functioning than their names imply, most likely that of EF.

✓ We then analyzed these nine EF symptoms in the context of the existing 18 DSM items to see if they were redundant or were in fact better at discriminating among these three groups. Our results showed that six of these EF symptoms and just one DSM-IV-TR inattention symptom (easily distracted) would be the best symptom list for identifying ADHD in adults. Adding two additional inattention symptoms would slightly enhance group classification thus yielding a set of nine symptoms that could be recommended for consideration for use in DSM-V for the diagnosis of adult ADHD.

✓ We further found that a total of six out of these nine best symptoms would be a useful diagnostic threshold accurately classifying 99% of Community controls, 92% of ADHD patients, and 53% of Clinical patients. Along with a review of the best childhood recollected DSM symptoms (mainly inattention) and the use of a revised age of onset of 14 to 16 years for symptoms producing impairment, both discussed in Chapter 5, these nine best symptoms and the threshold of six of these nine would comprise a better diagnostic algorithm for ADHD in adults than do the current DSM-IV-TR criteria. We offered these nine symptoms and this cutoff score in Table 7.5 as a better set of criteria for diagnosing ADHD in adults than is the DSM-IV-TR.

✓ We then examined the use of this symptom list in the Milwaukee Study and found that these nine items worked well at distinguishing children with

ADHD who retained their disorder at age-27 follow-up, though not quite as well as they did in the UMASS Study. We repeated the same analyses used in the UMASS Study to the original item pool but using the Milwaukee groups instead and found a largely similar though not identical set of eight items to work well in identifying the H+ADHD group from the other two groups.

✓ Both studies suggest that items which emphasize distractibility, impulsiveness, poor concentration or persistence, and problems with working memory and organization will be the best constructs for identifying adults with ADHD. Items reflecting hyperactivity proved much less useful for doing so in both studies.

✓ The results of this chapter indicate that clinicians need not use the current DSM-IV-TR symptom list to identify adults with ADHD. A smaller, more time-efficient list of nine symptoms based largely on the construct of impulse control and attention–EF is superior to the DSM-IV-TR in accurately classifying adults with ADHD from both Clinical and Community control groups.

✓ Our results also serve to inform clinicians that adults with ADHD are far more likely to complain of difficulties involving EF than they are of hyperactivity. Difficulties with impulsive decision making, stopping, starting, and organizing activities, persistence toward goals, and planning for future events will prove to be among the most significant complaints in identifying these adults with ADHD.

CHAPTER 8

Comorbid Psychiatric Disorders and Psychological Maladjustment

Just as do children and adolescents diagnosed with ADHD (Barkley, 2006), adults given a clinical diagnosis of ADHD have considerably higher rates of co-morbidity with certain other psychiatric disorders than would be expected from the base rates of those disorders in the population at large (Marks, Newcorn, & Halperin, 2001). Although there is some general consistency in the pattern of comorbidity seen in adults with ADHD compared to their childhood counter-parts, there are also some important differences, as discussed in this chapter.

Like children with ADHD, adults with the disorder have been found in prior studies to have a greater risk for comorbid oppositional defiant disorder (ODD) and conduct disorder (CD) than do either clinical control groups with-out a diagnosis of ADHD or normal, nonreferred adults. Approximately 24 to 35% of clinic-referred adults diagnosed with ADHD have ODD and 17 to 25% have CD, either currently or over the course of their earlier development (Barkley, Murphy, & Kwasnik, 1996; Biederman et al., 1993; Murphy & Barkley, 1996; Murphy et al., 2002; Spencer, 2004). These figures for clinic-referred adults are below those reported in studies of ADHD children, particu-larly studies of hyperactive children followed to adulthood, where levels of ODD and CD may be double or triple these rates reported for adults diagnosed with ADHD (see Barkley, 2006, for a review; Barkley et al., 1990; Fischer et al., 2002; Weiss & Hechtman, 1993). Among parents of children having ADHD who also meet criteria for ADHD, disruptive behavior disorders also occur significantly more often (McGough et al., 2005; Minde et al., 2003). For instance, one study found that 53% have had ODD and 33% have had CD at some time in their lives (Biederman et al., 1993), figures closer to those seen in follow-up studies of hyperactive or ADHD children. Antisocial personality disorder is often an associated adult outcome in a large minority of those children or adolescents who have both ADHD and CD; thus it is not surprising to find that 7 to 44% of clinic-referred adults diagnosed with ADHD also qualify for a diagnosis of this personality disorder (Biederman et al., 1993; Shekim et al., 1990; Torgersen, Gjervab, & Rasmussen, 2006). Even among those who do not qualify for this diagnosis, many receive higher than normal ratings on those personality traits associated with this personality disorder (Tzelepis, Schubiner, & Warbase, 1995).

Substance dependence and abuse are known to occur to a more frequent degree among hyperactive children or children with ADHD who develop CD by adolescence or antisocial personality disorder by adulthood (Barkley, 2006; Tercyak, Peshkin, Walker, & Stein, 2002). A recent study of a large general population sample likewise found an association between ADHD in adults and antisocial personality disorder (Kessler et al., 2006). Adults clinically diagnosed with ADHD seem to be no exception to this rule, linking ADHD with antisocial activities as well as with drug use disorders. Studies have found lifetime rates of alcohol dependence or abuse disorders ranging between 21% and 53% of adults diagnosed with ADHD, whereas 8 to 32% may manifest some other form of substance dependence or abuse disorder (Barkley, Murphy, & Kwasnik, 1996; Biederman, 2004; Biederman et al., 1993; Biederman et al., 1995; Minde et al., 2003; Murphy & Barkley, 1996; Murphy et al., 2002; Roy-Byrne et al., 1997; Shekim et al., 1990; Wilens, 2004). Tzelepis et al. (1995) reported that 36% of their 114 adults with ADHD had experienced dependence on or abuse of alcohol, 21% for cannabis, 11% for cocaine or other stimulants, and 5% for polydrug dependence. Moreover, at the point of their initial evaluation, 13% met criteria for alcohol dependence or abuse within the previous month. Likewise, Torgersen et al. (2006) found that 45% of their sample of 45 adults with ADHD in Norway had lifetime alcohol abuse (33% currently), 51% for cannabis (36% currently), 49% for amphetamines (33% currently), and 16% for opiates (4% currently). Parents of ADHD children who have ADHD have also been found to have elevated risks for substance use disorders, primarily involving alcohol (McGough et al., 2005; Minde et al., 2003).

More recently, cigarette smoking has been shown to have an association with increased symptoms of ADHD in a general population sample of adults (Kollins, McClellan, & Fuemmeler, 2005). This finding is consistent with longitudinal studies of ADHD children that find them to carry an increased risk for smoking by adolescence (Milberger, Biederman, Faraone, Chen, & Jones, 1997; Molina, Smith, & Pelham, 1999; Tercyak, et al., 2002; Whalen, Jamner, Henker, Delfino, & Lozano, 2002). The highest risks for substance use disorders appears to be among those adults with ADHD who may also have comorbid CD, antisocial personality disorder, or bipolar disorder (Wilens, 2004).

Approximately 25% of children with ADHD have an anxiety disorder (see Barkley, 2006; Tannock, 2000). Most studies of ADHD in adults likewise find an overrepresentation of these disorders. The corresponding figure among adults is 24 to 43% for generalized anxiety disorder and 52% for a history of overanxious disorder (Barkley et al., 1996; Biederman et al., 1993; Minde et al., 2003; Shekim et al., 1990). Torgersen et al. (2006) found that 13% of their adults with ADHD had lifetime panic disorder and 18% lifetime social phobia. But not all studies of ADHD in adults have found it to be associated with anxiety disorders. Several of our own prior studies (Murphy & Barkley, 1996; Murphy et al., 2002) did not find anxiety to be overrepresented in those clinical samples of adults with ADHD. Neither did Roy-Byrne et al. (1997) in comparison to a clinical control group. The prevalence of anxiety disorders among adults with ADHD who are relatives of clinically diagnosed ADHD children, however, is 20%, again suggesting some comorbidity with ADHD (Biederman et al., 1993). Parents of children with ADHD who themselves have ADHD likewise have significantly more anxiety disorders than do those parents in a control group (McGough et al., 2005; Minde et al., 2003). In conclusion, there is some inconsistency in findings concerning the comorbidity of ADHD in adults with adult anxiety disorders, but the weight of the evidence favors some association, as it does in childhood ADHD (Angold, Costello, & Eiraldi, 1999).

Major depression does seem to have some inherent affinity with ADHD in children, especially those having CD (Angold et al., 1999). Similarly, approximately 16 to 31% of adults meeting ADHD diagnostic criteria also have major depressive disorder (Barkley et al., 1996; Biederman et al., 1993; Roy-Byrne et al., 1997; Tzelepis et al., 1995). Indeed, one study of Norwegian adults with ADHD reported a lifetime prevalence of 53% and current prevalence of 9% for major depression (Torgersen et al., 2006). Dysthymia, a milder form of depression, has been reported to occur in 19 to 37% of clinic-referred adults diagnosed with ADHD (Murphy et al., 2002; Roy-Byrne et al., 1997; Shekim et al., 1990; Tzelepis et al., 1995). Some follow-up studies have not been able to document an increased risk for depression among hyperactive children followed to adulthood (Weiss & Hechtman, 1993). However, the Milwaukee follow-up study of a large sample of hyperactive children found a prevalence of 27% for major depression by young adulthood—a finding quite consistent with the studies on clinic-referred adults diagnosed with ADHD. Even so, a few studies, including one of our own, that compared clinic-referred adults with ADHD to adults seen at the same clinic without ADHD have not found a higher incidence of depression among the ADHD group (Murphy & Barkley, 1996; Roy-Byrne et al., 1997). Rucklidge and Kaplan (1997) reported one of the few studies of women with ADHD and found them to report more symptoms of depression, anxiety, stress, low self-esteem, and a more external locus of control than did women in the control group. They later found this to be true of men with ADHD (Rucklidge, Brown, Crawford, & Kaplan, 2007). But psychiatric diagnoses were not reported in these studies, making it difficult to compare to earlier research using such diagnoses. In a study of parents of ADHD children who also have ADHD, Minde et al. (2003) did not find a greater prevalence of major depression relative to a control group of parents (15% vs. 8%). The study, however, used small samples, limiting its representation of parents with ADHD and its statistical power to detect group differences. It also did not find elevated rates of antisocial personality disorder, which, as discussed above, might be a potential moderator between ADHD and depression. In contrast, the much larger study of parents with ADHD who also had children with ADHD by McGough et al. (2005) did find greater mood disorders than in their comparison group. In general, the weight of the evidence suggests a significant relationship between ADHD in adults and risk for depression, as it does in children with the disorder.

The relationship of ADHD in adults to bipolar disorder (BPD) has not been well studied. Follow-up studies of children with ADHD into adulthood typically do not report elevated rates of this disorder by adult outcome (Barkley, 2006; Barkley, Fischer, Smallish, & Fletcher, 2002). But other studies of children with ADHD have found an elevated risk for BPD (6–27%)(Barkley, 2006; Biederman, 2004). Studies by Biederman and colleagues have also reported an elevated risk for this disorder in clinic-referred adults (11–14%)(Biederman, 2004). In contrast, in the Norwegian sample studied by Torgersen et al. (2006), the prevalence was 7% for lifetime disorder and 2% currently. That figure is comparable to what is often found in follow-up studies of hyperactive/ADHD children into adulthood (Fischer et al., 2002) and is close to the base rate for the general population. The relationship of ADHD to BPD in adults is therefore open to some doubt; it is in need of more research before some confidence can be placed in this pattern of comorbidity.

Obsessive–compulsive disorder (OCD) was initially reported to occur in 14% of clinically diagnosed adults with ADHD (Shekim et al., 1990). However, Tzelepis et al. (1995) were unable to replicate this finding and reported only 4% of their adults met diagnostic criteria for OCD. Roy-Byrne et al. (1997) likewise reported a 4.3 to 6.5% prevalence rate, which was not significantly different from their clinical control group. Spencer (1997) found that OCD was more common (12%) only among those adults with a comorbid tic disorder, whereas the figure for those adults with ADHD without tics was approximately 2%. Thus, OCD does not appear to be significantly associated with ADHD in clinic-referred adults unless Tourette syndrome or tic disorders are also present.

To summarize, past research suggests a higher than expected association between ADHD in adults and comorbid ODD, CD, antisocial personality disorder, substance use disorders, and probably depressive disorders (major depression and dysthymia). The link between ADHD and substance use disorders is likely mediated by the association of ADHD with CD or antisocial personality, and so may be the link between ADHD and major depression. The relationship between adult ADHD and adult anxiety disorders is inconsistent in past research. The link between ADHD and bipolar disorder is even less well established, especially for adults with ADHD. There seems to be no elevated risk for OCD among adults with ADHD.

Comorbid Psychiatric Disorders

The UMASS Study Results

In the present UMASS Study, we evaluated comorbidity for psychiatric disorders using the Structured Clinical Interview for DSM-IV Disorders (SCID) (Spitzer, Williams, Gibbon, & First, 1995) (see sidebar). The results are shown in Table 8.1. We found that both the ADHD group and the Clinical control group were more likely to have experienced major depression either currently, in the past, or at any time in life compared to the clinical control group. The occurrence of depression in the ADHD group is comparable to that seen in some prior studies and is certainly elevated over that seen in the Community control group (Marks et al., 2004; Spencer, Wilens, Biederman, Wozniak, & Harding-Crawford, 2000). But it was not elevated over that seen in other non-ADHD patients presenting to the same clinic as the ADHD adults. It is therefore not clear from our results that major depression is a specific comorbidity for ADHD in adults or whether it reflects a nonspecific association with clinic-referral status. The fact that ADHD relatives of children with ADHD also have elevated rates of depression does suggest some familial/genetic association between the disorders, as does the literature on comorbidity between the disorders in epidemiological samples of children (Angold et al., 1999) and adults (Kessler et al., 2006). As discussed in Chapter 5, our Clinical control group certainly had elevated symptoms of ADHD relative to the Community control group, even though they were not eventually diagnosed in this study as having ADHD. The risk for major depression may therefore be elevated in adults having elevated levels of ADHD symptoms, even though those levels may not rise to that qualifying for the diagnosis on all diagnostic criteria or in clinical judgment. The results of Roy-Byrne et al. (1997) are supportive of such an interpretation, given that they also found equally elevated levels of major depression in their clinical control and ADHD groups. Thus there may be true comorbidity between these two dimensions of psychopathology, which would be consistent with both past research and the present findings of elevated rates of depression in both our ADHD patients and

Structured Clinical Interview for DSM-IV Disorders (SCID) (Spitzer et al., 1995)

This set of semistructured interviews is used to make Axis I and Axis II diagnoses from the DSM-IV-TR. The SCID provides an interview covering the diagnostic criteria for mood disorders (major depression, mania, dysthymia), psychotic and associated symptoms, psychoactive substance use disorders, anxiety disorders, somatoform disorders, eating disorders, and adjustment disorder. All disorders were evaluated for their lifetime occurrence. The SCID-II reviews diagnostic criteria for 12 current personality disorders (avoidant, dependent, obsessive–compulsive, passive–aggressive, histrionic, self-defeating, antisocial, borderline, etc.). Administration procedures followed those set forth in the manual associated with these interviews. Information on interjudge agreement for the diagnoses was not collected in this project. For this project, only those modules from the SCID pertaining to the following disorders were selected for review with participants: major depression, dysthymia, generalized anxiety disorder, bipolar disorder, obsessive–compulsive disorder, alcohol dependence, alcohol abuse, and cannabis dependence and abuse. These modules were selected because of past research by us (Murphy et al., 2002) showing an elevation in the occurrence of these disorders in adults with ADHD or because there appeared to be some controversy in the literature concerning its association with ADHD.

The Symptom Checklist–90—Revised (Derogatis, 1986)

This scale provides a Global Severity Index as well as *T*-scores for nine specific scales of maladjustment (e.g. anxiety, paranoid ideation, interpersonal hostility, depression). It was used here to evaluate comorbidity for various psychopathological dimensions in addition to the evaluation of psychiatric diagnostic categories provided by the DSM-IV-TR–based clinical interview (SCID).

Young Adult Behavior Checklist

We obtained ratings from both the participants and, where possible, from parents (chiefly mothers) about these participants using the Young Adult Behavior Checklist (YABCL; Achenbach, 2001). Like its childhood counterpart the Child Behavior Checklist, the young adult version contains 137 items pertaining to behavior problems scores as 0, 1, or 2, some of which form a social problems dimension. *T*-scores are generated relative to a normal control group on eight scales measuring psychological maladjustment. These are: anxiety–depression, withdrawn, somatic complaints, thought problems, attention problems, intrusive, aggressive, and delinquent.

TABLE 8.1. Comorbid Psychiatric Disorders by Group for the UMASS Study

Measure	ADHD N	ADHD %	Clinical N	Clinical %	Community N	Community %	χ^2	p	Pairwise contrasts
Major depression now	19	13	14	14	1	1	13.9	.001	1,2 > 3
Major depression past	33	23	18	19	8	7	10.7	.005	1,2 > 3
Major depression ever	52	36	32	33	9	8	27.0	< .001	1,2 > 3
Dysthymia now	37	25	13	13	0	0	32.9	< .001	1 > 2 > 3
Dysthymia past	2	1	3	3	0	0	3.5	NS	
Dysthymia ever	39	27	16	16	0	0	33.8	< .001	1,2 > 3
Generalized anxiety now	23	16	14	14	1	1	16.1	< .001	1,2 > 3
Generalized anxiety past	2	1	0	0	0	0	2.8	NS	
Generalized anxiety ever	25	17	14	14	1	1	17.5	< .001	1,2 > 3
Bipolar disorder now	3	2	4	4	0	0	4.5	NS	
Bipolar disorder past	0	0	0	0	0	0	—	NS	
Bipolar disorder ever	3	2	4	4	0	0	4.5	NS	
OCD now	3	2	7	7	0	0	10.2	.006	2 > 1,3
OCD past	1	1	2	2	0	0	2.6	NS	
OCD ever	4	3	9	9	0	0	13.1	.001	2 > 1,3
Alcohol dep./abuse now[S]	26	18	12	12	0	0	20.9	< .001	1,2 > 3
Alcohol dep./abuse past[S]	27	18	12	12	11	10	4.0	NS	
Alcohol dep./abuse ever[S]	53	36	24	25	11	10	22.9	< .001	1,2 > 3
Cannabis dep./abuse now[S]	21	14	9	9	2	2	11.9	.003	1,2 > 3
Cannabis dep./abuse past[S]	28	19	7	7	4	4	17.3	< .001	1 > 2,3
Cannabis dep./abuse ever[S]	49	34	16	16	6	6	31.6	< .001	1 > 2,3

Note. N = sample size endorsing this item; % = percent of group endorsing this item; χ^2 = results of the omnibus chi-square test; *p* = probability value for the chi-square test; pairwise contrasts = results of the chi-square tests involving pairwise comparisons of the three groups; OCD = obsessive–compulsive disorder; Dep. = dependence; [S] = main effect for sex.

Clinical controls. But the difference between ADHD and the Clinical controls does not rise to the level of significance.

In contrast, we did find an increased risk for current dysthymia in the ADHD group relative to both the Clinical and Community control groups. The Clinical control group also showed a higher risk for dysthymia than the Community control group but not to the degree shown in the ADHD group. Rates of past dysthymia were not significantly different among the groups, but because of the greater risk of current dysthymia, both the ADHD and Clinical groups had a significantly greater risk of having ever had dysthymia than did the Community group. Past studies found that 17 to 37% of adults with ADHD experienced dysthymia (see above), and our results accord with the higher end of this range

We also found an increased risk for current cannabis dependence and abuse disorders in our ADHD group compared to our Community control group, consistent with our prior study (Murphy et al., 2002). But this risk was also elevated in the Clinical control group, which did not differ from the ADHD group in this respect. The ADHD group did show an increased rate of past such disorders compared to both control groups. As a consequence, the ADHD group had an elevated risk for lifetime occurrence of these disorders compared to both control groups. Our findings suggest a specific comorbidity between ADHD and cannabis use disorders. As we discuss in Chapter 11, on health and lifestyle risks, the ADHD group had an increased likelihood of smoking, and that served to mediate this risk for greater cannabis use. In other words, it is among the adults with ADHD who smoke cigarettes that one is likely to find the increased risk for cannabis use as well.

There were two other disruptive behavior disorders that were prominent in the literature noted above on comorbidity with ADHD: ODD and CD. The SCID does not have modules for these particular disorders. But we did obtain reports of these symptoms on our self-report rating scales of retrospectively recalled childhood ADHD (see sidebar in Chapter 5). From these scales, we were able to determine if participants met symptom thresholds for these two disorders retrospectively at some time during childhood. For ODD, the total number of ODD symptoms was significantly different across groups, with the ADHD group having significantly greater symptoms relative to both control groups [ADHD: M = 3.7 (SD = 2.8), Clinical: M = 1.5 (2.1), and Community: M = 0.3 (0.8)]. There were no main effects or interactions for sex. The proportion of each group having ODD was ADHD = 50% (N = 71), Clinical = 18% (17), and Community = 2% (2) (χ^2 = 78.96, df = 2, p < .001). Consistent with all prior studies discussed above, the ADHD group had a markedly greater risk for ODD than did either of the two control groups, making it clear that ADHD and ODD are specifically associated with each other in the childhood histories of adults with ADHD. The Clinical control group also had a greater rate than the Community group but fell well below that seen in the ADHD group. The main effect for sex was also significant, with more males having ODD as children (31%) than females (20%), χ^2 = 5.2, df = 1, p = .022. Even so, there was no interaction of sex with group in these analyses.

Concerning past occurrence of CD, we found that 25% of the ADHD group and 16% of the Clinical control group qualified for this diagnosis retrospectively, while the rate for the Community control group was 7%. The ADHD and Clinical control groups did not differ significantly from each other in this respect, but both differed from the Community control group. Our results are certainly consistent with past studies comparing ADHD and community control samples, which found a higher risk for CD in association with ADHD. Yet they also suggest that this risk is elevated in non-ADHD clinic-referred samples, although not to the degree seen in ADHD samples. Again, this may have to do with the elevated occurrence of ADHD symptoms even in the Clinical control group. Epidemiological studies have also found an association of ADHD with these other disruptive disorders (Kessler et al., 2006; Secnik et al., 2005), as did the study of nonreferred ADHD adult relatives among ADHD children reported by McGough et al. (2005).

To summarize, for the most part, our results are relatively consistent with past studies on comorbidity. We found that relative to Community controls, ADHD was associated with an increased risk for depression, dysthymia, generalized anxiety disorder, alcohol and cannabis dependence and abuse disorders, and a childhood history of ODD and CD. But it was not associated with any higher risk for OCD or for bipolar disorder. Dysthymia, cannabis use disorders, and ODD were also significantly elevated in the ADHD group relative to the Clinical control group, implying that these disorders may be specifically associated with ADHD beyond their elevated association with clinic-referred adults not having ADHD.

Many studies examining comorbidity in any age group use treatment-seeking samples, like our study, which are typically biased toward finding elevated comorbidity relative to population levels. This is because each psychiatric condition that an individual has increases the odds of treatment seeking. Thus, our findings could be overestimates of actual population rates of comorbidity for ADHD generally. But they are representative of clinic-referred adults—the group most relevant to clinicians. Studies of epidemiological (community-derived) or nonreferred samples nevertheless are important in testing hypotheses about comorbidity with ADHD because they are free of such bias. Several such studies were discussed above in the context of our own findings and appear to support many of the associations found here between ADHD and certain other disorders. There is considerable agreement across these sources regarding adults with ADHD as to the elevated risk for anxiety disorders, antisocial personality disorder, ODD, and CD, as discussed above. All of this suggests that ADHD confers an inherently elevated risk for these disorders. The risk for depression in adults with ADHD is somewhat conflicting. We did not find elevated rates over our clinical control group but did relative to the Community control group. Other studies, including epidemiological ones, have documented some association between these two disorders, making it unlikely that the association is due merely to a referral bias to the study. The risk for substance use disorders is also elevated, yet it seems to be mediated largely by comorbidity for CD or antisocial behavior more generally.

We then examined comorbidity more globally as representing the risk between ADHD and comorbidity for any disorders examined here. The risk for lifetime comorbidity with any non-ADHD disorder is shown in Table 8.2. The adults with ADHD were significantly more likely to have at least one other non-

TABLE 8.2. Non-ADHD Lifetime Comorbidity Risk by Group for the UMASS Study

Measure	ADHD		Clinical		Community		χ^2	p	Pairwise contrasts
	N	%	N	%	N	%			
Had 1+ disorders[S]	117	80	64	66	22	20	95.7	< .001	1 > 2 > 3
Had 2+ disorders[S]	78	53	41	42	7	6	62.4	< .001	1,2 > 3
Had 3+ disorders[S]	57	39	19	20	4	4	45.2	< .001	1 > 2 > 3
Had 4+ disorders	30	25	11	11	0	0	25.6	< .001	1,2 > 3

Note. Sample sizes are ADHD = 146, Clinical = 97, Community = 109. N = sample size endorsing this item; % = percent of group endorsing this item; χ^2 = results of the omnibus chi-square test; p = probability value for the chi-square test; pairwise contrasts = results of the chi-square tests involving pair-wise comparisons of the three groups; [S] = main effect for sex.

ADHD disorder compared to both control groups (80% vs. 66 and 20%, respectively). A similarly high rate of global lifetime comorbidity was reported among the ADHD parents of children with ADHD by McGough et al. (2005). Our adults with ADHD were also more likely to have at least three or more disorders (39%) compared to the Clinical (20%) and Community (4%) control groups. All of this suggests that ADHD significantly increases the risk for having other lifetime comorbid psychiatric disorders. This is yet another demonstration that ADHD in adults is not benign.

Where sex effects were found males had significantly more comorbidity than females, as shown in Table 8.2. But within the ADHD and Clinical control groups, no significant sex differences were evident. Males in the Community control group, however, were significantly more likely to have at least 1+ non-ADHD disorder compared to females (31 vs. 10). The same was true for having at least 2+ (12 vs. 2), and for having at least 3+ (8 vs. 0) disorders. The significant main effect for sex differences, then, seems to be driven largely by the sex differences in the Community control group.

The results for global comorbidity suggest what has already been demonstrated in the literature on childhood comorbidity—disorders cluster together such that one disorder may increase the risk not only for a second disorder but for additional disorders as well (Angold et al., 1999). To examine the specific risks that one comorbid disorder with ADHD may convey for the risk for the other disorders studied here, we computed the conditional probabilities (expressed as percentages) for all other disorders given the presence of each disorder in turn. The results are shown in Table 8.3 and are for the ADHD group only. There is a discernible pattern of clustering among these disorders. For instance, not unexpectedly, MDD conveys an elevated risk for dysthymia and generalized anxiety disorder (GAD) as do both of the latter disorders for MDD. Dysthymia (DYS) conveys an additional elevated risk for OCD as does OCD for dysthymia. GAD conveys a specific elevated risk for bipolar disorder (BPD) and vice versa.

Caution must be exercised, however, in interpreting the results for the disorders having very low base rates in this sample, such as in OCD ($N = 4$) and BPD ($N = 3$). All of these can be considered internalizing disorders, and they obviously share liability for each other. Interestingly, they do not share liability for the drug abuse disorders, ODD, or CD. Nor do the latter disorders show an increased liability for the former internalizing disorders within our ADHD sample.

But like the internalizing disorders, the externalizing disorders show some increased liability for each other. Alcohol dependence or abuse disorders (ALC) convey an increased risk for cannabis dependence and abuse disorders (CAN) and vice versa as well as with ODD and CD. But CAN disorders shows an increased liability only with ALC disorders, as already noted. Both ODD and CD show liability for each other as well as for ALC disorders. These two- and three-way risk liabilities are not equally bidirectional, however. For example, nearly three-fourths of all CD patients have ODD, while only one-third of ODD patients have CD. This is consistent with the literature on children with these disorders (Loeber et al., 2000) indicating that while ODD shares a low but significant risk for CD, CD shows a markedly higher risk for comorbid ODD.

TABLE 8.3. Association of Psychiatric Disorders with Each Other Using ADHD Group Only

Disorder (%)	MDD	DYS	GAD	BPD	OCD	ALC	CAN	ODD	CD
MDD—Yes (N = 52)		42*	31*	4	6	42	36	49	26
MDD—No (N = 94)		18	10	1	1	33	32	51	24
DYS—Yes (N = 39)	56*		30*	3	8*	49	36	56	31
DYS—No (N = 107)	28		12	2	1	32	33	48	22
GAD—Yes (N = 25)	64*	48*		8*	4	48	32	62	37
GAD—No (N = 121)	30	22		1	2	34	34	48	22
BPD—Yes (N = 3)	67	33	67*		0	67	33	67	67
BPD—No (N = 143)	35	27	16		3	36	33	69	24
OCD—Yes (N = 4)	75	75*	25	0		50	75	50	33
OCD—No (N = 142)	34	25	17	2		36	32	50	25
ALC—Yes (N = 53)	41	36	23	4	4		60*	69*	40*
ALC—No (N = 93)	32	21	14	1	2		18	39	16
CAN—Yes (N = 49)	39	29	16	2	6	65*		61	31
CAN—No (N = 97)	34	26	17	2	1	22		45	22
ODD—Yes (N = 71)	35	31	21	3	3	51*	42		34*
ODD—No (N = 70)	37	24	13	1	3	23	27		14
CD—Yes (N = 34)	38	32	9	6	3	59*	41	72*	
CD—No (N = 103)	35	23	15	1	2	29	30	45	

Note. For each disorder present, the table shows the percentage having the other disorders for the UMASS Study. % = percent of each disorder having the other disorders; MDD = major depressive disorder; DYS = dysthymia, GAD = generalized anxiety disorder; BPD = bipolar disorder; OCD = obsessive–compulsive disorder; ALC = alcohol dependence or abuse disorders; CAN = cannabis dependence or abuse disorders; ODD = oppositional defiant disorder; CD = conduct disorder. ODD and CD are for childhood, retrospectively recalled. All other disorders are lifetime occurrence.

*$p < .05$.

Statistical analysis: Pearson chi-square.

We repeated these analyses using the entire sample. The results can be found in Table 8.4. Many of the same conclusions found for the ADHD sample hold for the entire sample. However, with the substantial increase in sample size, some relationships now become significant that were not previously so. The internalizing disorders continue to create an increased risk for each other, even more so with this added statistical power. Some internalizing disorders now increase the liability for drug use disorders as well as ODD and vice versa, but typically not for CD. The exception is BPD, which increases the risk for CD more than threefold (57% vs. 16%). And while drug-use disorders and ODD continue to show increased liability for each other, as shown in the ADHD group, they now convey liability for internalizing disorders to a small but significant degree, just as the latter had been shown to do with them. But again, those increases in liability remain relatively low. Overall, then, internalizing disorders show higher liability for each other than for drug-use and externalizing disorders and vice versa, just as had been seen in the ADHD group alone. But with added power, some of the smaller relationships across these two domains of disorders (internalizing and externalizing) now increase to significance, chiefly for drug-use disorders and ODD.

TABLE 8.4. Association of Psychiatric Disorders with Each Other Using Entire Sample

Disorder (%)	MDD	DYS	GAD	BPD	OCD	ALC	CAN	ODD	CD
MDD—Yes (N = 94)		32*	23*	5*	11*	36*	27	35*	22
MDD—No (N = 259)		10	7	1	1	21	18	23	14
DYS—Yes (N = 56)	54*		36*	2	7	41*	30*	44*	23
DYS—No (N = 297)	21		7	2	3	22	18	23	15
GAD—Yes (N = 41)	54*	49*		7*	5	37	27	47*	26
GAD—No (N = 312)	23	11		1	3	23	20	23	15
BPD—Yes (N = 7)	71*	14	43*		29*	27	14	43	57*
BPD—No (N = 346)	26	16	11		3	25	20	26	16
OCD—Yes (N = 13)	77*	31	15	15*		31	31	38	27
OCD—No (N = 340)	25	15	11	1		25	20	26	16
ALC—Yes (N = 88)	38*	26*	17	2	4		50*	48*	41*
ALC—No (N = 265)	23	12	10	2	3		10	19	8
CAN—Yes (N = 72)	35	24*	15	1	6	65*		48*	33*
CAN—No (N = 281)	25	14	11	2	3	22		20	13
ODD—Yes (N = 90)	35*	27*	20*	3	6	46*	38*		35*
ODD—No (N = 254)	24	12	8	2	3	17	15		10
CD—Yes (N = 55)	36	22	18	7*	5	62*	38*	57*	
CD—No (N = 276)	25	14	10	1	3	18	16	21	

Note. For each disorder present, the table shows the percentage having the other disorders for the UMASS Study. % = percent of each disorder having the other disorders; MDD = major depressive disorder; DYS = dysthymia; GAD = generalized anxiety disorder; BPD = bipolar disorder; OCD = obsessive–compulsive disorder; ALC = alcohol dependence or abuse disorders; CAN = cannabis dependence or abuse disorders; ODD = oppositional defiant disorder; CD = conduct disorder. ODD and CD are for childhood, retrospectively recalled. All other disorders are lifetime occurrence.
  * $p < .05$.
Statistical analysis: Pearson chi-square.

The Milwaukee Study Results

The rate of comorbidity for the various SCID disorders was substantially lower in the Milwaukee Study H+ADHD group than in the ADHD group in the UMASS Study. This is an important point, which was evident when one compared past studies of clinic-referred adults having ADHD with results of past longitudinal studies of children with ADHD as adults. Children with ADHD, even if they retain their ADHD into adulthood, show lower levels of comorbidity with other specific Axis I psychiatric disorders than do adults with ADHD seen in clinics. Such higher rates in the latter group could be related to referral status; as noted earlier, treatment-seeking adults often have a higher risk of comorbid disorders than do those not seeking treatment. As was evident in Chapter 4, most cases of hyperactive children in the Milwaukee Study were not currently in treatment, nor had most received any treatment since the last follow-up at age 21.

The significant comorbid risks are shown in Table 8.5. In keeping with other longitudinal studies of children with ADHD grown up, we failed to find any elevated risks specifically for major depressive disorder (MDD) or dysthymia. This is quite surprising, given that major depression was found to be more prevalent in the hyperactive group at the last follow-up (age 21) than in the Community control group. At that follow-up, we did not separate the groups into those with and without current ADHD to examine comorbidity because so few of the hyperactive group met criteria for ADHD by self-report (5%). Perhaps subdividing that hyperactive group here led to significantly smaller samples, with the attendant problem of reduced statistical power. To explore that possible problem, we recombined the hyperactive groups together for comparison to the control group on each specific mood disorder. The groups did not differ on MDD single episode, dysthymia, or MDD-NOS (not otherwise specified). But there was a slight yet significantly greater occurrence of MDD recurrent episode in the hyperactive than the control group (6% vs. 0%, $\chi^2 = 4.69$, $p = .03$). This rate is still well below the 27% found at the prior follow-up.

This lack of a robust association between MDD/dysthymia and ADHD disagrees with studies of clinic-referred adults with ADHD, where the occurrence of dysthymia in particular was often substantially greater than in control groups. But when we collapsed all possible SCID mood disorders together, the H+ADHD group did show a significantly greater likelihood of having at least one mood disorder, being four times more likely to do so than the H−ADHD group and six times more likely than the Community control group. We also discuss below the fact that the H+ADHD group had a significantly elevated risk for depressive personality disorder. Thus, even though the risk for MDD or dysthymia specifically was not found here, risk for any mood disorder was elevated, as was the specific risk for depressive personality disorder, both of which are in keeping with a link between ADHD and depression. The younger ages of

TABLE 8.5. Significant Current and Past SCID Diagnoses and Current and Childhood ODD and CD by Self-Report for the Milwaukee Study

Measure	H+ADHD N	H+ADHD %	H–ADHD N	H–ADHD %	Community N	Community %	χ^2	p	Pairwise contrasts
Axis I disorders—current									
Alcohol abuse	11	20.4	6	7.6	6	8.0	6.44	.040	1 > 2,3
Alcohol dependence	6	11.1	2	2	3	4	5.10	NS	
Cannabis abuse	5	9.3	5	6.3	5	6.7	0.46	NS	
Cannabis dependence	2	3.7	0	0.0	4	5.3	4.03	NS	
PTSD	10	18.5	5	6.3	1	1.3	13.39	.001	1 > 2,3
Social phobia	7	13.0	5	6.3	1	1.3	7.25	.027	NS
Specific phobia	9	16.7	11	14.1	3	4.0	6.23	.044	1,2 > 3
Generalized anxiety	6	11.5	1	1.3	2	2.7	8.66	.013	1 > 2,3
Any mood disorder	13	24.5	5	6.3	3	4.0	16.40	< .001	1 > 2,3
Any drug disorder	14	25.9	8	10.3	10	13.3	6.40	.041	1 < 2
Any anxiety disorder	24	46.2	17	22.7	7	9.3	23.06	< .001	1 > 2 > 3
Axis I disorders—past									
Any mood disorder	7	13.2	2	2.6	3	4.0	7.23	.027	1 > 2
Any drug disorder	28	53.8	41	53.2	30	40.0	3.50	NS	
Any anxiety disorder	4	7.7	8	10.7	3	4.0	2.43	NS	
Personality disorders—current									
Avoidant	8	14.8	1	1.3	1	1.2	15.96	< .001	1 > 2,3
Obsessive–compulsive	9	16.7	4	5.1	2	2.7	10.07	.006	1 > 2,3
Passive–aggressive	18	33.3	5	6.3	1	1.3	34.88	< .001	1 > 2,3
Depressive	8	14.8	4	5.1	0	0.0	12.79	.002	1 > 2 > 3
Paranoid	9	16.7	4	5.1	3	4.0	8.33	.015	1 < 2,3
Borderline	13	24.1	3	3.8	1	1.3	24.88	< .001	1 > 2,3
Antisocial	21	38.9	13	16.5	6	8.0	19.92	< .001	1 > 2,3
Any personality disorder	36	66.7	22	27.8	9	12.0	44.08	< .001	1 > 2 > 3
Disruptive disorders									
ODD current	26	47.3	13	16.3	3	4.0	38.27	< .001	1 > 2 > 3
ODD childhood	41	74.5	38	47.5	6	8.0	60.97	< .001	1 > 2 > 3
CD childhood	33	61.1	41	51.3	22	29.7	13.73	.001	1,2 > 3

Note. N = sample size endorsing this item; % = percent of group endorsing this item; χ^2 = results of the omnibus chi-square test; p = probability value for the chi-square test; pairwise contrasts = results of the chi-square tests involving pairwise comparisons of the three groups; PTSD = posttraumatic stress disorder; H+ADHD = hyperactive group that currently has a diagnosis of ADHD at follow-up; H–ADHD = hyperactive group that does not have a diagnosis of ADHD at follow-up; ODD = oppositional defiant disorder; CD = conduct disorder.
   Statistical analysis: Pearson chi-square.

our groups here in contrast to the UMASS Study and other studies of clinic-referred adults could be a factor in this disparity for specific mood disorders. Perhaps over time the milder levels of depression noted here in conjunction with ADHD could rise to the level of more specific mood disorders, such as MDD.

Also consistent with the UMASS Study and the larger literature on clinic-referred adults, we found a greater occurrence of GAD in the H+ADHD than in the Community control group. Unlike prior research of either clinic referred adults or children grown up, we also found a significantly higher risk for specific phobias and posttraumatic stress disorder (PTSD). But the H+ADHD and H–ADHD groups differed only in their rates of GAD and PTSD. Thus, growing up as a hyperactive (ADHD) child conveys a greater risk for specific phobias by adulthood, but persistent ADHD into adulthood further elevates the risk for GAD and PTSD beyond that conveyed by childhood hyperactivity status alone. Why PTSD would be more elevated in the H+ADHD group than the other two groups when this has not been reported in any prior studies is not immediately evident unless it was never specifically evaluated in the earlier literature—an issue we cannot discern from the methods published for other studies. But it was reviewed in the UMASS Study and was not found to be an elevated risk there.

Given the greater risk of GAD and PTSD in the H+ADHD group, it is not a surprise that they showed a markedly greater risk of having at least one or more anxiety disorders than both control groups, being twice as likely to do so than the H–ADHD group and five times more likely than the Community control group. This is certainly consistent with the association of ADHD with anxiety disorders in adults with ADHD seen in clinics. But it does not agree with prior follow-up studies of ADHD children into adulthood where no such elevated risk was evident (Mannuzza et al., 1993, 1998; Rasmussen & Gilberg, 2001; Weiss & Hechtman, 1993). Why this should be so is not immediately obvious to us. This elevated risk was not present at the last (age-21) follow-up, but then neither was the risk for current ADHD at that age, as discussed in Chapter 4. The increase in reporting this disorder may be due to the same process that has resulted in an increase in self-reported ADHD in our hyperactive group since that last follow-up—greater self-awareness or at least willingness to acknowledge other disorders than was earlier the case.

As in the UMASS Study, and consistent with much of the prior literature on adults with ADHD (whether clinic-referred or children grown up), we found no elevated rates of OCD or tic disorders in either hyperactive group relative to the control group. Nor did we find any elevated rates of BPD over the control group. Our studies lend further weight to the conclusions we drew above from the past literature and the UMASS Study that ADHD does not have a reliable or strong association with these particular disorders in adulthood.

More of the H+ADHD groups had a current alcohol abuse disorder. This is also in keeping with the past literature and the UMASS Study, where 18% of adults with ADHD had a current ALC or dependence disorder and 36% had a lifetime occurrence of those same disorders. We found that 20% of the H+ADHD group had a current ALC disorder, which was significantly greater than either the H–ADHD or Community control groups, who did not differ from each other (8% each). Many prior studies have found such an association of ADHD in adults, but the UMASS Study found that these disorders were also more common in their Clinical control adults who had other disorders, calling into question whether ALC disorders have a specific link to ADHD or just to adult outpatient psychopathology more generally. In contrast, cannabis abuse or dependence disorders were significantly more common in the ADHD group in the UMASS Study, which was not the case here. This suggests yet another difference between clinic-referred adults with ADHD and children growing up with ADHD at adult follow-up and calls into question any specific linkage of adult ADHD to cannabis abuse. Despite the much lower rates of these two drug use disorders in the Milwaukee Study ADHD sample than in the UMASS Study, the H+ADHD group did show a significantly greater risk for having at least one or more drug-use disorders relative to the H–ADHD group, although the difference between these two groups and the Community control group was only marginally significant. Such findings imply that drug-use disorders may be generically more likely to occur in conjunction with ADHD at adult outcome for children with the disorder even if no link to a specific drug use disorder is evident.

Our groups did not differ in their likelihood of having any past specific SCID disorder. When we looked at risk for the larger categories of disorders (mood, anxiety, and drug-use disorder clusters), we found only a significant elevation of risk for any mood disorder in the H+ADHD group compared to the H–ADHD group. Yet the difference between these two groups and the Community control group was only marginally significant. The risk for any anxiety disorder in their histories remained low and nonsignificant across all three groups, while the risk for any prior drug-use disorder was quite high (40–54%), although again not different among the groups. We found a high rate of drug use and its disorders earlier at the age-21 follow-up for both the Hyperactive and Control groups and concluded that while the rate of drug-use disorders in the former group was considerable, the markedly elevated rate in the Control group relative to the general population kept this difference from being significant.

As we did at the age-21 follow-up, we once again examined the risk for various current SCID personality disorders in our groups. Those for which significant group differences were evident are also shown in Table 8.5. The risk for any personality disorder was more than twice as great in the H+ADHD than H–ADHD group (67% vs. 28%) and was more than five times greater than in the Community control group (12%). Therefore persistent ADHD into adulthood has a high comorbidity with personality disorders. The most common was antisocial personality disorder, followed by passive–aggressive, and borderline personality disorders. OCD, paranoid, depressive, and avoidant disorders were also elevated to a small but significant extent in the H+ADHD group relative to the H–ADHD and Community control groups. Most of these specific personality disorders were also elevated in the Hyperactive group at the age-21 follow-up, but the current results show that it is largely current ADHD rather than a history of being hyperactive or having ADHD in childhood that is elevating these risks. Personality disorders were not evaluated in the UMASS Study or in other studies of clinic-referred adults to any great extent, making it difficult for us to draw comparisons between these adult-outcome results and those for clinic-referred adults with ADHD.

However, as in the UMASS Study, we found a higher occurrence of ODD and CD in the histories of both the hyperactive groups here compared to the Community control group, although the H+ADHD group had the highest risk for past and current ODD. As in studies of children, studies of adults with ADHD show a highly significant association of ADHD with ODD/CD either in childhood or at adult follow-up. This has been true whether samples were clinic-referred or epidemiological samples drawn from the community, as noted earlier.

In general, we found that the mean number of SCID disorders was significantly greater in the H+ADHD group ($M = 3.4$, $SD = 3.5$) than in the H–ADHD ($M = 0.9$, $SD = 1.5$) or control groups ($M = 0.8$, $SD = 1.9$) ($F = 22.39$, $p < .001$), with the latter two groups not differing from each other. It therefore appears that the persistence of ADHD into adulthood is associated with an elevated risk of comorbidity more generally than is the case for hyperactive children who no longer qualify for an ADHD diagnosis or the Community controls by adult follow-up. We found no differences among the groups in their risk for a past history of any SCID disorders, however.

As we did in the UMASS Study, Table 8.6 shows the risk for escalating levels of comorbidity (up to four additional disorders). As one would gather from the information presented above, more than 84% of the H+ADHD group had at least one other disorder, a level nearly twice that for the H–ADHD group and nearly four times that for the control group. Nearly 61% of the currently ADHD group had at least two other disorders, while 45% had three or more disorders, all of which were higher than in either control group. These levels are nearly identical to those found in the UMASS Study for clinic-referred adults with ADHD and once more illustrate the elevated risk that ADHD in adults conveys for having other psychiatric disorders, regardless of how the ADHD group is sampled (epidemiological, clinic-referred, or children grown up).

In the UMASS Study, we had sufficiently large samples of a number of specific SCID disorders that were elevated in the ADHD group to examine their co-occurrence or their risk conveyance for all other elevated disorders. But because the number of other SCID disorders in the Milwaukee Study was con-

TABLE 8.8. Significant Current and Past SCID Diagnoses and Childhood ODD and CD by Other-Report for the Milwaukee Study

Measure	H+ADHD N	H+ADHD %	H–ADHD N	H–ADHD %	Community N	Community %	χ^2	p	Pairwise contrasts
Axis I disorders—current									
Alcohol dependence	6	11.1	3	3.9	0	0.0	9.34	.009	1 > 3
Alcohol abuse	10	18.5	6	7.8	4	5.3	6.74	.034	1 > 3
Specific phobia	9	16.7	5	6.4	3	4.0	7.22	.027	1 > 3
Generalized anxiety	5	9.3	0	0.0	1	1.3	10.74	.005	1 > 2,3
Any mood disorder	5	9.3	4	5.1	2	2.7	2.72	NS	
Any drug disorder	12	22.2	12	15.6	5	6.7	6.51	.039	1 > 3
Any anxiety disorder	18	33.3	9	11.7	6	8.0	16.69	< .001	1 > 2,3
Axis I disorders—past									
Any mood disorder	4	7.4	1	1.3	2	2.7	3.85	NS	
Any drug disorder	19	35.2	26	33.8	16	21.3	3.91	NS	
Any anxiety disorder	3	5.6	4	5.2	1	1.3	2.07	NS	
Personality disorders—current									
Avoidant	10	18.5	4	5.1	2	2.7	12.25	.002	1 > 2,3
Passive–aggressive	18	33.3	15	19.2	2	2.7	21.50	< .001	1,2 > 3
Depressive	10	18.5	5	6.4	0	0.0	16.15	< .001	1 > 2 > 3
Paranoid	15	27.8	9	11.5	1	1.3	20.71	< .001	1 > 2 > 3
Narcissistic	4	7.4	7	9.0	0	0.0	6.76	.034	1,2 > 3
Borderline	16	29.6	10	12.8	0	0.0	25.10	< .001	1 > 2 > 3
Antisocial	15	27.8	12	15.4	2	2.7	16.63	< .001	1,2 > 3
Any personality disorder	32	59.3	28	35.9	8	10.7	34.12	< .001	1 > 2 > 3
Disruptive disorders									
ODD childhood	35	64.8	39	51.3	7	9.7	45.37	< .001	1,2 > 3
CD childhood	29	54.7	35	46.7	11	14.7	26.21	< .001	1,2 > 3

Note. N = sample size endorsing this item; % = percent of group endorsing this item; χ^2 = results of the omnibus chi-square test; p = probability value for the chi-square test; pairwise contrasts = results of the chi-square tests involving pair-wise comparisons of the three groups; PTSD = posttraumatic stress disorder; H+ADHD = Hyperactive group that currently has a diagnosis of ADHD at follow-up; H–ADHD = Hyperactive group that does not have a diagnosis of ADHD at follow-up. ODD = oppositional defiant disorder; CD = conduct disorder.
Statistical analysis: Pearson chi-square.

risks for these disorders were substantially lower than was seen for self-reported disorders. And generally the two hyperactive groups did not differ from each other except for GAD.

These other reports did not disclose any elevated risk for mood disorders that had been found in the self-reports. This was also true for any past mood disorders as well as past anxiety or drug-use disorders. Such results are not terribly surprising, given that mood disorders are likely to be more reliably reported by the participant experiencing the disorder than by those with whom they may socialize or reside. The collateral information did reveal an elevated risk for drug-use and anxiety disorders in connection with the H+ADHD group, which had also been documented by self-reports. A closer convergence of findings between these two sources was more evident in the current personality disorders for our groups. As found previously, passive–aggressive, borderline, and antisocial personality disorders were the most commonly seen in the H+ADHD group and differed significantly from the Community control group. But the H–ADHD group had elevated rates for these same disorders and did not differ from the H+ADHD group in rates of passive–aggressive and antisocial personality disorders. For the remaining personality disorders, the overall pattern was clear in showing the H+ADHD group to have the greatest risk for each of these other disorders and for an overall risk for any personality disorder, just as had been found in self-reported information. Unlike self-reported information, the other reports also showed that a childhood history of ODD was equivalently and significantly elevated in both hyperactive groups instead of just favoring the currently ADHD subset. But consistent with self-reports, the risk for CD was elevated in both hyperactive groups, who did not differ in this respect from each other. In short, our concerns about self-reported information appear to be somewhat assuaged by these findings. We did not find the tremendous disparity between self- and other-reported information that had been found for ADHD at the last follow-up. Perhaps that is because that disparity had also lessened by this follow-up as we noted in a previous chapter. Self-reports of ADHD are beginning to increase in frequency in the hyperactive groups and are beginning to converge on those levels reported by others. This gives us some hope that the same may hold true for self-reports of other psychiatric disorders as well, which seems to be suggested in the information presented above.

We examined at a rather coarse level the degree of agreement between self- and other-reported disorder categories in the SCID (i.e., if the disorder was self-reported, was it also other-reported?). The greatest agreement was for the risk for any personality disorder (72%, kappa = .46) and for any drug-use disorder (71%, kappa = .60). The risk for any anxiety disorder showed moderate to low agreement (45%; kappa = .39) and that for any mood disorder was quite low (18%; kappa = .12). Again, the lower agreements for the latter two disorders may have to do with the lessened visibility of mood states to others.

Psychological Maladjustment

The above research has approached the subject of comorbidity with ADHD from the psychiatric, categorical view of disorders. Another approach is the psychological, dimensional view, which examines differences between groups on more continuously scaled measures of these same domains of psychological maladjustment. At least four prior studies have taken this approach to evaluating their clinic-referred adults with ADHD, using variations of the Symptom Checklist–90—Revised (SCL-90-R; see sidebar). The study by Shekim et al. (1990) also reported results for this instrument, but not in comparison to any clinical or community control group. They did find that patients with ADHD and panic disorder have significantly higher scores on many of the scales of this instrument than did those without panic disorder. The results of the four prior studies using control groups are summarized in Table 8.9. Three of these four studies were conducted by us and found that clinic-referred adults with ADHD had significantly greater elevations on most if not all scales of the SCL-90-R relative to either clinical control groups or to a community control group. The exception is the study by Roy-Byrne et al. (1997), who compared cases of probable ADHD with possible ADHD and with no ADHD, all of whom had been seen at a psychiatric clinic. No differences were found among these groups on any of the SCL-90-R scales. It is difficult to explain this disparity, given that two of our own studies used such clinical comparison groups of adults seen at the same ADHD clinic that were not diagnosed with the disorder, yet we found differ-

TABLE 8.9. Summary Table of Prior Studies of Adults with ADHD on Dimensions of Psychological Maladjustment Having Significant Differences from Control Groups Using the SCL-90-R

Scale	Barkley et al. (1996)	Murphy et al. (1996)	Murphy et al. (2002)	Roy-Byrne et al. (1997)
Somatic	A>C	A>C	A>N	NS (A vs. C)
Obsessive–Compulsive	A>C	NS	A>N	NS
Interpersonal Sensitivity	A>C	A>C	A>N	NS
Depression	A>C	A>C	A>N	NS
Hostility	A>C	A>C	A>N	NS
Anxiety	A>C	A>C	A>N	NS
Phobic	A>C	A>C	A>N	NS
Paranoia	A>C	NS	A>N	NS
Psychoticism	A>C	NS	A>N	NS

Note. SCL-90-R = Symptom Checklist–90—Revised; A = ADHD sample; C = Clinical control sample; N = normal or Community control sample; NS = comparison of groups was not statistically significant.

ences in psychological maladjustment on this instrument. Using a different set of instruments, Ramirez and colleagues (Ramirez, Rosen, Deffenbacher, Hurst, Nicoletta, Rosencranz, & Smith, 1997) found adults with high ADHD symptom levels to express more anger and in more dysfunctional ways and to be more labile in anxious/depressed moods than those low in symptoms.

The UMASS Study Results

The UMASS Study used both the SCL-90-R by Derogatis (1986) and the Young Adult Behavior Checklist (self and other-report forms; see sidebar) by Achenbach to evaluate psychological and emotional maladjustment. The results for the SCL-90-R are shown in Table 8.10. Just as in our prior studies, we found that our adults with ADHD had significantly higher elevations on all of the scales of this instrument than did either the Clinical or the Community control groups. And while the Clinical control group was also significantly elevated on all scales relative to the Community group, they rated themselves as significantly less in their maladjustment than did the adults with ADHD. Thus, the previous study by Roy-Byrne et al. (1997) is truly the exception to the rule—adults with ADHD do manifest significantly more psychological maladjusted on most dimensions of such maladjustment than either community control adults or non-ADHD clinic-referred adults seen at the same clinic as the adults with ADHD.

TABLE 8.10. SCL-90-R Scales (*T*-Scores) by Group in the UMASS Study

	ADHD		Clinical		Community				Pairwise
Measure	Mean	SD	Mean	SD	Mean	SD	F	p	contrasts
Somatic	60.3	10.1	55.2	10.2	46.7	8.6	52.8	< .001	1 > 2 > 3
Obsessive–Compulsive	73.3	8.1	68.4	8.6	45.1	8.3	337.9	< .001	1 > 2 > 3
Interpersonal Sensitivity[A]	70.1	9.7	64.9	10.8	47.2	8.6	152.6	< .001	1 > 2 > 3
Depression	69.6	9.1	65.4	10.3	46.5	9.2	170.8	< .001	1 > 2 > 3
Anxiety[S]	65.8	11.2	61.8	10.9	42.2	7.6	156.6	< .001	1 > 2 > 3
Hostility[A]	64.6	10.7	58.7	10.7	44.5	6.4	119.0	< .001	1 > 2 > 3
Phobia[A,S]	59.8	11.0	53.0	10.5	46.6	4.6	47.2	< .001	1 > 2 > 3
Paranoia[A]	64.5	11.5	57.9	11.5	45.2	7.6	88.9	< .001	1 > 2 > 3
Psychoticism	66.8	10.2	61.7	11.4	48.0	7.5	102.0	< .001	1 > 2 > 3
General Severity Index[S]	70.2	9.0	65.0	9.6	43.6	9.6	232.3	< .001	1 > 2 > 3

Note. Sample sizes are ADHD = 142, Clinical control = 97, and Community control = 100. SD = standard deviation; F = F-test results of the analysis of variance (or covariance); p = probability value for the F-test; NS = not significant, [S] = significant main effect for sex (see text for details); [GxS] = Significant group × sex interaction (see text for details); [A] = age used as a covariate in this analysis.

Statistical analysis: Groups were initially compared using two-way (groups × sex) analysis of variance (or covariance as necessary). Where this analysis was significant (p < .05) for the main effect for group, pairwise comparisons of the groups were conducted, the results of which are shown in the last column.

We did find several sex differences on these scales, as shown in Table 8.10. Males across these groups reported significantly greater elevations on the Anxiety and Phobia scales than did females. But there was no significant interaction of the group factor with sex on these or any other scales.

For this project, we also obtained both self-reports and other reports (mainly from parents) on the Young Adult Behavior Checklist (see sidebar), an upward extension of the well-known Child Behavior Checklist. The results for the eight scales measuring psychological maladjustment for both sources of reports are provided in Table 8.11. For self-reports, we found that the adults with ADHD reported significantly greater elevations on all eight scales than did the Community control group, consistent with our earlier results for the SCL–90-R above. The ADHD group also had significantly greater elevations than the Clinical group on five of these scales, those being: anxiety–depression, attention problems, intrusiveness, aggression, and delinquency. Such results are quite concordant with the findings on comorbidity for psychiatric diagnoses reported above in showing elevated risks for anxiety, depression, and disruptive behavior disorders among adults with ADHD than in our control groups.

The findings for the smaller subset of cases on which we had the reports of others are also shown in Table 8.11. Again, the ADHD group had significantly greater elevations on all scales of maladjustment than did the Community control group, yet so did the Clinical control group. In this instance, the ADHD group differed from the Clinical control group in having only an elevated score on the aggression scale, but not on any of the seven other scales. Such a disparity with the self-reported information could simply be due to the lower statistical power involved in these comparisons as a consequence of the smaller sample sizes available here. Certainly the mean scores are in the same direction of showing greater elevations in the ADHD than in the Clinical control group on most other scales except the withdrawn scale. While these results for the ADHD group versus Community group certainly corroborate the self-reports on this same scale, they are not able to provide as fine a discrimination of the ADHD from the Clinical control group as did the self-reported information.

We found several sex differences in both sources of information. For the self-reported information, females reported slightly yet significantly higher scores on the anxiety–depression scale ($M = 60.5$, $SD = 12.2$) than did males (59.6, 10.4) and also on the delinquent scale (females: $M = 56.9$, $SD = 8.2$; males: $M = 56.3$, $SD = 7.7$). Such differences were driven largely by differences between females and males in the two clinical groups that were far less apparent in the control group. In both cases, the group × sex interaction was marginally significant ($p < .10$) supporting this interpretation of our findings.

We also found two significant interactions of sex with the group factor that must qualify the results for those scales. On the self-reports for the attention scale, females reported significantly greater symptoms than did males in both the

TABLE 8.11. Young Adult Self-Report and Other-Report Scales for the Adult Behavior Checklist by Group (T-Scores) in the UMASS Study

Measure	ADHD Mean	SD	Clinical Mean	SD	Community Mean	SD	F	p	Pairwise contrasts
Self-report scales									
Anxiety–Depression[S]	64.8	10.5	61.8	12.3	51.2	3.0	58.3	< .001	1 > 2 > 3
Withdrawn	60.2	8.4	58.8	8.7	52.3	5.2	27.0	< .001	1,2 > 3
Somatic Complaints	59.8	8.3	57.9	8.5	51.6	4.1	29.4	< .001	1,2 > 3
Thought Problems[A]	58.4	9.4	56.3	8.3	50.6	2.4	22.0	< .001	1,2 > 3
Attention Problems[S, GxS]	69.1	8.8	65.0	9.4	50.7	2.3	152.5	< .001	1 > 2 > 3
Intrusive[A]	58.4	8.2	56.2	7.3	50.7	2.1	28.9	< .001	1 > 2 > 3
Aggressive[A]	61.3	8.9	56.5	8.5	50.9	2.5	45.9	< .001	1 > 2 > 3
Delinquent[A,S]	59.6	8.5	57.3	7.8	51.5	3.3	30.5	< .001	1 > 2 > 3
Other-report scales									
Anxiety–Depression[S]	66.6	10.5	65.7	9.8	51.2	2.7	45.3	< .001	1,2 > 3
Withdrawn[A]	58.8	8.3	61.6	10.3	51.1	2.9	18.0	< .001	1,2 > 3
Somatic Complaints	59.8	8.1	58.1	6.7	52.0	4.5	18.2	< .001	1,2 > 3
Thought Problems[A]	59.4	8.6	58.1	8.4	50.7	2.8	21.6	< .001	1,2 > 3
Attention Problems[A]	67.4	9.4	65.9	9.1	50.9	2.6	54.0	< .001	1,2 > 3
Intrusive[A]	59.2	8.2	56.3	10.0	50.8	2.4	13.2	< .001	1,2 > 3
Aggressive[A, GxS]	62.4	7.6	58.7	6.3	50.6	1.7	48.7	< .001	1 > 2 > 3
Delinquent[A]	59.5	7.6	57.9	7.8	51.5	3.5	14.1	< .001	1,2 > 3

Note. Sample sizes for the self-report scales are ADHD = 120, Clinical control = 75, and Community control = 83. For the other-report scales they are ADHD = 76, Clinical control = 38, and Community control = 45. SD = standard deviation, F = F-test results of the analysis of variance (or covariance); p = probability value for the F-test; NS = not significant; [S] = significant main effect for sex (see text for details); [GxS] = significant group × sex interaction (see text for details); [A] = age used as a covariate in this analysis.

Statistical analysis: Groups were initially compared using two way (groups × sex) analysis of variance (or covariance as necessary). Where this analysis was significant (p < .05) for the main effect for group, pairwise comparisons of the groups were conducted, the results of which are shown in the last column.

ADHD and Clinical control groups while there were no significant sex differences in the Community control group. The pattern is shown in Figure 8.1. It suggests that females in both clinical groups may have been somewhat more severe in the attention problems than were males or than was the case for the Community control women. On the aggression scale from the other-report form, we also found a significant interaction of sex with group that is depicted in Figure 8.2. In this case, the females in the ADHD group were reported by others to be significantly more aggressive than the males in this group, while no sex differences were evident in the other reports from the two other control groups. Given that such findings of sex differences for the self- and other-reports are not evident on any of the other measures found in this project, it is difficult to interpret them with any degree of confidence. They could merely reflect chance occurrences in so large a project as this one, having collected many different measures for analysis.

TABLE 8.12. SCL-90-R Scales (*T*-Scores) by Group in the Milwaukee Study

Measure	H+ADHD		H–ADHD		Community		*F*	*p*	Pairwise contrasts
	Mean	SD	Mean	SD	Mean	SD			
Somatization	62.5	10.2	53.8	10.2	48.3	10.3	30.00	< .001	1 > 2 > 3
Obsessive–Compulsive	67.9	8.8	56.6	10.0	54.1	10.1	33.19	< .001	1 > 2,3
Interpersonal Sensitivity	66.4	12.3	54.5	11.4	54.0	10.8	22.69	< .001	1 > 2,3
Depression	65.8	11.1	54.2	9.8	52.0	11.0	29.60	< .001	1 > 2,3
Anxiety	63.6	9.6	52.5	11.1	50.2	10.7	27.24	< .001	1 > 2,3
Hostility	64.2	11.6	55.5	10.5	51.6	9.1	23.47	< .001	1 > 2 > 3
Phobic Anxiety	59.6	10.7	51.0	8.2	49.9	6.8	23.51	< .001	1 > 2,3
Paranoid Ideation	65.1	11.5	54.4	10.0	50.4	10.7	30.50	< .001	1 > 2 > 3
Psychoticism	60.9	11.9	52.9	10.5	49.9	9.2	17.75	< .001	1 > 2,3
General Severity Index	67.6	10.1	55.7	10.6	51.2	11.1	38.15	< .001	1 > 2 > 3

Note. Sample sizes are H+ADHD = 54, H–ADHD = 80, and Community control = 74. H+ADHD = hyperactive group that currently has a diagnosis of ADHD at follow-up; H–ADHD = hyperactive group that does not have a diagnosis of ADHD at follow-up.

Statistical analysis: Groups were initially compared using one-way (groups) analysis of variance. Where this analysis was significant (*p* < .05) for the main effect for group, pairwise comparisons of the groups were conducted, the results of which are shown in the last column. SD = standard deviation, *F* = *F*-test results of the analysis of variance, *p* = probability value for the *F*-test, NS = not significant.

bidity for categorical psychiatric disorders and illustrate the wide range of psychological difficulties associated with ADHD in adults. Whether one studies clinic-referred adults (UMASS Study) or hyperactive children grown up (Milwaukee Study), greater psychological maladjustment is linked reliably to the presence of ADHD over and above that seen in other outpatient disorders or in adults who were hyperactive as children but are no longer considered to have ADHD.

Suicidality

There are no prior studies on the prevalence of suicidal thinking, attempts, or completions (suicidality) among adults with ADHD. Two reasons would lead us to suspect that their occurrences would be higher in this group than in a community control group of adults. First, the higher than expected comorbidity between ADHD and dysthymia, and probably major depression, in clinic-referred adults as well as depressive personality disorder in children with ADHD grown up demonstrated above would automatically lead one to hypothesize a higher frequency of suicidality in adults with ADHD than in a normal population. Differences from Clinical control groups would be less certain depending upon the frequency of mood disorders within that particular control group.

The second reason is that two follow-up studies of hyperactive (ADHD combined type) children into adulthood have found suicidality to be higher than expected compared to control groups followed contemporaneously. In their excellent textbook *Hyperactive Children Grown Up*, Weiss and Hechtman (1993) briefly dealt with this issue in describing the results of their own longitudinal study of hyperactive children followed to adulthood. They indicated that the great majority of their hyperactive participants who made suicide attempts requiring psychiatric hospitalization were part of the approximately 10% who had significant psychiatric or antisocial disturbance at their 15-year follow-up (mean age 25). However, they did not present an actual incidence rate. In reviewing the published reports of the New York (Mannuzza et al., 1993, 1998) and Swedish (Rasmussen & Gillberg, 2001) longitudinal studies, we could find no consideration of such outcomes.

In contrast, two of us (Barkley & Fischer, 2005) reported results from the Milwaukee Study at the age-21 follow-up that focused on suicidality. At the young adult follow-up, we interviewed participants about 12 questions dealing with the topic of suicidality. At this follow-up (mean age 20.8 years, range 19–26), information was obtained from 149 of the Hyperactive group (94% of the original sample) and 76 of the Control group (90%) to address these questions. Six of the questions dealt with these issues during high school, and the same six were repeated again for functioning since leaving high school. The questions were: (1) Had they ever considered committing suicide? (2) If so, how many times? (3) If they had considered suicide, had they ever attempted suicide? (4) If so, how many times? (5) If they had attempted suicide, had they ever been hospitalized for an attempted suicide? (6) If so, how many times?

We have reproduced here the results from that study for the categorical questions (yes or no, questions 1, 3, and 5 above) in Table 8.13. Those results indicated that members of the Hyperactive group were twice as likely to have considered suicide as members of the Control group and more than seven times as likely to have attempted suicide. They were also more likely to have been hospitalized for such an attempt, which we took to be an indicator of severity of the attempt. After high school, the Hyperactive group was more than twice as likely to have considered suicide than the Control group, but it did not differ significantly from the Control group in either the percentage that had attempted suicide or been hospitalized after such an attempt. It is in high school, therefore, that the greatest risk for suicidal ideation, attempts, and hospitalizations after such attempts appears likely to arise in the Hyperactive group. Even so, an elevated risk of suicidal ideation remains in the Hyperactive group after leaving high school. Barkley and Fischer found that the elevated risks for suicidal thinking and attempts were chiefly mediated by the presence of major depression, although the presence of CD and, to a lesser

TABLE 8.13. Proportion of Hyperactive and Control Groups Endorsing Suicidality Questions at the Age 21 Follow-Up for the Milwaukee Study

Question	Hyperactive		Control		χ^2	Odds ratio	95% CI	p
	N	%	N	%				
In high school								
Considered suicide	53	36	17	22	4.09	1.92	1.01–3.62	.043
Attempted suicide	24	16	2	3	8.94	7.10	1.63–30.92	.003
Hospitalized	11	7	0	0	5.90	—	—	.015
Since high school								
Considered suicide	38	25	9	12	5.68	2.55	1.16–5.60	.017
Attempted suicide	9	6	2	3	1.26	2.4	0.5–11.3	NS
Hospitalized	7	5	1	1	1.68	3.70	0.45–30.61	NS

Note. Sample sizes by group are Hyperactive = 149 and Control = 76. N = number answering "yes" to this question; χ^2 = results of Cochran's chi-square test; odds ratio = common odds ratio for the Mantel–Haenszel Test; 95% CI = 95% confidence interval for the Mantel–Haenszel Test. From Barkley and Fischer (2005). Copyright 2005 by Guilford Publications. Reprinted by permission.

extent, the severity of ADHD in childhood made significant contributions to risk for suicidality.

With this exceptionally limited background of research in mind, we present the results for the UMASS Study of clinic-referred adults. As in the Milwaukee Study at age-21 follow-up, we asked participants whether they had ever considered suicide or attempted it prior to age 18 years of age and also after age 18 years. Our findings appear in Table 8.14. Here it can be seen that our groups did not differ in either suicidal ideation or attempts prior to 18 years of age, in con-

TABLE 8.14. Suicidal Thinking and Attempts before and after Age 18 Years for Each Group in the UMASS Study

Measure	ADHD		Clinical		Community		χ^2	p	Pairwise contrasts
	N	%	N	%	N	%			
Before age 18 years									
Suicidal thinking	37	25	16	16	16	15	5.1	NS	
Suicide attempt	9	6	4	4	2	2	2.8	NS	
After age 18 years									
Suicidal thinking	42	29	25	27	6	6	22.8	< .001	1,2 > 3
Suicide attempt	12	8	5	5	1	1	6.8	.033	1 > 3

Note. Sample sizes are ADHD = 145, Clinical = 94, Community = 108. N = sample size endorsing this item; % = percent of group endorsing this item; χ^2 = results of the omnibus chi-square test; p = probability value for the chi-square test; pairwise contrasts = results of the chi-square tests involving pair-wise comparisons of the three groups.

trast to the findings of the Milwaukee Study. We found that 15 to 16% of both control groups had considered suicide and 2 to 4% had made an attempt at suicide before age 18, in comparison to 25% of the ADHD group, who had considered it and 6% who had attempted it. After age 18, however, we found that more of both the ADHD and Clinical control groups had considered suicide (29% and 27%, respectively) more than was the case for the Community control group (6%). But the two former groups were not different from each other, implying that suicidal ideation, at least, was associated with outpatient psychopathology rather than specifically with ADHD in these adults. A significantly greater proportion of the ADHD group (8%), however, had also made a suicide attempt than of the Community control group (1%) since age 18. The Clinical control group fell between both of these groups in this case and was not significantly different from either of them. It therefore seems that unlike hyperactive children followed into young adulthood, clinic-referred adults with ADHD are not more likely to consider or attempt suicide before 18 years of age. After age 18 years, both ADHD and Clinical control groups show an elevated rate of suicidal thinking only but not attempts relative to a community group of adults. For hyperactive children at age 21, differences from control groups occur both before and after leaving high school, although the higher risk is clearly during their high school years. Despite the difference in patterns of results, it is of interest to note that the proportion of adults who were hyperactive as children and considered suicide after high school (25%) is very similar to that found for the ADHD group of adults here (29%), and both are markedly higher than in the Community control samples used in these studies (12% and 6%, respectively). But suicidality risk appears to be as elevated in non-ADHD outpatient referrals as in ADHD referrals, leaving us with the impression that a specific link of this behavior to ADHD is questionable, while a link to general psychopathology is more likely to exist.

We found no significant effects for sex on any comparison. However, we did find that in the ADHD group, females were more likely to consider suicide after age 18 than were males (43% vs. 22%). They were not more likely to attempt it, however, and they did not differ from males in either ideation or attempts before age 18. In the Clinical control group, females were more likely to consider suicide before age 18 than were males (27% vs. 9%). They did not differ from males in either suicidal thinking or attempts after age 18. There were no sex differences in the Community control group on any of these four measures of suicidality.

We turn now to the results of the Milwaukee Study at age-27 follow-up. We asked our participants whether they had considered or had attempted suicide in the 6 years (on average) since we had last evaluated them. Such a question does not reflect lifetime risk, which we studied at the age-21 follow-up, but only interim risk or risk going forward from age 21 to 27. We found that a significantly greater percentage of both hyperactive groups, once again, had considered suicide (38% and 24% respectively) in comparison to our control group (8%) (χ^2 = 17.15, p .001). Although the level of suicidal ideation was somewhat greater in the H+ADHD group than in the H–ADHD group, they did not differ statistically in this regard. There were not group differences in the risk of suicide attempts in the interim (13%, 9%, and 3%, respectively). Such findings are consistent with the age-21 follow-up in showing that after high school, only the risk of ideation is greater in the hyperactive children growing up, and it is not a function of whether or not ADHD has persisted to age 27. They are also in keeping with our results for clinic-referred adults in showing that risk for suicidality is nonspecific to ADHD status in adulthood but more to ongoing general psychological maladjustment.

What Predicts the Risk of Suicidality?

What factors in these samples, then, may have inflated the risk for suicidality in the clinical groups relative to the community control groups if it isn't current ADHD? Barkley and Fischer (2005) found that the risk of suicidal thinking and attempts was mediated by comorbidity for MDD and, to a lesser extent, CD. We examined this possibility in our UMASS Study. Using the entire sample, we determined what percentage of those who had either thought of or attempted suicide or had not thought of doing so had MDD (lifetime), dysthymia (lifetime), or CD (retrospective, childhood). These results are shown in Table 8.15. There is a striking though hardly surprising relationship with both MDD and dysthymia but far less so for CD. Perhaps this is because CD is not reflecting lifetime occurrence but just that in childhood. We found that more than three times as many people who had thought of suicide before age 18 years also had MDD compared to those who had not considered suicide. The same was true for those who had made a suicide attempt (73% vs. 25%). Dysthymia was somewhat less prevalent than MDD among those who had or had not considered or attempted suicide before age 18 years, but the pattern of risk was still similar, such that more than 2.5 times as many people who considered suicide or attempted it had this disorder compared to those who had not considered or attempted it. The prevalence of CD was not significantly higher in this age group among those who had or had not considered or attempted suicide. The results are even more striking for those who considered or attempted suicide after 18 years of age. Here more than four times as many people who considered or attempted suicide had MDD, and more than three times as many had dysthymia. CD was not related to suicidal thinking at this age but was related to attempts. More than twice as many attempters had CD than among nonattempters.

The same relationships were found when the ADHD group was considered separately (see lower half of Table 8.15). If anything, the associations between

TABLE 8.15. Percentage of All Participants and of ADHD Group Who Did or Did Not Report Suicidal Thinking or Attempts Who Also Had Major Depressive Disorder, Dysthymia, or Conduct Disorder for the UMASS Study

Behavior	%MDD			%DYS			%CD		
	No	Yes	χ^2	No	Yes	χ^2	No	Yes	χ^2
All participants									
Before age 18 years									
Suicidal thinking (%)	18	61	51.18*	12	32	16.37*	15	24	3.15
Suicide attempt (%)	25	73	17.40*	15	40	6.80*	16	29	1.49
After age 18 years									
Suicidal thinking (%)	15	71	93.30*	10	37	30.58*	16	21	1.08
Suicide attempt (%)	23	100	52.07*	14	50	16.48*	16	37	5.25*
ADHD-only group									
Before age 18 years									
Suicidal thinking (%)	25	70	24.35*	20	49	11.03*	20	39	4.89*
Suicide attempt (%)	35	67	3.76*	26	56	3.76*	24	37	0.68
After age 18 years									
Suicidal thinking (%)	22	71	31.01*	18	50	14.87*	27	21	0.48
Suicide attempt (%)	31	100	22.71*	24	67	10.00*	24	40	1.26

Note. MDD = major depressive disorder; DYS = dysthymia; CD = conduct disorder; No. = percent of those who did not engage in this behavior who had this disorder; Yes = percentage of those who engaged in this behavior who did have this disorder; χ^2 = results of the chi-square test.
* χ^2 significant at $p < .05$.
Statistical analysis: Pearson chi-square.

suicidality and MDD and dysthymia were even stronger than was the case for the entire sample of participations. We then examined all of the predictors (MDD, dysthymia, CD, and ADHD severity), jointly using logistic regression to determine which among them made a significant contribution to predicting suicidal thinking and suicide attempts after age 18. The results appear in Table 8.16. There it can be seen that MDD, dysthymia, and ADHD severity (number of symptoms from interview) all significantly contributed to the prediction of suicidal thinking. Only MDD significantly predicted a suicide attempt after age 18 (results not shown in table). Our results corroborate the findings of Barkley and Fischer (2005) in showing that the risk for suicidality among our participants was mostly a function of their higher comorbidity for MDD and dysthymia and to a far lesser extent their severity of ADHD. CD was not predictive of these outcomes after statistically controlling for these other disorders.

We undertook the same type of regression analysis using the entire Milwaukee sample and examining the extent to which current mood, anxiety, drug use, and antisocial personality disorders as well as severity of ADHD may have predicted the higher risk of suicidal thinking in our hyperactive groups since age 21. We found much the same results as above (see Table 8.17). Risk for suicidal ide-

TABLE 8.16. Prediction of Suicidal Thinking after Age 18 Years as a Function of Major Depression, Dysthymia, Conduct Disorder, and Severity of ADHD for the UMASS Study

Symptom	Beta	SE	Wald	p	Odds ratio	95% CI
Total ADHD symptoms (interview)	0.10	.04	7.16	.007	1.10	1.03–1.18
Major depressive disorder (lifetime)	2.53	.34	54.43	< .001	12.52	6.40–24.51
Dysthymia (lifetime)	0.81	.40	4.02	.045	2.25	1.02–4.98

Note. SE = standard error for beta; odds ratio = Exp(B); 95% CI = 95% confidence interval for the odds ratio.
Statistical analysis: Logistic regression using forward conditional entry method (constant included in equation).

ation since the age-21 follow-up was largely predicted by current mood disorder and, to a lesser extent, current anxiety disorder. In considering past SCID disorder categories, having any past mood disorder and severity of ADHD were associated with this risk. In summary, and hardly surprising, it is largely the existence of mood disorders that elevates suicidality risks in our samples, after which severity of current ADHD makes only a minor contribution. This likely explains why clinic-referred adults or hyperactive children grown up who currently have ADHD were not found to have an elevated risk for these events over clinical

TABLE 8.17. Prediction of Suicidal Thinking in Interim as a Function of SCID Disorder Categories (Mood, Anxiety, Drug, and Personality Disorders) and Severity of ADHD Symptoms in the Milwaukee Study

SCID categories	Beta	SE	Wald	p	Odds ratio	95% CI
From current SCID disorders						
Any current mood disorder	1.73	.574	9.03	.003	5.62	1.82–17.31
Any current anxiety disorder	1.40	.406	11.93	.001	4.07	1.83–9.01
Any drug disorder				NS		
Any personality disorder				NS		
Severity of ADHD (self-reported)				NS		
From past SCID disorders						
Severity of ADHD (self-reported)	0.16	.044	13.21	< .001	1.17	1.08–1.28
Any mood disorder	1.29	.622	4.27	.039	3.62	1.07–12.25
Any anxiety disorder				NS		
Any drug disorder				NS		

Note. SE = standard error for beta; odds ratio = Exp(B); 95% CI = 95% confidence interval for the odds ratio.
Statistical analysis: Binary logistic regression using forward conditional entry method (constant included in equation).

control groups who also had elevated rates of these events and of the mood disorders associated with them. It is not ADHD so much as comorbidity for mood disorders that creates these risks.

Conclusions and Clinical Implications

The present chapter has reviewed the literature on the nature of those comorbid psychiatric disorders and psychological maladjustments likely to exist with ADHD in adults. Our own results largely corroborate this literature, but with some important differences emerging as well.

✓ In general, there appears to be convincing evidence that ADHD increases the liability for certain other psychiatric disorders. More than 80% of our ADHD groups had at least one other disorder, more than 50% had two other disorders, and more than one-third had at least three other disorders, these being markedly higher than in our control groups in both studies.

✓ We found that the internalizing disorders of MDD, dysthymia, and anxiety disorders are more likely to occur in ADHD cases referred to clinics over that risk seen in the Community control group. But MDD and anxiety disorders are also significantly elevated in non-ADHD Clinical control patients seen at the same ADHD clinic and thus may not be as specifically linked to ADHD as to general outpatient psychopathology. Even so, both epidemiological studies in children (Angold et al., 1999) and adults (Kessler et al., 2006) find some association between ADHD and depression, which make it unlikely that our findings of a limited association are purely due to referral bias.

✓ The Milwaukee Study did not find an elevated risk for MDD specifically in those with persistent ADHD into adulthood but did find an elevated risk for mood disorders more generally and depressive personality disorder, both of which suggest some link between ADHD and level of depressive symptoms, even if not with fully syndromal MDD.

✓ It therefore seems to be dysthymia or depressive personality disorder that is most convincingly elevated in ADHD cases beyond the risk seen in Clinical control groups.

✓ The risks for bipolar disorder and OCD were not significantly elevated in the ADHD groups in either study and so are not reliable comorbid disorders with ADHD.

✓ We found that both the ADHD groups in our studies showed a greater risk for alcohol use disorders, while the clinic-referred adults (but not the hyperactive children grown up) also showed a greater risk for cannabis use disorders compared to Community controls. Our results suggest that alcohol use disorders and risk for any drug use disorder may be specifically linked to ADHD, although the level and type of drug use disorders probably have more to do with comorbid CD and antisocial personality disorder as well as local access to specific drugs than to ADHD per se.

✓ As in the prior literature on children and adults with ADHD, we found a markedly elevated risk for ODD, and to a lesser extent for CD, in our clinic-referred ADHD group and our hyperactive children as adults. Current ADHD was especially associated with a childhood history of ODD.

✓ Within our clinic-referred ADHD group, internalizing disorders increased the liability for each other but not for the externalizing disorders. The opposite also held true.

✓ However, when we reexamined our entire sample, the increased power for these comparisons revealed a smaller but significant cross-liability between internalizing disorders and drug use disorders and ODD but not typically for CD. The opposite pattern of cross-domain liability was also evident between the externalizing disorders. These disorders were more highly predictive of each other than of the internalizing disorders, but ODD and drug use disorders created a small but significant risk for mood and anxiety disorders.

✓ In examining comorbidity dimensionally using the SCL-90-R, adults with ADHD (whether clinic-referred or children grown up) showed elevations on all scales of psychological maladjustment relative to Community controls and on most of the scales relative to the Clinical controls. Our findings are consistent with all but one prior study in the literature on adults with ADHD using this instrument. There is clearly greater maladjustment of all types associated with ADHD than in clinical or community comparison groups. Such findings imply that ADHD is a more severe psychological disorder than many outpatient disorders seen in the same clinics.

✓ Such findings also extended to the internalizing and externalizing scales of the Young Adult Behavior Checklist, self-report version. However, on the other-report form, we found that both the ADHD and Clinical control group showed significant elevations on all scales compared to Community adults, but the two former groups typically did not differ from each other.

✓ We also studied the risk of suicidal ideation and attempts in our samples. We found that the ADHD group in the UMASS Study had only a slight but not significant increase in risk over the two control groups in both ideation (25% vs. 15–16%) and attempts (6 vs. 2–4%) prior to 18 years of age. But after age

18, both the ADHD and Clinical control groups reported elevated rates of suicidal thinking (27–29%) over that seen in the Community control group (6%). The ADHD group specifically also reported a greater risk of suicide attempts relative to the Community control group (8% vs. 1%). The Milwaukee study also found an elevated risk of suicidal thinking and attempts in the hyperactive groups, particularly before 18 years of age, and an ongoing risk of greater ideation (but not attempts) going forward to ages 21 and 27 follow-ups. But the two hyperactive subgroups did not differ in these risks, indicating that persistent ADHD into adulthood was not the major determinant of such risks.

✓ Subsequent analyses demonstrated that the greater risks of ideation and thinking reported here were largely mediated by the presence of MDD and, to a lesser extent, dysthymia, but was not especially related to the presence of comorbid CD.

✓ Clinicians need to be aware of and specifically assess for the high comorbidity of ADHD with other psychiatric disorders, particularly dysthymia, depression, ODD, conduct disorder, alcohol use disorders, and drug use disorders more generically. The elevated risk for suicidal ideation and attempts associated with the disorder is driven largely by comorbid mood disorders and not so much by ADHD specifically.

✓ Such comorbid disorders and psychological problems are highly likely to require separate treatment approaches than those usually aimed at the management of ADHD symptoms and their related impairments.

✓ ADHD in adults, particularly when seen in clinic-referred adults, is therefore likely to require polypharmacy more than is the case for childhood ADHD, given these higher risks for comorbid mood and anxiety disorders. While anti-ADHD drugs, such as stimulants and nonstimulant norepinephrine reuptake inhibitors, are clearly indicated for such cases, they are unlikely to address the risk for mood disorders evident here that are likely to require separate medical (i.e., antidepressant) and psychological (i.e., cognitive-behavioral) treatments in their own right. The elevated risk for anxiety disorders in both clinic referred ADHD adults and children with persistent ADHD in adulthood also suggests (1) that the nonstimulant atomoxetine may be of some benefit for these comorbid cases, in view of recent findings that it does not exacerbate anxiety and may reduce it to some extent, and (2) that cognitive-behavioral interventions having utility in management of anxiety disorders generally may be of some benefit for this comorbid population.

✓ Drug detoxification and rehabilitation programs will also be required for that subset of comorbid ADHD cases having drug use disorders, many of whom are also likely to have antisocial personality disorder or a history of CD. It is our opinion that early and aggressive treatment of the ADHD seen in these comorbid conditions at initial entry into detox or rehabilitation programs offers the best chance of assisting these individuals with their rehabilitation efforts. Ignoring it is highly likely to result in recurrent treatment failures due to the significant self-regulation and EF deficits we identified with this disorder in Chapter 7.

CHAPTER 9

Educational and
Occupational Functioning

$\mathbf{C}$linicians who specialize in evaluating and treating adults with ADHD often remark in trade books on the adverse impact the disorder seems to have had on the educational histories of these patients (Adler, 2006; Hallowell & Ratey, 1994; Wender, 1995). Authors of clinical textbooks have likewise noted this domain of impairment as one deserving of attention in the clinical evaluation of the adult ADHD patient (Goldstein & Ellison, 2002; Gordon & McClure, 1996; Triolo, 1999; Weiss et al., 2001). As demonstrated in Chapter 5, the educational domain of major life activities is among the three most impaired domains in adults with ADHD relative to Community control adults, while it is among the top two domains of impairment separating the ADHD group from the Clinical control adults. Here we examine the educational histories of the three groups in the UMASS Study more thoroughly to determine more precisely the sorts of impairments they experience in this domain of major life activities. We also evaluate this domain in the children with ADHD grown up in the Milwaukee Study for its convergence (or divergence) from that of the clinically referred adults with ADHD in the UMASS Study. Before doing so, we briefly review the previous research on this domain.

Background Research: Educational Functioning

It seems fair to say that nearly all clinic-referred children with ADHD are doing poorly at school, typically underperforming relative to their known levels of ability as determined by intelligence and academic achievement tests. Indeed, school

245

is one of the two settings of symptoms leading to impairment required in the DSM-IV criteria for a diagnosis of ADHD. These school difficulties are believed to be the result of the inattentive, impulsive, and restless behavior in the classroom associated with ADHD, the typically lower than average intelligence associated with the disorder (Rapport, Scanlan, & Denney, 1999), as well as of the higher comorbidity of ADHD with learning disabilities (Barkley, 2006; Tannock & Brown, 2000). These school performance problems do not appear to be the result of the conduct problems (social aggression) often associated with the disorder (Fergusson & Horwood, 1995; Rapport et al., 1999). Given these deficits in academic skills and behavior, it is not surprising to find that as many as 56% of ADHD children may require academic tutoring, approximately 30% may repeat a grade in school, and 30 to 40% may be placed in one or more special education programs. As many as 46% may be suspended from school, and 10 to 35% may drop out entirely and fail to complete high school (Barkley, DuPaul, & McMurray, 1990; Barkley, Fischer, et al., 1990; Barkley, Fischer, et al., 2006; Faraone et al., 1993; Szatmari, Offord, & Boyle, 1989; Weiss & Hechtman, 1993).

By adolescence, these chronic and cumulative experiences with school failure, learning disorders, school misbehavior, and sometimes lower intelligence begin to generate other adverse educational outcomes. For instance, the academic outcome of the hyperactive (ADHD) adolescents was considerably poorer in Barkley and Fischer's Milwaukee teen follow-up study than that of the normal adolescents followed concurrently. At least three times as many hyperactive (ADHD) children failed a grade (29.3% vs. 10%), had been suspended (46.3% vs. 15.2%), or been expelled (10.6% vs. 1.5%)(Fischer et al., 1990). Others have also identified such high educational risks in their longitudinal studies (Ackerman, Dykman, & Peters, 1977; Mendelson et al., 1971; Minde et al., 1971; Stewart, Mendelson, & Johnson, 1973; Weiss, Minde, Werry, Douglas, & Nemeth, 1971; Wilson & Marcotte, 1996). Among another sample of clinic-referred teenagers with ADHD, a similar risk for school retention and suspension was documented (Barkley, Anastopoulos, Guevremont, & Fletcher, 1991). Almost 10% of the hyperactive sample followed into adolescence had quit school at this follow-up point in the Milwaukee Study compared to none of the normal sample (Barkley, Fischer, et al., 1990). Fischer et al. (1990) also found that the levels of academic achievement were significantly below normal on standard tests of math, reading, and spelling, falling toward the lower end of the normal range (standard scores between 90 and 95).

Barkley and Fischer examined whether the presence of conduct disorder (CD) at follow-up within the hyperactive group accounted for these greater than normal rates of academic failure (Fischer et al., 1990). The results indicated that although hyperactivity alone increased the risk of suspension (30.6%

of pure hyperactives vs. 15.2% of controls) and dropping out of school (4.8% of pure hyperactives vs. 0% for controls), the additional diagnosis of CD greatly increased these risks (67.4% suspended and 13% dropped out). Moreover, the presence of CD accounted almost entirely for the increased risk of expulsion within the hyperactive group in that the pure hyperactive group did not differ from normal in expulsion rate (1.6% vs. 1.5%), whereas 21.7% of the mixed hyperactive/CD group had been expelled from school. In contrast, the increased risk of grade retention in the hyperactive group was entirely accounted for by their hyperactivity with no further risk occurring among the mixed hyperactive/CD group.

In general, it appears that academic performance difficulties in adolescence are associated with having persistent ADHD since childhood, whereas school disciplinary actions such as suspensions and expulsions are more closely linked to comorbid conduct problems or CD than to ADHD alone (Barkley, Fischer, et al., 1990; Fischer et al., 1990; Wilson & Marcotte, 1996). ADHD children with the lowest levels of adaptive functioning in childhood are also the most likely to have comorbid psychiatric disorders and academic impairments in adolescence (Barkley, Shelton et al., 2002; Greene, Biederman, Faraone, Sienna, & Garcia-Jetton, 1997; Wilson & Marcotte, 1996). Here "adaptive functioning" refers to the development of self-sufficiency as measured by such instruments as the Vineland Adaptive Behavior Scale.

These trends toward lower academic achievement and ability and greater grade retentions, suspensions, and expulsions evident in the adolescent years increase, such that by adulthood, the percentage of children with ADHD having difficulties in these areas is even greater than those percentages noted in adolescence and, of course, greater than those of control groups. Hyperactive children in follow-up studies into adulthood had less education, achieved lower academic grades, failed more of their courses, and were more often retained in grade, failed to graduate high school, and did not attend college than in control groups (Lambert & Hartsough, 1988; Mannuzza et al., 1993; Mannuzza et al., 1998; Weiss & Hechtman, 1993).

The Milwaukee Study (Barkley, Fischer, et al., 2006) found much the same results at the age 21 follow-up: more than three times as many Hyperactive than Community control group members had been retained in grade at least once (42% vs. 13%) during their schooling or had been suspended from high school at least once (60% vs. 18%). The Hyperactive group members had completed fewer years of education, and had a lower grade-point average (1.69 vs. 2.56 out of a possible 4.0) and class ranking in their last year of schooling (69th percentile vs. 49th percentile) than those in the Community control group. More of the Hyperactive group had also received special educational services while in high school relative to the Community control group. Of significant social and eco-

nomic impact, however, was the finding that 32% of the Hyperactive group had
failed to complete high school compared to none of the members of the Community control group. Substantially fewer hyperactive than control children had
ever enrolled in college (21% vs. 78%) or were currently attending at this follow-
up point (15% vs. 66%). In the Canadian follow-up study, approximately 20%
attempted a college program yet only 5% completed one, as compared to over
41% of Community control children (Weiss & Hechtman, 1993). These findings
demonstrate that the educational domain is a major one for impaired functioning
and reduced attainment for children growing up with ADHD.

As we have noted previously, children with ADHD followed into adulthood are not identical in their impairments to clinic-referred adults diagnosed
with ADHD. Studies of ADHD in children often find them to be significantly below those in control groups in their intellectual estimates, averaging
about 7 to 10 IQ points of difference (see above and Barkley, 2006). This does
not seem to be the case for clinic-referred adults with ADHD in prior studies.
For them, intelligence estimates seem to fall in the normal range and are comparable to control groups of clinic-referred adults (Barkley et al., 1996; Murphy &
Barkley, 1996; Murphy, Barkley, & Bush, 2002). Although Biederman and colleagues (Biederman et al., 1993) found that their adults diagnosed with ADHD
had IQ scores significantly below their control groups, the IQ scores for the
adults with ADHD were 107 to 110, nearly identical to the results of our own
studies of adults with ADHD. The adults with ADHD in the Biederman et al.
(1993) study therefore seem to differ significantly from the control groups only
by virtue of the fact that the control group had above-average IQs (110–113).

Adults diagnosed with ADHD do seem to have a higher risk for adverse
educational outcomes and lower academic functioning at some time during their
schooling, just as was found in children having ADHD and followed over development. Between 16% and 40% of clinic-referred adults have repeated a grade,
in keeping with the figures reported for ADHD in children discussed earlier in
this chapter (Barkley et al., 1996; Biederman et al., 1993; Murphy & Barkley,
1996). Up to 43% have also received some form of extra tutoring services in their
academic histories to assist them with their schooling (Biederman et al., 1993).
We found that 16 to 28% of young adult samples with ADHD had received special educational services in our prior studies (Barkley et al., 1996; Murphy et al.,
2002), a figure about half that found in hyperactive children followed to young
adulthood but still higher than normal. Consistent with these studies, Roy-Byrne
et al. (1997) also found clinic-referred adults with ADHD to have a significantly
greater frequency of achievement difficulties in school, to be more likely to suffer
grade retentions, and to be more likely to have received special educational services. A history of behavioral problems and school suspensions is also significantly
more common in clinic-referred adults with ADHD than in clinical control

groups (Murphy & Barkley, 1996). Yet young adults with ADHD seen in clinics are far more likely to have graduated high school (78–92%) and attended college (68%) than are clinic-referred children with ADHD followed to adulthood (see above), for whom the high school graduation rate is only about 64%. Some studies indicate that clinic-referred adults with ADHD may have less education than non-ADHD adults seen at the same clinic (Roy-Byrne et al., 1997), a finding consistent with adult follow-up studies of ADHD children (Mannuzza et al., 1993). We, in contrast, have not found this to be the case in two prior studies (Murphy & Barkley, 1996; Murphy et al., 2002). An exception is the study by Torgersen, Gjervan, and Rasmussen (2006) using a Norwegian sample ($N = 45$), which found that only 20% of their adults with ADHD had 12 or more years of education—a figure well below those of other studies of ADHD in adults. This Norwegian sample appears to reflect a far more severe disorder of ADHD than is typical of North American studies.

Concerning actual academic achievement skills, adults diagnosed with ADHD perform significantly less well on tests of math than do those in control groups (Biederman et al., 1993). Only those adults with ADHD who were relatives of ADHD children were found to be significantly lower on tests of reading in this study. As a consequence, more of the adults with ADHD qualified as reading-disabled (6%) than did Community control adults (0%). Others have also found clinic-referred adults with ADHD to perform less well on reading achievement tests than do control groups from the same clinic (Roy-Byrne et al., 1997). Yet the mean scores on both achievement tests in these studies were still within the normal range for these adults with ADHD. Again, the problem in these studies is the use of supernormal control groups and not subnormal functioning in the clinic-referred adults with ADHD. Studies of children with ADHD almost routinely found them to be below normal in their academic achievement skills (see Barkley, 2006; Rapport et al., 1999). The prevalence of actual learning disabilities in adults diagnosed with ADHD is well below that found in children with ADHD, ranging from 0 to 22% (Barkley et al., 1996; Biederman et al., 1993; Matochik, Rumsey, Zametkin, Hamburger, & Cohen, 1996; Torgersen et al., 2006).

All this suggests the following: adults with clinically diagnosed ADHD share some of the same types of academic difficulties in their histories as do children who were hyperactive or followed over development; however, their intellectual levels are higher, their high school graduation rates are higher, more are likely to have attended college, and their likelihood of having achievement difficulties or learning disabilities is considerably less in most respects than that seen in children with ADHD followed to adulthood.

This higher level of intellectual and academic functioning in clinic-referred adults with ADHD makes sense, given that they are self-referred to clinics in comparison to children with ADHD. This fact makes it much more likely that these adults have employment, health insurance, and a sufficient educational level to be so employed and insured. They could also be expected to have a sufficient level of intellect and self-awareness to perceive themselves as being in need of assistance for their psychiatric problems and difficulties in adaptive functioning. Children with ADHD brought to clinics by their parents are less likely to have these attributes by the time they reach adulthood. They are not as educated, are having considerable problems sustaining employment, are more likely to have had a history of aggression and antisocial activities, and are not as self-aware of their symptoms as are adults having ADHD who are self-referred to clinics (see earlier discussions and also Barkley, 2006). Only 3 to 5% of hyperactive children followed to adulthood in the Milwaukee Study endorsed sufficient symptoms to receive a clinical diagnosis of ADHD at age 21. That figure was 48% if their parents' reports were employed and 66% if a developmental reference (98th percentile) was used instead of the DSM criteria (Barkley et al., 2002), as noted in earlier chapters. This suggests that children with ADHD brought to clinics as children may have a more severe form of ADHD with earlier onset, or one that at least predisposes them to more severe impairments in school than do adults self-referred to clinics and diagnosed then as having ADHD.

Impaired Educational Settings

As reported in Chapter 6, adults with ADHD in the UMASS Study were significantly more likely to have reported being impaired in current educational activities, rated themselves as being so impaired in childhood school functioning, and were rated by others as such in their current and childhood educational adjustment than were either the Clinical or Community control adults in this study. These findings are reiterated in Table 9.1 along with additional findings on the specific school settings in which these adults were likely to be impaired. We asked others who knew the participants well to complete a rating scale with regard to ADHD symptoms manifested in school settings as children and the settings adversely affected by those symptoms (see sidebar, Chapter 6). As Table 9.1 indicates, adults with ADHD were rated by others as more likely to be impaired in all eight school situations than were Community control adults and were so rated in six of the eight situations compared to the Clinical control adults, these being classwork, homework, classroom behavior, recess and lunchroom activities, and overall time management at school. Only in school bus behavior and interactions with classmates did the ADHD group fail to separate significantly from the Clinical control group. In most settings, adults with ADHD were at least three times as likely to have been impaired as the Clinical control group and

TABLE 9.1. School Activities Rated by Others as Often Impaired by Group (from Rating Scales) in the UMASS Study

Measure	ADHD		Clinical		Community		χ^2	p	Pairwise contrasts
	N	%	N	%	N	%			
Current self-ratings									
Educational activities	127	89	62	70	1	1	172.5	< .001	1 > 2 > 3
Childhood self-ratings									
School	126	91	48	53	5	6	159.8	< .001	1 > 2 > 3
Current other-ratings									
Educational activities	87	63	40	56	2	3	84.8	< .001	1 > 2 > 3
Childhood other-ratings									
School	59	66	15	37	1	2	57.7	< .001	1 > 2 > 3
School ratings (others)									
Classwork	57	64	13	30	1	2	63.1	< .001	1 > 2 > 3
Homework	59	66	19	44	2	3	61.0	< .001	1 > 2 > 3
Classroom behavior	33	37	6	14	0	0	33.2	< .001	1 > 2 > 3
School bus behavior	12	15	2	5	0	0	11.3	.004	1 > 3
Interactions with classmates	31	35	2	5	0	0	37.9	< .001	1 > 3
Recess activities	23	27	3	7	0	0	24.0	< .001	1 > 2 > 3
Lunchroom activities	16	19	0	0	0	0	22.3	< .001	1 > 2,3
Time management	57	65	16	37	1	2	62.1	< .001	1 > 2 > 3

Note. N = sample size endorsing this item; % = percent of group endorsing this item; χ^2 = results of the omnibus chi-square test; p = probability value for the chi-square test; pairwise contrasts = results of the chi-square tests involving pairwise comparisons of the three groups.

vastly more so than the Community control adults. This is the first study of adults with ADHD to specifically document the settings most likely to be impaired in childhood school functioning and to have done so through the reports of others. What it shows is a nearly pervasive adverse impact of the disorder on school activities in the childhood histories of these adults.

Adverse Educational Outcomes (Categorical)

In the clinical interview with the adults in the UMASS Study (see sidebar, Chapter 5), we inquired not only about their level of education but also the frequency with which they had been suspended from school or been truant from school. We also inquired of them if they had ever been retained in grade, received special educational services or any other extra assistance, and had ever been diagnosed as having a learning disability or any behavioral disorders in school. We further asked if they had been punished more than others or felt as if they had more problems in school than others. The results for these categorical educational outcomes are shown in Table 9.2.

We did not find any differences among out groups in the proportions that had graduated from high school. This is consistent with other studies of clinic-referred adults with ADHD and, as noted above, discrepant from studies of children with ADHD followed to adulthood, where high school drop out rates may approach 30 to 40%. But significantly fewer of the adults with ADHD had graduated from college than in the two control groups, who did not differ from each other. More adults with ADHD reported that they had been retained in grade, had received special educational services or other assistance, and had been diagnosed with a learning disability or behavioral disorder in school compared to both control groups. These findings are depicted in Figure 9.1 and, again, are very consistent with previous studies of both clinic-referred adults and children with ADHD followed to adulthood. More adults with ADHD also reported that they believed they had been punished more than others and had more problems in school generally than others than was found in either control group.

There were main effects of sex on most of the outcomes reported in Table 9.2. All of these indicated that males were significantly more likely to experience adverse outcomes in schooling than were females (grade retentions, special education, other assistance, learning disorders, and punishment experiences). But there was no interaction of sex with group which would suggest that males and females with ADHD were not any different from each other than would be expected by these more general population sex differences.

TABLE 9.2. Educational Outcomes by Group for the UMASS Study

Measure	ADHD		Clinical		Community		χ^2	p	Pairwise contrasts
	N	%	N	%	N	%			
Graduated from high school	128	88	90	96	99	92	4.0	NS	
Graduated from college	43	30	58	62	58	54	27.5	< .001	1 < 2,3
Retained in grade[S]	36	25	7	7	5	5	25.6	< .001	1 > 2,3
Received special education[S]	51	35	9	10	12	11	31.3	< .001	1 > 2,3
Received other assistance[S]	69	48	28	30	11	10	40.8	< .001	1 > 2 > 3
Diagnosed learning disorder[S]	40	28	12	13	0	0	37.8	< .001	1 > 2 > 3
Diagnosed behavior disorder[S]	59	41	17	18	2	2	55.5	< .001	1 > 2 > 3
Punished more than others[S]	60	42	18	19	1	1	59.1	< .001	1 > 2 > 3
More problems with others	63	44	25	27	3	3	53.4	< .001	1 > 2 > 3

Note. N = sample size endorsing this item; % = percent of group endorsing this item; χ^2 = results of the omnibus chi-square test; p = probability value for the chi-square test; pairwise contrasts = results of the chi-square tests involving pairwise comparisons of the three groups; [S] = significant main effect for sex (see text for details).

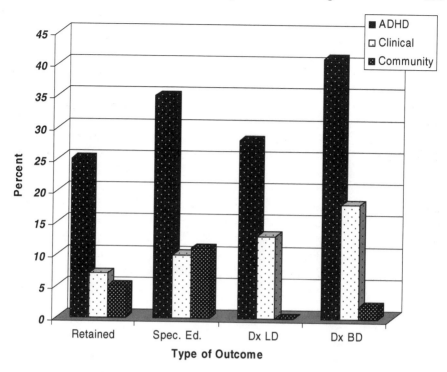

FIGURE 9.1. Percentage of each group experiencing various adverse educational outcomes in the UMASS Study. Retained = retained in grade; Spec. Ed. = placed in special education services; Dx LD = diagnosed with a learning disability; Dx BD = diagnosed with a behavior disorder.

We turn our attention now to the hyperactive children grown up in the Milwaukee Study and their educational outcomes. These appear in Table 9.3. As we had found at the earlier age-21 follow-up and in contrast to the clinic-referred adults above, both of the hyperactive groups, regardless of having current ADHD at age 27, were less likely to have graduated from high school (62–67%) than were members of the Community control group (99%) or the clinic-referred adults with ADHD in the UMASS Study. And far fewer of the hyperactive groups had attended college (9–20%) than had the control adults (68%). We depict these findings in Figure 9.2, which can be compared to those for the UMASS ADHD adult group in Figure 9.1.

In virtually all of these adverse educational outcomes, the two hyperactive groups experienced a higher likelihood of adversity than the control group, yet they did not differ from each other in these respects except in problems with others, where those with current ADHD had a significantly higher risk than the

TABLE 9.3. Educational Outcomes by Group from the Milwaukee Study

Measure	H+ADHD N	H+ADHD %	H–ADHD N	H–ADHD %	Community N	Community %	χ^2	p	Pairwise contrasts
Graduated from high school	34	61.8	54	67.5	74	98.7	31.25	< .001	1,2 < 3
Graduated from College	5	9.1	16	20.0	51	68.0	60.60	< .001	1,2 < 3
Retained in grade	26	47.3	25	31.3	11	14.7	16.40	< .001	1,2 > 3
Received special education	36	65.5	46	57.5	9	12.0	47.48	< .001	1,2 > 3
Received other assistance	23	41.8	18	22.5	10	13.3	14.23	.001	1 > 2,3
Diagnosed learning disorder	25	45.5	24	30.0	1	1.3	36.78	< .001	1,2 > 3
Diagnosed behavior disorder	28	50.9	32	40.0	5	6.7	34.01	< .001	1,2 > 3
Punished more than others	34	61.8	39	48.8	13	17.3	29.22	< .001	1,2 > 3
More problems with others	29	52.7	26	32.5	5	6.7	33.96	< .001	1 > 2 > 3
Ever suspended or expelled	39	70.9	55	68.8	16	21.3	45.15	< .001	1,2 > 3
Ever truant	42	76.4	61	76.3	52	69.3	1.21	NS	

Note. N = sample size endorsing this item; % = percent of group endorsing this item; χ^2 = results of the omnibus chi-square test; *p* = probability value for the chi-square test; pairwise contrasts = results of the chi-square tests involving pairwise comparisons of the three groups; H+ADHD = hyperactive group that currently has a diagnosis of ADHD at follow-up; H–ADHD = hyperactive group that does not have a diagnosis of ADHD at follow-up.

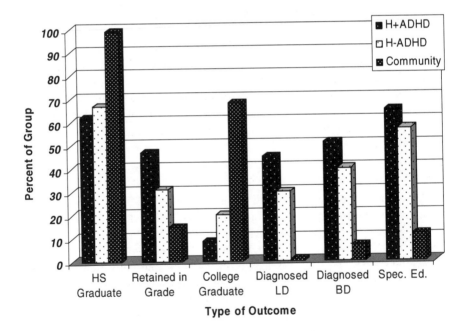

FIGURE 9.2. Percentages of each group experiencing various adverse educational outcomes in the Milwaukee Study. HS = high school; Spec. Ed. = placed in special education services; Diagnosed LD = diagnosed with a learning disability; Diagnosed BD = diagnosed with a behavior disorder; H+ADHD = Hyperactive group currently having ADHD; H–ADHD = Hyperactive group not currently having ADHD; Community = Community control group.

other two groups. All of this indicates that hyperactive children have a significantly worse educational career regardless of whether their ADHD persists to age 27 or not. They also experienced a higher prevalence of adversities in their schooling than even the clinic-referred adults with ADHD seen in the UMASS Study. Consider retention in grade, for instance—an outcome we found at age 21 to be principally related to having ADHD and not to CD. Almost twice as many H+ADHD cases had been retained in grade than clinic-referred adults with ADHD (47% vs. 25%). This was also the case for the percentage that had received special educational assistance (65% vs. 35%). Of course, most significant from a societal or economic standpoint is the considerably lower high school and college graduation rates for the hyperactive groups relative to the Community control group and to the higher rates seen in clinic-referred adults with ADHD in the UMASS Study. All of this suggests that children growing up as ADHD are more adversely affected in their educational careers than are clinic-referred adults with ADHD, even if their ADHD does not persist to age 27.

Educational Performance

Consistent with prior studies, the UMASS Study found that the adults with ADHD had significantly fewer years of education than both control groups, even though they averaged at least 2 years of education beyond high school. This information is shown in Table 9.4. Members of the ADHD group were also suspended more often and were truant more often from school than adults in either of our control groups. (Of note is that our Clinical control group had more years of education than our Community control group.) We found much the same results in the Milwaukee Study. Those findings are shown in Table 9.5. We found that both hyperactive groups had had fewer years of education, had been suspended more times from school, and had been truant from school more than our Community control group. Yet the two hyperactive groups did not differ from each other on these outcomes, and their level of education and number of school suspensions and truancy were all more adversely affected than seen in the adults in the UMASS Study. Again, this shows that it is growing up as a hyperactive/ADHD child that predisposes to greater educational adversity rather than persistent ADHD to age 27. We can therefore say that while clinic-referred adults with ADHD and children growing up with ADHD both have greater educational problems and lower attainment than Clinical or Community control groups, these problems are more severe in the children with ADHD as they grow up.

   In the UMASS Study, we also asked permission from our participants to obtain their elementary, high school, and college transcripts if available. From those transcripts, we coded the percentage of grades that were Ds, Fs, or Us

TABLE 9.4. Educational Functioning by Group for the UMASS Study

Measure	ADHD Mean	SD	Clinical Mean	SD	Community Mean	SD	F	p	Pairwise contrasts
From interview									
Education (years)[GxS]	14.2	2.2	16.3	2.8	15.4	2.7	15.0	< .001	1 < 3 < 2
No. of times suspended[S, GxS]	1.6	3.1	0.4	0.8	0.4	0.9	8.8	< .001	1 > 2,3
No. of times truant	18.8	33.9	8.5	15.2	5.1	10.4	8.0	< .001	1 > 2,3
Elementary school Transcript									
Percent D, F, and U grades	8.1	13.9	2.7	6.7	0.8	2.1	4.7	.01	1 > 2,3
Days absent[A]	10.4	7.8	10.0	7.9	7.5	4.2	2.4	NS	
High school Transcript									
Percent Ds	17.1	15.8	8.5	11.9	7.1	9.8	12.4	< .001	1 > 2,3
Percent Fs	6.6	10.3	1.7	3.6	1.5	4.0	11.2	< .001	1 > 2,3
Class ranking	36.2	24.6	54.4	29.0	65.0	25.3	13.0	< .001	1 < 2,3
Mean days absent/sem.	8.4	7.0	5.7	4.0	5.0	5.0	3.1	049	1 > 2,3
Verbal test percentile	63.1	26.9	72.2	25.4	69.0	24.8	1.29	NS	
Quantitative test percentile	62.5	31.6	69.5	28.9	66.5	26.9	0.6	NS	
Grade-point average[S]	2.2	0.7	2.7	0.7	2.9	0.7	19.2	< .001	1 < 3
College Transcript									
Percent Ds[GxS]	8.6	10.6	5.0	6.3	4.6	8.3	5.5	.005	1 > 2,3
Percent Fs	6.7	10.7	3.8	9.0	1.0	2.6	7.3	< .001	1 > 2 > 3
Percent withdrawals	7.5	11.2	2.5	4.3	5.1	11.6	3.9	.021	1 > 2
Grade-point average[S]	2.5	0.7	2.7	0.7	3.0	0.6	9.4	< .001	1 < 2 < 3
SAT verbal score	492.2	124.5	540.2	111.1	510.7	121.1	1.29	NS	
SAT quantitative score	491.8	127.5	547.0	119.1	532.3	121.2	2.1	NS	

Note. Sample sizes for interview reports are ADHD = 145, Clinical control = 94, and Community control = 108. For elementary school, they are 70, 44, and 33, respectively. For high school percent Ds and Fs, they are 116, 80, and 86. For class ranking, they are 52, 37, and 53. For days absent they are 44, 30, and 35. For Verbal and Quantitative Test Percentiles, they are 51, 31, and 41. For grade-point average, they are 115, 78, and 86. For college, percent Ds and Fs, they are 75, 75, and 69. For percent withdrawals, they are 74, 71, and 69. For grade-point average, they are 74, 73, and 68. For SAT scores, they are 42, 39, and 34. SD = standard deviation; F = F-test results of the analysis of variance (or covariance); p = probability value for the F-test; NS = not significant, [S] = significant main effect for sex (see text for details); [GxS] = significant group × sex interaction (see text for details); [A] = age used as a covariate in this analysis; percent D, F, and U grades = percentage of grades recorded on transcript that were D, F, or unsatisfactory; mean days absent/sem. = average number of days absent per semester.

Statistical analysis: Groups were initially compared using two-way (groups × sex) analysis of variance (or covariance as necessary). Where this analysis was significant ($p < .05$) for the main effect for group, pairwise comparisons of the groups were conducted, the results of which are shown in the last column.

TABLE 9.5. Educational Functioning by Group for the Milwaukee Study

Measure	H+ADHD		H–ADHD		Community		F	p	Pairwise contrasts
	Mean	SD	Mean	SD	Mean	SD			
Education (years)	12.2	2.2	12.8	2.1	15.8	2.3	52.49	< .001	1,2 < 3
No. of times suspended	16.6	34.0	14.5	50.5	1.3	4.4	3.80	.024	1,2 > 3
No. of times truant	93.2	162.1	71.9	119.1	23.5	76.9	5.94	.003	1,2 > 3

Note. Sample sizes are H+ADHD = 55, H–ADHD = 80, and Community control = 75. *SD* = standard deviation; *F* = *F*-test results of the analysis of variance (or covariance); *p* = probability value for the *F*-test; NS = not significant; H+ADHD = Hyperactive group that currently has a diagnosis of ADHD at follow-up; H–ADHD = Hyperactive group that does not have a diagnosis of ADHD at follow-up.

Statistical analysis: Groups were initially compared using one-way (groups) analysis of variance. Where this analysis was significant (*p* < .05) for the main effect for group, pairwise comparisons of the groups were conducted the results of which are shown in the last column.

(unsatisfactory). For elementary school and high school, we also coded the average number of days they were reported as having been absent from school per year on the transcript. On their high school transcript, we recorded their class ranking in their senior or last year of high school attended. For high school and college, we computed their grade-point average using a scale of 0 to 4 (grades of F to A). If reported in numerical scores, such as 90–100, 80–89, 70–79, we recoded them as 0 (50–59), 1 (60–69), and so on. If any verbal or quantitative test scores were available on the high school transcript, we recorded that information as well. We did likewise for the verbal and quantitative Scholastic Aptitude Test (SAT) scores that may have been recorded on college transcripts. All of this information is also reported in Table 9.3 for each group. On their elementary school transcripts, the ADHD group had a greater percentage of poor or failing grades than either control group, which did not differ from each other. The groups did not differ in their average number of days absent in elementary school.

In high school, once again, the adults with ADHD had a significantly greater percentage of grades of D and F on their transcripts and were ranked lower in their class standing than were adults in either of our control groups. Not surprisingly, then, we also documented a lower grade-point average for the ADHD group than the two control groups. Unlike the case during their elementary school period, we did find that the ADHD group had significantly more days absent from high school than adults in either of our control groups. Of note is that the Clinical and Community control groups did not differ in any of these respects.

Among those who attended college and allowed us to obtain their transcripts, we found results consistent with those noted above for high school. Once again, the percentage of unsatisfactory grades (Ds and Fs) was significantly higher for the ADHD group than for either of the control groups. The adults with ADHD had also withdrawn from more classes that they had initially registered for in college than had the Clinical control adults. Again, we found a significantly lower grade-point average among the adults with ADHD than was the case for either control group in college. The results for SAT scores did not differ across the groups, however.

This is the first study to our knowledge to document, through official archival records, the adverse impact of ADHD on education in clinic-referred adults in comparison to both a Clinical and a Community control group. Our extensive and detailed examination of school records corroborates the self-reports of these adults and the reports obtained from others (Table 9.1) with regard to the lower educational functioning of adults with ADHD. They do so across elementary, high school, and college educational histories. Despite having verbal and quantitative test scores comparable to those of the control groups in both high school and college, adults with ADHD received more unsatisfactory grades, had a lower overall grade-point average, received a poorer class ranking, and, in high school, had more days absent from school than adults in our other two groups. That ADHD in adults is associated with educational impairment and is more likely to be so than in other outpatient clinical disorders is readily apparent in the totality of these findings. The disorder exacts a considerable toll in the educational sphere that can be specifically attributed to ADHD and not just to outpatient psychiatric status.

There were some significant main effects for sex or significant interactions of sex with group membership in some of these findings, as indicated in Table 9.4. One of these was already described in Chapter 4, in dealing with years of education. Recall from there that males with ADHD had significantly less education than did females with ADHD, whereas the opposite pattern was evident in the Community control group. The sexes did not differ in the Clinical control group. School suspension rates also differed by sex across the groups (see Figure 9.3). Males in the ADHD group experienced more school suspensions than did females, whose suspension rates were low and comparable to those seen in females in the two control groups. In those groups, the difference between males and females was not significant. Males across all groups had a lower grade-point average than did females, with this difference being more obvious in the ADHD group. In college grades, we found a significant interaction of sex with group, as shown in Figure 9.4. Females with ADHD had a higher percentage of D's on their transcripts than did males with ADHD—a pattern that was the reverse of that seen in the Clinical control group. This was not the case for grades of F on this transcript, where no significant sex difference was evident, as shown in Table 9.4. In their college grade-point averages, males in general scored significantly lower than females. To summarize, males experienced more school suspensions and had lower high school and college grade-point averages than did females.

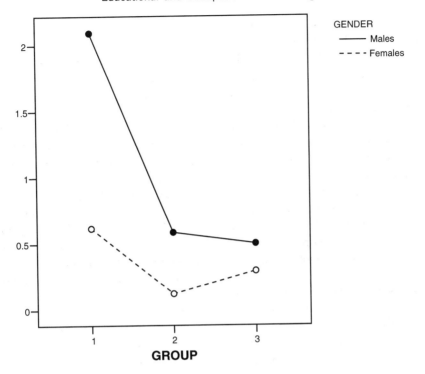

FIGURE 9.3. Illustration of the significant group × sex interaction on the raw scores for number of school suspensions (self-reported, interview). Scores are shown for each sex within each group. Group 1 = ADHD, 2 = Clinical control, 3 = Community control. Gender 1 = males and 2 = females.

The number of years of education, however, was significantly lower in males with ADHD, while the number of school suspensions was significantly higher in males than in females with ADHD. All of this suggests that males in general may have greater educational difficulties but that this may be especially so for males with ADHD.

Achievement Test Scores

Achievement tests were given to the participants in both studies (see sidebar) so as to evaluate single-word reading, written arithmetic, written spelling, reading comprehension, and reading rate. The results for the clinic-referred adults in the UMASS Study are shown in Table 9.6. It is immediately evident that the ADHD group scored significantly lower on four of the five achievement tests relative to the Community control group, the only exception being single word reading

Structured Clinical Interview of Impairments

For this project, we created an interview consisting of questions dealing with various domains of major life activities, including educational history, occupational history, antisocial activities, drug use, driving, money management, and dating and marital history. This interview was administered by a psychological technician holding a master's degree in psychology and trained in the evaluation of clinic-referred adults. The questions dealing with educational and occupational history are reported here.

Wide Range Achievement Test–III (Jastak & Jastak, 1996)

Reading, spelling, and math skills were briefly assessed with this widely used achievement test. Reading is assessed through single-word pronunciation that progresses until the participant either completes the list or gets 5 words wrong out of the previous 10. The spelling test consists of spelling to dictation in which the participant is given a word and must spell the word correctly in writing. The test progresses until all words are dictated or the point of 5 missed words out of the previous 10 is reached. The math test consists of a series of written math problems of progressively greater difficulty. All scores are converted from the raw test scores to both a standard score and a percentile score based on norms provided by the publisher.

Nelson–Denny Reading Test (Riverside Publishing Company, 1993)

This test evaluates comprehension for written passages. After reading the passages, the participant answers a series of multiple-choice questions about the content of the paragraph. Reading rate is also assessed. Raw scores are converted to percentiles based on norms provided by the publisher.

from the WRAT-III. Also, the ADHD group was significantly below the levels of skills of the Clinical control group on spelling, written math, and reading comprehension. The ADHD and Clinical control groups did not differ in their reading rate, however.

It is important here to recall that subsets of the ADHD and Clinical control groups were taking medication at study entry (Chapter 4). It is possible that such medications may have effects on these test results. We therefore compared those ADHD cases taking medication to those not doing so on all of these test scores. The groups did not differ significantly on any tests. We did the same for the adults in the Clinical control group, where we also found no differences between the medicated and unmedicated groups. These findings suggested that medication status had no detectable influence on these test scores and is unlikely to

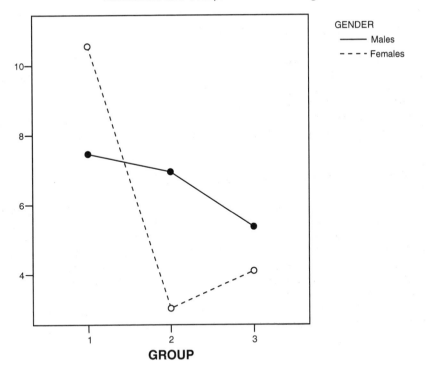

FIGURE 9.4. Mean percentage of D's on college transcript for each sex within each group. Group 1 = ADHD, 2 = Clinical control, 3 = Community control.

account for any group differences. We therefore reported the results for all participants in Table 9.6.

The results for the hyperactive children grown up are shown in Table 9.7. Like those of the UMASS Study, these results indicate that those with ADHD in adulthood have significantly lower achievement skills than do control groups. In this case, both hyperactive groups did more poorly in reading skills, but the H+ADHD group was even more impaired in spelling and math than were those in the H−ADHD group. Unlike our findings in the UMASS Study, we did not find differences among our groups on the Nelson–Denny Reading test. To summarize, whether one is studying clinic-referred adults with ADHD or children growing up with the disorder, it is associated with significantly lower academic achievement skills than are seen in other outpatient control groups or community control groups. There is evidence here as well that growing up as a child with ADHD has a more adverse impact on these skills in adulthood than is seen in clinic-referred adults, at least for basic skills assessed by the WRAT-III. Reading comprehension, in contrast, seems more impaired, for some unknown reason, in the clinic-referred adults with ADHD.

TABLE 9.6. Achievement Test Results (Percentiles) by Group for the UMASS Study

Measure	ADHD Mean	SD	Clinical Mean	SD	Community Mean	SD	F	p	Pairwise contrasts
WRAT-3									
Reading percentile	64.8	19.9	69.0	19.6	64.2	19.2	1.7	NS	
Spelling percentile[S]	54.5	23.6	65.6	20.7	64.4	19.5	6.1	.002	1 < 2,3
Math percentile[S]	49.3	24.6	61.5	25.5	56.3	23.1	6.8	.001	1 < 2,3
Nelson–Denny reading									
Comprehension percent	40.8	28.9	49.7	28.4	52.9	25.3	5.5	.004	1 < 2,3
Reading rate percentile	44.2	29.5	50.9	29.1	60.8	27.6	8.6	< .001	1,2 < 3

Note. Sample sizes for WRAT-3 are: ADHD = 143, Clinical = 92, Community = 108. For Nelson–Denny, they are ADHD = 126, Clinical = 87, Community = 108. SD = standard deviation; F = F-test results of the analysis of variance; p = probability value for the F-test; NS = not significant; [S] = significant main effect for sex (where this was found, females outperformed males).

Statistical analysis: Groups were initially compared using two-way (groups × sex) analysis of variance. Where this analysis was significant (p < .05) for the main effect for group, pairwise comparisons of the groups were conducted, the results of which are shown in the last column.

TABLE 9.7. Achievement Test Results (Standard Scores) by Group for the Milwaukee Study

Measures	H+ADHD Mean	SD	H–ADHD Mean	SD	Community Mean	SD	F	p	Pairwise contrasts
WRAT-3									
Reading	99.5	12.4	101.0	11.8	104.8	6.2	6.79	.001	1,2 < 3
Spelling	93.1	14.7	97.2	14.9	100.3	9.5	6.78	.001	1,3
Math	91.6	13.9	96.1	13.3	102.1	11.3	14.4	< .001	1 < 2 < 3
Nelson–Denny reading									
Reading vocabulary	222.8	27.8	223.7	28.1	225.7	14.3	0.73	NS	
Comprehension	209.1	26.8	211.2	27.4	215.1	20.0	1.71	NS	
Reading rate score	202.0	24.9	206.7	30.3	204.8	20.7	0.68	NS	

Note. Sample sizes for WRAT-3 are ADHD = 143, Clinical = 92, Community = 108. For Nelson–Denny, they are ADHD = 126, Clinical = 87, Community = 108. WRAT-3 scores are standard scores. Nelson–Denny scores are standard scores (M = 200, SD = 25). Means are estimated marginal means. SD = standard deviation; F = F-test results of the analysis of variance); p = probability value for the F-test; NS = not significant; H+ADHD = hyperactive group that currently has a diagnosis of ADHD at follow-up; H–ADHD = hyperactive group that does not have a diagnosis of ADHD at follow-up.

Statistical analysis: Groups were initially compared using one-way (groups) analysis of covariance with WAIS Vocabulary and Block Design serving as covariates. Where this analysis was significant (p < .05) for the main effect for group, pairwise comparisons of the groups were conducted, the results of which are shown in the last column.

Learning Disabilities

At a certain point, deficits in academic achievement skills rise to the level of being considered specific learning disabilities (SLDs). In view of their deficits in academic achievement skills noted above, it is not surprising that adults with ADHD may be more likely than Community control adults to have SLDs, as shown above. An SLD, however, is not simply failing to do one's work in school but is typically defined as a significant discrepancy between one's intelligence, or general mental abilities, and a specific area of academic achievement skills, such as reading, math, or spelling. The prevalence rates of SLDs can vary greatly as a function of whether and how this significant discrepancy between IQ and achievement is defined or whether another metric for SLD is used instead, such as a very low percentile score only on the achievement test. Only a few studies have examined the prevalence of learning disabilities (discussed above), and there is some disparity among studies. Some found only math disorders among adults with ADHD, while others found only reading disorders. Part of the problem in such studies is one of definition—how should a SLD be defined?

Several different formulas can be applied to define an SLD. For a review of the previous literature on SLDs in ADHD children using a variety of approaches, see the report by Semrud-Clikeman et al. (1992). One such formula used in past research with children having ADHD (Lambert & Sandoval, 1980) compared scores on intelligence tests with those on achievement tests for reading and math. An SLD was defined as a significant discrepancy between these scores. Such a discrepancy can be based on an absolute amount, say 20 points, or it can be based on the standard deviation (*SD*) or error of the tests, say 15 points or 1 *SD*, where both tests have a mean of 100 and an *SD* of 15. A problem with this IQ–achievement discrepancy approach is that it tends to overestimate the prevalence of learning disorders, especially in children performing normally in school and those who are intellectually above average or gifted. For instance, when Dykman and Ackerman (1992) defined a reading disorder as a discrepancy between IQ and achievement of only 10 points as well as a standard score on the reading test below 90, they found that 45% were so disordered. Likewise, when Semrud-Clikeman et al. (1992) required only a 10-point discrepancy between IQ and achievement, 38% of their ADHD children could be considered reading-disabled and 55% math-disabled (the rates for normal children were 8% and 33%, respectively). Such children may be performing perfectly adequately in school and on achievement tests, but because of their higher than normal levels of intelligence may have a significant discrepancy between their IQ and achievement test scores (e.g., IQ = 130, whereas Reading Standard Score = 100). Barkley (1990) previously reported on the prevalence of children with ADHD who had an SLD by this relatively simple criterion (15-point IQ–achievement discrepancy) using the results of one of his studies (Barkley, DuPaul, et al., 1990). The rates were 40% in reading, nearly 60% in spelling, and nearly 60% in math. However, the rates in the normal control group were 20%, 38%, and 35%, respectively, being defined as SLD. Clearly this illustrates the problem of overidentification noted above and is not a rigorous approach to defining SLD.

A second approach is to use a larger discrepancy (20 points). Frick and colleagues (Frick, Kamphaus, Lahey, Loeber, Christ, Hart, et al. 1991) estimated that 16% of ADHD children had a reading disability, whereas 21% had a math disability. The corresponding prevalence in their normal control group was 5% and 7%, respectively. Likewise, when Semrud-Clikeman et al. (1992) increased the required discrepancy to 20 points, 23% of the ADHD children could be considered reading-disabled and 30% math-disabled versus 2% and 22% of normal children, respectively.

A third approach is to define SLD as a score falling below 1.5 SDs from the normal mean on an achievement test (7th or 16th percentile, representing approximately 1.5 and 1 SDs below the mean, respectively), regardless of the child's IQ. This approach makes more sense, given the close association of IQ and academic achievement, and it is far less likely to diagnose normal children as having an SLD. But it may diagnose borderline mildly retarded children as such, because their achievement test scores would be consistent with their exceptionally low IQ scores and place them below this SLD cutoff point. Using this approach, Barkley (1990) found the following prevalence of SLD in the same children with ADHD used previously in his earlier calculations above, using the 7th percentile as the threshold for SLD: 21% in reading, 26% in spelling, and over 28% in math. For the normal children, these rates were 0%, 2.9%, and 2.9%, respectively. None of the children in this particular study were in the borderline range of IQ or lower (mental retardation); thus the rate of misclassifying ADHD children with so low an IQ score cannot be determined from this study. Obviously, this approach addressed the problem of overidentification of SLD in normal children and adults.

For the UMASS Study, we defined SLD by these three methods. First, we used a disparity of 1 SD between the IQ score (standard score) of our participants and their achievement test standard scores in reading, spelling, and math from the WRAT-III. We then applied a greater disparity of 1.5 SD to define SLD. Finally, we simply used the 14th percentile or lower on an achievement test (slightly lower than −1 SD below the mean). In this case, we were also able to compute SLDs for reading comprehension using the Nelson–Denny Reading Test, given that it provided percentile scores (but not standard scores based on a mean of 100 and an SD of 15, like the IQ and WRAT-III tests). We also had available scores for listening comprehension from the Learning and Memory Battery, discussed in Chapter 13, on neuropsychological deficits. We present these results in Table 9.8.

TABLE 9.8. SLD Diagnoses under Three Different Definitions for Each Group in the UMASS Study

Measure	ADHD N	ADHD %	Clinical N	Clinical %	Community N	Community %	χ^2	p	Pairwise contrasts
SLD by 1 *SD* disparity									
Reading disorder	8	6	7	8	8	7	0.5	NS	
Spelling disorderS	22	15	15	16	13	12	0.8	NS	
Math disorder	32	22	10	11	17	16	5.3	NS	
SLD by 1.5 *SD* disparity									
Reading disorder	3	2	3	3	1	1	1.3	NS	
Spelling disorderS	11	8	4	4	5	5	1.5	NS	
Math disorder	11	8	2	2	5	5	3.5	NS	
SLD by 14th percentile									
Reading disorder	4	3	2	2	2	2	0.2	NS	
Spelling disorderS	13	9	5	5	1	1	7.9	.02	1 > 3
Math disorder	15	10	6	6	5	5	3.2	NS	
Reading comprehension dis.	28	21	14	16	10	9	6.4	.041	1 > 3
Listening comprehension dis.S	55	41	23	26	15	14	21.7	< .001	1 > 2 > 3

Note. Sample sizes are ADHD = 143, Clinical = 92, and Community = 108 for SLD determined by WRAT-3 achievement tests. For the Nelson–Denny, they are ADHD = 132, Clinical = 89, and Community = 108. *N* = sample size endorsing this item; % = percent of group endorsing this item; χ^2 = results of the omnibus chi-square test; *p* = probability value for the chi-square test; pairwise contrasts = results of the chi-square tests involving pairwise comparisons of the three groups; S = Significant main effect for sex (see text for details); SLD by 1.5 *SD* disparity = diagnosed as specific learning disabled by having at least a 1.5 *SD* (22+ standard points) difference between IQ and that WRAT-3 achievement test; SLD by 1 *SD* disparity = diagnosed as specific learning disability by having at least a 1 *SD* (15+ standard points) difference between IQ and that WRAT-3 achievement test; SLD by 14th percentile = diagnosed as specific learning disability by being at or below the 14th percentile (< −1 *SD* from normative mean) on the WRAT-3 reading, spelling, and math subtests, Nelson–Denny reading comprehension test, and the Learning and Memory Battery Paragraph Free Recall subset retention score; dis. = disorder.

By the most liberal definition of SLD (1 *SD* disparity of IQ vs. achievement), we found that 6% of adults with ADHD had a reading disorder, 15% had a spelling disorder, and 22% had a math disorder. These percentages did not differ from those found in the other two groups. Indeed, this illustrates the problem of overidentification in normal controls discussed above, given that we found that 7 to 16% of our Community control group had an SLD by this definition. When we used a larger disparity of 1.5 *SD*, the proportion of each group having an SLD declined considerably (2–8% for ADHD, 2–4% for Clinical control, and 1–5% for Community control groups); but again the groups did not differ in this regard. In contrast, using the 14th percentile on an achievement test to define SLD, we found differences among our groups that are graphically depicted in Figure 9.5. The ADHD group had a significantly higher percentage of spelling, reading, and listening comprehension disorders

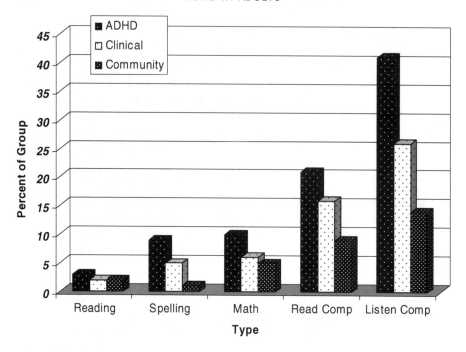

FIGURE 9.5. Percentage of each group in the UMASS Study having reading, spelling, math, reading comprehension, and listening comprehension disorders defined as 14th percentile or lower for test standardization sample. Groups do not differ in reading and math disorders (see Table 9.8). Comp = comprehension.

than did the Community control group. Differences between the ADHD and Clinical control groups, however, were not found, nor did the Clinical control group differ from the Community control group in these respects. Only on listening comprehension did we find a significantly greater occurrence among the ADHD group (41%) than the Clinical control group (26%), with the latter also differing from the Community control group (14%). Given that the 14th percentile on the tests was chosen to define SLD, we would have expected 14% of our normal Community control group to be so identified, which we did. These results suggest that spelling and comprehension problems (reading and listening) are SLDs for adults with ADHD compared to Community control adults, but only listening comprehension problems distinguish the ADHD group from the Clinical control adults. These rates of SLD are dramatically below those seen in children with ADHD, and in those children followed to adulthood. This seems to indicate that clinic-referred ADHD adults are not as likely to have SLDs as are children with ADHD.

Consistent with several prior studies discussed above, we documented a spelling disorder for adults with ADHD, but unlike these prior studies we were not able to identify a greater prevalence of reading or math disorders. That is not to say that adults with ADHD are functioning well in these academic areas. Above, we documented that such adults perform more poorly not only on spelling tests, but also on math and comprehension tests even if these deficits do not rise to the level of diagnosis required for an SLD. As far as we are aware, this is the first study of adults with ADHD to examine reading and listening comprehension abilities as possible SLDs associated with this disorder, apart from the more traditional examination of math, reading, and spelling SLDs. We have documented a significant adverse effect of adult ADHD on these comprehension tests. Such findings are important, given that comprehension of what is read or heard is a ubiquitous requirement of adult functioning across most domains of major life activities; therefore the impact of deficits in this area would be equally ubiquitous.

We found several main effects for sex. These were on spelling and listening comprehension disorders, where males were more likely to have these disorders than females ($p = .003$ and $.006$, respectively). Otherwise, there was no interaction of sex with the group factor. This indicates that where males and females with ADHD may differ in rates of these disorders, more general sex difference typical of the population at large are reflected.

Our results were not unexpected. Research in children with ADHD has documented problems with story comprehension. The topic has been studied extensively in ADHD children by Elizabeth Lorch and her colleagues, using television programs (see Lorch, O'Neil, Berthiaume, Milich, Eastham, & Brooks, 2004; Lorch, Milich, Sanchez, van den Broek, Baer, Hooks, et al. 2000). Both elementary-age and preschool-age children with ADHD demonstrate impaired recall of story information after watching televised stories. Particularly problematic was their recall of causal connections (Lorch et al., 2000; Lorch et al., 2004; Lorch et al. 1999; Sanchez, Lorch, Milich, & Welsh, 1999). Cued recall does not seem to be problematic, especially for simple details. But unassisted recall, particularly for deeper information such as knowledge of relations and causal connections, is more impaired by ADHD. Again, some research suggests that listening comprehension is also problematic in children with language impairments as well as those with ADHD, raising some questions about the Lorch research group's findings and their specificity to ADHD alone (McInnes, Humphries, Hogg-Johnson, & Tannock, 2003). But as Lorch's research implies, ADHD is certainly associated with higher-order problems in listening comprehension, which have shown some association with other working memory tasks (McInnes et al., 2003), and with the presence of distractors during TV viewing. This is an area ripe for further study in adults with ADHD, given our initial findings that comprehension, whether while reading or while listening, is an area of deficiency for clinic-referred adults with ADHD as well as their childhood counterparts.

As discussed earlier, we administered the WRAT-III to the H+ADHD and H–ADHD groups in the Milwaukee Study at age-27 follow-up. We used these results to define a SLD in this study as well. To save time, we did not calculate the three different definitions of SLD discussed above. Instead, we used only the most stringent of those definitions, that being a score on an achievement test falling at or below the 14th percentile. These findings are shown in Table 9.9. They indicate that, as with other measures of academic success, both hyperactive groups had significantly higher rates of learning disabilities than did the Community control group. Although the two hyperactive groups did not differ in their percentages of having reading and spelling disorders, those having current ADHD (H+ADHD) had significantly more math disorders than did those who no longer qualified as having ADHD (H–ADHD). Both hyperactive groups had significantly more members with a reading comprehension disorder than did the Community control group, but again the two former groups did not differ from each other in this respect. We depict these group differences in Figure 9.6, so that they can be more easily compared to those for the UMASS ADHD adult group in Figure 9.5. The percentages of SLDs in reading, spelling, and math for the hyperactive groups can be seen to be far greater than those in the UMASS Study adults with ADHD, while the percentage for reading comprehension is nearly identical to that in the UMASS Study. Once more, we show that children growing up with ADHD are more educationally impaired than are clinic-referred adults diagnosed with the disorder.

TABLE 9.9. SLD Diagnoses (14th Percentile or Lower) for Each Group in the Milwaukee Study

	H+ADHD		H–ADHD		Community				Pairwise
Measures	N	%	N	%	N	%	χ^2	p	contrasts
Reading disorder	10	19	11	14	1	1	11.39	.003	1,2 > 3
Spelling disorder	19	36	22	29	1	1	27.13	< .001	1,2 > 3
Math disorder	21	40	17	21	2	3	27.60	< .001	1 > 2 > 3
Reading comprehension	10	20	16	20	2	3	11.72	.003	1,2 > 3

Note. Sample sizes are H+ADHD = 52, H–ADHD = 79, and Community = 73. SLD was determined by WRAT-3 reading, spelling, and math, and Nelson–Denny Reading Comprehension standard scores falling at or below 84 (–1 *SD* or 14th percentile). N = sample size endorsing this item; % = percent of group endorsing this item; χ^2 = results of the omnibus chi-square test; p = probability value for the chi-square test; pairwise contrasts = results of the chi-square tests involving pairwise comparisons of the three groups. H+ADHD = hyperactive group that currently has a diagnosis of ADHD at follow-up; H–ADHD = hyperactive group that does not have a diagnosis of ADHD at follow-up.

Statistical analysis: Pearson chi-square.

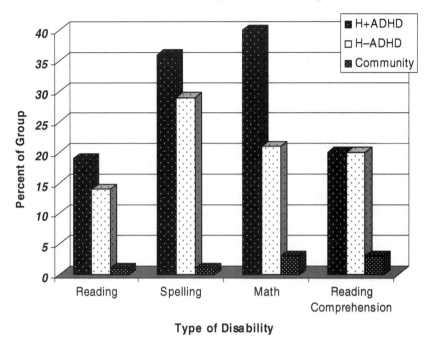

FIGURE 9.6. Percent of each group in the Milwaukee Study having reading, spelling, math, and reading comprehension disorders defined as falling at or below 14th percentile of the test normative sample. H+ADHD = Hyperactive group currently having ADHD; H–ADHD = Hyperactive group not currently having ADHD; Community = Community control group.

Predicting Adverse Educational Outcomes

As we did in the previous chapter, we selected those outcomes that appeared to be specific risks for the ADHD group in the UMASS Study relative to the Clinical and Community control groups and attempted to identify predictors (correlates, actually) that may have contributed to or been associated with these outcomes. We used the entire sample to do so. The ADHD group had a significant risk for having been retained in grade. We examined predictors of this categorical outcome using logistic regression. The results appear in Table 9.10. As this table indicates, risk of grade retention was predicted by greater severity of ADHD, lower IQ, and poorer spelling performance (WRAT-3). Level of reading, reading comprehension, math, severity of childhood ADHD, and diagnosis of ODD or CD made no significant contribution to this outcome.

Several educational outcomes that were specific to the ADHD group were dimensional in nature, these being fewer years of education and lower high school grade-point average. We used multiple regression to examine a set of predictors of these outcomes. The results are shown in Table 9.11. More years of education were predicted by lower levels of ADHD symptoms, better reading comprehension, a lower criminal diversity score (see Chapter 10), and better spelling ability. Level of IQ, basic reading ability, childhood CD severity, current anxiety, and current depression were not predictive of this particular educational outcome. For grade-point average in high school, we again found that lower levels of ADHD symptoms, higher IQ, better spelling ability, lower criminal diversity, and better reading comprehension and math abilities were all significantly predictive of a higher high school grade-point average. Such analyses give us some idea of the other individual characteristics, besides ADHD severity, that were contributing to these educational outcomes in our UMASS Study groups.

We used these same two forms of statistical analysis to examine predictors of several of the educational outcomes in the Milwaukee Study. We chose two categorical outcomes that were significantly more impaired in the hyperactive groups (H+ADHD and H–ADHD) than control group, these being having ever been retained in grade and whether or not they had graduated high school. We used sets of predictors from childhood study entry and teen and young adult (age 21) follow-up points, similar to those used in the UMASS Study. There were 14 predictors used in total. In this case, however, these predictors were not retrospectively recalled but had actually been collected at those age periods. The results for these analyses appear in Table 9.12. They show that risk for retention

TABLE 9.10. Predicting Risk of Grade Retention in the UMASS Study

Outcome/predictors (block entered)	Beta	SE	Wald	p	Odds ratio	95% CI
Retained in grade						
(1) No. of ADHD symptoms (interview)	.131	.036	13.53	< .001	1.14	1.06–1.22
(1) Age	–.006	.015	0.17	NS	0.99	0.96–1.02
(2) IQ (Shipley)	–.055	.024	5.36	.021	0.95	0.90–0.99
(2) Spelling (WRAT-3)	–.062	.017	13.83	< .001	0.94	0.91–0.97

NS: reading (WRAT-3), math (WRAT-3), reading comprehension (Nelson–Denny), no. of child ADHD symptoms (interview), ODD diagnosis (childhood ratings), CD diagnosis (childhood ratings)

Note. SE = standard error for beta; odds ratio = Exp(B); 95% CI = 95% confidence interval for the odds ratio; NS = not significant; WRAT-3 = Wide Range Achievement Test–3 standard score; Shipley = Shipley Institute of Living Scale IQ estimate; Nelson–Denny = Nelson–Denny Reading Comprehension Test standard score; ODD diagnosis = met DSM-IV criterion for oppositional defiant disorder on symptom threshold from self-reported childhood rating scale; CD diagnosis = met DSM-IV criterion for conduct disorder on symptom threshold from self-reported childhood rating scale.
Statistical analysis: Logistic regression using forced entry method at block 1 and forward conditional method at block 2. Used the entire sample (N = 353).

TABLE 9.11. Predicting Years of Education and High School Grade-Point Average in the UMASS Study

Outcome/predictors (step entered)	Beta	R	R²	R²Δ	F	p
Education (years)						
(1) No. of ADHD symptoms (interview)* and age (NS)	−.089 .304	.326	.106	.106	20.81	< .001
(2) Reading comprehension (Nelson–Denny)	.209	.493	.243	.137	62.94	< .001
(3) Math (WRAT-3)	.220	.542	.294	.051	25.23	< .001
(4) No. of crime types (lifetime)	−.162	.563	.317	.023	11.90	.001
(5) Spelling (WRAT-3)	.145	.576	.332	.015	7.61	.006

NS: IQ (Shipley), reading (WRAT-3), no. of CD symptoms (childhood), anxiety (SCL-90-R), depression (SCL-90-R)

Outcome/predictors (step entered)	Beta	R	R²	R²Δ	F	p
High school grade-point average						
(1) No. of ADHD symptoms and age (NS)	−285 −.055	.285	.081	.081	15.41	< .001
(2) IQ	.175	.488	.238	.157	72.06	< .001
(3) Spelling	.179	.541	.292	.054	26.57	< .001
(4) No. of crime types (lifetime)	−.187	.567	.322	.029	15.05	< .001
(5) Reading comprehension	.155	.581	.338	.016	8.56	.004
(6) Math	.110	.589	.347	.009	4.78	.030

NS: No. of ADHD childhood symptoms, reading (WRAT-3), no. of CD symptoms (childhood), anxiety (SCL-90-R), depression (SCL-90-R)

Note. R = regression coefficient; R² = percent of explained variance accounted for by all variables at this step; R²Δ = percent of explained variance accounted for by this variable added at this step; F change = results of F-test for the equation at this step; p = probability value for the F-test; * = this variable became nonsignificant when other variables were entered in the next step; beta = standardized beta coefficient; NS = not significant. Nelson–Denny = Nelson–Denny Reading Comprehension Test standard score; WRAT-3 = Wide Range Achievement Test-3 standard score; Shipley = Shipley Institute of Living Scale IQ estimate; SCL-90-R = Symptom Checklist–90—Revised T-score.

Statistical analysis: Multiple linear regression using forced entry method at step 1 and stepwise conditional method at subsequent steps. Used the entire sample (N = 353).

in grade was significantly predicted from five measures. From childhood, the severity of the CPRS-R Hyperactivity Index and childhood IQ were significant. From the teen follow-up, the number of ODD symptoms was inversely related to this risk—to our surprise, indicating that lower levels of parent-reported ODD were more likely to be associated with being retained. Level of math skills at the teen follow-up was also associated with risk of retention. Just one young adult measure was significant, and that was the number of ADHD symptoms reported by the parent by age 21. To summarize, it is severity of childhood ADHD and its persistence to age 21, along with lower childhood IQ and teen math achievement skills, that significantly increase risk for grade retention across the school careers of these participants. Levels of antisocial behavior (CD symptoms) and

TABLE 9.12. Predicting Risk of Grade Retention and High School Graduation in the Milwaukee Study

Outcome/predictors (block entered)	Beta	*SE*	Wald	*p*	Odds ratio	95% CI
Retained in grade						
Child CPRS-R Index	.087	.042	4.35	.037	1.09	1.00–1.18
Child IQ (final model)	−.039	.023	2.86	.091	0.96	0.92–1.00
Initial entry at block 1	−.054	.019	7.70	.007	0.95	0.91–0.98
Teen no. of ODD symptoms (parent)	−.496	.173	8.21	.004	0.61	0.43–0.85
Teen WRAT math score	−.097	.025	14.45	< .001	0.91	0.86–0.95
Age 21 no. of ADHD symptoms (parent)	.187	.090	4.36	.037	1.21	1.01–1.44

NS: Child WWPARS, CPRS-R conduct problem, and HSQ no. of settings scores, teen no. of ADHD and CD symptoms (parent), WRAT reading and spelling standard scores, and duration of childhood stimulant treatment, and young adult (age 21) no. of ADHD, ODD, and CD symptoms (self-reported).

Graduated from high school						
Child HSQ no. of settings (final model)	−.280	.199	1.98	.159	0.76	0.51–1.12
Initial entry at block 1	−.497	.145	11.82	.001	0.61	0.46–0.81
Teen no. of ADHD symptoms (parent)	−.301	.150	4.02	.045	0.74	0.55–0.99
Age 21 no. of CD symptoms (self)	−.925	.393	5.54	.019	0.40	0.18–0.86

NS: Child WWPARS, CPRS-R Index, and childhood IQ, Teen no. of ODD and CD symptoms (parent) and WRAT reading, spelling, and math scores, and duration of childhood stimulant treatment, and young adult (age 21) ADHD (parent and self-reported) and ODD (self) symptoms

Note. SE = standard error for beta; odds ratio = Exp(B); 95% CI = 95% confidence interval for the Odds Ratio; NS = not significant; WRAT = Wide Range Achievement Test standard score, CPRS-R = Conners Parent Rating Scale–Revised; WWPARS = Werry–Weiss–Peters Activity Rating Scale, HSQ = Home Situations Questionnaire number of problem settings; childhood IQ = Peabody Picture Vocabulary Test score; ADHD = attention deficit hyperactivity disorder (DSM-III-R); ODD = oppositional defiant disorder symptoms (DSM-III-R); CD = conduct disorder symptoms (DSM-III-R).

Statistical analysis: Binary logistic regression using three entry blocks for child, teen, and young adult measures, respectively, with forward conditional method of entry. Used the entire sample (*N* = 236). All results are for the final model across all three entry blocks unless a predictor became nonsignificant in the final model, in which case the results for its initial entry and block are shown as well.

social aggressiveness (ODD symptoms) are not predictive of this outcome, and the latter may actually be inversely related to it. Two of these significant predictors are similar to those found in the UMASS Study to predict this same outcome, those being severity of ADHD and IQ. The Milwaukee Study, though, is a far better predictor of this outcome, given its collection of measures at time points in the actual educational careers of these participants from childhood through adolescence and adulthood.

We also examined predictors of graduating from high school, as reported at age 27. We used the same set of 14 predictors as above. These results also appear in Table 9.12. Just three predictors were related to this outcome, those being the pervasiveness of childhood ADHD (HSQ scores), the severity of teen ADHD symptoms as reported by parents, and the severity of CD symptoms self-reported at age 21. That the CD symptoms enter the equation only after the age at which one typically graduates high school suggests that they may not be so much a predictor as an outcome associated with not completing high school. We say this because severity of conduct problems in childhood and specifically ODD and CD at teen follow-up around the time of high school were not predictive of high school graduation. This makes it clear that the likelihood of graduating or not from high school is largely related to ADHD especially in high school, but it may be associated with increased CD symptoms thereafter. Given that the groups in the UMASS Study did not differ in their high school graduation percentages, we did not examine that outcome for any predictors, so we cannot compare these Milwaukee Study results to the UMASS Study in this instance.

We did, however, examine predictors of the same two-dimensional educational outcomes that were used in the UMASS Study discussed above, these being years of education and high school grade-point average. We had collected the latter at the age-21 follow-up directly from high school transcripts, as in the UMASS Study. We explored the utility of the same set of 14 predictors used above for predicting grade retention and high school graduation. The results for these analyses are displayed in Table 9.13. Educational attainment was predicted by 6 of the 14 predictors. Those from childhood were severity of hyperactivity (WWPARS), IQ, and pervasiveness of behavioral problems (HSQ). From the teen follow-up measures, three more were significant: teen math achievement (WRAT) and the number of teen CD and ODD symptoms as reported by parents. Once more, teen ODD symptoms surprised us by being associated with more years of education, much as they had been associated with high school graduation. Higher levels of ODD symptoms were related to more years of education once teen CD symptoms had been controlled in the equation. This suggests that teen ODD symptoms that are independent of CD may actually make positive contributions to educational success. At the age-21 follow-up, just severity of CD symptoms predicted years of education. In total, these predictors accounted for nearly 44% of the variance in educational attainment, and most of

TABLE 9.13. Predicting Years of Education and High School Grade-Point Average in the Milwaukee Study

Outcome/predictors (step entered)	Beta	R	R^2	$R^2\Delta$	F	p
Education (years)						
Child WWPARS	−.239	.533	.284	.284	92.80	< .001
Child IQ	.186	.579	.336	.052	18.17	< .001
Child HSQ no. of settings	−.176	.592	.351	.015	5.35	.022
Teen WRAT Math	.189	.620	.384	.033	12.51	< .001
Teen no. of CD symptoms (parent)	−.195	.636	.404	.020	7.81	.006
Teen no. of ODD symptoms (parent)	.168	.645	.416	.012	4.68	.032
Age-21 no. of CD symptoms (self)	−.159	.662	.438	.021	8.70	.004

NS: Child CPRS-R Hyperactivity Index and conduct problem scores, teen no. of ADHD symptoms (parent) and WRAT reading and spelling scores, and duration of childhood stimulant treatment, Age-21 no. of ADHD (self and parent) and ODD (self) symptoms

	Beta	R	R^2	$R^2\Delta$	F	p
High school grade-point average						
Child CPRS-R Hyperactivity Index	−.224	.460	.211	.211	62.70	< .001
Child IQ	.150	.500	.250	.038	11.87	.001
Teen WRAT math	.233	.560	.313	.064	21.55	< .001
Teen no. of CD symptoms (parent)	−.126	.585	.342	.029	10.12	.002
Age-21 no. of CD symptoms (self)	−.199	.614	.377	.034	12.69	< .001

NS: Child CPRS-R conduct problem score and HSQ no. of settings, Teen no. of ADHD and no. of ODD symptoms (parent) and WRAT reading and spelling scores, and duration of childhood stimulant treatment, age-21 no. of ADHD (self and parent) and ODD (self) symptoms

Note. R = regression coefficient; R^2 = percent of explained variance accounted for by all variables at this step; $R^2\Delta$ = percent of explained variance accounted for by this variable added at this step; *F* = results of *F*-test for the equation at this step; *p* = probability value for the *F*-test; Beta = standardized beta coefficient; NS = not significant; WRAT = Wide Range Achievement Test standard score; CPRS-R = Conners Parent Rating Scale—Revised; WWPARS = Werry–Weiss–Peters Activity Rating Scale; HSQ = Home Situations Questionnaire number of problem settings; child IQ = Peabody Picture Vocabulary Test score; ADHD = attention-deficit/hyperactivity disorder (DSM-III-R); ODD = oppositional defiant disorder symptoms (DSM-III-R); CD = conduct disorder symptoms (DSM-III-R).

Statistical analysis: Multiple linear regression using three entry blocks for child, teen, and age-21 predictors, respectively, and stepwise conditional entry method. Used the entire sample (*N* = 236).

them make perfect sense. Table 9.13 also shows that high school grade-point average was also predicted by most of these same characteristics. Again, childhood hyperactivity (this time, the CPRS-R Hyperactivity Index score) and IQ were significant, as were teen math achievement (WRAT), teen CD severity, and young adult CD severity. Nearly 61% of the variance in high school grade-point average was explained by these predictors. Noteworthy here is that in none of these analyses did the length of time participants had spent on stimulant medication have an effect on the results. Our results imply that both educational attainment and high school grade-point average are best predicted by childhood ADHD severity, IQ, math achievement, and degree of antisocial behavior (CD) in adolescence and early adulthood. But once these are controlled, teen ODD symptoms may make a surprisingly positive contribution to educational attainment.

Occupational Functioning

Results from past studies suggest that as adolescents, individuals with ADHD are no different in their functioning in their jobs than are normal adolescents (Weiss & Hechtman, 1993). However, these findings need to be qualified by the fact that most jobs taken by adolescents are unskilled or semiskilled and usually held only part time and typically of limited duration (summer months). As ADHD children enter adulthood and take on full-time jobs that require skilled labor, independence of supervision, acceptance of responsibility, and periodic training in new knowledge or skills, their deficits in attention, impulse control, and regulating activity level—as well as their poor organizational and self-control skills—could begin to handicap them on the job. The findings from the few outcome studies that have examined job functioning suggest that this may be the case. Two prior studies examined occupational status by adulthood and reported their hyperactive groups to rank significantly lower than control groups (Mannuzza et al., 1993; Weiss & Hechtman, 1993). Employer ratings revealed significantly worse job performance in the hyperactive than the community control group (Weiss & Hechtman, 1993). More of the hyperactive group had also reported having been fired or laid off from employment than had members of the control group. The Milwaukee Study (Barkley, Fischer et al., 2006) obtained employer ratings of work performance at the young adult follow-up assessment and found that hyperactive participants were rated as performing significantly less well at work than were community control subjects.

Adults who grew up with ADHD are likely to have a lower socioeconomic status than their brothers or control subjects in these studies and to move and change jobs more often but to also have more part-time jobs outside their full-time employment. Employers have been found to rate these adults as less adequate in fulfilling work demands, less likely to be working independently and to complete tasks, and less likely to be getting along well with supervisors. They also do less well at job interviews than do normal individuals (Weiss & Hechtman, 1993). And these adults report that they find certain tasks at work too difficult. Finally, children with ADHD followed to adulthood are more likely to have been fired from jobs as well as to be laid off from work relative to control participants. In general, adults who grew up with hyperactivity/ADHD appear to have a poorer work record and lower job status than normal adults (Weiss & Hechtman, 1993). These findings were recently corroborated in the Milwaukee study at age-21 follow-up as well (Barkley, Fischer et al., 2006).

The above findings pertain to hyperactive/ADHD children followed into adulthood, some of whom no longer have the disorder. In contrast, all clinic-referred adults diagnosed with ADHD by definition have the disorder. As noted earlier, for these and other reasons the results of children with ADHD followed to adulthood may not be necessarily representative of clinic-referred adults diagnosed with the disorder. Although opinions abound on the topic in trade books on ADHD in adults, there is very little research on the occupational functioning of clinic-referred adults with ADHD. In one such study of 172 adults with ADHD, we (Murphy & Barkley, 1996) reported that such adults were more likely to have been fired from employment (53% vs. 31%), had impulsively quit a job (48% vs. 16%), and were more likely to report chronic employment difficulties (77% vs. 57%). The ADHD group also had changed jobs significantly more often than those in the control group (6.9 vs. 4.6). Similar findings were reported by De Quiros and Kinsbourne (2001) in that adults with ADHD reported more frequent job changes and poorer job performance than control adults. A notably poor picture for employment was reported by Torgersen et al. (2006) for their Norwegian sample, in which just 16% were employed at the time of referral—a figure well below that seen in studies using U.S. samples. The selection criteria used in that study suggests that this sample had severe ADHD and was also anti-social, so it likely does not correspond to the severity of ADHD seen in adult outpatient clinics. Yet the general pattern of employment difficulties is in keeping with the outcomes of follow-up studies of hyperactive children. But they are based on just three studies of clinic-referred adults, all covering this topic in a rather superficial manner. We therefore chose to examine occupational functioning in more detail in the UMASS Study.

The UMASS Study Results

As part of their initial interview (see sidebar, Chapter 4), participants were interviewed about their occupational history. We also, with permission, obtained ratings from their employers (see sidebar, Chapter 6). Employers were kept blind to the diagnostic status of the participants and were told only that we were conducting a survey of job satisfaction and performance and requested their cooperation in completing a short questionnaire for which they were reimbursed $20. The interviewer (K. R. M.) also completed the Social and Occupational Functioning Assessment Scale (see sidebar, Chapter 6) to provide a clinician summary rating of the current occupational, social, and academic functioning of the participant.

The groups did not differ in the proportions that were currently employed: ADHD = 73%, Clinical = 71%, and Community = 77%. But significantly more members of both the ADHD and Clinical control groups reported that they had problems getting along with others at work (30%, 18%, and 7%, respectively) and had difficulties with their behavior or work performance on the job (53%, 50%, and 5%, respectively). The results for the dimensional measures obtained in this study are shown in Table 9.14. The groups did not differ in the length of time they had held their current work positions, averaging between 4 and 5 years, nor did they differ in the average number of hours per week they reported working (38–43 hours). Interestingly, adults in the Clinical control group had significantly higher-status employment as determined on the Hollingshead Job Index than did participants in either the ADHD or Community control groups, who did not differ from each other. This was also true with regard to current annual salary. But on numerous other measures, the adults with ADHD showed greater occupational impairment and more adverse outcomes related to their employment than did Community control adults and, to a lesser extent, than those in the Clinical control group.

The adults with ADHD were rated by the clinician as functioning at a lower level than were those in both the Clinical and Community control groups. While the Clinical control group was also rated as more impaired, they were less so than the ADHD group. Both the ADHD and Clinical control groups had held more jobs since leaving high school than had the Community control group, even after controlling for the differences in age between these groups. And the longest time they had ever held a specific job was significantly lower for both of these groups than for the Community control group. The ADHD and Clinical control groups rated themselves as demonstrating significantly lower work quality than did participants in the Community control group but did not differ from each other in this regard. Participants reported the number of jobs on which they had experienced various difficulties, and we converted these to a percentage of the total jobs they had held since leaving high school. These findings are graphically depicted in Figure 9.7 and also appear in Table 9.14. As the figure shows, the adults with ADHD reported having trouble with others, behavior problems at work, being fired or dismissed from a job, quitting a job out of boredom, and being disciplined by their supervisor on the job in a higher percentage of the jobs they had held than did participants in both the Clinical and the Community control groups. The adults in the ADHD group also reported quitting more jobs over their own hostility in the workplace than did adults in the Community con-

TABLE 9.14. Occupational Functioning for Each Group on Dimensional Measures in the UMASS Study

Measure	ADHD		Clinical		Community		F	p	Pairwise contrasts
	Mean	SD	Mean	SD	Mean	SD			
From interview									
Clinician SOFAS rating[A, GxS]	60.7	7.0	68.6	10.3	87.6	6.9	315.4	< .001	1 < 2 < 3
Hollingshead Job Index[A]	38.1	26.8	54.1	31.3	42.3	26.7	64.9	.004	2 > 1,3
Time at current job (mos.)[S]	49.4	60.8	65.5	88.3	69.4	88.9	1.5	NS	
No. of jobs since high school[A, GxS]	7.6	7.0	8.6	7.5	5.0	3.8	10.3	< .001	1,2 > 3
Longest time held job (in months)[A,S]	65.9	63.2	84.1	88.3	97.0	91.6	3.9	.022	1,2 < 3
Hours worked Per Week[A,S]	42.4	15.6	43.1	12.1	38.4	13.7	1.8	NS	
Annual salary (K)[A,S,GxS]	32.6	25.8	48.1	38.0	25.8	15.5	9.5	< .001	2 > 1 > 3
Self-rated work quality	2.0	0.8	1.8	0.7	1.5	0.7	8.2	< .001	1,2 > 3
% Jobs trouble with others	32.8	37.7	19.7	28.3	12.4	23.3	13.8	< .001	1 >2 ,3
% Jobs behavior problems	44.6	41.2	32.4	36.6	2.4	7.1	42.7	< .001	1 > 2 > 3
% Jobs fired (dismissed)[S]	17.4	21.9	9.3	14.6	3.7	9.6	13.1	< .001	1 > 2 > 3
% Jobs quit for hostility[A]	17.3	26.5	11.5	23.4	4.9	11.0	7.94	< .001	1 > 3
% Jobs quit for boredom[A]	32.6	37.8	17.9	28.7	15.5	28.4	5.65	.004	1 > 2,3
% Jobs disciplined	11.1	23.4	2.4	5.3	0.6	2.3	16.3	< .001	1 > 2,3
From employer ratings									
Inattention score[S, GxS]	9.0	7.2	5.8	5.9	1.9	2.7	21.8	< .001	1 > 2 > 3
Hyperactive–imp. score[A]	7.1	5.3	7.4	6.0	3.1	4.2	12.8	< .001	1,2 > 3
Impair coworker relations[S]	0.7	0.7	0.7	0.8	0.4	0.7	3.4	.036	NS
Impair assigned work	1.1	1.0	0.7	0.8	0.3	0.6	13.0	< .001	1 > 2 > 3
Impair supervisor relations	0.7	0.8	0.6	0.6	0.3	0.6	2.39	NS	
Impair client relations[GxS]	0.7	0.9	0.5	0.8	0.3	0.7	3.0	NS	
Impair education at work	0.6	0.8	0.5	0.7	0.1	0.3	8.0	.001	1,2 > 3
Impair punctuality	0.9	1.1	0.6	1.0	0.2	0.5	7.7	.001	1 > 3
Impair time management	1.2	1.0	0.7	0.8	0.4	0.7	9.36	< .001	1 > 2,3
Impair equipment use	0.5	0.8	0.3	0.7	0.1	0.3	2.8	NS	
Impair vehicle use	0.3	0.7	0.1	0.4	0.0	0.2	3.32	.041	NS
Impair daily respons.[S, GxS]	1.0	0.9	0.6	0.8	0.3	0.6	9.3	< .001	1 > 2,3
Overall work performance	2.5	1.0	2.0	1.0	1.7	0.8	8.7	< .001	1 > 2,3

Note. Sample sizes are for SOFAS: ADHD = 145, Clinical control = 94, and Community control = 108; job index: 137, 87, 103, respectively; time on job: 104, 66, 83; no. of jobs since high school: 139, 91, 97; longest time held job: 142, 90, 105; hours worked: 105, 66, 81; salary: 105, 65, 79; self-rated work quality: 105, 66, 84; % jobs trouble with others: 141, 90, 104; % jobs behavior problems and % jobs quit for boredom: 138, 90, 96; % jobs fired: 139, 89, 97; % jobs quit for hostility and % jobs disciplined: 139, 90, 97; employer ratings: 39, 25, 50. SD = standard deviation; F = F-test results of the analysis of variance (or covariance); p = probability value for the F-test; NS = not significant; [S] = significant main effect for sex (see text for details); [GxS] = significant group × sex interaction (see text for details); [A] = age used as a covariate in this analysis; K = thousands of dollars; hyperactive–imp. = hyperactive–impulsive symptom score; Respons. = responsibilities. Work quality rated 1–5 (1 = excellent, 5 = poor); impair scores are rated 0–3 (0 = never or rarely, 3 = very often); overall work performance rated 1–5 (1 = excellent, 5 = poor).

Statistical analysis: Groups were initially compared using two way (group × sex) analysis of variance (or covariance as necessary). Where this analysis was significant (p < .05) for the main effect for group, pairwise comparisons of the groups were conducted the results of which are shown in the last column.

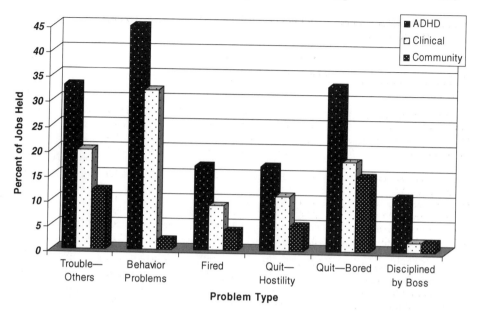

FIGURE 9.7. Percentage of jobs held in which various workplace problems occurred for each group in the UMASS Study.

trol group. Based on this self-reported information, our results clearly show that adults with ADHD have greater problems with occupational functioning than do those seen in the same clinic who are not diagnosed with ADHD or those from our Community control group. Just as ADHD was found to take a significant toll on educational functioning, so also does it adversely affect occupational functioning.

The results of the employer ratings are also shown in Table 9.14. Although the employers were blind to the diagnoses of our participants, they rated the adults with ADHD as having significantly greater problems with inattention in the workplace than was the case for either control group. Even though the Clinical control adults had higher symptom ratings in this domain than those in the Community control group, they still fell well below the adults with ADHD. Interestingly, employers rated both the ADHD and Clinical control adults as having more symptoms of hyperactive and impulsive behavior than adults in the Community control group. Compared to Community control adults, the adults with ADHD were rated as being more impaired by their symptoms in performing assigned work, pursuing educational activities at work, being punctual, using good time management, and managing their daily responsibilities. When compared to the Clinical control group, the ADHD group was again rated as more impaired in performing assigned work, in time management, and in performing daily responsibilities. As a consequence, the adults with ADHD were rated as having a poorer overall work performance level than were adults in either of the control groups. Such findings are important, as they corroborate the reports of the adults themselves, which showed that ADHD has a detrimental effect on occupational functioning and that this effect is greater than is seen in clinically referred adults who are not diagnosed with ADHD.

The foregoing results for employer ratings must be qualified by the exceptionally small samples within each group who granted permission to obtain employer ratings and who had those ratings returned to the project staff. Specifically, we had employer ratings for just 39 ADHD group members (27%), 25 Clinical control members (26%), and 50 Community control members (46%). We therefore needed to examine whether the proportion of participants in each group on whom we had employer ratings differed in any significant demographic or ADHD severity measures from those for whom we were not able to get such ratings, which may have biased the results reported above. We examined these subsets of participants within each group on age, sex, ethnic group, education, total current ADHD symptoms, age of onset of those symptoms, the total number of domains they reported as being impaired, their total childhood ADHD symptoms, and the clinician rating on the Social Occupational Functioning Assessment Scale (SOFAS) (see sidebar, Chapter 6). Within the ADHD group, we found no significant differences between these two subsets on any of these measures. In other words, those on whom we had employer ratings could be viewed as being representative of the entire ADHD group. For the Clinical control group, the only difference we found was that those on whom we had employer ratings were more likely to be female (67%) than those for whom we did not have such ratings (37%). Otherwise, the subset that had employer ratings available did not differ on age, education, ethnicity, or ADHD severity scores or on the SOFAS ratings than the subset without employer ratings. For the Community control group, we found no differences on any of these measures. To summarize, it appears that the subsets of participants within each group on whom employer ratings were available can be taken to be representative of the total group membership on key demographic and ADHD severity measures as well as clinician SOFAS ratings. The only exception to this is the gender representation in the Clinical control group, which was biased toward greater female representation.

Several main effects for sex were evident in Table 9.14, regardless of group. On average, males had held their current positions longer than females, had held their longest job significantly longer than females, and had worked more hours per week than females on average. But males were also fired from a higher percentage of their jobs than were females and were rated by their employers as being more impaired in their coworker relations than were females.

In several instances, the sex of the participant interacted significantly with his or her group assignment, warranting closer inspection of the results as a function of sex within each group. On the SOFAS clinician rating, males and females within the ADHD and Community control groups did not differ, but males in the Clinical control group were rated as functioning better than were females in this group. Similarly, males and females in both the ADHD and Community control groups did not differ in the number of jobs they had held since high school, but females in the Clinical control group reported holding significantly more such jobs than did males in that group. For average annual salary, males overall earned more money than females, but this was partly a function of their group. Males in the ADHD and Clinical control groups earned significantly more money than did females within those two groups, while the sex difference in the Community control group was far less apparent. On employer ratings of inattention at work, we found again that males and females in both the ADHD and Community control groups did not differ in this regard, while males in the Clinical control group were rated as having significantly more inattention symptoms than females in that group. This was also the case for employer ratings of impairment in daily responsibilities. Interestingly, in relations with clients, females with ADHD were rated by their employers as being significantly more impaired than were males in that group, but the opposite pattern of sex differences emerged in the other two control groups. We show this group × sex interaction in Figure 9.8. In general, then, it appears that most of the significant interactions of sex with group revealed that it was the Clinical control group in which such differences were most likely to be evident and not the other two groups. However, women with ADHD may have more difficulties in their relationships with clients or customers in their workplace than do men with the disorder.

Our results are consistent with both the literature on children with ADHD followed to adulthood and the more scant literature on clinic-referred adults with ADHD in finding numerous adverse events and greater impairment in the occupational functioning of adults with ADHD. These problems typically exceed the levels of impairment noted in adults having other, non-ADHD outpatient disorders as well as in Community control adults, once more attesting to the fact that ADHD in adults is a more impairing disorder than most others seen in outpatient settings.

The Milwaukee Study Results

We collected the same interview measures in the Milwaukee Study at the age-27 follow-up. However, we did not ask for permission to contact employers at this follow-up as we had done so at the age-21 follow-up. As noted earlier, that evaluation found the hyperactive group to be rated as having more ADHD and

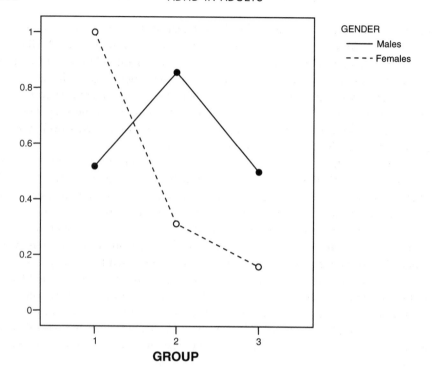

FIGURE 9.8. The mean employer ratings for how much ADHD symptoms impair relations with clients in the UMASS Study. Scores are for each sex within each group, depicting the significant interaction effect for group × sex on this measure. Group 1 = ADHD, 2 = Clinical control, 3 = Community control.

ODD symptoms in the workplace and to have lower workplace performance evaluations than the Community control group. At that follow-up, we did not examine subsets of the hyperactive group who currently had ADHD on these measures.

Unlike the results of the UMASS Study, we found that significantly fewer of the H+ADHD group at age-27 follow-up were currently employed compared to both the H–ADHD and Community control adults. The H+ADHD group also reported themselves more likely to have problems with others at work as well as difficulties with their behavior and workplace performance more generally compared to these other two groups. On such categorical measures of occupational functioning, it appears that children growing up as having ADHD whose ADHD persists to age 27 are more severely affected than are clinic-referred adults with ADHD, although both ADHD groups have more difficulties in that setting than others.

Table 9.15 shows the same information that appeared in Table 9.14 for the UMASS Study adults. Once more, we see that it is the H+ADHD group that is most impaired in these various indices of occupational success relative to both the H–ADHD and Community control groups. While both the H–ADHD and H+ADHD groups held lower-status jobs relative to our Community control group at this follow-up, the H+ADHD group rated themselves as having lower workplace performance quality than the other two groups. The three groups did not differ in their current annual salary or in the length of time they had held their current positions, but the two hyperactive groups reported working fewer hours per week than did the Community control group.

The H+ADHD group also had held more jobs since leaving high school. Given such a higher job turnover rate (which we also found in the UMASS Study), we again adjusted for this difference across groups in the questions dealing with workplace adjustment by computing the percentage of jobs held in which these problems had been reported to occur. The H+ADHD group experienced a greater percentage of jobs in which they had trouble getting along with others, had behavior problems, had been fired or dismissed from the job, or had been disciplined formally by their supervisors compared to both the H–ADHD and Community control groups. The group with current ADHD also reported quitting more jobs due to hostility vis-à-vis others than the community group, with the H–ADHD group placing between these two extremes but not differing significantly from either of the other groups. We illustrate these results in Figure

TABLE 9.15. Occupational Functioning for Each Group on Dimensional Measures in the Milwaukee Study

Measures	H+ADHD Mean	SD	H–ADHD Mean	SD	Community Mean	SD	F	p	Pairwise contrasts
Hollingshead Job Index[IQ]	35.2	19.8	42.4	20.6	51.7	27.3	7.05	.001	1,2 < 3
Time at current job (mos.)	22.7	22.8	27.0	29.7	30.8	26.5	1.20	NS	
No. of jobs since high school	4.9	5.4	3.5	2.0	2.5	1.4	8.92	< .001	1 > 2,3
Hours worked per week	43.3	14.0	44.4	9.6	49.2	12.8	4.23	.016	1,2 < 3
Annual salary (K)[IQ]	26.3	14.4	30.7	19.4	35.1	18.1	2.83	NS	
Self-rated work quality	2.0	0.7	1.6	0.6	1.5	0.6	7.17	.001	1 > 2,3
% Jobs trouble with others	25.7	30.8	6.9	16.2	6.2	21.0	13.58	< .001	1 > 2,3
% Jobs behavior problems	26.5	36.6	6.0	15.4	2.1	9.2	20.94	< .001	1 > 2,3
% Jobs fired (dismissed)	43.2	39.1	30.0	34.4	14.0	30.3	11.45	< .001	1 > 2 > 3
% Jobs quit for hostility	31.1	34.6	21.3	35.7	14.8	29.9	3.61	.029	1 > 3
% Jobs quit for boredom	30.5	40.1	25.1	38.8	25.8	37.6	0.33	NS	
% Jobs disciplined	28.1	34.0	8.1	22.2	3.1	15.6	17.77	< .001	1 > 2,3

Note. SD = standard deviation; F = F-test results of the analysis of variance (or covariance); p = probability value for the F-test; NS = not significant; k = thousands of dollars; [IQ] = WAIS-3 vocabulary and block design scores were used as covariates on these measures (where covariates were used, means are marginal means). Work quality was rated from 1 (excellent) to 5 (poor).

Statistical analysis: Groups were initially compared using one-way (groups) analysis of variance (or covariance as necessary). Where this analysis was significant (p < .05) for the main effect for group, pairwise comparisons of the groups were conducted, the results of which are shown in the last column.

9.9, which can be compared to the UMASS findings on these same measures, shown in Figure 9.5. Such a comparison suggests that children growing up with persistent ADHD may experience even more workplace adjustment problems than do clinic-referred adults having ADHD. While both groups have comparable rates of difficulty in getting along with others and having behavior problems at work, children whose ADHD continued to adulthood experience far more firings and disciplinary actions at work as a percentage of jobs held than do clinic-referred adults having this same disorder. All of this suggests that having ADHD in childhood may predispose toward lower occupational status regardless of the persistence of ADHD to age 27, most likely due to its adverse effects, as noted above, on educational success and eventual years of education attained. But persistent ADHD into adulthood appears to have a far more adverse impact on current job functioning than simply having had ADHD in childhood.

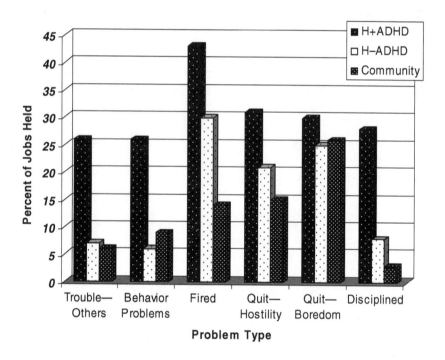

FIGURE 9.9. Percentage of jobs held in which various workplace problems occurred for each group in the Milwaukee Study. The groups did not differ in quitting jobs due to boredom. For all other problems, the Hyperactive group currently having ADHD (H+ADHD) had significantly more problems than the Community control group and, except for quitting over hostility, also exceeded the problems shown by the Hyperactive group no longer having ADHD (H–ADHD).

Predicting Occupational Outcomes

As we did for several significant educational outcomes, we also selected several occupational outcomes that were specifically problematic for the ADHD group in the UMASS Study in order to determine possible correlates of or contributors to these adverse outcomes. These outcomes were employer ratings of workplace performance and the percentage of jobs from which the participants had been dismissed or fired. These results appear in Table 9.16. Lower workplace performance ratings were significantly predicted by severity of self-reported ADHD symptoms and by employer ratings of severity of ADHD in the workplace. No other predictors were significant for this outcome. The percentage of jobs from which participants had been fired was also predicted by severity of self-reported ADHD currently, severity of childhood CD, and higher criminal diversity scores (see Chapter 10, on antisocial activity). Thus it seems that while severity of ADHD in clinic-referred adults is associated with both workplace performance and job dismissals, the extent of antisocial behavior and its diversity were also contributing factors to the latter adverse employment outcome.

TABLE 9.16. Predicting Occupational Outcomes for the UMASS Study

Outcome/predictors (step entered)	Beta	R	R^2	$R^2\Delta$	F	p
Employer-rated work performance						
(1) No. of ADHD symptoms*	.186	.187	.035	.035	6.36	.002
and Age (NS)	.051					
(2) Workplace ADHD—employer ratings	.588	.595	.354	.319	172.12	< .001
NS: IQ (Shipley), education (years), no. of CD symptoms (childhood), no. of crime types, depression, anxiety, hostility (SCL-90-R)						
Percent of job dismissals (firings)						
(1) No. of ADHD symptoms and	.337	.336	.113	.113	22.33	< .001
age (NS)	.066					
(2) No. of CD symptoms (childhood)	.192	.424	.180	.067	28.40	< .001
(3) No. of crime types (lifetime)	.171	.447	.200	.020	8.85	.003
NS: IQ, Education, No. of CD symptoms (childhood), no. of crime types, depression, anxiety, hostility						

Note. R = regression coefficient; R^2 = percent of explained variance accounted for by all variables at this step; $R^2\Delta$ = percent of explained variance accounted for by this variable added at this step; F = results of F-test for the equation at this step, p = probability value for the F-test; * = this variable became nonsignificant when other variables were entered in the next step; beta = standardized beta coefficient; NS = not significant; Shipley = Shipley Institute of Living Scale IQ estimate; SCL-90-R = Symptom Checklist 90—Revised T-score. Employer-rated work performance was rated as 1 (excellent) to 5 (very poor).
    Statistical analysis: Multiple linear regression using forced entry method at Step 1 and stepwise conditional method at subsequent steps. Used the entire sample (N = 353).

We did the same analyses for the Milwaukee Study samples. However, we did not have employer-rated workplace performance ratings at this follow-up so instead we substituted self-rated work performance quality, which was also significantly impaired in the H+ADHD group (see above). These results appear in Table 9.17. We also used a similar set of predictors to those used in the UMASS Study. Work performance was predicted by the number of current ADHD symptoms (self-reported), just as in the UMASS Study. But nonverbal IQ was important here as well, to our surprise. The participants' scores on the WAIS-III block design subtest was related to their work performance rating. The percentage of jobs from which participants had been fired was predicted by years of education and by the number of self-rated current ODD symptoms. Better-educated and less oppositional participants were less likely to be dismissed from their jobs. Both predictors make perfect sense. While ADHD, crime, and childhood CD symptoms had been associated with job dismissals in the UMASS Study adults, that was not the case here.

TABLE 9.17. Predicting Occupational Outcomes for the Milwaukee Study

Outcome/predictors (step entered)	Beta	R	R^2	$R^2\Delta$	F	p
Self-rated work performance						
No. of ADHD Symptoms (self)	.303	.320	.103	.103	23.80	< .001
WAIS-III Block Design Score	−.139	.349	.122	.019	4.49	.035
NS: WAIS-III Vocabulary score, years of education, no. of ODD symptoms now, no. of CD symptoms in childhood, no. of different crime types committed, and SCL-90-R depression, anxiety, and hostility scores						
Percent of jobs with dismissals (firings)						
Education (in years)	−.250	.336	.113	.113	26.50	< .001
No. of current ODD symptoms (self)	.221	.393	.154	.041	10.11	.002
NS: No. of ADHD symptoms (self), WAIS-III Vocabulary and Block Design scores, no. of CD symptoms in childhood, no. of different crime types committed, and SCL-90-R depression, anxiety, and hostility scores						

Note. R = regression coefficient; R^2 = percent of explained variance accounted for by all variables at this step; $R^2\Delta$ = percent of explained variance accounted for by this variable added at this step; F = results of F-test for the equation at this step, p = probability value for the F-test; beta = standardized beta coefficient; NS = not significant; WAIS-III = Wechsler Adult Intelligence Scale—3rd edition; CD = conduct disorder; ODD = oppositional defiant disorder; SCL-90-R = Symptom Checklist–90—Revised T-score. Self-rated work performance was rated as 1 (excellent) to 5 (very poor).
   Statistical analysis: Multiple linear regression using stepwise entry method. Used the entire sample (N = 210).

Conclusions and Clinical Implications

This chapter examined the educational and occupational histories and current workplace functioning of adults with ADHD—both those self-referred to clinics as adults and children with ADHD followed to age 27. The past research on this topic has been largely confined to follow-up studies of children with ADHD reevaluated in adulthood.

✓ What small literature does exist on the educational histories of adults with ADHD has suggested numerous adverse effects of the disorder in this domain of major life activities, consistent with the follow-up studies of children with ADHD but often suggesting somewhat less impairment in the clinic-referred adults.

✓ Compared to hyperactive or ADHD children followed over development, the intellectual levels of adults with ADHD are higher, their high school graduation rates are higher, they are more are likely to have attended college, and their likelihood of having achievement difficulties is considerably less in most respects than that seen in children with ADHD followed to adulthood.

✓ Nevertheless, the present UMASS project found that adults with ADHD rated themselves as being more impaired in educational settings than adults in the control groups. These ratings were corroborated by the ratings provided by others, which showed that ADHD was associated with impaired functioning in all of the specific educational situations we examined, including classwork, homework, class behavior, and behavior at recess and in the lunchroom as well as in overall time management.

✓ Although as many adults with ADHD had graduated high school as in the two control groups in the UMASS Study, fewer had graduated from college, resulting in the ADHD group having less years of education.

✓ More of the adults with ADHD reported having been retained in grade, received special education, and been diagnosed with learning disabilities or behavioral disorders while in compulsory schooling than did adults in either of the two control groups.

✓ The official school transcripts obtained on these participants revealed a similar pattern. The ADHD group had a significantly greater percentage of poor (D) or failing grades (F), on both their elementary school and high school transcripts. The ADHD group had a lower grade-point average and more days absent from school during high school than did the adults in either of the control groups.

✓ Similarly, among those participants who had attended college, the ADHD group had significantly more unsatisfactory grades and had withdrawn from more classes, as reflected on their college transcripts, than did the two control groups.

✓ Yet no differences were found in the high school standardized tests or in college SAT scores between the groups, suggesting that the problems of adults with ADHD in school may not simply be a function of low ability.

✓ Nevertheless, evidence of lower ability was also found on tests of educational achievement administered in this project. The ADHD group was found to be poorer in their arithmetic, spelling, and reading, and listening comprehension skills than were adults in the Community control group and were poorer in arithmetic, spelling, and reading comprehension relative to the Clinical control group.

✓ In contrast, the Milwaukee Study, on follow-up, found that having ADHD as a child was a more significant risk factor for most types of educational problems than was having persistent ADHD to age 27. Both hyperactive (child ADHD) groups were less educated, less likely to graduate high school, less likely to attend college, and more likely to have received various forms of educational assistance in school than the Community control group. Compared to clinic-referred adults, it is clear that children growing up with ADHD are even more adversely affected in their educational careers than are clinic-referred adults with the disorder, much as the earlier research literature might have implied.

✓ The prevalence of specific learning disabilities in each study was also computed and, when defined as falling at or below the 14th percentile on an achievement test, revealed that clinic-referred adults with ADHD were more likely to have spelling and comprehension disorders (reading and listening) than the Community control group, while only their listening comprehension disorders distinguished them from the Clinical control group. Noteworthy is that the most common area of deficiency or specific learning disabilities had to do with reading and listening comprehension—abilities established previously to be deficient in ADHD children and to be related to their working memory deficits. We return to this issue in Chapter 13, dealing with neuropsychological deficits associated with ADHD in adults, where working memory is shown to be deficient in these adults with ADHD.

✓ Children growing up with ADHD, however, regardless of its persistence to age 27, were more likely to have learning disabilities by this same definition than the control group, and a larger percentage did so relative to clinic-referred adults with the disorder. Having ADHD in childhood, regardless of its persistence to adulthood, is more likely to be associated with specific learning disabilities than is adult ADHD.

✓ In their occupational functioning, clinic-referred adults with ADHD were rated by a clinician as functioning at a lower level overall than adults in the other groups. They were also found to have experienced a number of problems in a higher percentage of their previous jobs than adults in the two control groups. These problems were related to getting along with others, demonstrating behavior problems, being fired, quitting out of boredom, and being disciplined by supervisors, all of which were more frequent in the work histories of the adults with ADHD than in either of the control groups.

✓ The Milwaukee Study, on follow-up, found much the same results, except that growing up as a child with ADHD was associated with lower job status and fewer current working hours per week regardless of its persistence into adulthood. Even so, we found that the group with persistent ADHD experienced even more difficulties in their current workplace functioning than did either the H–ADHD or the Community control group. This was also true in comparison to the clinic-referred adults with ADHD, where adults with ADHD persisting from childhood have a far more significant history of having been fired from their jobs or experiencing disciplinary actions than do clinic-referred adults with the disorder.

✓ Problems in the workplace were also independently corroborated in the UMASS Study through the ratings we obtained from the supervisors or employers of these participants. The ADHD group was rated as having significantly more symptoms of inattention in the workplace and as being more impaired in performing assigned work, pursuing educational activities, being punctual, using good time management, and managing daily responsibilities. We had found much the same result using a similar measure at the age-21 follow-up in the Milwaukee Study. Both projects provide direct evidence that ADHD has an adverse impact on workplace functioning not only via self-reports but also corroborated through employer-blinded ratings.

✓ The results presented here clearly demonstrate that ADHD in adults is associated with a number of adverse outcomes and more impaired functioning in their educational and occupational histories than is the case for normal adults or those diagnosed with other clinical disorders than ADHD. Being diagnosed as having ADHD in childhood has an even more adverse effect on one's educational career, eventual job status, and workplace adjustment (firings and disciplinary actions) than when ADHD is diagnosed in self-referred adults.

✓ Clinicians are likely to be asked to involve themselves in the educational impairments of those adults with ADHD still pursuing further education at the time of clinical evaluation. They may be asked to make recommendations concerning the need for and types of accommodations these adults are likely to require in those settings. In so doing, clinicians will need to familiarize themselves with the standards of evidence required under the American with Disabilities Act for obtaining such accommodations (see Gordon & Keiser, 1998).

✓ Clinicians may also be asked to involve themselves in workplace impairments and the types of accommodations that may be needed to deal with these impairments. Where they are untrained or uncomfortable in doing so, clinicians should refer their patients having such concerns to other professionals specializing in vocational assessment, accommodations, and rehabilitation for the expertise that may be required to address the workplace difficulties of adults with ADHD. Here again, familiarity with the appropriate aspects of the Americans with Disabilities Act will be required to obtain such accommodations.

✓ The pervasive adverse impact of ADHD in the workplace also indicates that long-acting ADHD medications will likely prove very useful for assisting adults with ADHD, much as they have done for the educational functioning of children with ADHD, and may be even more useful given the longer hours adults spend in their jobs than they were likely to spend in school settings as children. In fact, long-acting medications may even need to be further supplemented with immediate-release medications to provide the additional hours of coverage these adults are likely to require beyond that necessary to cover a child's school day. Behavioral interventions that have proven so useful in educational settings for ADHD children seem to us to be much less likely to be feasible or to be adopted in employment settings, making medication a more convenient and effective intervention component for adults with the disorder. Workplace accommodations may offer some additional benefits beyond medication for adults with ADHD, but no research is available to demonstrate their efficacy.

CHAPTER 10

Drug Use and Antisocial Behavior

Some information has been collected on drug use and abuse in both children with ADHD followed to adulthood and in clinic-referred adults with ADHD. There is also a growing body of evidence concerning their risks for antisocial activities. As discussed in Chapter 8, on comorbidity for psychiatric disorders, (as well as below), these two areas of functioning are related. The available literature shows that adults with ADHD have a higher than normal risk for problems in both domains. For instance, Chapter 8 discussed evidence that clinic-referred adults with ADHD have a greater frequency of drug-use disorders, specifically for alcohol and marijuana dependence and abuse, and that these are most common in persons with conduct disorder (CD). The reverse is also true—patients seen in drug abuse clinics also display a significantly elevated risk of ADHD (Kalbag & Levin, 2005).

Tobacco, Alcohol, and Drug Use

Much of the research on drug use among adults with ADHD comes from longitudinal studies of children with ADHD followed to adulthood (Weiss & Hechtman, 1993). That youth with ADHD are at higher risk for increased tobacco and alcohol use as adolescents and young adults has been demonstrated in several previous studies (see Tercyak, Peshkin, Walker, & Stein, 2002, for a review). Barkley's study with Mariellen Fischer in Milwaukee found a significantly greater number of hyperactive children as teens had smoked cigarettes or marijuana (Barkley, Fischer, et al., 1990). Greater use of alcohol and other substances was also documented at their young adult follow-up point (Barkley et al., 2004). The follow-up study by Hartsough and Lambert (1985) found only cigarette use to be greater in hyperactive than in normal adolescents. Borland and Heckman (1976) also found more of their hyperactive children as teens to be smoking cigarettes than their brothers at follow-up, all of which certainly points to a higher than normal risk for cigarette use among hyperactive children in adolescence that can probably be extrapolated upward to adulthood.

Subsequent follow-up studies have done much to refine our understanding of this risk. For instance, Milbergerand colleagues (1996) followed 6- to 17-year-olds with and without ADHD for 4 years and found that ADHD was specifically associated with a higher risk for initiating cigarette smoking even after controlling for social class, psychiatric comorbidity, and intelligence. Molina et al. (1999) reported, in a study of 202 adolescents, that ADHD was associated with increased use of all substances, including nicotine, but only when it was associated with comorbid CD. Yet they also found that it was the impulsive-hyperactive dimension of ADHD within this comorbid group that was most closely associated with this elevated risk of substance use. In partial agreement with these results, Burke, Loeber, and Lahey (2001) followed 177 clinic-referred boys with ADHD to age 15 and likewise found that 51% of these teens reported tobacco use, but that this risk was elevated only in the comorbid group of having CD. Differing from the study of Molina et al. (1999), these authors found that it was the inattention dimension that was specifically associated with a 2.2 times greater risk for tobacco use by adolescence, even after controlling for other factors known to be associated with such use (CD, poor parental communication, ethnicity, etc.). Tercyak, Lerman, and Audrain (2002) also confirmed this linkage not only with ADHD but also specifically its inattention symptoms with the risk for cigarette use by adolescence. Even mild levels of ADHD symptoms appear to elevate this risk for smoking (Whalen et al., 2002).

A recent study (Kollins et al., 2005) further cements the relationship of ADHD symptoms to increased risk of nicotine use. Kollins et al. used the National Longitudinal Study of Adolescent Health, a nationally representative sample, to examine whether ADHD symptoms were associated with increased smoking risk. They followed 15,197 adolescents into young adulthood. Analyses showed a linear relationship between inattentive and hyperactive–impulsive ADHD symptoms and lifetime likelihood of being a regular smoker (having smoked at least one cigarette per day for at least 30 days). Even when controlling for CD symptoms, each additional ADHD symptom significantly increased the risk for regular smoking. For those who did smoke, more symptoms were associated with an earlier age of smoking onset. ADHD symptoms are therefore a useful predictor of risk for smoking and an earlier onset of smoking even outside of a clinical setting. Given the stimulant-like action of nicotine on the dopamine transporter in the striatum of the brain and its similarity to the effects of methylphenidate on that site (Krause et al., 2002), these findings suggest that greater nicotine use among those with ADHD could be a form of self-medication.

Concerning alcohol use, Blouin, Bornstein, and Trites (1978), in a retro-spective study, were among the first to report that children with hyperactivity may be more at risk than control children for adolescent alcohol use (57% of hyperactives vs. 20% of the controls). Weiss and Hechtman (1993) also found somewhat more of their hyperactive participants, as teenagers, to have used alco-hol than did their control group, but this was not found at the adult follow-up. With the exception of the study by Hartsough and Lambert (1985), there is some consistency across studies in finding hyperactive children to be at somewhat higher risk for alcohol use in adolescence than normal children. These and other studies have also documented a greater frequency of use of other substances as well among adolescents with ADHD (Chilcoat & Breslau, 1999).

Given the well-known association of CD to risk of drug use, Barkley, Fischer, and colleagues (2004) subdivided their hyperactive group into those who did and did not have lifetime CD by young adulthood (self-reported) and com-pared them to the control group for their frequency of use of various drugs. Results found significant group differences for 9 of the 11 drug-use activities sur-veyed. In all cases, it was the hyperactive group having CD that accounted for these differences, there being no significant differences between the hyperactive alone and control groups in any form of drug use.

Most studies concur with the Milwaukee Study in finding that the elevated risk for alcohol and substance use and abuse in adolescence is to be found primar-ily among hyperactive or ADHD children who had conduct problems in child-hood or frank CD (August, Stewart, and Holmes, 1983; Barkley, Fischer, et al., 1990; Biederman et al., 1997; Chilcoat & Breslau, 1999; Claude & Firestone, 1995; Flory, Lynam, Milich, Leukefeld, & Clayton, 2001; Gittelman et al., 1985; Kuperman et al., 2001; Lynskey & Fergusson, 1995; Mannuzza et al., 1993; Molina et al., 1999; Wilson & Marcotte, 1996). Likewise, youth diagnosed with alcohol dependence have a markedly higher incidence of ADHD and CD, with the developmental sequence being a progression from initial alcohol or tobacco use moving on to marijuana and finally to other street drugs (Kuperman et al., 2001). Such findings are quite consistent with studies of community samples in showing that CD but not ADHD is associated with greater risk for substance use, dependence, and abuse (Armstrong & Costello, 2002). Once again, it may be the attention symptoms and associated EF deficits seen in ADHD that are most pre-dictive of later tobacco and other substance-use problems (Tapert, Baratta, Abrantes, & Brown, 2002). Such a greater use of drugs among youth with combined ADHD and CD may contribute to further problems with learning, memory retention, and attention (Tapert, Granholm, Leedy, & Brown, 2002).

Studies of the drug use patterns of clinic-referred adults with ADHD have been few in number and less consistent in their findings. Generally they indicate a significant relationship between ADHD and substance abuse (Kalbag & Levin, 2005). As noted in Chapter 8, these adults are more prone to be diagnosed as having drug dependence or abuse disorders, particularly for alcohol and marijuana. Other studies using self-reported information also find adults with ADHD to rate themselves as more likely to abuse drugs (De Quiros & Kinsbourne, 2001; Murphy & Barkley, 1996), primarily marijuana, cocaine, and psychedelics (Murphy & Barkley, 1996). However, the frequency of alcohol use often presents a mixed picture. De Quiros and Kinsbourne (2001) did not find a greater frequency of alcohol use or bouts of intoxication in their ADHD than in their control group. Neither did we in an earlier and considerably smaller study (Barkley et al., 1996). That study did not find any greater use of either alcohol or various forms of illegal drugs but was likely limited in its statistical power due to very small samples (ADHD = 25; control = 23). But in our later study of considerably larger samples, we found that the ADHD group reported consuming significantly more alcoholic drinks per week, having gotten drunk significantly more often in the previous 3 months, and having used illegal drugs more often in those 3 months than had the members of our control group (Barkley, Murphy, et al., 2002). The study of Norwegian adults with ADHD also found higher rates of alcohol use disorders as well as for cannabis, amphetamines, and opiates (Torgersen et al., 2006), as reported in Chapter 8.

The UMASS Study Results

As part of their initial interviews, participants in our study were queried about their use of various substances. The results of that interview are shown in Table 10.1 and are graphically illustrated in Figure 10.1. A higher percentage of both the ADHD and Clinical control groups had smoked at some time in their lives than was the case for the Community control group. Also, more members of the ADHD group were current smokers than the Community control group, but neither of those groups differed significantly from the Clinical control group, which placed part way between the results for these other two groups. Therefore, while our results partially replicated earlier follow-up studies of children with ADHD into adolescence and adulthood showing an increased risk of smoking in adults with ADHD relative to community adults, this was not the case relative to adults having other clinical disorders. This implies a nonspecific risk for smoking among outpatient disorders rather than a specific one for ADHD.

TABLE 10.1. Proportion of Each Group Using Various Substances in the UMASS Study

Measure	ADHD		Clinical		Community		χ^2	p	Pairwise contrasts
	N	%	N	%	N	%			
Smoked tobacco	100	70	54	58	46	43	18.9	< .001	1,2 > 3
Currently smokes tobacco[S]	32	22	16	17	9	8	8.5	.014	1 > 3
Currently uses alcohol[S]	73	50	59	63	60	56	3.6	NS	
Used marijuana[S]	116	80	68	72	57	53	22.2	< .001	1,2 > 3
Used cocaine[S]	57	39	22	23	19	18	15.9	< .001	1 > 2,3
Used heroine[S]	8	5	4	4	1	1	3.7	NS	
Used LSD[S]	56	39	21	22	20	18	14.4	.001	1 > 2,3
Used prescribed drugs illegally[S]	31	21	14	15	10	9	6.9	.032	1 > 3
Treated for alcohol abuse[S]	25	17	10	11	2	2	15.5	< .001	1,2 > 3
Treated for drug abuse[S]	12	8	6	6	0	0	9.0	.011	1,2 > 3

Note. N = sample size endorsing this item; % = percent of group endorsing this item; χ^2 = results of the omnibus chi-square test; p = probability value for the chi-square test; pairwise contrasts = results of the chi-square tests involving pairwise comparisons of the three groups; [S] = significant effect of sex on this measure (males more likely than females on all measures).

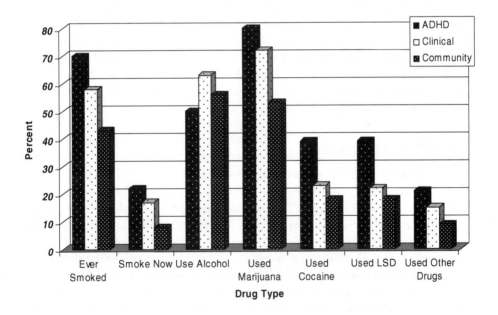

FIGURE 10.1. Percent of each group using various types of drugs in the UMASS Study.

We did not find any group differences concerning the percentage of each group that currently used alcohol (50–63% across groups). But we did find that more of the ADHD and Clinical control groups had been treated for alcohol abuse than members of the Community control group, consistent with the higher frequency of alcohol abuse disorders we reported in Chapter 8. Marijuana users were more common in both the ADHD and Clinical control groups relative to the Community control group. But ADHD was specifically associated with a greater number of cocaine and LSD users as well as users of prescription drugs on an illegal basis compared to both of our control groups. Consequently, it is not surprising that a greater number of both the ADHD and Clinical control groups had been treated previously for a drug-use disorder than occurred in the Community control group. To summarize, more adults with ADHD were likely to have been past or current smokers; to be users of marijuana, cocaine, LSD, or prescription drugs, and to have been treated for previous alcohol and drug use disorders than was the case in the Community control group. Such results are consistent with the prior literature discussed above that ADHD elevates the risk for various drug-use problems over that of community control groups (De Quiros & Kinsbourne, 2001; Murphy & Barkley, 1996). But the Clinical control group also showed some elevated risks for some drug use problems, primarily past tobacco use and current marijuana use. The ADHD group differed from that clinical group chiefly in having more members who had tried cocaine and LSD, implying that these may be the specific risks associated with ADHD in clinic-referred adults, whereas abuse of other drugs may simply be related to outpatient disorders more generally.

As noted earlier, it appears to be the subset of those with ADHD who also had CD that had an increased risk for drug use. We therefore compared those in the ADHD group who qualified for a diagnosis of CD in childhood based on their retrospective reports of their CD symptoms to those who did not, in the proportion having ever used each type of drug. The groups did not differ in any drug-use category except for cocaine, where those who had CD were twice as likely to have tried cocaine compared to those without CD (62% vs. 31%, $\chi^2 = 10.37$, $p = .001$). Thus, at least in our clinic-referred adults with ADHD, the presence of retrospectively reported CD in childhood does not account entirely for the elevated proportion of ADHD adults who had tried various substances. Of course the link of drug use and abuse to current CD may still exist, but we were not able to examine it, as we had not collected information dealing specifically with CD symptoms in the prior 6 months.

There were a number of measures on which we found significant main effects for sex. In each instance, males regardless of group were more likely than females to have used these particular substances. We also examined the effect of sex within each group. Within the ADHD group, we found that more males than females used marijuana, cocaine, LSD, and prescription drugs and had been treated for alcohol abuse. Within our Clinical control group, we found no sex differences in the proportion using any drugs. In the Community control group, more males used alcohol, LSD, and prescription drugs. Thus it seems that the overall sex differences we found for drug use were driven largely by males in both the ADHD and Community control groups.

Lambert and Hartsough (1998) previously argued that stimulant drug treatment among children with ADHD may increase their risk of using nicotine or cocaine as adolescents or young adults. Many other studies, however, have not found such a connection (Barkley, Fischer, et al., 2003; Wilens, Faraone, Biederman, & Gunawardene, 2003). Nevertheless, we deemed it worth examining whether those participants in the ADHD and Clinical control groups who were currently medicated with stimulants might be more likely to be smoking or using cocaine. We compared those who were stimulant-treated to those who were not in both groups and found no differences between them in any category of drug use. Our results conflict with those reported by Lambert and Hartsough, of a connection between stimulant use and drug use at least in adulthood, but these results are consistent with the vast majority of the earlier studies that found no such relationship.

The frequencies of drug use for each drug type within each of our groups are shown in Table 10.2. These frequencies are only for those participants who reported having ever used each of these substances. Among those who had ever used tobacco, the groups did not differ in the length of time during which they had been tobacco users. Likewise, the groups did not differ in the average number of cigarettes they smoked per day if they were current smokers, although there was a marginally significant ($p < .10$) elevation among the ADHD group

TABLE 10.2. Frequency of Drug Use for Each Group among Those Using Each Drug Type in the UMASS Study

Measure	ADHD		Clinical		Community		F	p	Pairwise contrasts
	Mean	SD	Mean	SD	Mean	SD			
Years used tobacco[A]	9.5	8.4	10.7	9.8	11.0	9.7	0.1	NS	
Cigarettes/day	17.7	11.1	10.6	10.2	11.1	8.4	3.1	NS	
Alcoholic drinks/week[S]	9.4	10.8	6.8	6.6	4.7	4.6	3.2	.044	1 > 3
Marijuana use[S]	1038.1	1574.1	402.1	654.4	252.8	561.4	7.9	< .001	1 > 2,3
Cocaine use	93.3	143.3	18.3	30.4	25.0	35.9	2.4	NS	
LSD Use[S]	18.0	27.5	13.9	23.4	19.1	30.2	0.2	NS	
Prescribed drug use	31.2	40.3	19.7	30.3	30.0	39.3	0.6	NS	

Note. Sample sizes for each drug are shown in Table 10.1. SD = standard deviation; F = F-test results of the analysis of variance (or covariance); p = probability value for the F-test; NS = not significant, [S] = significant main effect for sex (see text for details); [GxS] = significant group × sex interaction (see text for details); [A] = age used as a covariate in this analysis.

Statistical analysis: Groups were initially compared using two way (group × sex) analysis of variance (or covariance as necessary). Where this analysis was significant ($p < .05$) for the main effect for group, pairwise comparisons of the groups were conducted the results of which are shown in the last column.

relative to smokers in the two control groups. Among users of alcohol, we found that the adults with ADHD consumed more drinks per week on average than did participants in the Community control group. The Clinical control group did not differ from either of these groups in this respect. But among marijuana users, the frequency of use was significantly greater among the adults with ADHD than in either of the two control groups. The groups did not differ in their frequencies of using cocaine, LSD, or illegal prescription drugs among those who had ever used these substances. The greater use of alcoholic beverages and marijuana by the ADHD group certainly concurs with our two earlier studies (Barkley, Murphy et al., 2002; Murphy & Barkley, 1996). It disagrees with the earlier report by De Quiros and Kinsbourne (2001) that found no elevated rate of alcohol use in adults with ADHD, but that disparity could be due to their use of considerably smaller samples (ADHD = 48, control = 40), thereby limiting their statistical power to detect such differences.

Because of the previously established link between the presence of CD in those with ADHD and their greater risk for substance use, we subdivided the ADHD group into those who did and did not qualify for a diagnosis of CD in childhood. While these two groups did not differ in their consumption of cigarettes, cocaine use, or heroin use, those having CD used marijuana and LSD more often than those who did not. The CD group was also marginally more likely to drink more alcoholic beverages per week ($p = .052$) and to use prescription drugs illegally ($p = .056$) more often than those adults with ADHD who did not have CD retrospectively as children. These results are more in keeping with past research than was our earlier analysis of these same groups concerning the proportions that had ever tried these drugs at least once. The presence of CD appears to account for the significantly higher frequency of some drugs used by the ADHD group relative to the control groups. Therefore, while the presence of childhood CD may not account for whether an adult with ADHD ever tries a particular substance at least once, it does in many instances seem to contribute to the frequency with which he or she may subsequently continue to use that drug.

We again compared those participants in the ADHD and Clinical control groups who were treated with stimulants to those who were not being so treated and, once again, found no significant differences in their frequencies of use of these substances. We therefore find no support for the assertion that stimulant treatment increases the risk of drug use or abuse, especially for other stimulants such as tobacco or cocaine.

Predicting Drug Use Risk

Ever having tried cocaine or LSD were both drug-use risks specifically associated with the ADHD group in the UMASS Study. We examined a set of predictors of these outcomes, the results of which appear in Table 10.3. Risk for cocaine

TABLE 10.3. Predicting Drug Use Categorical Outcomes in the UMASS Study

Outcome/predictors (block entered)	Beta	S	Wald	p	Odds ratio	95% CI
Ever tried cocaine						
(1) No. of ADHD Symptoms*	.088	.025	12.61	< .001	1.09	1.04–1.15
(1) Age	.010	.001	0.76	NS	1.01	0.99–1.03
(2) IQ	−.045	.017	6.93	.008	0.96	0.92–0.99
(2) No. of crime types (lifetime)	.692	.124	31.30	< .001	2.00	1.57–2.55

NS: Sex, no. of child ADHD symptoms, no. of CD symptoms (childhood), currently smoke cigarettes, depression, anxiety, on stimulants at study entry, ever treated with psychiatric drugs

Ever tried LSD						
(1) No. of ADHD symptoms*	.092	.025	13.60	< .001	1.10	1.04–1.15
(1) Age	−.027	.012	5.18	.023	0.97	0.95–1.00
(2) Sex (male)	.673	.329	4.17	.041	1.96	1.03–3.74
(2) No. of crime types (lifetime)	.616	.129	22.85	< .001	1.85	1.44–2.38
(2) Currently smoke cigarettes	.872	.371	5.53	.019	2.39	1.16–4.95

NS: IQ, no. of child ADHD symptoms, no. of CD symptoms (childhood), depression, anxiety, on stimulants at study entry, ever treated with psychiatric drugs

Note. SE = standard error for beta; odds ratio = Exp(B); 95% CI = 95% confidence interval for the odds ratio; NS = not significant; * = this variable became nonsignificant when other variables were entered in the next block; Shipley = Shipley Institute of Living Scale IQ estimate; SCL-90-R = Symptom Checklist–90—Revised T-score; CD diagnosis = met DSM-IV criterion for conduct disorder on symptom threshold from self-reported childhood rating scale; no. of crime types = number of 10 different crime types ever committed.
Statistical analysis: Logistic regression using forced entry method at Block 1 and forward conditional method at Block 2. Used the entire sample (N = 353).

use was related to higher ADHD symptoms, lower IQ, and greater criminal diversity scores (number of different crimes ever committed; see below). In contrast, risk for LSD use was predicted by severity of ADHD symptoms, younger age, being male, higher criminal diversity scores, and being a current smoker.

We also found that clinic-referred adults with ADHD used more marijuana and drank more alcoholic beverages per week. For these dimensional outcomes, we used multiple regression to evaluate a set of predictors that could be reasonably associated with these risks. The results of those analyses are shown in Table 10.4. For marijuana use, once more, severity of ADHD was significantly predictive of this outcome but, not surprisingly, so was having a higher criminal diversity score (number of crime types—see below), and having a lower IQ. For frequency of alcohol use per week, a different set of predictors became evident. Severity of ADHD was predictive of this outcome, as expected, but so was being

TABLE 10.4. Predicting Drug Use Frequencies in the UMASS Study

Outcome/predictors (step entered)	Beta	R	R^2	$R^2\Delta$	F	p
Frequency of marijuana use						
(1) No. of ADHD symptoms	.224	.223	.050	.050	9.12	< .001
and age (NS)	.024					
(2) No. of crime types (lifetime)	.272	.358	.128	.078	31.39	< .001
(3) IQ (Shipley)	−.170	.395	.156	.028	11.57	.001
NS: Sex, Education, no. of CD symptoms, no. of impaired domains, depression, anxiety, hostility (SCL-90-R)						
Typical no. of alcoholic drinks/week						
(1) No. of ADHD symptoms	.175	.193	.037	.037	6.80	.001
and age (NS)	−.065					
(2) Sex (female)	−.188	.262	.069	.031	11.68	.001
(3) No. of impaired domains	−.300	.299	.089	.021	7.96	.005
(4) Hostility	.186	.327	.107	.018	6.91	.009
NS: education, IQ, no. of CD symptoms, no. of crime types, depression, anxiety						

Note. R = regression coefficient; R^2 = percent of explained variance accounted for by all variables at this step; $R^2\Delta$ = percent of explained variance accounted for by this variable added at this step; F = results of F-test for the equation at this step; p = probability value for the F-test; Beta = Standardized Beta Coefficient; NS = not significant; Shipley = Shipley Institute of Living Scale IQ estimate; SCL-90-R = Symptom Checklist–90—Revised T-score.

Statistical analysis: Multiple linear regression using forced entry method at Step 1 and stepwise conditional method at subsequent steps. Used the entire sample (N = 353).

male, having fewer domains of impairment, and having a higher hostility score on the SCL-90-R. Why the lower level of impairment would be associated with greater frequency of alcohol use per week is not immediately obvious, as one might have expected the inverse relationship.

The Milwaukee Study Results

We used the same interview concerning drug use in the UMASS Study in the Milwaukee Study as well.

Risk for Drug Use

The results concerning whether or not a participant had ever tried each of the various substances are reported in Table 10.5. It is apparent here that hyperactive children were at greater risk of being a current tobacco or alcohol users and of ever having gotten drunk, but whether or not their ADHD had persisted to age 27 made little difference here. And while the H+ADHD group had a signifi-

TABLE 10.5. Drug Use Categories by Group on Categorical Measures in the Milwaukee Study

Measures	H+ADHD N	H+ADHD %	H−ADHD N	H−ADHD %	Community N	Community %	χ^2	p	Pairwise contrasts
Smoked tobacco	46	85	58	73	49	65	6.36	.042	1 > 3
Currently smokes tobacco	30	62	45	66	17	30	18.01	< .001	1,2 > 3
Currently uses alcohol	32	60	48	61	59	79	7.07	.029	1,2 < 3
Ever used alcohol	44	80	63	81	66	92	4.47	NS	
Ever gotten drunk	28	54	40	51	54	72	7.74	.021	1,2 < 3
Drink caffeine	51	93	71	91	61	85	2.49	NS	
Used marijuana	27	50	30	38	23	31	4.97	NS	
Used cocaine	9	17	6	8	4	5	5.22	NS	
Used heroine	2	4	2	2	2	3	0.17	NS	
Used LSD	5	9	4	5	1	1	4.38	NS	
Used speed (methamphetamine)	2	4	3	4	3	4	0.18	NS	
Used prescribed drugs illegally	7	13	3	4	0	0	11.74	.003	1 > 2,3
Considers him- or herself alcoholic	12	22	14	18	12	16	0.82	NS	
Told by others he or she was an alcoholic	15	28	22	28	17	23	0.72	NS	
Lost a job due to alcoholism	4	7	0	0	1	1	8.19	.017	1 > 2
Treated for alcoholism	9	17	8	10	7	9	1.87	NS	
Considered him- or herself a drug abuser	13	24	7	9	4	5	11.49	.003	1 > 2,3
Told by others he or she was a drug abuser	18	33	12	15	8	11	11.50	.003	1 > 2,3
Lost a job due to drug abuse	3	6	3	4	1	1	1.80	NS	
Treated for drug abuse	10	18	10	13	7	9	2.34	NS	

Note. Sample sizes are H+ADHD = 54, H−ADHD = 78, and Community controls = 75. N = sample size endorsing this item; % = percent of group endorsing this item; χ^2 = results of the omnibus chi-square test; p = probability value for the chi-square test; pairwise contrasts = results of the chi-square tests involving pairwise comparisons of the three groups *Statistical analysis:* Pearson chi-square.

cantly greater percentage that had ever smoked tobacco than the community group, the H–ADHD group placed between these two extreme groups and did not differ significantly from either. Noteworthy here is that the groups did not differ in the percentage who had ever tried any of the other illegal drugs listed in this table except that the H+ADHD group had significantly more members who had illegally used a prescription drug compared to the other two groups. The latter finding agrees with the results for the UMASS Study in showing some association between current ADHD and illegal prescription drug use. And it is consistent with Weiss and Hechtman's (1993) findings at their adult follow-up of hyperactive children.

The remainder of these results appear to be somewhat at odds with those for the ADHD group in the UMASS Study. A higher percentage of the Milwaukee Study's H+ADHD group appear to have tried tobacco, currently use tobacco, and currently use alcohol than the clinic-referred adults with ADHD in the UMASS Study. But a greater percentage of the UMASS study adults with ADHD have tried marijuana and cocaine. The proportions of the Milwaukee Study's ADHD group using the other drugs are relatively low and comparable to the adults with ADHD in the UMASS Study. Yet the UMASS Study's ADHD group differed from its control group in some of these respects, especially for marijuana, cocaine, and LSD use. We also found that more of the H+ADHD group considered themselves to have a drug abuse problem and had been told by others that they were drug abusers than was the case in the other two groups. This suggests that while few differences emerged here in the proportion of each group that had ever tried the illegal drugs listed, the H+ADHD group may be using these drugs more often.

Frequency of Drug Use

We examined that issue next. The frequencies of using various drugs are shown in Table 10.6. The frequency of using most drugs was very low and did not differ among the groups, and so these rates are not shown in the table. We do show those for which either there were significant differences or there had been in the UMASS Study. As in that study, the results here are for drug use frequencies only for that subset of participants who had tried the drug at least once. This resulted in such small sample sizes for the groups that some comparisons simply could not be tested (i.e., no or so few members having tried a given substance) by a para-

TABLE 10.6. Drug Use Frequencies for Each Group (If Ever Had Used That Substance) for the Milwaukee Study

Measures	H+ADHD Mean	SD	H–ADHD Mean	SD	Community Mean	SD	F	p	Pairwise contrasts
Years used cigarettes[VIQ]	9.2	4.8	8.4	4.8	7.4	8.7	0.79	NS	
Cigarettes/day[VIQ,PIQ]	11.3	15.7	8.7	9.9	5.8	6.7	2.90	NS	
Alcoholic drinks/week	16.0	19.1	8.3	8.3	7.3	7.7	6.43	.002	1 > 2,3
No. of drunken episodes	10.9	12.9	5.3	10.0	6.1	11.8	2.22	NS	
Caffeine drinks/day	4.0	4.0	4.4	4.2	2.3	2.7	6.41	.002	1,2 > 3
Marijuana use	124.7	149.9	96.0	107.9	63.6	88.1	1.64	NS	
Cocaine use	21.9	34.5	23.8	47.2	4.7	6.8	0.40	NS	
Speed use	3.5	2.1	22.3	25.8	3.3	2.1	1.50	NS	

Note. Sample sizes: See Table 10.5 for number of participants in each group that had used each substance as those sample sizes served as the sample sizes here for each substance. SD = standard deviation; F = F-test results of the analysis of variance (or covariance); p = probability value for the F-test; NS = not significant; [VIQ] = Verbal IQ subtest used as a covariate in this analysis; [PIQ] = Nonverbal performance IQ subtest used as a covariate in this analysis.

  Statistical analysis: Groups were initially compared using one-way (groups) analysis of variance (or covariance as necessary). Where this analysis was significant ($p < .05$) for the main effect for group, pairwise comparisons of the groups were conducted, the results of which are shown in the last column.

metric analyses. As this table shows, the number of years participants had been smoking and their frequency of cigarette use per day did not differ among our three groups in this study. Nor did the frequencies differ for marijuana, cocaine, or speed. This latter result is likely due to the small sample sizes compounded by the substantially skewed and kurtotic distributions for these frequencies in which there were high-use outliers in each group, causing standard deviations to be as large or larger than mean scores. Nevertheless, we did not find the greater use of marijuana in the ADHD group specifically or hyperactive group more generally, as had been found in the UMASS Study adults with ADHD. We did find that the H+ADHD group consumed more alcoholic drinks per week than either the H–ADHD or Community control group, in keeping with the greater incidence among them of alcohol use disorders found in Chapter 8 and consistent with the findings in the UMASS Study regarding adults with ADHD. Both hyperactive groups appeared to use caffeinated beverages more often each day than the community group—but caffeine use was not studied in the UMASS project. A pattern here suggests itself: the Milwaukee Study's hyperactive groups appear to be using the less expensive and legally available substances more than are adults in the UMASS Study who have ADHD, whereas those adults are using more expensive and illegal drugs such as marijuana and LSD more often than the Milwaukee Study groups. Given that the UMASS Study adults are older, on average, by at least 5 to 10 years, and have a higher income, they may have more money available to expend on these more expensive illegal substances. Thus, the drugs most likely to be abused by the two ADHD groups across these projects are those which they find to be most available and affordable. It is interesting to note as well that differences between the hyperactive and Community control groups in drug use were much more evident at the age-21 follow-up than at this later follow-up point, perhaps suggesting either a declining frequency of use in the hyperactive group with age relative to controls or an increasing rate of use among the controls over this period.

Relationship of Childhood Stimulant Treatment with Lifetime Drug Use by Age 27

We and others have previously reviewed the literature concerning the risk that childhood stimulant treatment may pose for later drug use and abuse, especially for nonprescription stimulants such as nicotine or cocaine (Barkley et al., 2003; Wilens et al., 2003). We had also reported on evidence from the Milwaukee study concerning such relationships at the age-21 follow-up (Barkley et al., 2003). We did so given concerns raised in research by Lambert and Hartsough (1998; Lambert, 2002) that found such apparent relationships, particularly for stimulant treatment and risk for nicotine and cocaine use by adolescence and young adulthood. Fourteen other studies have examined such relationships in various ways, and not one has produced evidence of such relationships (see Barkley et al., 2003; Wilens et al., 2003). We took this opportunity once more to use the Milwaukee Study to evaluate these potential relationships at the age-27 follow-up. Certainly the greater time since the last follow-up should have allowed such relationships to emerge, given that it is considered the peak age period for such drug use and abuse.

We correlated duration of childhood stimulant treatment as reported by parents at the teen follow-up to reported drug use frequency at adult follow-up using the entire sample. This included length of time smoking cigarettes, number of cigarettes currently smoked (per day) if smoking, number of drinks currently consumed (per week), and how many times they had ever used marijuana, cocaine, heroine, LSD, speed, or illegal prescription drugs. All but one were not significant; the one was current cigarette use ($r = .178$, $p = .034$). But when we reanalyzed these correlations using only the hyperactive group—which is the more appropriate group to study here, given that rarely did a control child take stimulants—none of the correlations were significant or even close to being so. It is because none of the control group took stimulants in childhood that the relationship between stimulant treatment duration and smoking frequency became significant.

We then compared those who had been treated with stimulants in childhood to those who never been so treated on whether they had ever tried these substances, using the entire sample. No significant findings emerged. We repeated these analyses again using just the hyperactive group. Surprisingly, and contrary to Lambert's findings, those who had *never* been treated with a stimulant were *more* likely to have tried speed (9% vs. 1%) ($p = .045$) and were *more* likely to have used a prescription drug illegally (23% vs. 2%) ($\chi^2 = 11.70$, $p = .001$). This actually supports the meta-analytic review by Wilens et al. (2003) that treatment of ADHD with stimulants in childhood and adolescence could have a protective effect against some types of drug use or abuse.

Finally, we repeated the analyses above, but this time comparing those treated for less than a year to those treated for more than a year, first using the entire sample. We did so because this is the manner in which Lambert and Hartsough (1998) had grouped their study participants for their own analyses. Again, no comparisons reached or approached significance. Once again, we repeated these analyses just using the hyperactive group. We found the same result as above for ever having used a prescription drug illegally; those treated for less than a year had a greater risk for this drug-use category than did those treated for longer than a year (12% vs. 2%) ($\chi^2 = 4.25$, $p = .039$). Again, therefore, we have disproved Lambert and Hartsough's hypothesis that childhood stimulant exposure is related to later drug use.

Antisocial Activities

Although the association of childhood ADHD and conduct problems with adolescent CD and substance use have become increasingly well established (Loeber et al., 2000; see also above discussion), the risks for antisocial activities in young adulthood are less certain. Only a handful of studies of clinically diagnosed ADHD or hyperactive children exist that have followed them into adulthood to evaluate their ongoing risks for antisocial activities at this developmental stage. There seem to be only four follow-up studies that used large clinic-referred samples, had control groups, retained at least 50% or more of their original samples into adulthood, and examined for antisocial behavior by young adulthood. These consist of the Montreal follow-up study (clinical $N = 103$) conducted by Weiss and Hechtman (1993), the New York City longitudinal study of two separate cohorts ($Ns = 101, 94$) conducted by Mannuzza, Klein, Bessler, Malloy, and LaPadula (1998; Mannuzza et al., 1993), the Los Angeles study ($N = 89$) conducted by Satterfield and Shell (1997), and the Swedish follow-up study ($N = 50$) conducted by Rasmussen and Gillberg (2001).

These studies found that antisocial personality occurred in a significant minority of children with ADHD by adulthood compared to control children (Montreal = 23% vs. 2.4% of controls; New York = 27% vs. 8% in late adolescence; 12%–18% vs. 2%–3% in adulthood; Sweden = 18% vs. 2.1%) (Mannuzza et al., 1993, 1998; Rasmussen & Gillberg, 2001; Weiss, Hechtman, Milroy, & Perlman, 1985). Criminal arrests have also been shown to be higher among hyperactive children followed to adulthood (Babinski, Hartsough, & Lambert, 1999; Rasmussen & Gillberg, 2001; Satterfield & Schell, 1997). These results show that at least some children with ADHD are at risk for antisocial activities, arrests, and even antisocial personality disorder by adulthood. While documenting arrest rates and antisocial disorders by adulthood is certainly informative, more precise information on the specific forms of antisocial activities would help to further clarify the nature and risks for maladjustment of the adult outcome of this disorder.

This led Barkley and Fischer to use their Milwaukee young adult follow-up of hyperactive (H) children to evaluate specific antisocial activities (Barkley et al., 2004). At the age-21 follow-up, they found that more of the H group had committed a variety of antisocial acts and more who had been arrested for doing so (corroborated through official arrest records) than had the Community control (CC) group. Their findings are shown in Table 10.7. The H group were found to have rated higher on the frequency of property theft, disorderly conduct, assault with fists, carrying a concealed weapon, and illegal drug possession; they also had more arrests. This study extended the results of prior follow-up studies in several important respects.

TABLE 10.7. Proportion of Hyperactive and Control Groups That Ever Committed Various Antisocial Activities by Young Adulthood or Were Arrested (Self-Reported and Official Records) in the Milwaukee Study at Age 21

Activity	Hyperactive		Control		χ^2	p	Eta
	%	(No.)	%	(No.)			
Stole property	85	(125)	64	(47)	12.19	< .001	.235
Stole money	50	(73)	36	(26)	3.89	.049	.133
Broke into a home	20	(29)	8	(6)	4.83	.028	.148
Disorderly conduct	69	(101)	53	(39)	4.92	.026	.150
Assault with fists	74	(109)	52	(38)	10.74	.001	.221
Assault with a weapon	22	(32)	7	(5)	7.76	.005	.188
Robbery or mugging	4	(6)	0	(0)	3.06	NS	.118
Set serious fires	15	(22)	5	(4)	4.21	.04	.138
Carried concealed weapon	38	(56)	11	(8)	17.41	< .001	.281
Forced sexual activity	1	(1)	0	(0)	0.50	NS	.048
Had sex with prostitute	2	(3)	0	(0)	1.51	NS	.083
Took money to have sex	2	(3)	0	(0)	1.51	NS	.083
Ran away from home	31	(45)	16	(12)	5.10	.024	.152
Illegal drug possession	52	(76)	42	(31)	1.66	NS	.087
Illegal drug sales	24	(35)	20	(15)	0.29	NS	.037
Ever arrested (self-reported)	54	(79)	37	(27)	5.48	.019	.158
Arrested 2+ times	39	(58)	12	(9)	16.95	< .001	.278
Arrested 3+ times	27	(40)	11	(8)	7.55	.006	.185
Misdemeanor arrest (official)	24	(35)	11	(8)	5.02	.025	.151
Felony arrest (official)	27	(40)	11	(8)	7.42	.006	.183

Note. Samples sizes are Hyperactive = 147 and Control = 73. % = percent of group; (No.) = number committing this act; χ^2 = chi-square; p = probability associated with the chi-square statistic; eta = effect size; official = derived from the official state crime records. From Barkley, Fischer, Smallish, and Fletcher (2004). Copyright 2004 by the Association for Child Psychology and Psychiatry. Reprinted by permission.

- It identified a wider range of offenses among the hyperactive group than had been previously reported.
- It unearthed two relatively robust underlying dimensions to these antisocial activities, which we called *predatory-overt* and *drug-related,* that each accounted for more than 20% of the variance in antisocial activities. Additional factors were discovered pertaining to sexual deviance-theft, fire-setting, and sexual assault. But each accounted for less than 10% of the variance, comprised mainly of just one or two antisocial actions each, and those actions occurred relatively infrequently, leading us to view those factors as not particularly reliable or stable.
- It found that the hyperactive group differed primarily from the control group only on the *drug-related* antisocial dimension, while not on the *predatory–overt* dimension. Such a distinction in the nature of antisocial activities toward which hyperactive children may be predisposed had not been previously reported.
- It found that this group difference in *drug-related* antisocial activities was related to severity of ADHD in childhood, adolescence, and adulthood after con-

trolling for the contribution of both ADHD and severity of conduct problems at the earlier developmental period. Only severity of childhood conduct problems made an additional significant contribution to predicting this form of young adult antisocial behavior beyond severity of childhood ADHD. Severity of teen CD and adult CD made no significant additional contributions to this dimension of adult antisocial behavior after controlling for severity of childhood conduct problems. All this implies that it is severity of ADHD that may be the principal risk factor for determining the frequency of *drug-related* antisocial behavior committed by young adulthood.

• Other longitudinal studies have found that severity of childhood ADHD symptoms was specifically associated with risk for later drug use apart from the better established association of childhood conduct problems with later drug use (Babinski et al., 1999). To our knowledge, however, this is the first time that ADHD has been linked to these drug-related antisocial activities and that such a contribution is apart from any made by severity of childhood, teen, or adult conduct disorder.

• Finally, the Milwaukee study was able to extend prior follow-up research on hyperactive children by evaluating the degree to which severity of teen CD and teen drug use contributed independently from each other to later antisocial activity by adulthood. Such an examination was initiated primarily to explore previous suggestions (Brook, Whiteman, Finch, & Cohen, 1996) that teen drug use may contribute additional risk to antisocial activities by young adulthood apart from its well-known affiliation with severity of teen CD. The study results supported this hypothesis, but only for certain types of young adult antisocial activities. Drug use did not contribute independently to the *predatory–overt* dimension of antisocial activities by young adulthood apart from severity of teen CD. Teen CD, however, was significantly predictive of this dimension of antisocial behavior by young adulthood, in keeping with numerous prior longitudinal studies finding such a linkage (Brook et al., 1996; Satterfield & Schell, 1997; Loeber et al., 2000). In contrast, it was teen substance use that was significantly predictive of the *drug-related* dimension of antisocial behavior by young adulthood apart from any contribution of teen CD to this dimension. Teen drug use, in fact, seemed to mediate the link of teen CD to this form of young adult criminal behavior. These results are quite consistent with the findings of Brook et al. (1996) that teen drug use contributes additional risk for later young adult delinquency apart from teen delinquency. These results also are in keeping with those of Ridenour et al. (2002), showing that adolescent drug use before 18 years of age significantly increased the risk of adult antisocial behavior. The Milwaukee Study findings go further in showing that, at least among its groups, teen drug use contributed chiefly to the dimension of *drug-related* antisocial activities rather than that of *predatory–overt* antisocial behavior.

As reported in Chapter 8, clinic-referred adults with ADHD may have a higher likelihood of antisocial personality disorder that would be consistent with these childhood ADHD follow-up studies. We had previously reported that adults with ADHD were also more likely to have been arrested than control adults (40% vs. 12%), particularly if they had the combined type of the disorder as opposed to the inattentive type (Murphy, Barkley, & Bush, 2002), though this was not the case in an earlier, smaller study (Barkley et al., 1996). Nevertheless, even that smaller study found that adults with ADHD had been arrested significantly more often than control adults. Torgersen et al. (2006), in their study of 45 Norwegian adults with ADHD, also reported high rates of arrests and sentencing (47%). Our small study is also only one of two we could identify that examined specific antisocial activities in the histories of clinic-referred adults with ADHD (Barkley et al., 1996). It found that a greater percentage of the ADHD group had stolen others' property, stolen others' money, and engaged in disorderly conduct than did the control group. The groups did not differ in the proportions who had engaged in breaking and entering, assault, running away from home as a child or teen, illegal drug possession, or selling illegal drugs. However, the frequency with which the two groups engaged in these antisocial activities differed on a number of these behaviors. The adults with ADHD had higher reported frequencies of stealing property, stealing money, disorderly conduct, running away from home, and illegal drug possession. The total number of antisocial acts was also greater in the ADHD than control group. Torgersen et al. (2006) also found elevated rates of violent crime (24%), theft (27%), and drug-related crime (18%) in their Norwegian sample of adults with ADHD. Such findings are certainly in keeping with earlier reports of a greater risk for antisocial personality disorder among clinic-referred adults with ADHD.

Given the relationship of adult ADHD to adult antisocial personality disorder (Chapter 8), one would not be surprised to find ADHD over represented in adult prison populations. We are aware of just two published studies on the issue (Eyestone & Howell, 1994; Rasmussen, Almvik, & Levander, 2001). In the first study, a random sampling of 102 inmates in the Utah State Prison was employed (Eyestone & Howell, 1994). Results indicated that 25.5% of those inmates evaluated qualified for a diagnosis of adult ADHD. This diagnosis required that they have self-reported significant symptoms of the disorder since childhood and meet DSM-III-R criteria for ADHD. Of interest in the study was its finding of a strong association of adult ADHD to major depression in this population, where the prevalence of disorder was also 25.5%. The overlap of the two disorders was 47%, with evidence that increasing severity of ADHD symptoms was associated with increasing risk for major depression. These authors also cited an unpublished master's thesis by Favarino that was reported to have found a similar prevalence rate for adult ADHD in a prison population. The more recent study by

Rasmussen et al. (2001), conducted in a representative Norwegian prison population ($N = 82$), used the Wender Utah Rating Scale for determining childhood retrospective reports of ADHD and found 46% met the recommended cutoff score for probable ADHD while another 18% surpassed the threshold, suggestive of further screening for the disorder. For current ADHD, the study used the Brown scales for adult ADHD and found that 30% met the recommend threshold for the disorder and another 16% had a sufficiently high level of symptoms to warrant further evaluation. In short, adults with ADHD are more likely to engage in antisocial activities and to be diagnosed with antisocial personality disorder while adults who engage in antisocial activities, especially as reflected in adult prisoners, are more likely to have ADHD than would be expected by chance alone.

The UMASS Study Results

The present projects interviewed their participants concerning whether or not they had engaged in various antisocial activities in their life. We also had them rate themselves with regard to symptoms of CD as children and adolescents and we had someone who knew them well do the same (typically parents) (see sidebar).

Structured Clinical Interview of Impairments

As reported in Chapter 6, we created an interview consisting of questions dealing with various domains of major life activities, including educational history, occupational history, antisocial activities, drug use, driving, money management, and dating and marital history. This interview was administered by a psychological technician holding a master's degree in psychology and trained in the evaluation of clinic-referred adults. The questions dealing with antisocial activities and drug use are reported here.

ADHD Rating Scale for Adults (Barkley & Murphy, 2006)

This scale was completed twice by adults in this study, once for current functioning, which dealt with ADHD symptoms and domains of impairment, and also again concerning childhood functioning. The retrospective childhood rating scale also contained the 12 symptoms of conduct disorder (CD) from the DSM-IV. Participants indicated whether or not they had ever engaged in any of these activities as children or adolescents. This same rating scale was obtained from parents of these participants whenever possible or from others who knew them well.

The proportion of each of our three groups that had ever engaged in 10 different antisocial activities is shown in Table 10.8, along with their reports of whether they had ever been arrested or sent to jail. The findings are graphically depicted in Figure 10.2. To our knowledge, no study of clinic-referred adults with ADHD has examined their antisocial activities so specifically. We found that the ADHD group differed significantly from both of the control groups in at least 7 of these 12 categories. More members of the ADHD group had engaged in shoplifting, stealing without confronting a victim, breaking and entering, assaults with fists, carrying an illegal weapon, being arrested and more had been sent to jail. Further, more adults with ADHD had sold drugs illegally in comparison to the Community control group. The Clinical control group did not differ from either of these two groups on this outcome. We found no significant group differences for robbing someone, assault with a weapon, setting fires intentionally, or forced sexual activity. The most common form of antisocial activity for the adults with ADHD was shoplifting (53%) followed by assaulting someone with their fists (35%), and selling illegal drugs (21%). These were also proportionally the most common activities in the two control groups as well but not to the degree they had occurred among members of the ADHD group.

Main effects for sex were evident in 7 of the 12 outcomes; in all instances males were more likely to have engaged in these activities than were females regardless of group. In examining within group sex differences specifically, we found that, for the ADHD group, more males engaged in shoplifting, assaulting with fists, carrying illegal weapon, and selling drugs; more had also been arrested and been in jail than had females. For the Clinical controls, more males had sold more drugs and been jailed. For the Community controls, more males had engaged in shoplifting and assaults with fists than did females.

From the above information, we created a measure reflecting criminal diversity that represented the number of different crime categories an individual had committed, formed by summing across the above 10 crimes except being arrested or jailed. We found that the adults with ADHD had higher criminal diversity scores ($M = 1.6$, $SD = 1.7$) than did adults in either control group (Clinical: $M = 0.8$, $SD = 1.0$; Community: $M = 0.6$, $SD = 1.0$), who did not differ from each other. Comparing males only, the adults with ADHD differed from males in both control groups, who again did not differ from each other. Comparing females only, the group main effect was marginal ($< .09$) and showed only females with ADHD differing from those in the control groups. There was a significant interaction of group with sex that is shown in Figure 10.3. Within each group, ADHD males ($M = 2.0$, $SD = 1.8$) differed from females ($M = 0.9$, $SD = 1.2$) and community males ($M = 0.9$, $SD = 1.0$) differed from females ($M = 0.4$, $SD = 0.9$), but clinical controls did not differ by sex (Ms: 0.9 vs. 0.6, SDs = 1.1 and 0.8).

TABLE 10.8. Categories of Crime Ever Committed by Each Group in the UMASS Study

Measure	ADHD		Clinical		Community		χ^2	p	Pairwise contrasts
	N	%	N	%	N	%			
Shoplifted[S]	77	53	34	37	33	31	14.5	.001	1 > 2,3
Stole money without confronting	25	17	6	6	6	6	11.4	.003	1 > 2,3
Robbed someone of money	2	1	1	1	1	1	0.1	NS	
Breaking and entering	12	8	1	1	3	3	8.0	.019	1 > 2,3
Assaulted with fists[S]	51	35	11	12	16	15	23.4	< .001	1 > 2,3
Assaulted with a weapon	11	8	5	5	2	2	4.2	NS	
Set fires intentionally[S]	5	3	0	0	1	1	4.6	NS	
Carried a weapon illegally[S]	18	12	2	2	0	0	20.6	< .001	1 > 2,3
Forced sexual activity	4	3	0	0	0	0	5.6	NS	
Sold drugs illegally[S]	31	21	12	13	7	6	11.5	.003	1 > 3
Arrested[S]	60	42	18	19	17	15	25.1	< .001	1 > 2,3
Jailed[S]	39	27	8	9	9	8	21.4	< .001	1 > 2,3

Note. Sample sizes for these comparisons are ADHD = 144, Clinical control = 92, and Community control = 108. N = sample size endorsing this item; % = percent of group endorsing this item; χ^2 = results of the omnibus chi-square test; p = probability value for the chi-square test; pairwise contrasts = results of the chi-square tests involving pairwise comparisons of the three groups; [S] = significant effect of sex on this measure (males more likely than females on all measures).

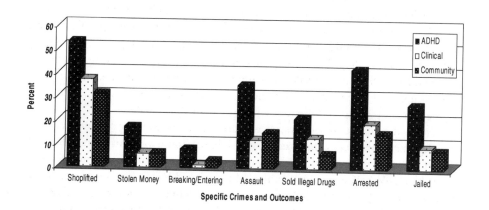

FIGURE 10.2. Percent of each group that engaged in various criminal activities in the UMASS Study.

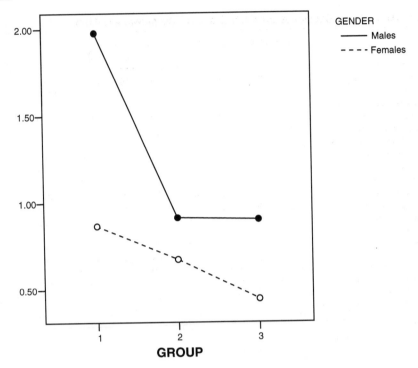

FIGURE 10.3. Graphical illustration of the diversity of crimes committed by each sex within each group from the UMASS Study.

The Milwaukee Study Results

We collected this same information at the age-27 follow-up of our Milwaukee sample. The proportions of each group that had ever committed each form of criminal activity are shown in Table 10.9. As is evident here, both hyperactive groups were more likely to have committed acts of breaking and entering, assaulting others with their fists, and carrying illegal weapons and both had been arrested and jailed more often than the Community control group. These findings are illustrated in Figure 10.4 and can be contrasted with Figure 10.2 from the UMASS Study. Clearly, children with ADHD as they grow up are at significant risk for these forms of criminal activity and their legal consequences, whether or not their ADHD has persisted to age 27. However, in other instances, the H+ADHD group was the only one to differ from the other two groups. This occurred for stealing property, assaulting others with a weapon, selling drugs, or engaging in disorderly conduct. Thus, ADHD that persists until age 27 seems to convey additional risks for these forms of antisocial behavior. The most common forms of criminal activity associated with those

TABLE 10.9. Crime Categories for Each Group in the Milwaukee Study

Measures	H+ADHD N	H+ADHD %	H−ADHD N	H−ADHD %	Community N	Community %	χ^2	p	Pairwise contrasts
Stole other's property	41	74	46	58	34	45	11.11	.004	1 > 2,3
Stole others' money	26	47	33	42	21	28	5.65	NS	
Robbed someone of money	4	7	2	2	1	1	3.72	NS	
Breaking and entering	8	14	12	15	2	3	7.69	.021	1,2 > 3
Assaulted with fists	23	42	26	33	12	16	11.09	.004	1,2 > 3
Assaulted with a weapon	16	29	5	6	2	3	25.46	< .001	1 > 2,3
Set fires intentionally	6	11	7	9	4	5	1.41	NS	
Carried a weapon illegally	22	40	16	20	6	8	19.60	< .001	1 > 2 > 3
Forced sexual activity	1	2	0	0	0	0	2.81	NS	
Possessed illegal drugs	37	67	48	61	36	48	5.26	NS	
Sold drugs illegally	22	40	21	27	14	19	7.31	.026	1 > 3
Engaged in disorderly conduct	26	47	27	34	18	24	7.66	.022	1 > 3
Arrested	40	73	41	52	25	33	19.77	< .001	1 > 2 > 3
Jailed	32	58	36	46	18	24	16.33	< .001	1,2 > 3

Note. Sample sizes for these comparisons are H+ADHD = 55, H−ADHD = 79, and Community control = 75. N = sample size endorsing this item; % = percent of group endorsing this item; χ^2 = results of the omnibus chi-square test; p = probability value for the chi-square test; pairwise contrasts = results of the chi-square tests involving pairwise comparisons of the three groups; H+ADHD = hyperactive group that currently has a diagnosis of ADHD at follow-up; H−ADHD = hyperactive group that does not have a diagnosis of ADHD at follow-up.
Statistical analysis: Pearson chi-square.

who were hyperactive as children and whose ADHD persisted into adulthood were stealing property (74%), followed by illegal drug possession (67%), assaulting others with fists (42%), engaging in disorderly conduct (47%), selling drugs (40%), and carrying illegal weapons (40%). Nearly three-fourths of the H+ADHD group had been arrested and more than half had served some time in jail. The figures were only somewhat lower for the H−ADHD group (52% and 46% respectively). The proportions of these groups engaging in these offenses is substantially greater than was seen in the UMASS adult ADHD group, often being at least double the percentages of the latter study. The only exception was for assaulting others with fists where, both of these ADHD groups were nearly equivalent. Percentages for being arrested and jailed in the Milwaukee Study H+ADHD group were twice the levels seen in the UMASS ADHD group. Our impression is that children with ADHD as they grow up are at considerably greater risks for various antisocial activities than are self-referred adults seen in clinics at adulthood. Both ADHD groups are certainly more antisocial than control groups in many instances, but childhood ADHD conveys more risk in this respect, especially if it persists to age 27. A recent 30-year study by Satterfield and colleagues using official arrest records also found this to be the case, but that it was childhood conduct problems that conveyed this risk more than ADHD (Satterfield et al., 2007).

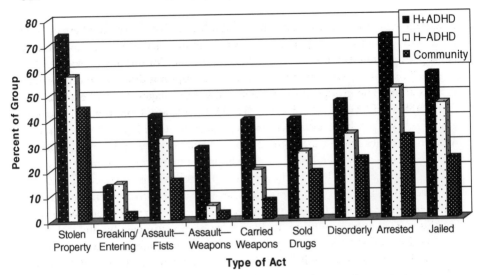

FIGURE 10.4. Percent of each group in the Milwaukee Study that ever engaged in various forms of antisocial activity (lifetime). Categories reflect those in which one or typically both hyperactive groups differed from the Community control group. H+ADHD = hyperactive group that had a diagnosis of ADHD at follow-up. H–ADHD = hyperactive group that did not have a diagnosis of ADHD at follow-up.

Once more, we created the same crime diversity score as we had done above for the UMASS Study adults. Because IQ correlated significantly with this measure ($rs = -.29$ for verbal and $-.17$ for spatial), we covaried it in our analysis of group differences. The H+ADHD group ($M = 4.25$, $SD = 2.83$) had committed significantly more crime types than either the H–ADHD ($M = 3.07$, $SD = 2.47$), or the Community control group ($M = 2.03$, $SD = 2.33$; $F = 18.17$, $df = 2/203$, $p = .041$), who did not differ from each other. This finding replicates that for the UMASS ADHD adult group and suggests that persistent ADHD into adulthood is associated with a significantly increased diversity of antisocial activity. We also found, not surprisingly, that males across all groups in the study ($M = 3.11$, $SD = 2.57$) had committed a greater diversity of crimes than females ($M = 2.09$, $SD = 2.33$; $F = 33.67$, $df = 1/203$, $p = .015$), although sex did not interact with group in this analysis. This finding also replicates that found in the UMASS Study, where sex differences could be tested more powerfully than in the Milwaukee Study.

Victimization

We asked several additional questions in the Milwaukee project only concerning whether or not the participants had experienced physical or sexual abuse, although we imposed no standard definition on those terms, leaving it to the participant's judgment what they considered abusive. We found that more members of both hyperactive groups had experienced physical abuse relative to the Community control group (H+ADHD = 30%, H–ADHD = 25%, Community control = 11%, χ^2 = 8.09, p = .017) with the two hyperactive groups not differing in this form of victimization. The groups did not differ in the percentages that had experienced sexual abuse (H+ADHD = 15%, H–ADHD = 13%, and Community control = 4%; χ^2 = 5.08, p = NS), although the percentages for the H groups were three to four times higher than in the control group. As noted previously, our samples of females in each group were small, severely limiting our power to examine the effect of sex on our measures. But we thought it important to examine sex differences in this case, given previous reports that females with ADHD may be more likely to experience sexual abuse. Comparing males versus females in the hyperactive group, females were significantly more likely to have been victimized by physical abuse (47% vs. 24%) (χ^2 = 4.63, p = .031). For sexual abuse, the differences were 21% versus 12%, but this was not significant. We found no evidence that the ADHD subsets of the hyperactive group differed on these measures either within males or within the females, so current ADHD had nothing to do with interacting with gender to produce the above group differences.

CD Symptoms in Childhood

We also collected the self-reports of the adults in each project with regard to the percentage endorsing each of the symptoms of CD (DSM-IV; American Psychiatric Association, 20000) recalled from their childhood and adolescent years between 5 and 18 years of age.

The UMASS Study Results

The results for the UMASS Study self-reports are shown in Table 10.10. Those on which the ADHD group differed significantly from both the Clinical and Community control groups are shown in Figure 10.5 as well. As the table shows, more adults with ADHD had engaged in many of the antisocial activities represented here than was the case for either of the control groups. Specifically, adults with ADHD were more likely to have bullied others, initiated fights, used a weapon against someone, been physically cruel to others or cruel to animals, destroyed others property, engaged in breaking and entering, often lied to avoid obligations, stolen nontrivial items, often stayed out past parental curfews, ran away from home, and been truant from school than adults in the Community control group. In 8 of these 12 activities, the adults with ADHD also were more likely to do them than adults in the Clinical control group. Worth noting here, however, is that only a minority of adults in any group, including the ADHD group, had ever engaged in these antiso-

TABLE 10.10. Percentage of Each Group Showing Each Conduct Disorder Symptom (DSM-IV) in Childhood (Self-Reports) in the UMASS Study

Measure	ADHD		Clinical		Community		χ^2	p	Pairwise contrasts
	N	%	N	%	N	%			
Often bullied others[S]	40	28	13	14	7	7	20.6	< .001	1 > 2,3
Often initiated physical fights[S]	31	22	5	5	4	4	24.1	< .001	1 > 2,3
Used weapon to harm others	13	9	4	4	2	2	6.5	.039	1 > 3
Physically cruel to people[S]	24	17	9	10	3	3	12.8	.002	1,2 > 3
Physically cruel to animals[S]	18	13	7	7	2	2	9.7	.008	1 > 3
Stolen while confronting victim	5	3	2	2	1	1	1.8	NS	
Forced sexual activity	1	1	0	0	1	1	0.8	NS	
Deliberately set fires[S]	7	5	5	5	2	2	1.9	NS	
Destroyed others' property[S]	32	23	13	14	6	6	13.9	.001	1,2 > 3
Breaking and entering[S]	23	16	7	7	6	6	8.5	.014	1 >2 ,3
Often lied to obtain favors or avoid obligations (conning)[S]	49	35	23	25	2	2	39.0	< .001	1,2 > 3
Stole nontrivial items	61	43	27	29	21	20	15.8	< .001	12,3
Often stayed out late past parental curfew[S]	56	39	21	23	12	11	25.6	< .001	1 > 2 > 3
Ran away from home	23	16	4	4	4	4	15.1	.001	1 > 2,3
Often truant from school	45	32	16	17	12	11	16.1	< .001	1 > 2,3
CD diagnosis[S]	34	25	14	16	7	7	14.1	.001	1,2 > 3

Note. Sample sizes for these comparisons are ADHD = 142, Clinical control = 93, and Community control = 106. N = sample size endorsing this item; % = percent of group endorsing this item; χ^2 = results of the omnibus chi-square test; p = probability value for the chi-square test; pairwise contrasts = results of the chi-square tests involving pairwise comparisons of the three groups; [S] = significant effect of sex on this measure (males more likely than females on all measures).
    Statistical analysis: Pearson chi-square.

cial activities. The most common activities committed by at least one-third of the ADHD group were stealing nontrivial items (43%), staying out past curfew (39%), often lying to avoid obligations (35%), and being truant from school (32%). Note that all are nonviolent offenses. These were proportionately the most common activities committed by adults in the other two groups as well. More of the ADHD group members qualified for a diagnosis of CD (3+ symptoms out of 15) based on these reports than did the Community control group. But the ADHD group did not differ significantly from the Clinical control group in this respect, although the difference was marginally significant ($p < .10$). Where sex differences were evident, males, of course, were more likely to have engaged in these activities than females regardless of group.

Based on these reports, we created a total CD symptom score that was a simple sum of all CD items endorsed by the adult. In a sense, it is comparable to the criminal diversity score we created above. To do so, we ensured that the item met the DSM decision rule to be counted as a symptom: staying out past curfew (before age 13), running away (2+ times), and truancy (before age 13).

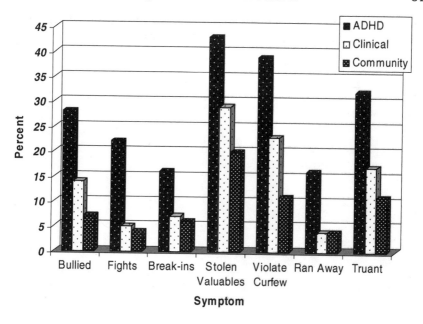

FIGURE 10.5. Percent of each group reporting various symptoms of CD occurring in childhood in the UMASS Study. Symptoms depicted are those on which the ADHD group differed significantly from the Clinical control and Community control group.

The groups differed significantly on this measure, with the ADHD group having a higher score (more CD symptoms) than either of the two control groups. The mean scores for each group were ADHD: $M = 1.7$, $SD = 2.5$; Clinical control: $M = 1.1$, $SD = 1.8$; and Community control: $M = 0.5$, $SD = 1.6$, $F = 6.2$, $df = 2/325$, $p = .002$. Pairwise contrasts showed ADHD > Clinical > Community. Not surprisingly, a significant main effect for sex was also found: $F = 9.61$, $df = 1/325$, $p = .002$—in which males had higher mean scores ($M = 1.5$, $SD = 2.3$) than females ($M = 0.6$, $M = 1.5$) regardless of group.

We also examined the reports of others who knew our participants well (typically parents) who completed this same scale. Their results are shown in Table 10.11. The group differences are neither as numerous nor as sizable as those based on the self-reports. This would be expected, given that much antisocial activity occurs outside of the supervision of parents. Here we found that the adults with ADHD were more likely to have destroyed property, lied to obtain favors, stolen nontrivial items, stayed out past curfew, and run away from home relative to the Community control group. Such results are consistent with the findings from self-reported behavior discussed above, even though the group differences are of a lower magnitude. In all of these respects, however, the ADHD group did not differ from the Clinical control group.

TABLE 10.11. Percentage of Each Group Showing Each Conduct Disorder Symptom (DSM-IV) in Childhood as Reported By Others in the UMASS Study

Measure	ADHD N	ADHD %	Clinical N	Clinical %	Community N	Community %	χ^2	p	Pairwise contrasts
Bullied others	16	17	4	9	5	7	4.1	NS	
Initiated physical fights	11	12	3	7	3	4	3.0	NS	
Used weapon to harm others	5	5	1	2	0	0	4.1	NS	
Physically cruel to people	5	5	1	2	1	1	2.0	NS	
Physically cruel to animals	1	1	0	0	0	0	1.2	NS	
Stolen while confronting victim	1	1	0	0	0	0	1.2	NS	
Forced sexual activity	1	1	0	0	0	0	1.2	NS	
Deliberately set fires	2	2	0	0	0	0	2.4	NS	
Destroyed others' property	9	10	1	2	1	1	6.3	.043	1 > 3
Breaking and entering	6	6	0	0	1	1	4.9	NS	
Lied to obtain favors or avoid obligations (conning others)^S	25	27	6	14	2	3	16.6	< .001	1,2 > 3
Stole nontrivial items	15	16	4	9	0	0	12.1	.002	1,2 > 3
Stayed out late past parental curfew	22	24	5	11	7	10	6.0	.049	1 > 3
Ran away from home	11	12	0	0	2	3	8.7	.013	1 > 2,3
Truant from school	15	16	4	9	5	7	3.1	NS	

Note. Sample sizes for these comparisons are ADHD = 92, Clinical control = 44, and Community control = 67. N = sample size endorsing this item; % = percent of group endorsing this item; χ^2 = results of the omnibus chi-square test; p = probability value for the chi-square test; pairwise contrasts = results of the chi-square tests involving pairwise comparisons of the three groups; ^{S} = significant effect of sex on this measure (males more likely than females on all measures).
Statistical analysis: Pearson chi-square.

To summarize, by their own reports, more adults with ADHD were likely to have committed various antisocial acts than were adults in the control groups; they also committed a more diverse array of such activities. The most common antisocial acts were largely of a nonviolent nature (shoplifting, stealing, lying, violating parental curfews, being truant, etc.), but a small subset of adults with ADHD committed some violent actions and more of them did so than control adults. The same was true with regard to self-reported CD symptoms from their childhood years. Not unexpectedly, the reports of parents about these adults did not reveal as many group differences but still showed the ADHD adults to differ from the Community control adults in these nonviolent activities. They did not, however, differ from the Clinical control group in these respects when we were using the reports of others.

The Milwaukee Study Results

We had the same information available from the same surveys used in the UMASS Study in the Milwaukee Study follow-up. The results for self-reported symptoms of CD retrospectively recalled from ages 5 to 18 years are shown in

Table 10.12. In general, where group differences are apparent, more members of both hyperactive groups had committed various antisocial acts than had the community control group, and they often did not differ from each other in those percentages. This is visually depicted in Figure 10.6. Both hyperactive groups had bullied others, initiated physical fights, lied (conned) to obtain favors, stayed out past curfew, ran away from home, and had been truant than had the Community group. The H+ADHD group differed from the H–ADHD group in only three types of activities, those being using a weapon to harm another, having lied to obtain favors, and stealing nontrivial items. Thus, ADHD in childhood and adolescence contributes to a significantly elevated risk for various types of antisocial activity regardless of whether such ADHD persists into adulthood. As a result, more members of both hyperactive groups qualified for a diagnosis of CD (having 3+ symptoms) retrospectively than did members of the control group.

The reports of others who knew the participants well are displayed in Table 10.13. On average, the percentages of each group reported to have had each of these various CD symptoms is somewhat lower than that found in self-reports, as we had seen in the UMASS Study. But they were not drastically lower, implying

TABLE 10.12. CD Symptoms (DSM-IV) Self-Reported in Childhood for Each Group in the Milwaukee Study

Measures	H+ADHD		H–ADHD		Community		χ^2	p	Pairwise contrasts
	N	%	N	%	N	%			
Often bullied others	17	31	22	27	7	9	10.98	.004	1,2 > 3
Often initiated physical fights	12	22	19	24	7	9	6.02	.049	1,2 > 3
Used weapon to harm others	15	28	9	11	4	5	13.96	.001	1 >2,3
Physically cruel to people	12	22	17	21	8	11	3.84	NS	
Physically cruel to animals	12	22	8	11	7	9	4.91	NS	
Stolen while confronting victim	4	7	3	4	0	0	5.33	NS	
Forced sexual activity	2	4	1	1	0	0	3.05	NS	
Deliberately set fires	4	7	8	10	2	3	3.31	NS	
Destroyed others' property	18	33	16	20	20	27	3.05	NS	
Breaking and entering	16	30	19	24	10	13	5.13	NS	
Often lied to obtain favors or avoid obligations (conning)	29	54	24	30	11	15	22.14	< .001	1 > 2 > 3
Stole nontrivial items	36	67	38	47	25	34	13.53	.001	1 > 2,3
Often stayed out late past parental curfew	31	57	42	52	18	24	17.93	< .001	1,2 > 3
Ran away from home	17	31	17	21	7	9	9.76	.008	1,2 > 3
Often truant from school	24	44	35	44	12	16	16.41	< .001	1,2 > 3
CD diagnosis (3+ symptoms)	33	61	41	51	22	30	13.72	.001	1,2 > 3

Note. Sample sizes for these comparisons are H+ADHD = 54, H–ADHD = 80, and Community control = 74. N = sample size endorsing this item; % = percent of group endorsing this item; χ^2 = results of the omnibus chi-square test; p = probability value for the chi-square test; pairwise contrasts = results of the chi-square tests involving pairwise comparisons of the three groups; H+ADHD = hyperactive group that had a diagnosis of ADHD at follow-up; H–ADHD = hyperactive group that did not have a diagnosis of ADHD at follow-up.
Statistical analysis: Pearson chi-square.

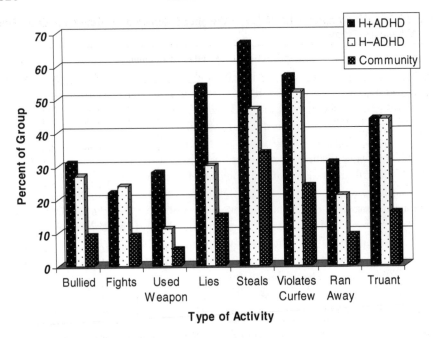

FIGURE 10.6. Percent of each group reporting various symptoms of CD occurring in childhood in the Milwaukee Study. Symptoms depicted are those on which the hyperactive groups differed significantly from the Community control group. H+ADHD = hyperactive group that had a diagnosis of ADHD at follow-up. H–ADHD = hyperactive group that did not have a diagnosis of ADHD at follow-up.

reasonable agreement between these sources in this domain of human behavior. The correlation of self-reported CD symptoms with other reported CD symptoms for childhood was .63 (p .001). The degree of agreement on who met the CD diagnostic criteria was 78% of those who were reported by others as having CD and who also had it by self-report (kappa = .500, $p < .001$), and 64% of those who self-reported met CD diagnostic criteria according to others. Group differences existed in 11 of the 15 antisocial activities; in nearly all but one of these, the hyperactive groups did not differ from each other, yet both differed from the Community control group. Only in physical cruelty to people did we find the H+ADHD group alone differing from the Community control group, yet even here the H–ADHD group did not differ from either, falling between these other two groups. The pattern essentially replicates that of self-reported information in showing that it is growing up as a child with ADHD that is the risk for these activities and not whether that ADHD has persisted to age 27. Once again, we found that more members of both hyperactive groups would have qualified for a retrospective diagnosis of CD by others' reports than the control group (47–55% vs. 15%).

TABLE 10.13. CD Symptoms (DSM-IV) in Childhood Reported by Others for Each Group in the Milwaukee Study

Measures	H+ADHD N	H+ADHD %	H–ADHD N	H–ADHD %	Community N	Community %	χ^2	p	Pairwise contrasts
Often bullied others	19	35	20	26	8	11	11.41	.003	1,2 > 3
Often initiated physical fights	16	30	18	23	7	9	9.04	.011	1,2 > 3
Used weapon to harm others	13	24	9	12	2	3	13.98	.001	1,2 > 3
Physically cruel to people	12	22	12	16	5	7	6.51	.039	1 > 3
Physically cruel to animals	5	9	8	10	4	5	1.38	NS	
Stolen while confronting victim	3	6	0	0	0	0	8.57	.014	Not viable
Forced sexual activity	3	6	3	4	1	1	1.80	NS	
Deliberately set fires	3	6	7	9	1	1	4.53	NS	
Destroyed others' property	17	31	20	26	6	8	12.42	.002	1,2 > 3
Breaking and entering	11	20	16	21	5	7	7.07	.029	1,2 > 3
Often lied to obtain favors or avoid obligations (conning)	26	48	31	40	4	5	34.30	< .001	1,2 > 3
Stole nontrivial items	24	45	23	30	10	13	16.07	< .001	1,2 > 3
Often stayed out late past parental curfew	26	48	33	43	17	23	10.63	.005	1,2 > 3
Ran away from home	11	20	15	19	4	5	8.09	.017	1,2 > 3
Often truant from school	25	46	31	41	9	12	21.65	< .001	1,2 > 3
CD diagnosis (3+ symptoms)	29	55	35	47	11	15	26.21	< .001	1,2 > 3

Note. Sample sizes for these comparisons are H+ADHD = 54, H–ADHD = 77, and Community control = 75. N = sample size endorsing this item; % = percent of group endorsing this item; χ^2 = results of the omnibus chi-square test; p = probability value for the chi-square test; pairwise contrasts = results of the chi-square tests involving pairwise comparisons of the three groups; H+ADHD = hyperactive group that had a diagnosis of ADHD at follow-up; H–ADHD = hyperactive group that did not have a diagnosis of ADHD at follow-up.
Statistical analysis: Pearson chi-square.

When we contrast these findings with those from the UMASS Study (see Tables 10.10 and 10.11), it is evident that children diagnosed as having ADHD carry a considerably higher risk of committing these various antisocial acts than do adults who are self-referred to clinics and then diagnosed, whether using self- or other-reported information. Both ADHD groups in these two projects are more likely to be antisocial than Community control groups, but the risk is greater in the clinically-referred children diagnosed with ADHD (hyperactivity) growing up, whether or not their ADHD is persistent to age 27. This was evident in 10 of the 15 CD symptoms. Only the symptoms of bullying others, initiating physical fights, stealing while confronting a victim, forced sexual activity, and fire setting seem not to differ across these studies for these ADHD groups. In the latter three instances, this is likely because less than 10% of the ADHD groups had ever committed these offenses. In short, having ADHD is a risk factor for antisocial activities and for being arrested and jailed for them, whether ADHD was diagnosed in childhood or adulthood. But being clinically referred and diagnosed as having ADHD in childhood carries an even greater risk for later antisocial activities and its legal consequences than does being self-referred and diagnosed in adulthood. By and large, these results are very consistent with the previous literature, which has found a significant association between ADHD and antisocial activities, whether in children with ADHD followed to adulthood or in clinic-referred adults diagnosed with ADHD.

Predicting Significant Antisocial Outcomes

We found that certain antisocial outcomes were specifically more likely to apply to adults with ADHD in the UMASS Study than to the other two control groups. Among these, we chose as the most important and most general representation of those outcomes to be the diversity of criminal activity (number of different crime types) and the number of arrests. We used multiple linear regression analyses to examine a set of possible predictors of these outcomes, the results of which appear in Table 10.14. As that table indicates, the number of types of criminal activity in which our participants had engaged during their lifetimes was predicted by higher current ADHD symptoms, younger age, the severity of their

TABLE 10.14. Predicting Antisocial Outcomes in the UMASS Study

Outcome/predictors (step entered)	Beta	R	R^2	$R^2\Delta$	F	p
No. of crime types (lifetime)						
(1) No. of ADHD symptoms	.301	.332	.110	.110	21.67	< .001
& Age	−.122					
(2) No. of CD Symptoms (childhood)	.416	.552	.305	.195	97.89	< .001
(3) Sex (female)	−.167	.576	.332	.027	14.05	< .001
(4) Education (years)	−.123	.588	.345	.013	7.08	.008
NS: IQ (Shipley), depression, anxiety, hostility (SCL-90-R)						
No. of arrests						
(1) No. of ADHD symptoms*	.239	.241	.058	.058	10.83	< .001
and age (NS)	−.017					
(2) No. of CD symptoms (childhood)	.288	.493	.243	.185	85.03	< .001
(3) No. of crime types (lifetime)	.211	.541	.292	.050	24.41	< .001
(4) Education	−.134	.565	.319	.026	13.43	< .001
(5) IQ	−.134	.576	.332	.013	6.82	.009
(6) Sex (female)	−.112	.586	.343	.011	6.00	.015
NS: depression, anxiety, hostility						

Note. R = regression coefficient; R^2 = percent of explained variance accounted for by all variables at this step; $R^2\Delta$ = percent of explained variance accounted for by this variable added at this step; F = results of F-test for the equation at this step; p = probability value for the F-test; * = this variable became nonsignificant when other variables were entered in the next step; beta = standardized beta coefficient; NS = not significant; Shipley = Shipley Institute of Living Scale IQ estimate, SCL-90-R = Symptom Checklist–90—Revised T-score.

    Statistical analysis: Multiple linear regression using forced entry method at Step 1 and stepwise conditional method at subsequent steps. Used the entire sample (N = 353).

retrospectively reported childhood CD symptoms, being male, and having less education. The frequency of arrests was best predicted by severity of current ADHD symptoms, severity of retrospectively reported childhood CD symptoms, lower level of education, the diversity of crimes in which they had previously engaged (number of crime types), lower IQ, and being male. That the diversity of one's committed crimes would predict arrest frequency is not surprising. In both of these outcomes, the number of retrospectively recalled childhood CD symptoms explained (predicted) the greatest percentage of variance in severity of the outcome. Such a finding is quite consistent with research on childhood CD—it is a major determinant of risk for later criminality and arrests (Loeber et al., 2000).

The Milwaukee Study provides a far better test of what predictors may be associated with the severity of later crime and arrests. That is because it does not rely on information reported retrospectively from childhood. The study actually collected measures not only in childhood but at adolescence and age 21. Thus the predictors it studies can be considered true predictors of future risk rather than current correlates or retrospective estimates of earlier behavior. We examined a set of 17 predictors of the same two measures of crime diversity and arrest frequency analyzed above in the UMASS Study. Many of those predictors are comparable to the ones used in the UMASS Study analyses. We did not use the SCL-90-R measures of anxiety, depression, or hostility this time as they were of no value in the UMASS analyses. Specifically, from childhood, we used the CPRS-R Hyperactivity Index Score, WWPARS hyperactivity score, HSQ number of problem settings, CPRS-R conduct problems score, and the child's IQ at study entry. At adolescence, we selected parent reports of teen ADHD, ODD, and CD symptoms along with teen-reported stressful life events and number of antisocial symptoms (out of 30 possible) for the teen's father as reported by the mother. At age 21, we again selected the number of ADHD, ODD, and CD symptoms that were self-reported; ADHD symptoms reported by parents; years of education by this follow-up; and IQ. The results for the analyses of the Milwaukee Study information are shown in Table 10.15. We included the father's level of antisocial conduct as a predictor because past research has found this to be a significant predictor of children's later antisocial activities (Loeber et al., 2000) and because it was significantly elevated in both our hyperactive groups (H+ADHD = 4.4, SD = 5.8; H–ADHD = 4.3, SD = 5.4; Community control = 0.9, SD = 2.7; F = 9.95, df = 2/145, p < .001).

For crime diversity, we found that five predictors were able to account for an impressive 48% of the variance in lifetime criminal diversity scores. These were pervasiveness of childhood ADHD and behavior problems (HSQ), the number of teen CD symptoms, the number of illegal drugs the teen had reported trying by teen follow-up, the number of CD symptoms reported at age 21, and years of education obtained by age 21. That the number of CD symptoms evi-

TABLE 10.15. Predicting Antisocial Outcomes in the Milwaukee Study

Outcome/predictors (step entered)	Beta	R	R²	R²Δ	F	p
No. of crime types (lifetime)						
Child HSQ no. of settings (parent)	.016	.281	.079	.079	20.10	< .001
Teen no. of CD symptoms (parent)	.091	.421	.177	.098	27.74	< .001
Teen no. of different drugs ever tried (self)	.127	.457	.209	.032	9.37	.002
Age-21 no. of CD symptoms (self)	.491	.677	.459	.250	106.65	< .001
Age-21 years of education (self)	−.193	.695	.482	.024	10.49	.001

NS: Child CPRS-R Hyperactivity Index or conduct problems scores (parent), WWPARS (parent), child IQ (PPVT); teen no. of ADHD and no. of ODD symptoms (parent) and stressful life events (self); age-21 no. of ADHD symptoms (self and parent); no. of ODD symptoms (self).

Outcome/predictors (step entered)	Beta	R	R²	R²Δ	F	p
No. of arrests						
Child WWPARS hyperactivity (parent)	.013	.235	.055	.055	13.63	< .001
Child CPRS-R conduct problems (parent)	.011	.266	.071	.016	3.89	.050
Teen no. of different drugs ever tried (self)	.112	.336	.113	.042	11.08	.001
Teen no. of CD symptoms (parent)	.003	.365	.133	.021	5.48	.020
Age-21 no. of CD symptoms (self)	.512	.610	.372	.238	87.31	< .001
Age-21 years of education (self)	−.194	.629	.396	.024	9.12	.003
Age-21 no. of ODD symptoms (self)	−.108	.637	.406	.010	3.89	.050

NS: Child HSQ no. of settings (parent, CPRS-R Hyperactivity Index (parent), child IQ (PPVT); teen no. of ADHD and no. of ODD symptoms (parent) and stressful life events (self); age-21 no. of ADHD symptoms (self and parent).

Note. R = regression coefficient; R² = percent of explained variance accounted for by all variables at this step; R²Δ = percent of explained variance accounted for by this variable added at this step; F = results of F-test for the equation at this step; p = probability value for the F-test; beta = standardized beta coefficient; NS = not significant; HSQ = Home Situations Questionnaire number of problem settings; CD = conduct disorder (DSM-III-R); CPRS-R = Conners Parent Rating Scale—Revised; WWPARS = Werry–Weiss–Peters Activity Rating Scale; PPVT = Peabody Picture Vocabulary Test; ADHD = attention-deficit/hyperactivity disorder (DSM-III-R); ODD = oppositional defiant disorder (DSM-III-R).

Statistical analysis: Multiple linear regression using three entry blocks for child, teen, and young adult measures and stepwise entry method at each block. Means substituted for any missing data. Used the entire sample (N = 235).

dent at earlier follow-up points would predict lifetime crime diversity at age 27 is not surprising, given the substantial literature showing that earlier and ongoing antisocial activities predict the risk for later such activities. The finding that diversity of teen drug use (number of different drugs tried) would also predict later antisocial behavior beyond that provided by earlier antisocial behavior is consistent with earlier findings (noted above) that teen drug use interacts with teen antisocial behavior to produce an interactive spiraling effect over time, in that each activity (drug use and crime) increases the risk for the other activity. That years of education is significantly associated with lifetime criminal diversity is also hardly surprising, but—as noted in the last chapter concerning predictors of high school graduation—it is not clear that crime is predicting less education; rather, those who get less education may be subsequently more likely to engage in criminal activities. Our sense is that this is much like teen drug use, in that these factors are interactive or produce a spiraling effect over time. We base this on the fact that earlier levels of antisocial activity in childhood and adolescence were already statistically controlled in these equations by the time years of education entered as a significant predictor. This would indicate that low education is making an independent contribution to crime diversity beyond that accounted for by earlier crime diversity. Unlike the findings of other studies, low IQ did not make significant prediction of this outcome once education had entered the equation, perhaps suggesting that earlier findings of its association with antisocial behavior may be partly or even largely due to its association with low education. Our significant predictors are rather similar to those seen in the UMASS Study for this outcome of crime diversity, but the Milwaukee results give us greater confidence that they are true predictors and not just correlates.

There were seven significant predictors for the number of arrests self-reported by age 27; these accounted for 41% of the variance in arrest frequency. Many, not surprisingly, are the same as those predicting criminal diversity above. Several are not and require additional comment. Notice that childhood hyperactivity (WWPARS scores) made an independent contribution to lifetime arrests independently of that contribution made by childhood conduct problems (CPRS-R scores). Others have found the same (Loeber et al., 2000), in that severity of childhood hyperactivity makes some contribution to later antisocial activities and arrest rates. Satterfield et al. (2007), however, found that only childhood conduct problems prdicted these outcomes in their 30-year follow-up of hyperactive children. Also worth noting is the finding, once again, that level of ODD symptoms (this time at age 21) makes a positive or protective contribution to risk of being arrested once severity of CD currently and earlier in development is controlled in these equations. We found the same thing for predicting high school graduation in the last chapter. As we noted then, severity of ODD that is *independent* of severity of CD may not be an adverse characteristic of a teen or young adult but a healthy one. We believe this may show that argumen-

ADHD IN ADULTS

tativeness, stubbornness, and even defiance that is *not* associated with antisocial behavior may not be an adversity during development but a sign of healthy independence from others and authority more generally and a willingness to openly reason, debate, argue, and otherwise challenge parental authority.

Conclusions and Clinical Implications

This chapter has reviewed the evidence for an association of ADHD in adults with drug-use disorders and with various antisocial activities.

✓ The previous literature on children with ADHD followed to adulthood indicated that they carry an elevated risk both for later substance use and abuse as well as for many forms of antisocial activities and their legal consequences (arrests, jail). In both instances, the presence of CD in childhood or adolescence greatly elevates these risks and, in some cases, accounts for them entirely. However, ADHD does convey some elevated risk for nonviolent activities—such as drug use, possession, or sale—and may convey an elevated risk for tobacco and alcohol use even in the absence of CD.

✓ What little research exists on clinic-referred adults with ADHD likewise suggests a greater likelihood of drug use disorders and antisocial personality disorder. But prior studies have not examined rates of drug use or specific forms of antisocial activities in as much detail as has the literature on children with ADHD followed to adulthood. The present UMASS project did so.

✓ We found that more adults with ADHD were likely to have been past or current smokers; to be users of marijuana, cocaine, LSD, or prescription drugs; and to have been treated for previous alcohol and drug-use disorders than was the case in the Community control group. Such results are certainly consistent with the prior literature that ADHD elevates the risk for various drug-use problems.

✓ But the Clinical control group also showed some elevated risks for some drug-use problems, primarily past tobacco use and current marijuana use. The ADHD group differed from the clinical group chiefly in having more members who had tried cocaine and LSD.

✓ We compared those in the ADHD group who qualified for a diagnosis of CD in childhood (based on their retrospective reports of their CD symptoms) to those who did not qualify in the proportion having ever used each type of drug. The groups did not differ in any drug-use category except for cocaine, where those who had CD were twice as likely to have tried cocaine compared to those without CD.

✓ Concerning the frequency of drug use, we found that adults with ADHD were marginally more likely to smoke more cigarettes and to drink more alcohol and use more marijuana than were adults in both of our control groups in the UMASS Study.

✓ We once more compared the ADHD group with CD to those without CD in childhood. While these two groups did not differ in their consumption of cigarettes, cocaine use, or heroin use, those having CD used marijuana and LSD more often than those who did not. The CD group was also marginally more likely to drink more alcoholic beverages per week and to use prescription drugs illegally more often than those adults with ADHD who did not have CD as children.

✓ As in past studies of children with ADHD grown up, we found that the presence of CD appears to account for the significantly higher frequency of some drugs used by the ADHD group relative to the two control groups. Therefore, while the presence of childhood CD may not account for whether an adult with ADHD ever tries a particular substance at least once, we found that it does, in many instances, seem to contribute to the frequency with which he or she may subsequently continue to use that drug.

✓ The findings from the longitudinal Milwaukee Study largely corroborated the UMASS Study in finding a greater risk for being a smoker, using alcohol, getting drunk, or using illegal prescription drugs among both hyperactive (childhood ADHD) groups at age 27. It also found a greater frequency of caffeine use for those groups than for the control group. This study shows, however, that it is largely being referred and diagnosed as ADHD in childhood that is related to risk for later substance use and abuse than whether or not that ADHD is persistent to age 27. The ADHD groups in both projects appear to be more likely to abuse both legal and illegal substances. It seems that the children with ADHD growing up may carry a greater risk for using alcohol and tobacco, while clinic-referred adults with ADHD seem more likely to use marijuana, cocaine, and LSD. As in the UMASS Study, we did find that a high proportion of the hyperactive groups in the Milwaukee Study had tried marijuana and a high frequency of its use if they had. But problematic in the Milwaukee Study was that the Community control group in this case had also tried this and other drugs and used them often (if they had done so at all), resulting in no group differences between the hyperactive and control groups. As we had found at the earlier age-21 follow-up, it is this elevated frequency of certain forms of drug use by our Community control group that resulted in our nonsignificant results and not merely a low frequency of such drug use by the hyperactive groups.

✓ The Milwaukee Study also found no evidence (again) that treatment with stimulants in childhood was associated with increased drug use or abuse in any category of illegal drugs. In fact, some evidence showed that being treated with stimulants as a child reduced the likelihood of using certain drug types, such as speed (amphetamines) or illegally obtained prescription drugs.

✓ As for their antisocial activities, a proportionally higher percentage of adults in the ADHD group in the UMASS Study had committed 7 of the 12 categories of antisocial behavior than had the Clinical and Community control groups. More members of the ADHD group had engaged in shoplifting, stealing without confronting a victim, breaking and entering, assaults with fists, carrying an illegal weapon, being arrested, and being sent to jail. And more adults with ADHD had sold drugs illegally in comparison to the Community control group. The Clinical control group did not differ from either of these two groups on this outcome.

✓ The most common forms of antisocial activity for the adults with ADHD were shoplifting (53%), followed by assaulting someone with their fists (35%), and selling illegal drugs (21%).

✓ The risk for childhood (retrospectively recalled) CD symptoms was also examined using self and other reports and also corroborated this higher risk of antisocial activity in the adults with ADHD in the UMASS Study. While much of this risk for antisocial behavior was mediated by the presence of a childhood history of CD (established retrospectively), even the non-CD subset of those having ADHD still committed more antisocial acts than the control groups. Such results are in keeping with follow-up studies of children with ADHD into adulthood in suggesting that the presence of childhood CD significantly elevates the risk of later antisocial behavior while not accounting for that risk entirely in those with ADHD.

✓ Like the UMASS Study, the Milwaukee Study continued to find markedly higher proportions of the hyperactive group to have committed various antisocial acts than the Community control group. In most cases, this elevated risk was not related to whether or not the ADHD had persisted to age 27. Thus, ADHD in both projects is clearly associated with a greater risk of antisocial activity than in control groups; however when ADHD occurs in children and leads to early clinic referral and diagnosis, it appears to be associated with an even greater risk for later antisocial acts, arrests, and being jailed than is seen in clinic-referred adults with ADHD.

✓ In both projects, lifetime criminal diversity and arrest frequency were likely to be predicted by childhood hyperactivity or ADHD as well as earlier levels of CD symptoms. The Milwaukee Study also found that diversity of teen drug use makes an independent contribution to both of these outcomes. This implies a spiraling effect over time between teen antisocial behavior and teen drug use in which each contributes to the maintenance and increase in the other at later developmental stages. We also found much the same for level of education, such that it makes an independent contribution to crime diversity and arrest frequency beyond that made by earlier severity of antisocial behavior. Such analyses inform us that it is not so much severity of ADHD that is associated with crime and arrest rates, although childhood hyperactivity makes a small contribution to risk (about 7–8%). Additional and greater contributions are made by childhood conduct problems, teen antisocial activity and drug use, and education, whereas persistence of ADHD across development did not contribute to these outcomes.

✓ Clinicians are advised that a significant minority of adults with ADHD seen in clinical settings are likely to have a past history of substance-use disorders and antisocial activities and that both may be ongoing at the time of clinical presentation. Both may require interventions that may be independent of those being implemented for the management of ADHD (Kalbag & Levin, 2005). In most cases, we recommend treating the ADHD first in order to determine the extent to which it may be contributing to any ongoing drug use or antisocial activities prior to engaging in rehabilitation efforts, which may be directly aimed at these latter problems. We predicate this recommendation on the fact that medication treatment of ADHD among substance abusers or antisocial individuals is likely to assist with their rehabilitation, whereas leaving their self-regulation deficits untreated may well contribute to risk for relapse or recidivism, respectively.

✓ Where the clinician is untrained or uncomfortable in addressing these drug use and antisocial difficulties, he or she should certainly refer ADHD patients to other professionals expert in these domains of rehabilitation for co-management of their cases.

✓ Clinicians working with adults with ADHD may find themselves embroiled in criminal or other legal proceedings related to the increased risks of these adults for drug-use disorders and antisocial activities. They should be prepared to seek expert legal advice concerning such involvement. There may also be increased issues of personal safety for clinicians in dealing with the antisocial subset of adults with ADHD, warranting the taking of preventive measures in the clinical settings where these adults are to be evaluated and treated.

CHAPTER 11

Health, Lifestyle,
Money Management, and Driving

Apart from the major life activities of education and occupational functioning likely to be affected by ADHD in adults, as shown in Chapter 9, other domains of adaptive functioning also seem likely to be adversely affected by the disorder, such as maintaining personal health, personal lifestyle and routine habits, the management of money and related assets and liabilities, and the operation of motor vehicles. We are aware of no past studies of clinic-referred adults with ADHD that have focused on their health, lifestyle concerns, and money management as domains of major life activities that may be impaired from their disorder. In contrast, research on driving risks associated with ADHD in adults has been much more abundant and is discussed later in this chapter.

Health and Lifestyle

Research has shown that one's lifestyle is a significant contributor to health and longevity. McGinnis and Foege (1993) determined that half of all deaths in the United States were the result of nongenetic factors, such as tobacco use (19%), diet and activity (14%), alcohol (5%), firearms (2%), sexual behavior (1%), driving (1%), and use of illicit drugs (1%). Similarly, Wigle and colleagues (Wigle, Semenciw, McCann, & Davies, 1990) determined that 50% of all premature deaths in Canada were preventable through lifestyle changes in domains similar to those identified above by McGinnis and Foege. Our own research and prior studies reviewed in earlier chapters suggest a higher than normal risk for drug use and abuse among adults with ADHD in conjunction with increased antisocial acts. Those greater lifestyle risks would certainly affect the health status of these

330

adults and may even pose problems for the management of their finances and driving.

But another reason to suspect that adults with ADHD may have problems in their health and lifestyle domains of daily life activities comes from the very nature of their symptoms, particularly the impaired inhibition and self-regulation that is at the very heart of their disorder (Barkley, 1997; Nigg, 2001). The diminished regard for the future consequences of one's behavior that characterizes many adolescents and adults with ADHD would also predict a reduced concern for health-conscious behavior, such as exercise, proper diet, and moderation in using legal substances (caffeine, tobacco, and alcohol) throughout life (Barkley, Fischer, et al., 1990; Milberger et al., 1997). Such symptoms of ADHD can be construed as comprising part of that dimension of personality known as conscientiousness—an aspect of personality that has been linked to health problems and even to life expectancy (Friedman et al., 1995). Recent research has also shown that poor executive functioning is associated with higher body mass index (BMI) (Gunstad et al., 2007), indicating that adults with ADHD may be at greater risk for higher BMI due to their executive deficits. Concern over life expectancy in ADHD is not hypothetical or unfounded. Swensen and colleagues have recently found that adults with ADHD are more than twice as likely to die prematurely from their misadventures than are control cases (Swensen et al., 2004).

The follow-up study by Friedman and colleagues (Friedman, et al., 1995) of Terman's original sample of highly intelligent children demonstrates the link between low childhood conscientiousness (high impulsivity) and shortened life expectancy. Most of those participants are now in their 80s or older, and more than half of them were deceased at the time of follow-up (pre-1995). The follow-up study indicated that the most significant childhood personality characteristic predictive of reduced life expectancy by all causes was related to the impulsive, undercontrolled personality characteristics known as low conscientiousness. Individuals classified as falling into the lowest quartile on this set of characteristics lived an average of 8 years less than those who did not (73 vs. 81 years). Deaths among the study participants were most often due to cardiovascular disease or cancer, the two most common killers in the United States today. Friedman et al. (1995) provided data to show that low childhood impulse control or conscientiousness is linked to these killing agents via their impact on lifestyle, such as smoking, drinking, exercise, weight, and cholesterol management, among other lifestyle choices. Given that adults defined as having ADHD typically fall well below the threshold in the Friedman study (25th percentile), often in the lowest 5 to 7%, the risk for reduced longevity in those with ADHD would seem to be even greater than that found among Terman's participants. This conclusion would seem to be further supported by the fact that Terman's participants were also intellectually gifted and came from families of above-average or higher

socioeconomic backgrounds. Both of these factors would probably have conveyed a greater advantage toward longer life expectancy than would be the case
for intellectually normal children or adults with ADHD, who tend to come from
middle or lower socioeconomic backgrounds. Thus, there is some reason to suspect that health, lifestyle, and life expectancy may be adversely affected as a function of ADHD.

The UMASS Study Results

The UMASS Study examined health and lifestyle concerns in clinic-referred
adults using questions aimed at these domains in the initial interview dealing with
possible impairments as well as the Skinner Computerized Lifestyle Assessment
(Skinner, 1994) (see sidebar). The latter self-administered computer assessment
covers a variety of domains of one's lifestyle and expresses results in each domain
as being a strength, concern, or risk. The results for this lifestyle assessment
appear in Table 11.1, where we have shown the percentage of each group scoring within the range of either concern or risk in each lifestyle domain. For those
domains on which significant group differences were evident, the results are
graphically depicted in Figure 11.1 as well.

As shown in the table and figure, the groups did not differ in the percentage
scored as having a concern or risk in the lifestyle domains of nutrition, eating
habits, caffeine use, physical activity, or body weight. However, the ADHD
group included a higher percentage of individuals reporting problems in 9 out of
16 areas assessed. These areas were sleep, social relationships, family interactions,
tobacco use, nonmedical drug use, medical/dental care, motor vehicle safety,
work and leisure, and emotional health. The Clinical control group differed from
the Community control group in just three domains, these being sleep, work and
leisure, and emotional health. Again, our most important comparisons concern
the ADHD group and the Clinical control group, as this shows the specificity of
health concerns for ADHD and not just being clinically referred. The ADHD
group had more members with concerns/risks in nonmedical drug use, motor
vehicle safety, and emotional health. Obviously, adults with ADHD are leading
lifestyles that pose greater concerns/risks for more of them across many more
lifestyle domains than is seen in Community adults. But illicit drug use, driving,
and emotional health are areas in which adults with ADHD differ specifically
from other clinic-referred adults who do not have ADHD.

The results concerning the use of tobacco and nonmedical drugs are consistent with our findings reported in Chapter 10, and the results of other studies
that indicate elevated drug use in certain drug categories and a greater risk for
drug use dependence and abuse disorders among adults with ADHD. The findings for risks in the specific domain of motor vehicle safety are quite consistent
with the literature as well as our results, discussed below, in identifying this

Structured Clinical Interview of Impairments

As reported in Chapter 6, we created an interview consisting of questions dealing with various domains of major life activities, including educational history, occupational history, antisocial activities, drug use, driving, money management, and dating and marital history. This interview was administered by a psychological technician holding a master's degree in psychology and trained in the evaluation of clinic-referred adults. The questions dealing with health, money management, and driving are reported in this chapter.

Skinner Computerized Lifestyle Assessment (Skinner, 1994; Multi-Health Systems, Inc., North Tonawanda, NY)

This is a computer-administered self-report software program that questions adults about their behavior in a variety of lifestyle domains and then scores and reports these results as either a strength, a concern (needing some additional effort to change this pattern of behavior), or a risk (requiring immediate attention to change this behavior pattern). The domains evaluated are nutrition, eating habits, caffeine use, physical activity, body weight, sleep, social relationships, family interactions, tobacco use, alcohol use, nonmedical drug use, medical/dental care, motor vehicle safety, sexual activities, work and leisure, and emotional health. These domains are assessed using questions taken from a variety of more specialized instruments developed previously by Skinner and others (see manual). For instance, the questions related to alcohol use include those from the Michigan Alcoholism Screening Test. For this study, we scored whether or not each domain was reported as a concern or risk according to the software printout report for each participant. The entire assessment takes approximately 20 to 30 minutes. Internal consistency (Chronbach's alpha) of the scales is reported to be high—for instance .90 or higher for the alcohol screening items. Test–retest reliability over a 3- to 4-week period was acceptable, ranging from .66 (nutrition) to .99 (weight), with a median of .85. Validity has been evaluated by comparing results against physician interviews regarding seven of the lifestyle domains evaluated here, with agreement over lifestyle concerns being .92 and kappa being .74.

Department of Motor Vehicle (DMV) Records

With permission of our participants, we applied for the official driving record from the current state DMV. From this record, we coded the frequency of license suspensions or revocations, speeding citations, vehicular crashes, and the total number of citations. Official driving records are not necessarily more accurate than self-reports and should not be viewed as a gold standard in driving research. The two sources are certainly correlated significantly but share less than 36% of their variance. For instance, in the prior study of adults with ADHD and driving (Barkley, Murphy, et al., 2002), the correlation between self-reported accidents and those on the DMV record was $r = .41$ ($p < .001$) with self-reports yielding higher accident frequencies than did the DMV record. The same was true for self-reported traffic citations, where the correlation in that study was $r = .39$ ($p < .001$) and self-reports once again gave higher citation frequencies than did DMV records. Arthur and colleagues (Arthur et al., 2001) also found only moderate correlations between self-reported information and DMV records (.48 for crashes and .59 for citations). Previous research also shows that self-reported crash involvement and moving violations are not inferior to official archival records. Numerous limitations plague state DMV record keeping, often resulting in higher frequencies of events being self-reported than are found in archival data, with the higher self-reported events likely reflecting adverse events never reported to or recorded by DMV officials. For instance, in Wisconsin, only crashes resulting in damage greater than $1,000 are recorded on the official driving record. Another reason that self-reports can differ from official DMV records is that we obtained DMV records only from the state in which the subjects currently resided, and their self-reports may include driving infractions from other states in which they had lived in the past. There is also a stronger relationship of self-report information to other predictors known to be related to driving risks (Arthur et al., 2001). Thus, both sources of information need to be included in driving studies, but archival data are not necessarily superior or more accurate than self-reported data in reflecting participant histories of adverse driving outcomes.

TABLE 11.1. Health and Lifestyle Concerns/Risks by Group (Skinner Computerized Lifestyle Assessment) for the UMASS Study

Measure	ADHD N	ADHD %	Clinical N	Clinical %	Community N	Community %	χ^2	p	Pairwise contrasts
Nutrition	64	48	39	45	44	44	0.4	NS	
Eating habits[S]	63	48	40	46	41	41	1.0	NS	
Caffeine use	53	41	37	43	28	29	4.8	NS	
Physical activity	54	41	43	51	41	41	2.4	NS	
Body weight	78	59	46	54	63	64	1.7	NS	
Sleep	62	47	33	38	19	19	19.2	< .001	1,2 > 3
Social relationships	43	33	18	21	14	14	11.1	.004	1 > 3
Family interactions	17	20	7	13	3	4	9.6	.008	1 > 3
Tobacco use[S]	32	24	16	19	11	11	6.6	.037	1 > 3
Alcohol use[S]	45	34	22	26	26	26	2.5	NS	
Nonmedical drug use[S]	38	29	13	15	13	13	10.5	.005	1 > 2,3
Medical/dental care	109	83	62	72	62	63	11.7	.003	1 > 3
Motor vehicle safety[S]	84	64	43	50	41	41	12.1	.002	1 > 2,3
Sexual activities	72	54	42	49	42	42	3.3	NS	
Work and leisure	85	64	57	66	25	25	43.5	< .001	1,2 > 3
Emotional health	57	43	24	28	0	0	55.8	< .001	1 > 2 > 3

Note. N = sample size endorsing this item; % = percent of group endorsing this item; χ^2 = results of the omnibus chi-square test; p = probability value for the chi-square test; pairwise contrasts = results of the chi-square tests involving pairwise comparisons of the three groups; [S] = significant effect of sex on this measure (males more likely than females on all measures).
Statistical analysis: Pearson chi-square.

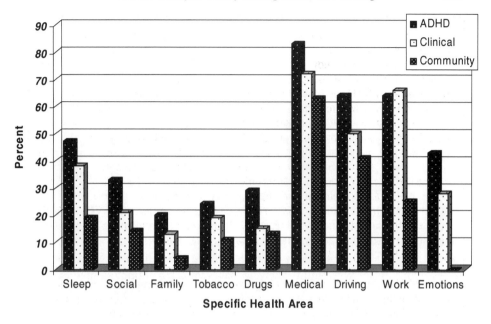

FIGURE 11.1. Percent of each group scoring in the risk or concern range on the Skinner Health and Lifestyle Interview from the UMASS Study. The figure depicts those health and lifestyle areas on which the ADHD group differed from the Community control group.

domain as uniquely elevated among adults with ADHD relative to both of our control groups. The findings for emotional health here are likewise corroborated by our findings in Chapter 8, dealing with increased psychological difficulties and greater emotional problems in the ADHD group compared to our two control groups (i.e., SCL-90-R scores). And the greater risks in the domain of social and family functioning are further corroborated in Chapter 12. All this is to say that the findings of concerns/risks here for adults with ADHD fit consistently into a larger nomological network of other measures of these same or related constructs.

It is possible that medication treatment at the time of study entry may have biased the results of those adults in our two clinical groups (ADHD vs. Clinical controls). We compared those in the ADHD group on medication at the time of study entry to those off medication on all 16 domains. Those on meds were significantly more likely to have lifestyle concerns in the physical domain (61% vs. 34%, $p = .005$), in the tobacco use domain (40% vs. 18%, $p = .007$), and work domains (81% vs. 58%, $p = .012$). For Clinical controls, those on medication did not differ from those off medication in any respects. Even so, just to be prudent we reanalyzed the three Skinner domains on which a difference existed within the ADHD group for those on and off medication. We compared our three groups using just those who were off medication. Results for the physical domain remained nonsignificant, as previously reported. The tobacco domain became nonsignificant, suggesting that it was the medicated ADHD subset that was driving this group difference from community controls. The work and leisure domain remained significant, and the pattern for post hoc comparisons stayed the same despite removing the medication-treated participants. In short, medication status did not influence the results for 15 of the 16 lifestyle domains, but it did affect the domain of tobacco use.

We detected some sex differences in these results. In general, regardless of group, males were more likely than females to have concerns/risks in the domains of eating habits, tobacco and alcohol use, nonmedical drug use, and motor vehicle safety. Within the ADHD group, males were more likely to have motor vehicle safety risks, and work/leisure concerns. In the Clinical control group, females were more likely to have social, sexual, and work concerns than males, while males were more likely to have concerns about nonmedical drug use. In the Community control group, males were more likely to have concerns about nonmedical drug use, medical/dental, and motor vehicle safety. Such a pattern suggests that the group status did not interact with sex to produce, within our groups, qualitatively different patterns of sex differences differing from the overall differences we found between men and women regardless of group.

The Milwaukee Study Results

Health and Lifestyle Domains

A major aim of the Milwaukee Study was to conduct a more in-depth exploration of health and medical status at the age-27 follow-up and of medical histories to that time. While that study also used the Skinner Computerized Lifestyle Assessment, it also collected detailed information on health and medical illnesses and conducted lab work on blood and urine samples. Thus it gives a more complete picture of the health risks that may be associated with ADHD, at least in children growing up with the disorder. The results for the Skinner assessment are shown in Table 11.2, which can be compared directly to Table 11.1 for the UMASS Study. Those domains of health in which either of the hyperactive groups differed from the control group are shown in Figure 11.2, which can also be contrasted with Figure 11.1 for the UMASS Study. As this figure illustrates, a higher percentage of the H+ADHD group had concerns about eating habits, sleep problems, social relations, tobacco use, nonmedical drug use, and emotional health than did the Community group. This H+ADHD group differed specifically from its sister group without ADHD (H−ADHD) in the domains of eating habits, sleep, and emotional health. We can conclude from this that childhood ADHD predisposes to a wider array of health concerns and risks than does

TABLE 11.2. Skinner Health and Lifestyle Concerns by Group for the Milwaukee Study

Measures	H+ADHD		H–ADHD		Community		χ^2	p	Pairwise contrasts
	N	%	N	%	N	%			
Nutrition	37	68	40	52	36	50	4.98	NS	
Eating habits	48	89	54	70	42	58	14.01	.001	1 > 2,3
Caffeine use	17	31	17	23	15	21	2.04	NS	
Physical activity	30	57	35	46	25	35	5.67	NS	
Body weight	40	74	54	71	41	57	4.55	NS	
Sleep	28	52	25	32	10	14	20.90	< .001	1 > 2 > 3
Social relationships	19	35	23	30	12	17	6.10	.047	1 > 3
Family interactions	6	24	3	6	3	6	5.40	NS	
Tobacco use	31	57	42	54	25	35	8.31	.016	1,2 > 3
Alcohol use	32	59	37	49	41	57	1.70	NS	
Nonmedical drug use	24	45	25	32	17	24	6.52	.038	1 > 3
Medical/dental care	48	89	65	85	62	86	0.33	NS	
Motor vehicle safety	41	76	56	73	52	73	0.18	NS	
Sexual activities	35	65	40	52	33	46	4.54	NS	
Work and leisure	27	50	23	30	29	40	5.23	NS	
Emotional health	17	32	7	9	2	3	24.30	< .001	1 > 2,3

Note. N = sample size endorsing this item; % = percent of group endorsing this item; χ^2 = results of the omnibus chi-square test; p = probability value for the chi-square test; pairwise contrasts = results of the chi-square tests involving pairwise comparisons of the three groups.
   Statistical analysis: Pearson chi-square.

ADHD that persists to age 27. Even the hyperactive group that was no longer considered to have ADHD had more concerns in the areas of sleep and tobacco use than did the Community control group.

   Given the substantial research on driving risks associated with ADHD and that it arose as a concern in the UMASS Study ADHD group as well, we were surprised to see that it was not a significant area of concern here relative to the control groups. In a post hoc analysis, we broke out those members of each group who placed in the more serious "risk" category on this health inventory rather than the less serious bracket of a "concern." We compared individuals in the risk category against those coded as having no risk (categories rated as just concerns or strengths). The group comparison results do not change for any domain of health except for driving. It now becomes a significant group difference ($\chi^2 = 6.55$, $p = .038$) in which the H+ADHD group (33%) manifests a greater percentage having driving risks than the H–ADHD (16%) and controls (18%), which do not differ from each other. Thus, as in the UMASS Study and other research, persistent ADHD into adulthood is associated with elevated driving risks as reflected on this health survey.

   When we contrast these results against those from the UMASS Study, we can conclude that ADHD, whether in clinic-referred adults or in children growing up, conveys an increased risk for health concerns, particularly in sleep, social functioning, tobacco use, and emotional health. The two groups of adults with ADHD across these projects differ in several important respects, however. Con-

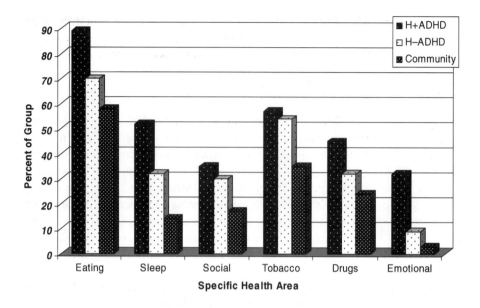

FIGURE 11.2. Percent of each group scoring in the risk or concern range on the Skinner Health and Lifestyle Interview for the Milwaukee Study. The figure depicts those health and lifestyle areas on which the hyperactive groups differed from the community control group. H+ADHD = hyperactive group that currently has a diagnosis of ADHD at follow-up; H–ADHD = hyperactive group that does not have a diagnosis of ADHD at follow-up.

cerns about eating habits arise in a substantially greater percentage of those with persistent ADHD from childhood to adulthood (H+ADHD) than in the clinic-referred adults. Both ADHD groups show similar percentages of concerns in the domains of sleep, social relations, tobacco, driving, and emotional health. In contrast, clinic-referred adults with ADHD showed a greater percentage of concerns relative to their control groups in the additional domains of family interactions, medical/dental, and work/leisure beyond that level seen in the children with ADHD grown up. Perhaps that is due to their being a somewhat older sample than that of the Milwaukee Study, where there is greater time for the former group to experience such concerns or at least to become more aware of them. But another possibility suggests itself as well. Interestingly, it is not that the hyperactive groups in the Milwaukee study did not have high percentages with such concerns but that the Community control group did as well, making these comparisons nonsignificant. Recall that we found a similar problem with regard to drug use in this control group. The Milwaukee Community control group, comprising children volunteered by their parents for this longitudinal study, may represent a somewhat different cross section of the general population than might the adults in the UMASS Community control group, who may be more typical of adults likely to volunteer in adulthood for such research projects.

Personal and Family Medical History

We questioned participants about whether or not they, their parents, their siblings, and their grandparents had ever experienced any of the following medical problems: diabetes, thyroid problems, vitamin deficiencies, anemia or leukemia, cancer, stroke, high blood pressure, heart attack or heart surgery, blood clots, bleeding tendencies, mental health problems, substance abuse problems, kidney disease, peptic ulcers, colitis, gallstones, liver disease, pancreatitis, urinary tract problems, prostate problems, seizures, head trauma, cataracts, emphysema, bronchitis, tuberculosis, rheumatic fever, arthritis, bone fractures, gout, and allergies. The groups differed in just a few of these numerous medical categories:

1. Cancer in grandparents was significantly less common in the H–ADHD (33%) than in the other two groups (50–54%).
2. High blood pressure was marginally more common ($p = .057$) in H+ ADHD (44%) than in the other two groups (26–28%).
3. Mental health problems in parents were more common in the H+ADHD group (31%) than in the other two groups (14% each).
4. Peptic ulcers were more common in the parents of both H groups (11% and 10%) than in the control group (0). It was also especially common for siblings to have greater peptic ulcer risk, but this was true only of the H+ADHD group (24%) compared to the H–ADHD group (12%) and the Community control group (1%).
5. Emphysema was marginally less common ($p = .061$) in the H–ADHD group (19%) than in the H+ADHD group (31%) and Community controls (37%).
6. Bronchitis was marginally more common ($p = .059$) in the siblings of members of the H+ADHD (30%) group than in the H–ADHD or Community control groups (19% and 13%). But it was significantly more common ($p = .04$) in the grandparents of the H+ADHD (20%) group compared to the H–ADHD and Community control groups (6% and 9%).
7. Arthritis was significantly more common ($p = .003$) in the parents of H+ADHD group (20%) than in either the H–ADHD or Community control groups (5% and 4%).

To summarize, persistent ADHD to adulthood may be associated with greater problems with high blood pressure, parental mental health, parental and sibling risk for peptic ulcers, grandparental bronchitis, and parental arthritis. While these results are interesting, great caution must be used in evaluating them, given the large number of statistical tests done to evaluate these 32 illness categories for the participants and their parents, siblings, and grandparents. Our few significant findings could simply reflect chance and not a reliable association with ADHD. If we count up the number of medical illnesses experienced only by the participants and ignoring relatives, we find that the groups do not differ in the number of illnesses they endorsed out of these 32 in their own personal histories (H+ADHD = 2.3, SD = 1.5; H–ADHD = 1.8, SD = 1.5, and Community = 2.3, SD = 1.6; F = 2.08, p = NS).

We inquired of these participants whether they had ever had surgery, broken bones, allergies, a chronic medical problem, or been hospitalized for nonsurgical reasons. The groups did not differ in the first four areas, but the H+ADHD group was nearly twice as likely to have been hospitalized for nonsurgical reasons (53%) compared to the H–ADHD and control groups (29 and 21% respectively) (p = .001). Both hyperactive groups had a significantly greater percentage that had ever experienced a serious injury (60% and 59%) and an accidental poisoning (11% and 14%) than had the control group (42% for injury, 3% for poisoning) (p = .05 for both). The groups did not differ in the percentage currently taking prescription drugs (23–40%) or using over-the-counter medications (71%–80%). These findings are consistent with earlier research showing hyperactive/ADHD children to be at higher risk for accidental injuries and poisonings as well as nonpsychiatric hospitalizations and emergency room admissions (Barkley, 2001, 2006).

We also examined group differences in the frequency of each of the above medical problems. The groups did not differ in the frequencies of surgical procedures, serious injuries, broken bones, allergies or chronic medical problems, or in their use of prescription or over-the-counter medications. The H+ADHD group had been hospitalized for nonsurgical reasons more often (0.87) than the other two groups (0.47, and 0.31, respectively). And while the omnibus test for frequency of accidental poisonings was significant (p = .045), none of the pairwise contrasts were so; there was a marginally significant (p = .058) finding suggesting that both hyperactive groups may have had a slightly higher occurrence of poisonings than the Community control group.

Current Medical Health Complaints

We employed a standard interview common to the life insurance industry to evaluate our participants for their current medical or general health concerns. This interview covered 59 complaints that are listed in Table 11.3. We found the hyperactive groups to differ from the Community control group in 26 or nearly half of these comparisons. In general, it is the group in which ADHD has per-

TABLE 11.3. Current Medical Complaints by Group (Self-Reported) for the Milwaukee Study

Measures	H+ADHD N	H+ADHD %	H–ADHD N	H–ADHD %	Community N	Community %	χ^2	p	Pairwise contrasts
Significant weight change in past year	32	58	29	37	27	37	7.14	.028	1 > 2,3
Fever or chills	7	13	4	5	7	10	2.45	NS	
Night sweats	11	20	3	4	2	3	15.59	< .001	1 > 2,3
Heat or cold intolerance	19	34	12	15	6	8	15.09	.001	1 > 2,3
Dental problems	26	47	21	27	15	21	10.99	.004	1 > 2,3
Changes in vision	10	18	9	11	7	10	2.16	NS	
Wear glasses	22	40	38	49	33	44	1.00	NS	
Eye problems	5	9	3	4	6	8	1.79	NS	
Ear or hearing problems	9	16	11	14	4	6	4.22	NS	
Ear pain or ringing	19	34	9	11	7	10	16.29	< .001	1 > 2,3
Other ear problems	1	2	5	6	2	3	2.19	NS	
Nose or sinus problems	22	40	29	37	14	19	7.83	.020	1,2 > 3
Hay fever	19	34	31	40	28	39	0.40	NS	
Nosebleeds	7	13	7	9	5	7	1.25	NS	
Other nasal problems	1	2	4	5	2	3	1.21	NS	
Throat irritation	18	33	8	10	9	12	13.14	.001	1 > 2,3
Hoarseness	12	22	8	10	4	6	8.23	.016	1 > 3
Neck swelling	6	11	3	4	2	3	4.63	NS	
Shortness of breath	26	47	16	20	9	12	21.46	< .001	1 > 2,3
Problematic cough	21	38	25	32	10	14	10.69	.005	1,2 > 3
Wheezing or asthma	15	27	17	22	8	11	5.60	NS	
Other problems with lungs	1	2	1	1	2	3	0.44	NS	
Chest pain or tightness	21	38	22	28	11	15	8.66	.013	1 > 3
Skipped heartbeats or palpitations	12	22	8	10	9	12	3.80	NS	
Heart murmur	6	11	3	4	3	4	3.49	NS	
High blood pressure	6	11	4	5	2	3	3.86	NS	
Need to sleep with head elevated	10	18	5	6	3	4	8.53	.014	1 > 2,3
Trouble breathing	6	11	1	1	5	7	5.66	NS	
Pain in legs when walking	12	22	8	10	5	7	6.88	.032	1 > 3
Swelling of legs or ankles	5	9	3	4	3	4	2.06	NS	
Other heart problems	0	0	0	0	2	3	3.73	NS	
Heartburn or vomiting	5	9	3	4	2	3	2.97	NS	
Difficulty swallowing	38	69	41	53	23	32	17.61	< .001	1,2 > 3
Stomach pain	3	5	1	1	1	1	2.87	NS	
Constipation or diarrhea	14	25	12	15	7	10	5.76	NS	
Bloody or black stools	11	20	12	15	12	17	0.50	NS	
Rashes or itching	5	9	7	9	2	3	2.86	NS	
Moles	21	38	15	19	9	12	12.55	.002	1 > 2,3
Other skin problems	5	9	6	8	6	8	0.83	NS	
Excessive urination	8	14	8	10	7	10	0.84	NS	
Nighttime urination	9	16	7	9	1	1	9.27	.010	1,2 > 3
Painful or burning urination	16	29	11	14	7	10	9.02	.011	1 > 2,3
Difficulty starting urination	3	5	0	0	1	1	5.20	NS	
Weak urine stream	6	11	3	4	1	1	6.38	.041	1 > 3

(continued)

TABLE 11.3. *(continued)*

Measures	H+ADHD N	H+ADHD %	H−ADHD N	H−ADHD %	Community N	Community %	χ^2	p	Pairwise contrasts
Leaking urine when coughing	2	4	2	3	3	4	0.30	NS	
Blood in urine	3	5	4	5	1	1	1.88	NS	
Any sexual dysfunction	2	4	2	3	0	0	2.40	NS	
Painful or swollen joints	2	4	1	1	0	0	2.89	NS	
Stiffness in joints	18	33	15	19	7	10	10.51	.005	1 > 3
Back pain	27	49	28	36	14	19	12.56	.002	1,2 > 3
Unusual hair growth	35	64	46	59	30	42	7.24	.027	1,2 > 3
Bruise easily	20	36	12	15	6	8	17.05	< .001	1 > 2,3
Other bleeding problems	7	13	2	3	1	1	10.09	.006	1 > 2,3
Weakness in arms or legs	3	5	1	1	0	0	5.14	NS	
Numbness or loss of feeling	6	11	3	4	1	1	6.38	.041	1 > 3
Headaches	20	36	12	15	4	6	20.85	< .001	1 > 2 > 3
Dizziness or fainting spells	31	56	36	46	26	36	5.19	NS	
Fatigue	7	13	8	10	5	7	1.22	NS	
Depression or anxiety	20	36	7	9	10	14	17.66	< .001	1 > 2,3

Note. Sample sizes are H+ADHD = 55; H−ADHD = 78; Community controls = 72. *N* = sample size endorsing this item; % = percent of group endorsing this item; χ^2 = results of the omnibus chi-square test; *p* = probability value for the chi-square test; pairwise contrasts = results of the chi-square tests involving pairwise comparisons of the three groups. *Statistical analysis:* Pearson chi-square.

sisted into adulthood that has a greater percentage of its cases voicing such concerns than either the H−ADHD or Community control groups. This was true for significant weight changes in the past year, night sweats, heat or cold intolerance, dental problems, pain or ringing in the ears, throat irritation, shortness of breath, sleeping with bed elevated, concerns about moles, painful or burning urination, bruising easily, other bleeding problems, headaches, and depression or anxiety. The H+ADHD group differed only from the Community control group in several additional complaints, these being throat hoarseness, pain in the legs when walking, weak urine stream, and numbness or loss of feeling. In a few areas, the hyperactive group that no longer had ADHD at age 27 (H−ADHD) complained more than Community control adults about sinus problems, problematic cough, difficulty swallowing, nighttime urination, back pain, and unusual hair growth. But the H+ADHD group also had more members making such complaints than the control group, with the two hyperactive groups not differing in this respect.

We computed the number of these 59 problems endorsed by members of each group. We compared the groups (controlling for nonverbal IQ, which was significantly related to this score) and found that the H+ADHD group had significantly more such complaints (*M* = 12.3, *SD* = 7.0) than the H−ADHD group (*M* = 8.4, *SD* = 4.7), which had more such concerns than the Community control group (*M* = 6.1, *SD* = 5.9; *F* = 24.75, *df* = 2/204, *p* < .001). Being a child with ADHD in this study is therefore associated with a higher number of current medical complaints than in the Community control group, but those with persistent ADHD have more such complaints than those who no longer have ADHD by age 27.

While this may well suggest a greater likelihood of legitimate health problems associated with having been hyperactive as a child, it is likely not lost on the educated reader that many of these complaints can fall within the psychosomatic domain or what is now called somatoform disorders. It may prove helpful to recall that, 35 years ago, the parents of hyperactive children were found to have a higher percentage of Briquette's syndrome or hysteria than the normal population (Cantwell, 1972; Morrison, 1980)—a syndrome that evolved into psychosomatic and then somatoform illnesses. We did not find a greater incidence of somatoform disorders in the psychiatric evaluations of these individuals (Chapter 8), however, with 2% or fewer of participants in these groups qualifying for such a diagnosis.

It is also possible that these complaints could be related to anxiety or depression and their associated psychiatric disorders, both of which were low but significantly elevated in the hyperactive groups (Chapter 8). This possibility is quite plausible, given that the total number of health complaints correlated significantly with self-reported levels of somatization ($r = .62$, $p < .001$), depression ($r = .47$, $p < .001$), anxiety ($r = .44$, $p < .001$), and phobic anxiety ($r = .41$, $p < .001$) from the SCL-90-R scale (see sidebar, Chapter 8), using the entire sample ($N = 203$). Regressing all four of the SCL-90-R scales onto the number of current health complaints showed that somatization and phobic anxiety were the scales significantly predictive of medical complaints, accounting for 38% of the variance in those complaints, with 37% being attributable to just the somatization scale. But then the above list of 59 health problems can itself be considered a somatization scale, hence the significant association between it and the SCL-90-R scale of that name. We repeated the regression analysis removing that scale and found that both the depression and phobic anxiety scales were now predictive of total health complaints, accounting for 24% of the variance (depression = 22% and phobic anxiety = 2%) (F for depression = 58.26, $p < .001$; F for phobic anxiety = 33.25, $p < .001$). These findings support the hypothesis that the greater number of medical complaints in the two hyperactive groups may well be a function, at least in part, of their elevated levels of depression and anxiety.

Exercise

One question we asked of our participants was whether or not they exercised frequently. We found that a significantly smaller percentage of the H+ADHD group reported doing so (44%) than did the other two groups (H–ADHD = 65%, Community control = 69%), which did not differ from each other. We had found this to be true at the age-21 follow-up, where the hyperactive groups reported that they exercised less often than our control group (Fischer & Barkley, 2006). If this pattern continues forward in life, we can hypothesize a greater likelihood of later life health problems in the hyperactive than in the control groups, especially in those having persistent ADHD.

Physical Exam and Lab Studies

As part of this study, we conducted physical exams on the participants, recording routine parameters of height, weight, body mass index, blood pressure, and temperature. We also drew blood and took urine samples for routine lipid profiles and urinalysis. From these findings, we were also able to compute future cardiovascular risks using the results of the Framingham Heart Study and other prior research on risk prediction. Our results appear in Table 11.4. Our groups did not differ in height or weight at age 27, similar to the findings of Weiss and Hechtman (1993) in their Canadian follow-up study of hyperactive children. But we did find that the group with persistent ADHD had a significantly greater body mass index than the Community control group, with the H–ADHD group placing between these two and not differing significantly from them. Both hyperactive groups had significantly lower HDL cholesterol than the Community control group, while only the H+ADHD group had a greater HDL:total cholesterol ratio, both of which are risk factors for future cardiovascular disease (Devroey, Vantomme, Betz, Vandevoorde, & Kartounian, 2004). But LDL:HDL ratios are now thought to possibly be a better indicator of when to initiate treatment for low HDL levels (Devroey et al., 2004) and those ratios did not differ among our groups. The results from the urinalyses found that the H+ADHD group had a significantly higher specific gravity than Community control adults, while both hyperactive groups had an elevated ratio of white blood cells per high-power field. Such elevations, although significant, are small and are difficult to interpret in view of current or future health risks. The groups did not differ in the presence or absence of respiratory problems on the physical exam: 10% versus 4% versus 4%, $\chi^2 = 2.22$ (NS). Nor did they differ in the percentage whose blood work results showed abnormal findings for viral antibodies for hepatitis or HIV or bacterial antibodies for syphilis (most of which were absent in all three groups or very rare).

The results for other urine studies that code as abnormal or not are shown in Table 11.5. We found that only the two hyperactive groups had more members with abnormal leukocyte esters than our Community control group. The meaning of this is unclear. The urine toxicology panels were negative for all drugs, with typically only 0 to 3 subjects in total showing positive for opiates, amphetamines, phencyclidine, phenothiazines, barbiturates, and benzodiazepines. There also were no group differences in screen positives for cannibis; however, the pro-

TABLE 11.4. Results of Physical Examination and Blood and Urine Tests by Group for the Milwaukee Study

Measure	H+ADHD Mean	SD	H–ADHD Mean	SD	Community Mean	SD	F	p	Pairwise contrasts
Height (centimeters)	177.7	10.6	176.8	9.7	178.4	7.3	0.60	NS	
Weight (kilograms)	94.8	28.9	93.0	22.7	88.2	24.0	1.17	NS	
Body mass index	30.4	9.1	29.5	6.7	27.3	5.4	3.32	.038	1 > 3
Systolic blood pressure	125.2	12.8	128.1	12.2	125.7	11.9	1.06	NS	
Diastolic blood pressure	78.6	10.9	78.3	8.8	75.4	9.5	2.18	NS	
Pulse	67.4	10.8	68.6	12.4	64.9	11.5	1.91	NS	
Temperature	97.9	0.6	97.9	0.7	97.7	0.8	1.95	NS	
Lipid profiles									
Total cholesterol	191.8	42.3	187.1	49.6	185.0	35.4	0.36	NS	
HDL	42.7	9.5	45.4	12.5	50.8	13.6	6.94	.001	1,2< 3
Total/HDL ratio	4.7	1.4	4.5	2.1	3.9	1.5	3.03	.050	1 > 3
LDL	107.5	32.1	105.9	33.5	102.2	29.5	0.42	NS	
LDL/HDL ratio	2.6	0.9	2.5	1.0	2.2	1.1	2.68	NS	
Triglycerides	201.6	109.7	159.4	101.6	172.9	126.6	2.13	NS	
Urinalysis									
Specific gravity	1.020	.0063	1.019	.0071	1.017	.0074	3.88	.022	1 > 3
Ph	6.34	0.83	6.45	0.80	6.55	0.79	1.05	NS	
WBC/HPF	1.08	0.84	1.00	0.71	0.65	0.68	6.14	.003	1,2 > 3
RBC/HPF	0.54	0.90	0.66	0.98	0.36	0.57	2.36	NS	
Framingham CHD risks									
Total CHD risk points	1.61	5.5	0.52	6.48	−0.45	4.97	1.86	NS	
5-year CHD risk percent	1.22	0.51	1.11	0.35	1.04	0.21	3.60	.029	1 > 3
10-year CHD risk percent	2.71	1.38	2.57	1.07	2.25	0.74	3.06	.049	1 > 3
Total CHD risk points with no age correction	4.83	4.34	3.97	4.54	1.98	4.11	6.89	< .001	1,2 > 3
5-year CHD risk percent with no age correction	1.45	0.82	1.32	0.64	1.15	0.43	3.40	.036	1 > 3
10-year CHD risk percent with no age correction	3.37	1.93	3.09	1.54	2.53	1.10	4.78	.009	1,2 > 3
Atherosclerosis risks									
Total risks—Berenson method (0–4)	1.51	1.21	1.37	1.10	1.12	1.04	1.76	NS	
Total risks—our method (0–6)	2.53	1.49	2.25	1.25	1.81	1.20	4.73	.014	1 > 3

Note. Sample sizes are H+ADHD = 52, H–ADHD = 77, Community controls = 70 for height, weight, body mass, and temperature. For blood pressure and pulse, they are H+ADHD = 51, H–ADHD = 75, and Community controls = 70. For cholesterol lipids panels, they are H+ADHD = 50, H–ADHD = 77, and Community controls = 69. SD = standard deviation; F = F-test results of the analysis of variance (or covariance); p = probability value for the F-test; NS = not significant; H+ADHD = hyperactive group that currently has a diagnosis of ADHD at follow-up; H–ADHD = hyperactive group that does not have a diagnosis of ADHD at follow-up; HDL = high-density lipids; LDL = low-density lipids; WBC/HPF = white blood cells per high-power field; RBC/HPF = red blood cells per high-power field; CHD = coronary heart disease; atherosclerosis risks = body mass index, systolic blood pressure, LDL, and triglycerides all at or above 75th percentile for control group plus current smoker and no regular exercise (range 0 to 6 risks).

Statistical analysis: Groups were initially compared using one-way (groups) analysis of variance. Where this analysis was significant (p < .05) for the main effect for group, pairwise comparisons (Student–Newman–Keuls tests) of the groups were conducted, the results of which are shown in the last column.

TABLE 11.5. Categorical Urine Laboratory Results for the Milwaukee Study

Measures	H+ADHD N	H+ADHD %	H–ADHD N	H–ADHD %	Community N	Community %	χ^2	p	Pairwise contrasts
Glucose abnormal	2	4	2	3	2	3	0.17	NS	
Ketones abnormal	4	8	2	3	2	3	2.43	NS	
Proteins abnormal	3	6	5	6	1	1	2.38	NS	
Leukocyte ester abnormal	11	21	14	18	3	4	8.59	.014	1,2 > 3
Bacteria abnormal	7	13	11	14	5	7	1.99	NS	

Note. Sample sizes are H+ADHD = 52; H–ADHD = 77; and Community controls = 69. N = sample size endorsing this item; % = percent of group endorsing this item; χ^2 = results of the omnibus chi-square test; p = probability value for the chi-square test; pairwise contrasts = results of the chi-square tests involving pairwise comparisons of the three groups; H+ADHD = hyperactive group that currently has a diagnosis of ADHD at follow-up; H–ADHD = hyperactive group that does not have a diagnosis of ADHD at follow-up.
  Statistical analysis: Pearson chi-square.

portion of subjects in each group screening positive was still impressive: 23% versus 20% versus 13%, χ^2 = 2.15 (NS). This suggests that a significant minority of our participants had used marijuana around the time of their evaluation in this study.

Future Risk for Heart Disease

We used the information from these exams and lab studies to develop a risk assessment for our participants for future coronary heart disease (CHD). Future risk of CHD has been repeatedly linked to several health and lifestyle characteristics, with the most frequent being smoking, blood pressure, serum cholesterol (and specifically HDL:LDL and HDL:total ratios), body mass index, diabetes, and frequency of exercise (Goldbourt, Yaari, & Medalie, 1993; Kannel & Larson, 1993; Rosolova, Simon, & Sefrna, 1993). We first used the Framingham Heart Study risk tables to do so. The study by Kannel and Larson (1993) provides tables to compute risk points for each subject, using sex, age, body mass index, HDL cholesterol, total cholesterol, systolic blood pressure, smoking, and diabetes. We had information on all of these parameters for most of the Milwaukee Study participants. We did the initial CHD risk points calculation following those tables, including their age correction. Given how young our sample is, however, this served to subtract 1 to 2 points for males and 11 to 12 for females. Therefore we also computed these risk points without the age correction, which essentially treats the males as if they were ages 32 to 33 and females as if they were age 40. This allows us to say what their future CHD risk would be if the current lifestyles and medical findings for these participants were to continue at a somewhat later age (5 or so years later for males and 13 or so for females), when no age correction would be done.

Results using the standard tables and risk points with the appropriate age correction did not reveal a significant difference in total points among the groups. But when these points were converted to risk for future CHD, the percent risks for both 5- and 10-year periods were significantly greater in the H+ADHD than the Community control group, with the H–ADHD group falling between them and not differing from either. Thus, persistent ADHD to age 27 is associated with a slight yet significant increase in 5- and 10-year CHD risk. While the percent risks are low in absolute terms, this is the result of the very young age of these samples. When we remove the age correction, treating the groups as if they were somewhat older (5 years for males, 12 for females), we can see that if the current health findings carried forward to those ages, both hyperactive groups would have greater risk point totals and both would have significantly elevated risk percentages for CHD in the subsequent 10 years. The H+ADHD group would have an elevated risk percentage for the next 5-year period as well. Again, the increase in percentage of risk over the Community control group remains small in absolute terms. Our point, though, is that growing up with ADHD is becoming associated with risk for CHD in future years, even if at a small magnitude of risk at the present time. Persistent ADHD to adulthood may carry a somewhat higher risk, but it does not differ from the risk seen in the H–ADHD group. To our knowledge, this is the first study either of hyperactive children followed to adulthood to study their medical risk profiles and particularly their risk for future CHD.

Berenson et al. (1998) developed a profile for determining risks for atherosclerosis in young people (ages 1–39) based on autopsies of those dying of accidental injuries. He used a range of 0 to 4 based on body mass index (BMI), systolic blood pressure, LDL levels, and triglycerides, all being at or above the 75th percentile for his control group. We made these calculations using the 75th percentile for our own Community control group. The results for this four-point risk profile are shown in Table 11.4, where no differences in our groups on this profile were evident. However, Berenson also examined the additional contribution of smoking. To quote from that study:

The mean percentage of the intimal surface covered by lesions in patients with different numbers of risk factors (0, 1, 2, and 3 or 4) . . . included body-mass index, systolic blood ressure, serum triglyceride concentration, and serum LDL cholesterol concentration. In subjects with 0, 1, 2, and 3 or 4 risk factors, 19.1 percent, 30.3 percent, 37.9 percent, and 35.0 percent, respectively, of the intimal surface area was involved with fatty streaks in the aorta (P for trend = 0.01). In the coronary arteries, 1.3 percent, 2.5 percent, 7.9 percent, and 11.0 percent, respectively, of the intimal surface was involved with fatty streaks (P for trend = 0.01), and 0.6 percent, 0.7 percent, 2.4 percent, and 7.2 percent was involved with collagenous fibrous plaques (P for trend = 0.003). The extent of fatty-streak lesions in the coronary arteries was 8.5

times as great in persons with three or four risk factors as in those with none (P = 0.03), and the extent of fibrous-plaque lesions in the coronary arteries was 12 times as great (P = 0.006). ... The mean (+/-*SE*) percentage of the intimal surface involved with fibrous-plaque lesions in the aorta was higher in smokers than in non-smokers (1.22+/-0.62 percent vs. 0.12+/-0.07 percent, P = 0.02), as was the percentage involved in fatty-streak lesions in the coronary vessels (8.27+/-3.43 percent vs. 2.89+/-0.83 percent, P = 0.04) (p. 1654).

Others have also found that these five factors as well as level of regular exercise can create a better profile of current and future atherosclerosis risk than does the 4-point profile (Batalla, Hevia, Reguero, Cubero, & Cortina, 2000; Stamler, Dyer, Shekelle, Neaton, & Stamler, 1993). We therefore computed a 6-point risk profile, adding smoking and lack of regular exercise to Berenson's 4-point scale. Using this expanded risk profile, we found that the H+ADHD group has a significantly greater point total and hence greater risk for current and future atherosclerosis of the coronary vessels.

In general, the hyperactive and control groups are not that much different in their current medical status; what differences we found, while significant, are relatively small. Those with persistent ADHD have more current medical complaints than other groups, especially in females, but these seem more reflective of the higher levels of depression, phobic anxiety, and likelihood of somatization more generally rather than of greater physical illness or disorder. However, those differences in current physical status, though minor now, do produce an increase in predicted current and future risk for both atherosclerosis and CHD more generally, especially if these patterns were to continue forward unchanged for another 5 to 13 years (depending on sex). Those risks remain quite small for the moment, largely due to the young age of our study participants. But if they were unchanged over the next few decades, such physical findings and lifestyles would be associated with an escalating risk of CHD and mortality generally in the group with persistent ADHD.

Sex Differences

Given that there were only five females in the control group, we elected to examine for sex differences just within the hyperactive group. No areas of concern on the Skinner Computerized Lifestyle Assessment differed between males and females. On the 59 current medical complaints, females were more likely than males to complain of these nine problems:

- Weight change in the past year (75% females vs. 41% males) (p = .005).
- Vision problems (30 vs. 11.5) (.029).

- Wheezing or asthma (45 vs. 20) (.017).
- Sleeping with bed head elevated (25 vs. 9) (.035).
- Swelling of legs/ankles (30 vs. 2) (.001).
- Bloody or black stools (35 vs. 14) (.023).
- Blood in urine (30% vs. 1%) (.001).
- Bleeding problems (20 vs. 4) (.011).
- Dizziness or fainting (75 vs 46) (.017).

We examined the total number of current medical complaints using a 2 (H+ADHD vs. H–ADHD) × 2 (sex) analysis of covariance (IQ as a covariate), and found not only the original main effect for group (H+ADHD greater than H–ADHD), but also a main effect for sex (females greater than males) ($F = 4.71$, $df = 1/124$, $p = .032$). These findings, however, are qualified by the fact that we also found a significant interaction of group with sex ($F = 5.25$, $df = 1/124$, $p =.024$). Females in the H+ADHD group had significantly more complaints (19.4) than males in that group (12.6) while there was no sex difference within the H–ADHD group (females = 8.5 vs. males = 8.4). Thus it is chiefly women with persistent ADHD that account for these sex differences in current medical complaints, having more than twice the number of complaints as women or men who had ADHD as children but no longer do at age 27 and 50% more such complaints than men with persistent ADHD.

We compared the hyperactive males versus females on the physical exam and lab results. Females had significantly higher BMIs (36.9 vs. 28.9) and temperatures (98.1 vs. 97.8) and were shorter, of course. Lipid profiles were not different. Females had significantly higher WBC/HPF ratios (1.39 vs. 0.97; $F = 4.78$, $p = .031$) and ratios of red blood cells per high-power field (1.56 vs. 0.46; $F = 24.61$, p .001) but no differences in specific gravity or Ph. Males had higher Framingham coronary heart disease (CHD) risk points (2.63 vs. –9.64), as expected, given that females were credited with greater points off their risk for their sex. As a consequence, the 10-year CHD risks were higher in males (2.73) than in females (2.00), while the 5-year risks were not different. The two other atherosclerotic risk totals were not different. Despite having higher BMIs, females who were hyperactive as children may have lower CHD risks at age 27 than males, owing largely to the sex differences in such risks in the general population.

Childhood Stimulant Treatment and Adult Height and Weight

Stimulant medication treatment of children with ADHD is known to produce a slight retardation of growth in height and weight, at least for the first year or two of treatment (Connor, 2006). But no evidence of long-term effects on growth into adulthood has been demonstrated to our knowledge (see Weiss &

Hechtman, 1993 for an earlier review of studies on this issue). We had information from the adolescent follow-up on the number of months the hyperactive children had been treated with stimulants as reported by parents. We correlated the duration of childhood stimulant treatment with current height, weight, and BMI from our physical exam. No correlations were significant or even close to being so (range .016–.031) whether using the entire sample or just using the hyperactive group (range −.060 to +.059), which is the more appropriate group to study here. Next we compared those who had ever been treated with stimulants versus those who had never been so treated on these same measures, and again there were no significant differences, whether using the entire sample or just the hyperactive group. Surprisingly, those who had never been treated were shorter in height than those who had been treated. This might pertain to physicians being reluctant initially in the 1970s and 1980s to put hyperactive children already short of stature on stimulants for fear of growth-suppression effects. These data provide no evidence of long-term suppression of growth into adulthood in height, weight, or BMI in children treated with stimulants regardless of treatment duration. They are in complete agreement with the Weiss and Hechtman (1993) longitudinal study of hyperactive children, where likewise no such effects were found.

Money Management

No research appears to exist on the specific money management problems that may be associated with ADHD in clinic-referred adults. De Quiros and Kinsbourne (2001) did report two items from their Adult Problem Questionnaire that pertain to money matters, which were rated as occurring more often in their ADHD than in their control group. These were frequently going on shopping sprees and having trouble sticking to a budget. As noted earlier, given the poor impulse control and self-regulation associated with the disorder, problems with handling money would be reasonable to anticipate in adults with ADHD.

Only one study of children with ADHD (hyperactivity) followed to adulthood has reported results for financial management at follow-up. Using the Milwaukee Study follow-up at age 21, we found that significantly more of the Community control group than the hyperactive (ADHD) group had ever had a credit card, but otherwise the groups did not differ in the proportion ever having had a car loan, other bank loans, or currently owing money to others (Barkley, Fischer, Smallish, & Fletcher, 2006). Significantly fewer members of the ADHD group had a savings account, and more of the ADHD group reported having trouble saving money to pay their monthly bills. The groups did not differ in their current annual salary amounts. Although the average savings for the ADHD group were lower than those of the Community control group, this difference was not significant. Of those who had owned credit cards, taken out current car loans, or had other bank loans outstanding, the groups did not differ in the amounts of these debts. But the ADHD group owed significantly more money to other individuals than did the Community control group. Given that the participants in this study had an average age of approximately 21 years, there may not have been enough time since leaving school for differences in financial status and management issues to have become apparent. Even so, this study suggests that there may be some impact of ADHD on financial management in early adulthood, albeit a relatively minor one.

The UMASS Study Results

The results for the current UMASS Study concerning the percentage of each group experiencing 12 different money management problems appear in Table 11.6. These were derived from the initial interview concerning possible impairments associated with the disorder. We found no overall sex differences in any of these 12 areas. More adults with ADHD reported more problems in eight of the 12 areas of money management we surveyed than did adults in the Community control group. The ADHD group had a higher proportion of its members reporting problems with managing money, saving money, buying on impulse, nonpayment of utilities resulting in their termination, missing loan payments, exceeding credit card limits, having a poor credit rating, and not saving for retirement. Relative to the Community control group, the adults with ADHD appear to be having relatively pervasive problems with the management of their finances. These findings are consistent with the far less comprehensive report of De Quiros and Kinsbourne (2001), discussed above, which found a greater likelihood of shopping sprees and poor adherence to a budget in their adults with ADHD.

There were also problems in the ADHD group that occurred to a greater percentage of them than occurred with even the Clinical control group. Those comparisons give a better picture of the risks associated specifically with ADHD and not just outpatient referral status. The ADHD group was more likely to have trouble saving money, buying on impulse, not paying their utilities, and not saving for retirement. While the Clinical controls also had difficulties in five of these areas compared to the Community control group, they were less likely to have such difficulties than the ADHD group, particularly in saving money and buying on impulse. Those four areas of money management in which the ADHD group differed from both the Clinical and Community control groups are illustrated in Figure 11.3. This figure makes it clearer that ADHD is associated with some rather specific financial problems having to do with deferred gratification (saving

TABLE 11.6. Money Management Problems by Group in the UMASS Study

Measure	ADHD		Clinical		Community		χ^2	p	Pairwise contrasts
	N	%	N	%	N	%			
Trouble managing money	97	67	53	57	16	15	72.3	< .001	1,2 > 3
Difficulty saving money	94	65	47	50	19	18	57.3	< .001	1 > 2 > 3
Problems buying on impulse	90	62	44	47	13	12	65.4	< .001	1 > 2 > 3
Ever missed paying rent	34	23	18	19	16	15	2.9	NS	
Had utilities turned off for nonpayment of bills	46	32	16	17	14	13	14.5	.001	1 > 2,3
Missed loan repayment	83	57	50	53	29	27	25.2	< .001	1,2 > 3
Exceeded credit limits on cards	68	47	38	40	31	29	8.6	.013	1 > 3
Wrote check with insufficient funds to cover the amount	92	63	60	64	60	56	2.0	NS	
Had a vehicle repossessed	10	7	3	3	4	4	2.2	NS	
Declared bankruptcy	8	6	5	5	9	8	2.4	NS	
Have a poor credit rating	34	26	17	19	7	7	14.3	.001	1,2 > 3
Not saving for retirement	101	71	48	52	45	42	22.0	< .001	1 > 2,3

Note. Sample sizes for the comparisons on interview information are ADHD = 144; Clinical control = 93; Community control = 108. N = sample size endorsing this item; % = percent of group endorsing this item; χ^2 = results of the omnibus chi-square test; p = probability value for the chi-square test; pairwise contrasts = results of the chi-square tests involving pairwise comparisons of the three groups.

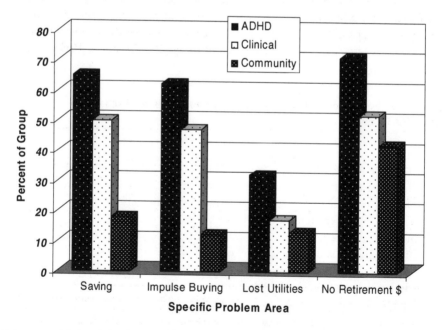

FIGURE 11.3. Percent of each group having various money management problems in the UMASS Study. These are the measures on which the ADHD group differed significantly from the Clinical control and the Community control groups. $ = savings.

and putting money away for retirement), impulse buying, and probably organization and meeting deadlines (nonpayment of utilities resulting in their termination).

We also collected some answers to five financial questions having to do with the frequency with which our subjects may have experienced a money problem. We also computed a money problem diversity score by summing the number of different problem areas in which a participant reported a problem across the 12 areas, as reported in Table 11.6. These frequency data appear in Table 11.7. In all six measures, the adults with ADHD reported these difficulties more often did the adults in our Community control group. Money difficulties were also more common in the ADHD than in the Clinical control group in at least four of these six areas, those being missing rent payments, missing utility payments, missing loan payments, and having more total money problems. Missing loan payments was the most common problem reported across groups, although it was significantly more common among the ADHD group members than in the other two control groups. Only one sex difference was evident, and this showed that, regardless of group, females reported having written checks without sufficient funds more often than did males ($M = 7.4$ vs. 4.7, respectively; $SDs = 14.4$ vs. 9.7; $F = 8.3$; $df = 1/318$; $p = .004$).

These difficulties with money management are not surprising in view of the problems with inhibition, executive functioning, and self-regulation documented in earlier chapters. They are also consistent with some of the financial problems emerging in hyperactive children followed to age 21 (Fischer & Barkley, 2006)

TABLE 11.7. Frequency of Money Management Problems for Each Group in the UMASS Study

Measure	ADHD Mean	ADHD SD	Clinical Mean	Clinical SD	Community Mean	Community SD	F	p	Pairwise contrasts
Missed rent payment	2.3	6.1	0.8	1.9	0.5	1.4	6.2	.002	1 > 2,3
Missed utility payment	1.4	3.8	0.5	1.2	0.2	0.5	7.5	.001	1 > 2,3
Missed loan payment	10.3	16.4	6.2	10.4	1.1	2.6	17.6	< .001	1 > 2 > 3
Exceeded credit limits	3.3	6.4	3.9	9.2	0.7	1.5	7.5	.001	1,2 > 3
Written checks without sufficient funds[S]	8.0	14.7	7.5	13.3	1.9	3.0	11.1	001	1,2 > 3
Total no. of problem areas	5.4	2.5	4.4	2.5	2.4	2.2	44.1	< .001	1 > 2 > 3

Note. Sample sizes for self-reports, depending on measure, are ADHD = 120–135, Clinical control = 80–84, Community control = 98–105. SD = standard deviation; F = F-test results of the analysis of variance (or covariance); p = probability value for the F-test; NS = not significant; [S] = significant main effect for sex; total no. of problem areas = total number of different money management problems reported across all items in prior table of categorical problems.

  Statistical analysis: Groups were initially compared using two-way (groups × sex) analysis of variance (or covariance as necessary). Where this analysis was significant ($p < .05$) for the main effect for group, pairwise comparisons of the groups were conducted, the results of which are shown in the last column.

noted above. To our knowledge, however, this is the first study of clinic-referred adults to actually examine the impact of ADHD on specific problem areas related to financial management. The disorder does seem to have an adverse impact on some aspects of this important domain of daily life activity, such as saving money, buying on impulse, and repaying debts. Such problems appear to be greater than in children with ADHD followed to young adulthood, discussed above, but we believe this likely has to do with the relatively young age of that follow-up (age 21) relative to the adult age groups studied here. With advancing age, there arise greater opportunities for problems with finances to become apparent, probably making it easier to detect the effects of ADHD on this domain of major life activity.

The Milwaukee Study Age-27 Results

We collected virtually the same information on financial status and money management issues from the Milwaukee Study participants at the age-27 follow-up. These can be observed in Table 11.8. In all but one of the 13 money issues, the H+ADHD group had a significantly larger percentage of cases having that problem than in the Community control group. The exception was for writing checks with insufficient funds, where no group differences were found. In seven of these problem areas, the H+ADHD group also had a higher risk than the H–ADHD group, these being trouble managing their money, buying on impulse, missing rent and credit card payments, exceeding credit card limits, not having a savings account, and having a poor credit rating (self-reported). In some areas, the two hyperactive groups had more participants with problems than did the Community control group, but they did not differ from each other, suggesting that having been a hyperactive/ADHD child carried some risk for financial problems even if ADHD had not persisted to this follow-up. These areas were difficulty saving money, having utilities turned off for nonpayment, having a vehicle repossessed, declaring bankruptcy, and not saving for retirement. This was also evident in other problem areas where the H–ADHD group fell below the level of risk for the H+ADHD group yet remained at higher risk than the Community controls, as in managing money, buying on impulse, missing rent payments, and having a poor credit rating. In summation, both hyperactive groups had a higher percentage of many of these financial problems than did the control group, suggesting that growing up with ADHD from childhood is a risk factor for financial difficulties even if that ADHD does not persist to age 27. But where it does persist, it increases the risks of financial difficulties even more. Those problem areas in which the H+ADHD group differed from both the H–ADHD and Community control groups are visually depicted in Figure 11.4, which can be contrasted with that for the UMASS Study in Figure 11.3.

TABLE 11.8. Money Management Problems by Group for the Milwaukee Study

Measures	H+ADHD N	H+ADHD %	H–ADHD N	H–ADHD %	Community N	Community %	χ^2	p	Pairwise contrasts
Trouble managing money	39	71	33	41	15	20	33.89	< .001	1 > 2 > 3
Difficulty saving money	35	65	43	54	14	19	32.11	< .001	1,2 > 3
Problems buying on impulse	42	78	36	45	18	24	36.61	< .001	1 > 2 > 3
Ever missed paying rent	17	31	13	16	4	5	15.70	< .001	1 > 2 > 3
Had utilities turned off for nonpayment of bills	23	43	26	33	8	11	18.03	< .001	1,2 > 3
Missed credit card payment	28	58	26	37	29	39	6.22	.045	1 > 2,3
Exceeded credit limits on cards	28	64	27	39	33	45	6.98	.031	1 > 2,3
Wrote check with insufficient funds to cover the amount	37	70	50	63	38	51	5.21	NS	
Had a vehicle repossessed	6	15	8	13	1	1	7.96	.019	1,2 > 3
Declared bankruptcy	5	9	15	19	3	4	8.90	.012	1,2 > 3
Do not have a savings account	33	61	31	39	20	27	15.61	< .001	1 > 2,3
Not saving for retirement	42	76	53	66	34	45	14.16	.001	1,2 > 3
Have a poor credit rating	29	54	26	32	6	8	32.42	< .001	1 > 2 > 3

Note. Sample sizes for the comparisons on interview information are H+ADHD = 55; H–ADHD = 80; Community control = 75 for all categories except for: car repossession, where Ns = 40, 61, 69, respectively; exceeding credit card limits, where Ns = 44, 70, and 73, respectively; and missing a credit card payment, where Ns = 48, 71, and 74, respectively. N = sample size endorsing this item; % = percent of group endorsing this item; χ^2 = results of the omnibus chi-square test; p = probability value for the chi-square test; pairwise contrasts = results of the chi-square tests involving pairwise comparisons of the three groups; H+ADHD = hyperactive group that currently has a diagnosis of ADHD at follow-up; H–ADHD = hyperactive group that does not have a diagnosis of ADHD at follow-up. A poor credit rating was categorized as a self-report of a 4 or 5 credit rating (poor or very poor).
    Statistical analysis: Pearson chi-square.

In comparison to the clinic-referred adults with ADHD in the UMASS Study, the percentages here for the H+ADHD group are nearly identical with one exception. That was the larger percentage of the latter group that had not yet begun saving for retirement—a difference that likely arises from the young age of the Milwaukee sample as compared with that used in the UMASS Study. Overall, this is a striking replication of findings across two different methods of ascertaining ADHD in adults, suggesting that the disorder is strongly associated with financial management problems. What the Milwaukee Study adds to this conclusion is that the risks for financial problems are also higher in those who had had ADHD as children, even if their ADHD does not persist fully to age 27.

Those measures of financial status that were dimensional in nature are shown in Table 11.9. Both hyperactive groups were earning less money per month than was the Community control group, yet the groups did not differ from each other in terms of income. While a significant difference among the three groups in the amount they had saved was evident, the pairwise contrasts

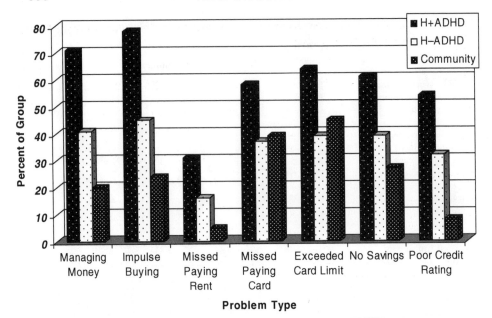

FIGURE 11.4. Percent of each group having various money management problems in the Milwaukee Study. These are the measures on which the H+ADHD group differed significant from the H–ADHD and the Community control groups. H+ADHD = hyperactive group that currently has a diagnosis of ADHD at follow-up; H–ADHD = hyperactive group that does not have a diagnosis of ADHD at follow-up.

were all nonsignificant. It is clear from the means that the hyperactive groups have saved far less than the Community control group, with the H+ADHD group saving the least. The sizable standard deviations across all groups explain the inability of the parametric tests to find significance due to such non-normality of the group distributions.

A better index here of propensity to save is probably the ratio of money currently saved to total annual income, as it controls in part for the greater income being received by the control group, who therefore have the potential to save more. This figure is also shown in Table 11.9 and clearly shows that the two hyperactive groups are saving proportionately less as a function of their annual income than are the control participants (3% vs. 4% vs. 11%, respectively).

The frequency with which various money problems had occurred to these groups did not differ across them except for exceeding their credit limit on their credit cards, which the H+ADHD group seemed to have done more often than the other two groups. The H+ADHD group also reported having a significantly poorer credit rating than both other groups, yet the H–ADHD group also reported a poorer rating than the Community control group. As we did in the

TABLE 11.9. Monthly Income, Savings, and Frequency of Money Management Problems by Group for the Milwaukee Study

Measure	H+ADHD		H–ADHD		Community		F	p	Pairwise contrasts
	Mean	SD	Mean	SD	Mean	SD			
Monthly income ($)	1945	1377	2448	1627	3089	1659	6.74	.001	1,2 < 3
Total savings ($)	1454	2520	2879	5889	6054	11,116	3.08	.049	NS
Savings: salary ratio	.03	.09	.04	.10	.11	.20	6.23	.002	1,2 < 3
Missed rent payment[IQ]	1.6	7.0	0.4	2.0	0.5	0.6	1.69	NS	
Utilities turned off for nonpayment[IQ]	0.8	1.9	0.7	1.5	0.4	0.9	0.88	NS	
Missed credit card payment	4.8	7.7	3.0	8.3	2.5	8.4	1.27	NS	
Exceeded credit limits	3.3	6.2	1.0	2.0	1.5	2.7	5.94	.003	1 > 2,3
Written checks without sufficient funds	5.4	8.8	3.7	6.4	2.8	5.4	2.36	NS	
Credit rating[IQ]	3.3	1.4	2.7	1.3	2.0	1.0	14.60	< .001	1 > 2 > 3
No. of money problems[IQ]	6.8	2.3	4.8	2.3	3.0	2.4	31.78	< .001	1 > 2 > 3

Note. SD = standard deviation; F = F-test results of the analysis of variance (or covariance); p = probability value for the F-test; NS = not significant; H+ADHD = hyperactive group that currently has a diagnosis of ADHD at follow-up; H–ADHD = hyperactive group that does not have a diagnosis of ADHD at follow-up; no. of money problems = total no. of the 13 different categorical money problems reported in next table as occurring at least once. Credit rating was scored on a 1–5 Likert scale, where 1 = excellent, 2 = good, 3 = fair, 4 = poor, and 5 = very poor.

Statistical analysis: Groups were initially compared using one-way (groups) analysis of variance or covariance. Where this analysis was significant (p < .05) for the main effect for group, pairwise comparisons (Student–Newman–Keuls tests) of the groups were conducted, the results of which are shown in the last column. [IQ] = both the Verbal and Performance IQ subtests served as covariates in these analyses. Where this occurred, means for that measure were estimated marginal means given the covariates.

UMASS Study, we created a sum of the number of different money problems experienced by the participants. Here again the persistently ADHD group (H+ADHD) had significantly more such problems than the other two groups, but the H–ADHD group also had more than the Community control group. Such findings suggest that clinic-referred children with ADHD as they develop into adulthood have significantly more financial problems than do Community control children, but the greatest money problems will be found in those children whose ADHD persists to age 27. Those money problem scores for the H+ADHD group are also quite similar to the number of financial problems seen in the UMASS clinic-referred adults with ADHD, again providing some corroboration that the disorder is associated with greater financial difficulties regardless of how adults with ADHD may be ascertained.

Unlike the UMASS Study, we went into detail with the Milwaukee participants on the extent to which they engaged in various gambling activities and the size of their wagers. We did so believing that the impulse control problems experienced by the hyperactive groups might make them more susceptible to the ubiquitous opportunities for gambling now available in the United States. We found little evidence for this hypothesis. The groups did not differ in the percentage that had ever bet money (73–80%), and specifically bet at state lotteries (73–78%), racetracks (25–37%), sports (47–56%), card games (48–67%), and slot machines (71–78%). There was also no difference in how often they played the state lottery, averaging less than four times per year across the groups and $3 to $5 per bet. There also were no group differences in the frequency with which the groups had engaged in racetrack betting, betting on sports, and betting at slot machines or in how much they spent each time, lost in a day, and the largest amount they had ever lost for those activities. They also did not differ in the number of different types of betting activities they had ever engaged in. But the groups differed in how often they had bet at cards (M = 109, 75, and 12; F = 3.92; df = 2/91; p = .023), with only the H+ADHD group differing from the Community control group. The groups also differed in how much they had lost in total at playing cards ($685, $133, and $151, respectively; F = 3.85; df = 2/89, .025), and again it was the H+ADHD group that differed from both the H–ADHD and control groups. So hyperactivity generally and ADHD specifically is not associated with elevated levels of gambling except perhaps for card playing. We should not be surprised at this finding for several reasons. First, the New York follow-up study (Mannuzza et al., 1993, 1998) reported that their hyperactive group was no more likely to be diagnosed with pathological or addictive gambling-related disorders than was the control group. Second, research conducted while this study was under way has found that excessive gambling is related principally to antisocial personality and not to ADHD (Raylu & Oei, 2002).

We therefore divided the entire sample into those who did (N = 40) and did not have current antisocial personality disorder (ASPD, N = 167) according to the SCID interview (see Chapter 8) and compared them on the percentages that had ever engaged in any of our gambling activities. The groups did not differ in whether or not they had bet at the racetrack, at cards, or at slot machines, but significantly more of those having ASPD had bet on sporting events (77% vs. 46%, χ^2 = 9.57, p = .002). Nor did they differ in the frequency with which they engaged in three of these activities (lottery, sports, cards), but those with ASPD played slot machines more often than those who did not (M = 31 vs. 11, p .001). But numerous differences were found in how much they bet each time, their largest bets, and how much they had lost in total to date at these activities. Those with ASPD spend more on state lottery tickets on average, had lost the most in a single bet and in total for this activity, had lost more in total at sporting events, bet more on average when playing cards, had lost the most in a single bet and in total losses for card games; spent more on average playing slot machines; and had lost more in single bets on those machines. These findings confirm earlier studies showing that adults with ADHD are not more prone to gambling than the general population but that those who may have ASPD are more likely to bet on sporting events, play slot machines more often, and bet and lose significantly more amounts of money at most of these activities.

Predicting Financial Problems

We chose to evaluate what set of predictors may have made a significant contribution to the financial problems of our groups. The criterion we selected to predict was the number of money problem areas experienced by participants, described above as the money problem diversity score. We chose this as it provided a single omnibus index of financial problems. We then used regression analysis with the entire sample from the UMASS Study to evaluate a set of potential predictors of this outcome, as shown in Table 11.10. We found that the severity of ADHD symptoms made a significant contribution to this money problem index, but so did the number of childhood CD symptoms retrospectively recalled, though of a much smaller magnitude than the degree of variance explained by ADHD severity. Education, IQ, criminal diversity, and the SCL-90-R scales of depression, anxiety, and hostility made no significant contribution to this index. Thus, ADHD largely accounts for the degree of financial difficulties of these participants, explaining nearly 21% of the variance in the diversity of such problems.

We conducted the same type of analysis for the Milwaukee Study groups. Those results are shown in Table 11.11. We used 13 predictors from childhood, adolescence, and young adulthood (age 21) in the regression analysis of the number of different money problems. Results showed that five predictors were significant and accounted for nearly 24% of the variance. These were severity of childhood hyperactivity, pervasiveness of childhood ADHD and behavior problems, the number of CD symptoms at adolescent follow-up, and the number of ADHD symptoms (self-reported) and years of education at the age-21 follow-up. Such results confirm and further clarify the results of the group comparisons above for this measure. Childhood hyperactivity and its pervasiveness predict current money problems, which is not surprising, as they were used to form these initial groups at childhood entry. But beyond that, the severity of teen CD symptoms and, later, the severity of ADHD symptoms at age 21 make additional contributions. This shows that persistence of ADHD to age 21 is a further predictor of financial problems besides initial childhood disorder, but that CD symptoms may further accentuate that influence. Years of education is not an unexpected predictor, given its link to occupational status and hence income. These results are in keeping with those predictors found for this same outcome in the UMASS Study (ADHD and childhood recalled CD) in finding both ADHD and earlier CD symptoms to be related to extent of current financial problems.

TABLE 11.10. Predicting Significant Financial and Driving Problems in the UMASS Study

Outcome/predictors (step entered)	Beta	R	R^2	$R^2\Delta$	F	p
No. of money problem areas						
(1) No. of ADHD symptoms	.451	.456	.208	.208	45.97	< .001
and age (NS)	−.038					
(2) No. of CD symptoms (childhood)	.101	.466	.217	.009	4.13	.043
NS: education (years), IQ (Shipley), no. of crime types, depression (SCL-90-R), anxiety (SCL-90-R), hostility (SCL-90-R)						
No. of vehicular crashes (self-reported)						
(1) No. of ADHD symptoms*	.190	.243	.059	.059	10.96	< .001
and age	.173					
(2) No. of speeding tickets (self-reported)	.318	.396	.157	.098	40.41	< .001
(3) Credit rating (self-reported)	.173	.427	.182	.025	10.82	.001
(4) Hostility	.158	.442	.195	.013	5.62	.018
NS: education, IQ, no. of CD symptoms, no. of crime types, average no. of alcoholic drinks per week, depression, anxiety						
No. of speeding citations (self-reported)						
(1) No. of ADHD symptoms	.264	.275	.076	.076	14.33	< .001
and age	.109					
(2) No. of crime types (lifetime)	.171	.351	.123	.048	19.02	< .001
(3) No. of CD symptoms (childhood)	.129	.368	.135	.012	4.77	.030
NS: education, IQ, average no. of alcoholic drinks per week, depression, anxiety, hostility, credit rating						
No. of citations on DMV record						
(1) No. of ADHD Symptoms	.192	.243	.059	.059	10.95	< .001
and age*	−.130					
(2) No. of crime types (lifetime)	.252	.337	.113	.055	21.46	< .001
(3) Credit rating (self-reported)	.226	.396	.157	.043	17.93	< .001
(4) Anxiety	−.166	.412	.170	.013	5.39	.021
NS: education, IQ, no. of CD symptoms, average no. of alcoholic drinks per week, depression, hostility						

Note. R = regression coefficient; R^2 = percent of explained variance accounted for by all variables at this step; $R^2\Delta$ = percent of explained variance accounted for by this variable added at this step; F = results of F-test for the equation at this step, p = probability value for the F-test; * = this variable became nonsignificant when other variables were entered in the next step; beta = standardized beta coefficient; NS = not significant; Shipley = Shipley Institute of Living Scale IQ estimate, SCL-90-R = Symptom Checklist-90—Revised T-score; DMV = Department of Motor Vehicles. Credit rating is self-reported as 1 (excellent) to 5 (very poor).
   Statistical analysis: Multiple linear regression using forced entry method at Step 1 and stepwise conditional method at subsequent steps. Used the entire sample (N=353).

TABLE 11.11. Predicting Significant Financial and Driving Problems in the Milwaukee Study

Outcome/predictors (step entered)	Beta	R	R^2	$R^2\Delta$	F	p
No. of money problem areas						
Child WWPARS Hyperactivity (parent)	.178	.388	.150	.150	41.42	< .001
Child HSQ no. of settings (parent)	.097	.407	.166	.015	4.24	.040
Teen no. of CD symptoms (parent)	.113	.431	.186	.020	5.80	.017
Age-21 no. of ADHD symptoms (self)	.154	.463	.214	.028	8.27	.004
Age-21 education in years (self)	−.180	.486	.236	.022	6.76	.010
NS: Child CPRS-R Hyperactivity Index and conduct problems score (parent) and IQ (PPVT); teen no. of ADHD and ODD symptoms (parent); age-21 no. of ADHD symptoms (parent), no. of ODD and CD symptoms (self)						
No. of different driving problems						
Child CPRS-R Hyperactivity Index (parent)	.007	.183	.033	.033	8.08	.005
Teen no. of ADHD symptoms (parent)	.157	.244	.060	.026	6.47	.012
Age-21 education in years (self)	−.181	.291	.085	.025	6.34	.012
NS: Child CPRS-R conduct problems score (parent) and IQ (PPVT); teen no. of ODD and CD symptoms (parent); age-21 no. of ADHD symptoms (self and parent); no. of ODD and CD symptoms (self)						

Note. R = Regression coefficient, R² = percent of explained variance accounted for by all variables at this step, R²Δ = percent of explained variance accounted for by this variable added at this step; F = results of F-test for the equation at this step; p = probability value for the F-test; beta = standardized beta coefficient; NS = not significant.

   Statistical analysis: Multiple linear regression using stepwise entry at each of three entry blocks (child, teen, and age 21). Used the entire sample.

Driving Risks

Weiss and Hechtman (1993) were the first to note an association of hyperactivity in childhood with increased car accidents by adolescence and adulthood. Numerous studies have since documented the greater risk that teens and adults with ADHD have in operating a motor vehicle (Barkley, 2004; Barkley & Cox, 2007). Such studies have focused on teens and adults who have high levels of ADHD symptoms identified in epidemiological samples, in children with ADHD (hyperactivity) followed to adulthood, and in clinic-referred teens and adults with ADHD. These studies indicate that problems with driving are more frequent in all three of these samples. In particular, studies of clinic-referred teens and adults with ADHD show those adults to be more likely to have received citations, especially for speeding, and to receive more such citations, to be more likely to have a vehicular crash, to have more such crashes in which they are at fault, and to be more likely to have their licenses suspended or revoked. These findings were also largely corroborated in the official driving records of these same participants. More recent studies continue to underscore the high risks of driving associated with ADHD in adults (Fried et al., 2006). Adults with ADHD are also more prone to road rage (anger, hostility, and aggression while driving) and to use their vehicles more aggressively when angered or thwarted (Richards, Deffenbacher, Rosen, Barkley, & Rodricks, 2006). As shown in our prior study (Barkley, Murphy, et al., 2002), these difficulties did not appear to be a function of the comorbid conditions likely to be associated with ADHD in adults, such as anxiety, depression, or conduct disorder. Research has also shown that some of the cognitive deficits related to driving performance in adults with ADHD may be more detrimentally affected by alcohol consumption than is the case among normal drivers (Barkley, Murphy, O'Connell, Anderson, & Conner, 2006).

Hampering efforts at treating these driving problems, however, are the findings from a related area of research. Adults with ADHD, like children with ADHD, do not evaluate their own behavior and performance deficits in the same way as do non-ADHD individuals. They may view themselves as functioning better than they actually do in various tasks and major life activities. This is not to say they have an inflated or grandiose view of their functioning or task performance relative to the general population. Instead, they seem to judge themselves as likely to be somewhat above average—the same as would a non-ADHD adult. The difference between those with ADHD and others is the disparity between these self-appraisals and their actual performance, which is often well below normal. This finding was first demonstrated in adults with ADHD by Knouse and colleagues, using driving performance as the task for both self-appraisals and actual functioning (Knouse et al., 2005). Knouse found that adults with ADHD do not judge themselves as being any different in their driving performance than do non-ADHD control adults—both groups tend to judge themselves as being slightly better than average. But the actual driving histories and performance of the adults with ADHD is worse than normal; thus the disparity between their self-appraisals and actual functioning is greater (Knouse et al., 2005). As Knouse noted in her paper, the implication of such a finding is that adults with ADHD are unlikely to recognize their deficient driving and therefore are less likely to engage in any treatment for it. Should that treatment be imposed or coerced upon them, one can readily predict that high rates of noncompliance would occur, given their view that there is nothing wrong and thus no need for a remedy. The first step in engaging treatment is acknowledging that a problem exists which requires treatment, and this is a step that adults with ADHD may be less likely to take.

The UMASS Study Results

The UMASS Study also surveyed participants concerning their driving histories. Where possible and with permission, we obtained their official driving records from the state DMV as well. The mean number of years of driving experience (self-reported) was 18.4 (ADHD: M = 15.7, SD = 10.9; Clinical: M = 21.0, SD = 12.6; Community: M = 19.6, SD = 11.9). The groups differed significantly in this respect (p = .002), with the ADHD group having less experience than the two control groups owing to their somewhat younger age. When age served as a covariate, the groups no longer differed in driving experience. We therefore used age as a covariate in any analysis in which it was found to be significantly correlated with any measure of driving risk. The percentages of each group that had experienced these various adverse events are shown in Table 11.12. We have cast the significant group differences in graphic form in Figure 11.5. As in prior studies, we found that adults with ADHD were more likely to have had their licenses suspended or revoked, to have driven without a valid driver's license, to have crashed while driving, to have been at fault in such a crash, and to have been cited for speeding and even reckless driving compared to the Community control group. De Quiros and Kinsbourne (2001) also found higher self-reported reckless driving in their study of adults with ADHD. These elevated risks were also found in the official DMV records of our participants. Comparisons with our

TABLE 11.12. Driving-Related Adverse Events by Group for the UMASS Study

Measure	ADHD		Clinical		Community		χ^2	p	Pairwise contrasts
	N	%	N	%	N	%			
Self-reported in interview									
License suspended/revoked[S]	53	37	12	13	15	16	23.9	< .001	1 > 2,3
Driven without valid license[S]	44	31	19	21	14	13	11.7	.003	1 > 3
Crashed while driving	130	91	77	84	80	74	12.8	.002	1 > 3
Cited for speeding[S]	122	85	69	75	73	68	11.2	.004	1 > 2,3
Cited for reckless driving[S]	25	17	8	9	1	1	19.1	< .001	1,2 > 3
Cited for driving while intox.[S]	16	11	8	9	4	4	4.6	NS	
At fault or caused a crash[S]	77	54	44	48	32	30	15.1	.001	1,2 > 3
DMV records									
License suspended/revoked[S]	36	29	11	13	10	10	14.9	.001	1 > 2,3
Cited for speeding[S]	70	56	37	44	34	35	10.2	.006	1 > 3
Crashed while driving[S]	44	35	25	30	19	20	6.8	.034	1 > 3
Any DMV citation[S]	98	79	60	71	46	47	25.6	< .001	1,2 > 3

Note. Sample sizes for the comparisons on interview information are ADHD = 142; Clinical control = 92; Community control = 108. For DMV records, sample sizes are ADHD = 124; Clinical control = 84; Community control = 97. N = sample size endorsing this item; % = percent of group endorsing this item; χ^2 = results of the omnibus chi-square test; p = probability value for the chi-square test; pairwise contrasts = results of the chi-square tests involving pairwise comparisons of the three groups; [S] = significant effect of sex on this measure (males more likely than females on all measures); intox. = intoxicated; DMV = Department of Motor Vehicles.

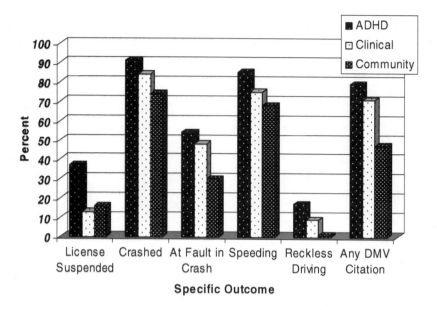

FIGURE 11.5. Percentage of each group experiencing various adverse driving outcomes by self-report and for ever having been cited on the record from the Department of Motor Vehicles (DMV) for the UMASS Study.

Clinical control group may help to show which driving risks were specific to ADHD. There we found that the ADHD group was more likely to have their license suspended/revoked and to have been cited for speeding. But it should also be borne in mind that even the Clinical control group was more prone to inattention than the Community group (Chapter 3) and that inattention has been found in studies of epidemiological samples (Barkley & Cox, 2007) to elevate the risk for various adverse driving outcomes. One would therefore expect our Clinical control group to have had more driving problems than the Community control group, which was found to be the case for reckless driving, being at fault in a crash, and having any citations on their DMV records.

Some sex differences were evident in these comparisons of self-reports, but not on the DMV measures. In all cases of sex differences, males suffered these adverse events more than females. Within the ADHD group, males were more likely to self-report having their licenses suspended, to have driven without a valid license, to have been cited for speeding and reckless driving, and to be at fault in a crash. On DMV records, males were more likely to have license suspensions and to have at least one DMV entry. Within the Clinical controls, males self-reported only more license suspensions. For the Community control group, males had more license suspensions and were more likely to be cited for speeding based on self-reported information. Thus, it would seem that adult males with ADHD have a greater likelihood of experiencing these adverse driving outcomes than any other group.

Again, the issue of medication status at study entry needs to be examined. Evidence shows that taking stimulants has a beneficial effect on driving (Barkley & Cox, 2007), as does taking atomoxetine (Barkley, Anderson, & Kruesi, 2007). Therefore we compared those participants on medication at the time of study entry to those off medication in the ADHD group on the above self-reported categorical measures. There were no significant differences. Then we did the same for the Clinical control group. Again there were no differences. This tells us that the above findings on driving are not a consequence of medication status. We repeated this same procedure for the DMV categorical outcomes. Here we did find that the ADHD participants on medication were *more* likely to have had a speeding ticket than those off medication (72% vs. 50%, $p = .023$). No other measures were significant. No differences were significant when we made this same comparison within the clinical controls. Given this difference for speeding in adults with ADHD, we reanalyzed that measure for any group differences after removing those on medication at study entry. The originally significant difference on this DMV measure was no longer significant. This suggests that the group difference on likelihood of ever having gotten a speeding ticket as recorded on the DMV record was accounted for mainly by the medicated subset of ADHD participants. Yet this was not the case for any of the other self-reported or DMV-recorded driving problems.

We also studied the frequency with which our participants had experienced these various driving outcomes. Those findings are shown in Table 11.13. Those group differences which were significant are graphed in Figure 11.6. For self-reported events, reckless driving and driving under the influence (DUI) citations were not analyzed, given the very low frequency in the two control groups. Of the nine frequency measures reported here, the ADHD group reported significantly more such adverse events on six of these outcomes and in each case differed significantly from both of the control groups, which did not differ from each other. Specifically, adults with ADHD had more license suspensions/revocations, more crashes, more speeding citations, and were held to be at fault in more such crashes than either the Clinical or Community control adults were. On the DMV record, the adults with ADHD again had more speeding citations and more total citations. Here, crash frequency did not differ, but as others have noted (Arthur et al., 2001; see sidebar), DMV records are not likely to be the more objective or more accurate method of recording driving risks. In any case, these findings once again agree with the results of previous studies of driving in showing clinic-referred adults with ADHD to have more specific elevated risks for various adverse driving outcomes than do other adults. These problems are seen at all theoretical levels of driving, including basic cognitive functions, such

TABLE 11.13. Frequency of Adverse Driving Events for Each Group for the UMASS Study

Measure	ADHD		Clinical		Community		F	p	Pairwise contrasts
	Mean	SD	Mean	SD	Mean	SD			
Self-reported									
License suspended or revoked[S,GxS]	0.8	1.4	0.2	0.8	0.2	0.5	6.9	.001	1 > 2,3
Driven without valid license[S]	48.1	220.6	33.6	120.1	0.3	0.9	1.7	NS	
Crashes[A]	3.1	3.5	2.2	1.7	2.2	2.3	5.1	.006	1 > 2,3
Speeding citations[S]	6.1	7.9	3.5	5.7	2.2	5.1	7.3	.001	1 > 2,3
Crashes at fault	1.2	1.8	0.8	1.2	0.5	1.1	4.3	.014	1 > 2,3
From DMV records									
License suspended/revoked[A,S]	0.8	1.8	0.3	1.0	0.3	1.3	1.8	NS	
Speeding citations[S]	1.6	2.2	0.7	1.2	0.7	1.2	6.1	.003	1 > 2,3
Crashes	0.6	0.9	0.4	0.7	0.3	0.7	2.8	NS	
Total citations[A,S]	4.4	6.1	2.2	2.9	1.7	3.3	5.33	.005	1 > 2,3

Note. Sample sizes for self-reports are ADHD = 142, Clinical control = 92; Community control = 108. For DMV records they were ADHD = 124; Clinical control = 84; Community control = 97. *SD* = standard deviation; *F* = *F*-test results of the analysis of variance (or covariance); *p* = probability value for the *F*-test; NS = not significant; [S] = significant main effect for sex; [GxS] = significant group × sex interaction (see text for details); [A] = age used as a covariate in this analysis.

Statistical analysis: Groups were initially compared using two way (group × sex) analysis of variance (or covariance as necessary). Where this analysis was significant ($p < .05$) for the main effect for group, pairwise comparisons of the groups were conducted, the results of which are shown in the last column.

as reaction time, attention, inhibition, and motor coordination; tactical operation of the vehicle, such as steering, braking, turn signal use, speed; and strategic operation, such as negotiating the vehicle in traffic and the goals for which the vehicle is being used (Barkley, 2004; Barkley & Cox, 2007).

A few sex differences were detected on these measures. The significant main effect for sex and the group by sex interaction found on license suspensions is shown in Figure 11.7. This graph shows that males were more likely to experience this outcome than females, with the greatest sex difference being in the ADHD group. In other words, females in all groups had a lower and comparable level of these events across groups. Males, especially those with ADHD, are more likely to experience this adverse event. The significant sex difference on driving without a valid license showed that males had a greater frequency than females (M = 49 vs. 15). The difference on speeding showed a greater frequency for males than for females as well (5.7 vs. 2.2).

As before, the possible biasing effect of medication treatment at study entry requires some examination here. We compared those on and off medication within the ADHD group and again within the Clinical control group on these self-reported frequency measures. No significant differences were evident for either group. Thus medication status does not seem to have biased these results.

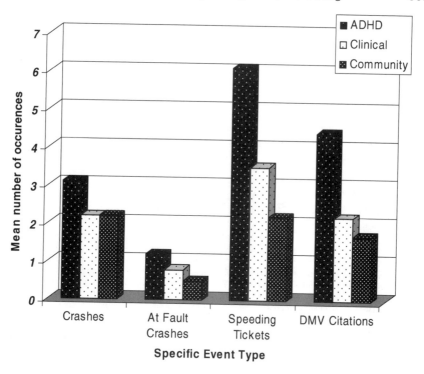

FIGURE 11.6. Mean frequency of various adverse driving events by group in the UMASS Study. Adults with ADHD had significantly more of these adverse events than the two control groups.

However, on the DMV frequency measures, we found that those with ADHD on medication had significantly more speeding tickets (2.5 vs. 1.2, $p = .005$) and total DMV citations (6.7 vs. 3.5, $p = .006$) and marginally more accidents (0.8 vs. 0.5, $p = .083$) than those not on medication. No such differences were found in the Clinical control group. Nevertheless, the difference within the ADHD group led us to reanalyze these measures, removing all participants who had been on medication at the time of study entry. The findings for license suspensions and crashes remained nonsignificant, as before. The findings for speeding and total citations remained significant, as before, and the post hoc pairwise contrast patterns were the same. So, the initial group differences are not likely to be due to medication status.

As a point of interest, given the beneficial effects of stimulants on driving performance (Barkley & Cox, 2007), we compared those on and off stimulants at study entry on the frequency of their DMV driving problems, outlined above. To our surprise, those taking stimulants had dramatically more speeding tickets

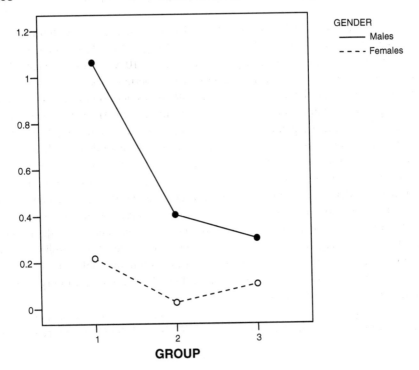

FIGURE 11.7. Frequency of license suspensions and revocations (self-reported) for each sex within each group, depicting the significant group × sex interaction for this measure in the UMASS Study.

(4.1 vs. 1.4) and total citations (11.7 vs. 3.9) (both $p < .001$). We also did the same for the driving events self-reported above. Only one difference emerged, and that was on license suspensions, where treated participants had significantly more suspensions than those who were not treated (1.7 vs. 0.7, $p = .023$). This certainly does not mean stimulants do not improve driving, as these measures are historical and cumulative and are not events going forward in time from when treatment was initiated. It is certainly possible that such driving risks actually resulted in these people being treated with stimulants by their treating clinicians. This finding was not observed among the Clinical controls, where all comparisons of stimulant-treated versus untreated were not significant.

The Milwaukee Study Results

We did not conduct as detailed an analysis of driving problems in the Milwaukee Study, given that we had done so at the age-21 follow-up (Fischer, Barkley,

Smallish, & Fletcher, 2007). But we did collect the same interview information as we had done above in the UMASS Study. Our groups did not differ in their years of driving experience, having approximately 10 years on average. The results for the percentage of each group that had experienced the various adverse driving outcomes are shown in Table 11.14. We focus here on just those types of driving problems found to be elevated in association with ADHD in prior studies. We found the frequencies of these adverse events to be highly skewed because some members of the hyperactive groups were outliers with extreme scores. These nonnormal distributions posed problems for doing parametric analyses of these frequency measures. Therefore, instead of analyzing the frequency measures, we determined the score that was at or above the 75th percentile for the Community control group on the measures of license suspensions, speeding, reckless driving, driving while intoxicated, and crash frequency. We then computed the percentage of each group that met or exceeded this threshold. The group comparisons on these measures are also shown in Table 11.14. Those measures on which the hyperactive groups differed from the Community control group are portrayed in Figure 11.8.

More members of the hyperactive groups were likely to have experienced many of these adverse outcomes than were members of the Community control

TABLE 11.14. Adverse Categorical Driving Outcomes for Each Group in the Milwaukee Study

Measures	H+ADHD N	H+ADHD %	H–ADHD N	H–ADHD %	Community N	Community %	χ^2	p	Pairwise contrasts
Currently have a license	42	76	65	81	72	96	11.36	.003	1,2 < 3
License suspended/revoked	30	57	45	57	27	36	7.84	.020	1,2 > 3
License suspended/revoked 2+	19	34	25	31	12	16	6.97	.031	1,2 > 3
Drove without a valid license	31	57	51	64	26	35	14.07	.001	1,2 > 3
Cited for speeding	45	83	62	77	60	81	0.73	NS	
Cited for speeding 5+	15	27	17	21	20	27	0.86	NS	
Cited for reckless driving	17	31	7	9	10	13	12.50	.002	1 > 2,3
Cited for reckless driving 2+	6	11	2	2	2	3	6.21	.045	1 > 2,3
Cited for driving intoxicated	6	11	11	14	12	16	0.68	NS	
Cited for driving intoxicated 2+	3	5	2	2	7	9	3.36	NS	
Involved in a crash	30	54	42	52	28	37	5.00	NS	
Involved in 2+ crashes	16	29	16	20	5	7	11.50	.003	1,2 > 3
If crashed, judged at fault	14	47	22	52	13	46	0.33	NS	
If crashed, did you hit and run?	4	13	3	7	2	7	0.98	NS	

Note. Sample sizes for these comparisons are H+ADHD = 54, H–ADHD = 80, and Community control = 74. N = sample size endorsing this item; % = percent of group endorsing this item; χ^2 = results of the omnibus chi-square test; p = probability value for the chi-square test; pairwise contrasts = results of the chi-square tests involving pairwise comparisons of the three groups; H+ADHD = hyperactive group that currently has a diagnosis of ADHD at follow-up; H–ADHD = hyperactive group that does not have a diagnosis of ADHD at follow-up.
Statistical analysis: Pearson chi-square.

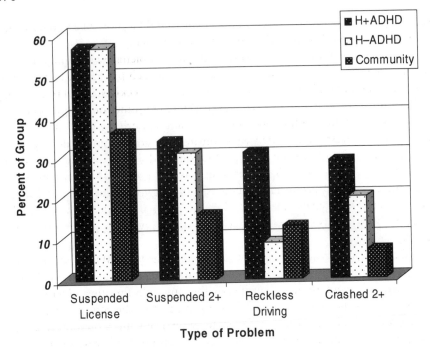

FIGURE 11.8. Percentage of each group in the Milwaukee Study experiencing various adverse driving events. 2+ = event happened two or more times; H+ADHD = hyperactive group that currently has a diagnosis of ADHD at follow-up; H–ADHD = hyperactive group that does not have a diagnosis of ADHD at follow-up.

group, thus replicating and extending our results from the age-21 follow-up. Fewer members of the hyperactive groups were likely to have a current license, probably owing to the fact that more members of both groups had their licenses suspended or revoked at some time in the driving careers. More of them were also likely to have had their licenses suspended at least two or more times. Although the groups did not differ in the percentage that had ever had a crash in their driving history, more of both hyperactive groups had been involved in at least two or more such crashes. Of interest was the finding that more than twice as many of the H+ADHD group had been cited for reckless driving than those in the other two groups, and more of them had been cited at least two or more times for this infraction. Contrary to the UMASS Study, we did not find a greater proportion of the hyperactive groups to have been cited for speeding, nor did we find them to have a higher frequency of that type of citation. Where driving risks are found, as in crashes and license revocations, it is growing up as a child with ADHD that appears to be the risk factor here, regardless of its persis-

tence to this present follow-up. But persistent ADHD is more likely to be associated with reckless driving and its repeated occurrence.

We created an omnibus measure of driving problems by summing the total
number out of the 13 outcomes we measured that each participant had reported
experiencing: suspensions, no valid license, speeding, reckless, illegal turns, illegal
right of way, not stopping, expired tags, parking, tailgating, other violations, and
accidents. This reflected the total number of different driving problems they had
experienced at least once. When we compared the groups on this driving problems score, we found that the H+ADHD group had significantly more problems
(M = 5.2, SD = 2.7) than the Community control group (M = 3.8, SD = 2.4),
with the H–ADHD group falling between these two groups and not differing
from either of them (M = 4.6, SD = 2.3; F = 5.28, df = 2/205, p = .006). Thus
it seems that it is persistent ADHD that is associated with the greater diversity of
driving problems.

Compared to the UMASS clinic-referred adults with ADHD, the hyperactive groups in this study had a lower percentage experiencing crashes (54% vs.
91%), but they were found to have nearly the same risks for other adverse driving
events, such as speeding (83% vs. 85%). Again, part of the reason the groups in
the Milwaukee Study were not found to differ from the Community control
group was the relatively high percentage in that group also having some of these
adverse events compared to Community control adults in the UMASS Study.

Predicting Adverse Driving Outcomes

As with other domains of impairment that we found to be specific to ADHD in
prior chapters and above for money management problems, we wished to see
what other factors besides ADHD may have contributed to the driving outcomes
that were rather specific to the ADHD group. To do so, we chose three outcomes for this examination, these being the number of vehicular crashes (self-
reported), the number of speeding citations (self-reported), and the total number
of citations from the DMV record. We chose a set of 12 possible predictors to
study using multiple regression analyses. Although most of these predictors are
obvious ones for study, a person's credit rating may not seem as if it is related to
driving problems. But it is routine for auto insurers in the United States to
request a person's credit rating as part of their determination of an individual's
driving risk, given actuarial evidence that they are related to each other. The
results of these analyses appear in Table 11.10.

The best predictors for the number of self-reported crashes were severity of
ADHD, older age, the number of self-reported speeding tickets one had
received, a poorer credit rating (self-reported), and higher levels of hostility. Our
results corroborate the findings of auto insurance companies that one's credit rat-

ing, even if self-reported, has a significant relationship with risk for auto crashes. Severity of ADHD is an understandable predictor, given that driver inattention is among the most common causes of auto crashes, as noted above. Age has a small but significant relationship, most likely because the older one is, the more likely it is that he or she will have experienced a vehicular crash due to increasing miles driven with increasing age. And certainly the extent of one's history of speeding citations is a sensible predictor, given the known relationship between propensity for speeding and risk of vehicular crashes (see above). Greater hostility is likely predictive of crash risk due to its probable association with road rage. Education, IQ, childhood CD severity, lifetime criminal diversity, weekly alcohol consumption, depression, and anxiety were not related to this outcome.

The number of speeding citations was predicted by severity of ADHD, older age, diversity of criminal activities, and severity of childhood CD symptoms. Again, these predictors make some sense. The inattentive and especially impulsive behavior associated with ADHD is understandably related to speeding citations, given that we found excessive speeding with a vehicle to be among the best symptoms for predicting ADHD in adults (Chapter 7). And given that speeding is a form of law violation, the relationship of criminal behavior and childhood conduct problems to this driving outcome is likewise understandable, as both reflect a propensity to break rules and laws of social conduct. Education, IQ, frequency of weekly alcohol use, depression, anxiety, hostility, and one's credit rating were not related to this specific outcome.

The total number of citations on the DMV record was again predicted by severity of ADHD, but it was also predicted by younger age, criminal diversity, a poorer credit rating, and lower anxiety levels. Once more, a poorer credit score appears to predict driving citation risk on the DMV records, just as it did for crash risk. The other predictors are sensible ones given that impulsiveness, youth, a propensity for rule violations, low anxiety (e.g., fearlessness), and irresponsibility (money management) would all seem to have some relationship to one's risk of violating driving laws.

For the Milwaukee Study, we explored possible child, teen, and young adult predictors that might potentially be related to the diversity of driving problems scores. Given so few differences between those groups in driving problems, we chose to focus on just this omnibus indicator of driving problems. The results for this analysis are shown in Table 11.11. Just three predictors were significant and accounted for only 8% of the variance in this omnibus driving problems score. Those predictors were severity of childhood hyperactivity (CPRS-R), severity of teen ADHD, and years of education received by age 21. It therefore appears to be persistence of ADHD from childhood through adolescence that is chiefly associated with the diversity of driving problems by age 27—findings consistent with those found for the UMASS Study of clinic-referred adults with ADHD.

Conclusions and Clinical Implications

This chapter concentrated on several domains of adaptive functioning or major life activities for adults with ADHD, many of which had not been previously studied. These domains include risks associated with health and lifestyle, problems with money management, and driving-related adverse events.

✓ The diminished regard for the future consequences of one's behavior that characterizes many adolescents and adults with ADHD led us to predict a reduced concern for health-conscious behavior, such as exercise, proper diet, and moderation in using legal substances (caffeine, tobacco, and alcohol) throughout life, with associated greater health and safety concerns in these various lifestyle areas. That is precisely what we were able to document.

✓ A higher percentage of the adults with ADHD in the UMASS Study reported problems in sleep, social relationships, family interactions, tobacco use, nonmedical drug use, medical/dental care, motor vehicle safety, work and leisure, and emotional health than did the Community control group. But illicit drug use, driving, and emotional health are areas in which adults with ADHD differed specifically from other clinic-referred adults who do not have ADHD.

✓ The Milwaukee Study found similar though not identical elevations in lifestyle and health risks, with eating habits, sleep, social relations, tobacco use, nonmedical drug use, and emotional health also being concerns for a significantly greater percentage of those hyperactive children having persistent ADHD to age 27 (H+ADHD group) compared to the Community control group. But even those hyperactive children whose ADHD did not persist to adulthood had more members reporting concerns about sleep and tobacco use than the Community control group.

✓ All of this suggests a less healthy lifestyle in adults with ADHD, whether clinic-referred or children grown up, that could have implications for their later risks for cancer and cardiovascular disease, accidental injury and death, and possibly a shorter life expectancy as a consequence. Several of these hypotheses were further supported in the Milwaukee Study, in which the hyperactive group had a significantly greater risk for injury, nonsurgical hospitalizations, and poisonings and experienced more such events than the Community control group. We also identified a slight but significantly higher risk lipid profile and a greater risk for coronary heart disease (CHD) over the next 5 and 10 years, mainly for the H+ADHD group compared to the Community control group. That group also reported less regular exercise than the other groups, while both hyperactive groups were more likely to be smokers and consumers of alcohol than the Community control group. If such trends continue over the next decade, it will become more evident that individuals with persistent ADHD into adulthood carry a higher risk of future heart disease (and possibly cancer) than the general population.

✓ The Milwaukee Study conducted a more detailed medical history of its participants and found a significantly greater number of current health complaints in the H+ADHD group relative to the H–ADHD group, but they also had more such complaints than the Community control group. We found such complaints to be significantly associated with elevated levels of somatization, depression, and phobic anxiety, implying that they may be more indicative of psychiatric rather than medical problems. Females with persistent ADHD had more such complaints than males in that group and than males and females in the nonpersistent ADHD group, who did not differ, intimating that females with ADHD may carry an elevated risk for psychosomatic complaints.

✓ The Milwaukee Study was also able to show that taking stimulant medication in childhood and the duration of that treatment had no significant impact on adult height, weight, or body mass index, indicating no long-term adverse effects of these ADHD medications on these physical parameters.

✓ The adults with ADHD reported problems in 8 of the 12 areas of money management we surveyed to a greater extent than did the adults in the Community control group. The ADHD group had a higher proportion of its members reporting problems with managing money, saving money, buying on impulse, nonpayment for utilities—resulting in their termination, missing loan payments, exceeding credit card limits, having a poor credit rating, and not saving for retirement. Relative to the normal control group, the adults with ADHD appeared to be having relatively pervasive problems with the management of their finances.

✓ Four areas of money management were specifically more elevated in the ADHD group than in either the Clinical or Community control groups, these having to do with deferred gratification (saving and putting money away for retirement), impulse buying, and meeting financial deadlines (nonpayment of utilities resulting in their termination).

✓ On all six frequency measures of money management, the adults with ADHD reported more difficulties more often than did the adults in our Community control group. Money difficulties were also more common in the ADHD than in the Clinical control group in at least four of these six areas, those being missing rent payments, missing utility payments, missing loan payments and having more total money problems.

✓ The Milwaukee Study also documented numerous financial problems associated with the hyperactive group, though these were the most common in that group whose ADHD had persisted until age 27. Thus, both the UMASS and Milwaukee Studies have found a clear, robust, and specific relationship of adult ADHD to a diversity of financial problems, regardless of how adult ADHD patients were ascertained (clinic-referred or children followed to adulthood).

✓ Driving problems have been reported in many previous studies of clinic-referred adults as well as in children with ADHD followed to adulthood and even in epidemiologically derived community samples having elevated symptoms of inattention or ADHD. These studies indicate a variety of increased risks associated with ADHD and related to driving. Our findings in the UMASS Study were similar, especially with regard to clinic-referred adults. Such risks do not seem to be due to the common comorbid disorders associated with ADHD.

✓ Clinic-referred adults with ADHD were more likely to have had their licenses suspended or revoked, to have driven without a valid drivers' license, to have crashed while driving, to have been at fault in such a crash, and to have been cited for speeding and even reckless driving compared to the Community control group. Several of these risks were also documented on official DMV records. The ADHD group also had more license suspensions/revocations, more crashes, more speeding citations, and were held to be at fault in more such crashes than either the Clinical or Community control adults. On the DMV record, the adults with ADHD again had more speeding citations and more total citations.

✓ The Milwaukee Study found similar though less robust differences between the hyperactive and control groups, perhaps in part because they were younger and had less driving experience than adults in the UMASS Study. But as in the UMASS Study, children who were hyperactive experienced a higher risk for frequent crashes, a greater risk for reckless driving and more citations for such driving, and a greater risk for license suspensions and revocations.

✓ We also found that these driving risks were associated not only with the severity of ADHD, but also with other factors such as age, more diverse criminal activity, poorer credit ratings, greater hostility (e.g., road rage), and low levels of anxiety (e.g., fearlessness), depending upon the driving outcome being predicted.

✓ Our findings certainly add to the considerable and growing body of evidence that ADHD is associated with substantially elevated driving risks (Barkley & Cox, 2007). Fortunately, recent studies have also shown that driving performance can be improved by stimulants and by atomoxetine (Barkley, Anderson, & Kruesi, 2007; Barkley & Cox, 2007). The driving performance problems noted in adults with ADHD may be made differentially worse by the consumption of alcohol.

✓ Apart from their obvious focus on ADHD and comorbid psychiatric disorders, clinicians need to pay more attention to the health and lifestyle risks likely to be present in adults diagnosed with ADHD. Primary care clinicians in particular need to be better trained to recognize ADHD in adults as a significant risk factor leading to lifestyles and health behavior choices that place individuals at greater risk for later CHD. These health and lifestyle risks will likely increase the need for various medical management and health improvement measures beyond just those interventions aimed at the management of ADHD itself. They are also likely to warrant referral to other medical and health professionals who are expert in the management of these health risk and lifestyle problem areas, such as smoking cessation programs, dietary management, and exercise regimens.

✓ Clinicians may also need to become aware of community resources, such as banks or credit unions, that help address the money management problems likely to exist in the adaptive functioning of adults with ADHD. Debt reorganization, credit counseling, budgeting advice, cognitive-behavioral treatments for impulse buying, and the like, may be needed for some adults with ADHD. Although there is no research on the issue, it is likely that ADHD medications may be as helpful in improving the money management problems of adults with the disorder as they have proven to be in other areas of symptom management and adaptive functioning.

✓ It is also crucial that clinicians recognize the increased driving risks associated with ADHD in adults and the hazards they pose to themselves and others by their driving impairments. These appear to be treatable risks that likely respond to the common ADHD medications currently recommended for adults and children with the disorder (stimulants and atomoxetine). What may be needed, however, is greater attention to the timing of when these adults are likely to drive to ensure that adequate levels of medication are in use to address their driving risks at those hours, such as late-night driving, when earlier doses, even of extended-release compounds, may be dissipating.

✓ Clinicians are likely to become embroiled in legal proceedings that may be related to these increased driving problems and should either be prepared to do so or to refer these adults to other professionals having greater expertise in serving as expert witnesses in such proceedings. Fortunately, the driving performance of adults with ADHD has been shown to improve with medication management, at least those aspects of poor driving likely to derive from ADHD itself.

CHAPTER 12

Sex, Dating and Marriage, Parenting, and Psychological Adjustment of Offspring

Previous chapters have demonstrated a greater likelihood of deficits in self-regulation and EF, psychiatric comorbidity, educational and occupational difficulties, psychological maladjustment, antisocial activities and drug use, and other adaptive impairments (driving, money management, and unhealthy lifestyles) in adults with ADHD, whether ascertained through clinic referrals or through following children to adulthood. One should not be surprised to find, therefore, that such factors—along with the very symptoms of ADHD itself—would have an adverse impact on dating relationships, marriages, or cohabiting relationships, parenting of offspring, and even offspring psychological adjustment. Indeed, given the high genetic contribution to ADHD (Barkley, 2006; Nigg, 2006), one would expect to find a higher incidence of ADHD among the biological offspring of adults with ADHD (Biederman et al., 1992; Faraone & Doyle, 2001; Minde et al., 2003). This would also be expected to further adversely affect parenting behavior and even marital adjustment even if the parent did not have ADHD (Fischer, 1990; Harvey, 1998; Johnston & Mash, 2001).

Sexual Activity

Little research exists on the dating and sexual activities of adults with ADHD, using either clinic-referred adults or in studies of children growing up. Barkley and Fischer were the first to report a pattern of early initiation (1 year earlier on average) and riskier sexual activity (more partners, less use of contraception) in their hyperactive group by the young adult follow-up (age 21) of the Milwaukee groups (Barkley, Fischer et al., 2006). This riskier pattern of conduct led to a markedly increased risk for teen pregnancy (38% vs. 4%) and sexually transmitted diseases (STDs) (17% vs. 4%) among the hyperactive as compared with the control group. More recently, others have demonstrated a similar pattern of sexual conduct in young male adults with a history of childhood ADHD (Flory, Molina, Pelham, Gnagy, & Smith, 2006) in which childhood ADHD was associated with earlier initiation of sexual activity and intercourse, more sexual partners, more casual sex, and more partner pregnancies. Both longitudinal studies found that these risks were further elevated by higher levels of conduct problems, but such problems did not account for the separate contribution made by ADHD.

We did not examine these areas of sexual activity in the UMASS Study of clinic-referred adults. However, we continued to collect detailed interview information about these domains at the age-27 follow-up of the Milwaukee Study groups. As noted above, the hyperactive group had already engaged in far higher rates of risky sexual behavior and had more members with teen parenthood and STDs. We asked first about sexual orientation. The groups differed slightly but significantly in the percentage identifying themselves as heterosexual (93%, 99%, 99%), with somewhat more of the H+ADHD group identifying themselves as bisexual (7% vs. 1% and 0%) but not as homosexual (0%, 0%, 1%) ($\chi^2 = 9.69$, $p = .046$). The groups did not differ in the percentages experiencing any of the sexual problems we reviewed, such as premature ejaculation or impotence in males or in inability to climax, exhibitionism, cross dressing, or voyeurism. They did differ in the proportion reporting having a lack of sexual desire at least sometimes or more often (49% vs. 25% and 24%) ($\chi^2 = 19.73$, $p = .003$), with the persistently ADHD group (H+ADHD) having a higher percentage with such difficulty than the other two groups. All but one of the 210 participants had experienced sexual intercourse by this follow-up. We had earlier reported that the hyperactive group had started having sexual intercourse about a year earlier, on average, than our control group (15 vs. 16) (Barkley et al., 2006). The groups did not differ in the percentage currently using birth control during sex (31%, 27%, and 24%) or in those who used it often or nearly always (51%, 53%, and 50%). But the groups differed in the number of lifetime sex partners, with the H+ADHD group ($M = 17$, $SD = 22$) having more such partners than the control group ($M = 8$, $SD = 9$) but not differing from the H–ADHD group ($M = 13$, $SD = 19$; $F = 4.15$, $df = 2/204$, $p = .017$). We reexamined this finding to see if gender was a significant factor, and it was not. The groups did not differ in the number of sex partners they had had during the past year (one to two), or in the frequency of intercourse in the past year (about monthly).

At this follow-up, the groups did not differ in the percentage reporting ever having had a STD (16%, 16%, and 8%), remaining at about the same proportion in the hyperactive groups as they did at age 21. But group differences were found in how many had ever been tested for HIV (73%, 67%, and 44%) ($\chi^2 = 13.39$, $p = .001$) with more members of both hyperactive groups having been so tested than the controls. Fortunately only one participant tested positive (H+ADHD group). Even so, this suggests that the hyperactive groups have continued to lead riskier sexual lives than the Community control group over this follow-up period. IQ was significantly related to both the number of STDs they had contracted in their lives ($r = -.54$) and their frequency of HIV testing ($r = -.20$) if they had ever had an STD or been tested for HIV. It therefore served as a covariate in the analysis of these frequencies. Among this small subset of participants having a STD, the groups did not differ in their frequency (1.1 to 1.8 times). This was also true for the frequency of HIV testing ($M = 2$–3 times).

Several measures of parenthood are shown in Table 12.1. It is obvious in this table that the pattern found at age 21 has continued—significantly more members of both hyperactive groups have either gotten pregnant in the case of females or gotten someone else pregnant in the case of males. The percentages here are more than triple those of the Community control group. Note that the representation of females is quite low in our study, so the finding is not consid-

TABLE 12.1. Marital, Dating, and Parental Status by Group for the Milwaukee Study

Measures	H+ADHD N	H+ADHD %	H–ADHD N	H–ADHD %	Community N	Community %	χ^2	p	Pairwise contrasts
Marital status									
Single	37	67	52	65	41	55	4.58	NS	
Married	16	29	26	32	32	43			
Divorced or separated	2	4	2	3	2	3			
Marital quality fair–poor	6	35	1	4	3	9	9.55	.008	1 > 2,3
Had an extramarital affair	5	28	1	4	2	6	8.25	.016	1 > 2,3
If single, dating someone now	24	62	36	65	24	50	2.66	NS	
Dating quality fair–terrible	10	42	12	33	2	8	7.65	.022	1,2 > 3
Have biological children	28	51	37	46	10	13	25.76	< .001	1,2 > 3
Live with biological children	20	71	25	68	8	80	0.60	NS	
Females: Ever pregnant?	7	78	10	100	1	20	11.44	.003	1,2 > 3
Males: Got someone pregnant?	33	72	35	51	16	23	28.01	< .001	1 > 2 > 3

Note. Sample sizes for the comparisons on interview information are H+ADHD = 55, H–ADHD = 80, Community control = 75. N = sample size endorsing this item; % = percent of group endorsing this item; χ^2 = results of the omnibus chi-square test; p = probability value for the chi-square test; pairwise contrasts = results of the chi-square tests involving pairwise comparisons of the three groups; H+ADHD = hyperactive group that currently has a diagnosis of ADHD at follow-up; H–ADHD = hyperactive group that does not have a diagnosis of ADHD at follow-up. Marital quality was rated as 1 = excellent, 2 = good, 3 = fair, and 4 = poor, while dating quality used this same Likert scale but with a 5 = terrible, or about to break up.

Statistical analysis: Pearson chi-square.

ered very reliable until replicated; however, it suggests a high rate of early pregnancy among both hyperactive groups, both for females and males. For the hyperactive females, the average number of pregnancies was 2.5 to 2.7; for the single pregnant control female, there was only one. The difference is not significant because one cannot use a parametric test with just one control subject. For the males, it was 2.3, 1.9, and 1.6 for those who had ever gotten someone pregnant, suggesting a similar trend, although this was not significant (owing to large SDs of 1.5, 1.4, and 0.7). Not surprisingly, more members of the hyperactive groups are the biological parents of offspring than is the case for the control group. The H+ADHD group, however, had more children ($M = 1.1$, $SD = 1.4$) than the H–ADHD group ($M = 0.8$, $SD = 1.0$), who have had more children than the control group ($M = 0.2$, $SD = 0.6$) ($F = 13.60$, $df = 2/297$, $p < .001$). Thus, degree of ADHD is clearly related to not just early parenthood but to having more children as well. The groups did not differ in the percentages who were currently residing with their children.

This pattern of being younger parents than average in the hyperactive groups was also found in their parents at childhood study entry. Then we found that the ages of the mothers of the hyperactive children were significantly younger ($M = 31.2$, $SD = 5.4$) than the mothers of the control children ($M = 34.2$, $SD = 4.7$; $F = 16.54$, $p < .001$), which was also true for their fathers hyperactive $M = 33.7$, $SD = 6.2$, control $M = 36.1$, $SD = 4.6$; $F = 8.46$, $p = .004$). This pattern was evident in the parents of both the hyperactive group whose ADHD had not persisted to age 27 and the group with persistent ADHD (mothers' ages $M = 30.4$ vs. 31.5; fathers' ages $M = 33.2$ vs. 34.1).

Dating and Marriage

Longitudinal studies of children with ADHD followed to young adulthood have not typically reported differing rates of marriage, separation, or divorce (Weiss & Hechtman, 1993), most likely owing to the relatively young age of the children at adult follow-up (typically 20–30 years of age). In the Weiss and Hechtman (1993) study, just 29% of their participants were married at the young adult follow-up (mean age = 25 years). As is evident in Table 12.1, we also did not find any group differences in the percentages of our groups who were currently married or separated/divorced. The majority of all groups were still single at this follow-up (55%–67%). It is therefore possible that the lack of differences among the groups in divorce rates is simply the result of the relatively young age of these groups and their low likelihood of marriage for now. That marital difficulties are in the offing for the hyperactive group with persistent ADHD (H+ADHD) is evident in the self-reported quality of their current marital relationship, if married, and in the proportions having extramarital affairs (see Table 12.1), both of which are markedly higher than in the H–ADHD and Community control groups. We found no differences in the percentage of our groups who were currently dating someone if they were currently unmarried. Nor did we find any differences in the number of people they had dated in the past 5 years (two), in the average length of that dating relationship (3 years), or in the longest time they had dated someone continuously (3.5 years). But both hyperactive groups had a higher percentage reporting fair to poor quality in their dating relationships, being four to five times higher than the percentage in the Community control group.

That ADHD in adults might eventually be associated with higher percentages of separation and divorce has been suggested in other studies. Using an older sample of adults, Biederman and associates (Biederman et al., 1993) were among the first to report a higher incidence of separation and divorce among adults with ADHD, whether clinic-referred and diagnosed (28%) or as nonreferred adult relatives of children with ADHD who subsequently met criteria for disorder in a research study (36%). Murphy and Barkley (1996), also using an older sample than in the Milwaukee Study, replicated these marital risks in a large study of clinic-referred adults in comparison to a clinical control group of adults without ADHD seen at the same clinic. They also found a marginally significant reduction in self-reported marital satisfaction on the Locke–Wallace Marital Adjustment Test ($p < .08$) and lower but nonsignificant spouse reports on this same instrument. In a more comprehensive study, albeit with small samples of adults with ADHD ($N = 33$) and control adults ($N = 26$), Minde et al. (2003) found marital and family functioning to be more impaired in the ADHD than control group regardless of the sex of the ADHD parent. As in the study by Murphy and Barkley (1996), self-reported marital adjustment was lower in the ADHD than control adults, with 58% falling in the maladjusted range of their measure (vs. 25% for the control group). Yet their spouse reports on this same measure were not different from those of spouses of the control group members. These authors, however, did not find higher rates of separation or divorce in the ADHD group despite having a comparable divorce/separation rate (27%) to that found in the Biederman et al. (1993) study above. Another study of ours also did not find a higher divorce rate (Murphy et al., 2002). The weight of the evidence therefore suggests that whether or not divorce/separation rates are higher in adults with ADHD, difficulties in marital satisfaction and functioning are evident.

This is not surprising, given that adults with ADHD rate themselves as becoming more easily angered, having frequent temper outbursts, having more unstable personal relationships, breaking off those relationships over trivial matters, and having difficulty maintaining friendships (De Quiros & Kinsbourne, 2001; Murphy & Barkley, 1996). Relationship and marital problems would also be expected from the difficulties with impulsiveness, attention, self-regulation, and EF evident in Table 7.5, listing new symptoms for the evaluation of ADHD.

Furthermore, surely the greater likelihood and diversity of financial difficulties demonstrated here in the ADHD groups (Chapter 11) would be expected to weigh heavily on marital relations.

In the UMASS Study, our results for the marital status of our three groups are presented in Table 12.2. The two clinic-referred groups were less likely to have ever been married than were members of the Community control group. Members of the ADHD group specifically were significantly less likely to be currently married (vs. being currently single) than were those of the Community control group, but they did not differ significantly from the Clinical control group. Among those who were currently married, the ADHD group also had a higher percentage who rated the quality of their marriage as poor relative to the Community control group. The Clinical control group, once again, did not differ from either of these other two groups. There was no difference in the incidence of divorce among our groups. In that sense, our results disagree with the earlier reports of higher divorce rates by Biederman et al. (1993) and from our own earlier study (Murphy & Barkley, 1996) but agree with the report of Minde et al. (2003) and another of our large studies (Murphy et al., 2002). The disparity in findings across these studies is not readily explained at this time and leaves open to doubt whether ADHD in adults is associated with a greater likelihood of divorce. Less in doubt is the consistently greater proportion of ADHD groups reporting poorer quality of their marital relationships. Yet even here the majority of all groups are not reporting such difficulties.

We examined sex differences in these marital status categories. Comparisons of males to females within each group showed no differences for ever being married or being currently married between males and females with ADHD, but females were more likely to have been divorced (21 vs. 7%) ($p = .013$). There were no differences in the Clinical control group between males and females on any marital status comparisons. For Community controls, more females had been

TABLE 12.2. Marital Status by Group in the UMASS Study

Measure	ADHD		Clinical		Community		χ^2	p	Pairwise contrasts
	N	%	N	%	N	%			
Ever married (or never married)	65	45	47	50	69	64	9.2	.010	1,2 < 3
Married currently (or single)	47	32	39	41	53	49	7.3	.026	1 < 3
Ever divorced (or not)	17	12	8	8	15	14	1.4	NS	
Marital quality rated as poor	8	17	3	7	1	2	7.7	.022	1 > 3

Note. Sample sizes are ADHD = 145, Clinical control = 94, Community control = 108. For quality of marriage, samples are ADHD = 47, Clinical control = 44, and Community control = 53. N = sample size in the clinical range; % = percent of group endorsing this item; χ^2 = results of the omnibus chi-square test; p = probability value for the chi-square test; pairwise contrasts = results of the chi-square tests involving pairwise comparisons of the three groups.

married (72% vs. 54%) (p = .047), but there were no differences in being currently married or being divorced. Comparing just the males across the groups, there were no differences in the marital status categories analyzed above. Comparing females, more Community control females had been married (72%) than ADHD (53%) or Clinical control females (44%), who did not differ between themselves. Similarly, more Community control females were currently married compared to the ADHD and Clinical groups (57% vs. 30% and 37%, respectively). Females did not differ in the proportions who were divorced (ADHD = 15% vs. Clinical = 21% and Community = 7%, respectively). As for the duration of marriage, the average length of time participants had been in their current marriage did not differ across groups when controlling for age. (Marginal M: ADHD = 14.2, Clinical = 12.9, Community = 14.7 years.) And there were no sex differences in the percentage of participants who rated the quality of their marriage as poor. All this suggest that females with ADHD may be less likely to marry than other females or than males with the disorder.

We collected the Lock-Wallace Marital Adjustment Test (Locke & Wallace, 1959) on our participants and on a smaller sample of current spouses of our participants. The results for this measure and its statistical analyses are reported in Figure 12.1. As that figure shows, both the ADHD and Clinical control groups reported significantly lower marital satisfaction than did the Community control group. In fact, the average scores for both the ADHD and Clinical control groups fell within the range believed to reflect marital dysfunction (< 100). The same results were observed for spousal reports on this same measure. Our results agree with our earlier report (Murphy & Barkley, 1996) and that of Minde et al. (2003) of greater marital dissatisfaction in the adults with ADHD compared to adults from a Community control sample. But unlike those studies, we also found greater dissatisfaction in the reports of their spouses. Nevertheless, the present study shows that such marital dissatisfaction, whether in self- or spousal reports, is not specific to just the ADHD group but also can be found in clinic-referred adults who are not diagnosed as having ADHD. That is hardly surprising, given that adults in the Clinical control group are also experiencing significant psychiatric disorders and psychological maladjustment (Chapter 8) as well as higher than normal levels of ADHD symptoms (Chapter 5), which would be expected to have some impact on marital relationships.

To summarize, longitudinal studies of ADHD in children followed into young adulthood have not documented differences in marriage or divorce probabilities, but those studies have not gone past the late 20s to early 30s of their participants. Studies of clinic-referred adults or those ascertained by other means (parents of ADHD children) present a more mixed picture, with some finding higher divorce rates and others, including our UMASS Study here, not doing so. We did find that females with ADHD were less likely to be married than other females or than males with ADHD. Both of our studies and earlier ones, how-

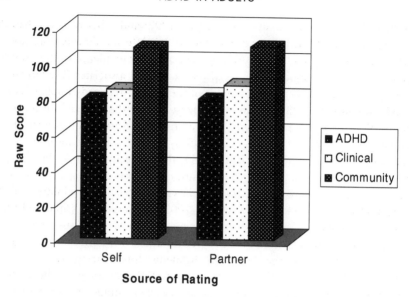

FIGURE 12.1. The Locke–Wallace Marital Adjustment Test scores for participant self-ratings and ratings from current partners for each group in the UMASS Study. Higher scores reflect greater satisfaction. The omnibus group comparison was significant for both self-ratings ($F = 10.7$, $df = 2/137$, $p < .001$) and partner ratings ($F = 11.1$, $df = 1/132$, $p < .001$). For both measures, pairwise comparisons showed that the ADHD and Clinical control groups did not differ, while both differed significantly from the Community controls. Means (SDs) by group for self-ratings were ADHD = 79 (35), Clinical = 85 (32), Community = 109 (34). For partner ratings, they were ADHD = 80 (35), Clinical = 88 (29), Community = 110 (30). Sample sizes for self-ratings were ADHD = 46, Clinical = 43, Community = 51. For partner ratings, they were: ADHD = 48, Clinical = 41, Community = 46. There was no main effect for sex of participant or for the group × sex interaction.

ever, have found that clinic-referred adults with ADHD and children growing up with persistent ADHD to age 27 rate the quality of their marital relations as less satisfactory or, if not married, the quality of their dating relationships as more likely to be poor than do comparison groups.

Psychological Morbidity of Offspring

ADHD is a highly heritable disorder (Nigg, 2006). Children with the disorder have significantly elevated rates of ADHD among their biological relatives (Biederman et al., 1992; Faraone & Doyle, 2001) and adults with the disorder have a significantly greater incidence (41%) of ADHD among their own siblings

(Manshadi, Lippman, O'Daniel, & Blackman, 1992) and other relatives than do adults without ADHD (Murphy & Barkley, 1996). We should therefore not be surprised to learn that adults with ADHD have a higher incidence of the disorder among their own biological offspring. Biederman and associates (Biederman et al., 1995) found that 57% of the offspring of their clinic-referred sample of adults with ADHD also met DSM diagnostic criteria for the disorder. More recently, Minde et al. (2003) found a similarly elevated risk to offspring in that 43% of the children of their adult ADHD group met DSM-IV criteria for the disorder. Consistent with studies of children with ADHD, the offspring with ADHD in this study were also more likely to have oppositional defiant disorder (47% vs. 6%) and either a mood or anxiety disorder (34% vs. 6%) relative to children of the non-ADHD control adults. Minde et al. (2003) also used the Child Behavior Checklist (Achenbach, 2001) to assess the psychological maladjustment of the offspring in this study. The ADHD children of adults with ADHD had significantly elevated scores on the Attention Problems, Internalizing, Externalizing, and Total Problems scales than did the non-ADHD offspring of the ADHD adults or than children of the control adults. Teacher ratings on this same scale found the children with ADHD of adults with ADHD to also be rated significantly higher on all but the Internalizing scale of the four scales noted above. The children who did not have ADHD yet who were offspring of adults with ADHD did not differ from the children of control adults on any of these four CBCL scales for either parent or teacher measures. All of this suggests not only a higher risk for ADHD but also for more general maladjustment among the offspring of adults with ADHD, at least those offspring who also have ADHD.

We also examined offspring risk for ADHD and psychological maladjustment in the UMASS Study as well as ratings of parenting stress. We did not do so in the Milwaukee Study, given the low number of children born to the control group at this follow-up and the relatively young age of those who had been born to all our participants, which would make it difficult to assess psychiatric morbidity. In the UMASS Study, we used the Disruptive Behavior Disorders Rating Scale, the Behavior Assessment System for Children, and the Parenting Stress Scale (see sidebar). The average number of children the participants had per group was 0.8 (SD = 1.2) for ADHD, 1.0 (1.3) for Clinical controls, and 1.0 (1.2) for Community controls. This difference was not significant, nor was there a main effect for sex or an interaction of group with sex. The sample sizes for the offspring on which we collected data were ADHD = 56, Clinical controls = 34, and Community controls = 26. There were no group differences in gender representation of the offspring (percent males by group: ADHD = 52%, Clinical controls = 51%, and Community controls = 49%). The mean ages of the parents and offspring for each group are shown in Table 12.3, along with the results for these various rating scales. The groups did not differ in either of these ages.

Locke–Wallace Marital Adjustment Test (Locke & Wallace, 1959)

This widely used rating scale evaluates marital satisfaction using 15 multiple-choice items. These items include the initial overall happiness in the marriage, followed by 14 items that examine the degree of agreement on specific issues such as finances, recreation, affection, friends, sex relations, conduct, life philosophy, dealing with in-laws, and mutual problem-solving, among others. The scale was used here to evaluate the quality of the relationship between currently cohabiting adult partners, whether married or not. Numerous studies attest to its validity and utility in distinguishing distressed from nondistressed couples (O'Leary & Arias, 1988). The single raw score was employed here to assess relationship satisfaction in the participants and in their cohabiting partners. The developers recommend that scores below 100 signify maladjustment.

Disruptive Behavior Disorders Rating Scale (DBDRS) (Barkley & Murphy, 2006)

The DBDRS contains the symptoms for ADHD, oppositional defiant disorders, and conduct disorder as they appeared in the DSM-IV. The ADHD and ODD items are rated on a four-point Likert scale (0–4) representing (1) not at all or rarely, (2) sometimes, (3) often, and (4) very often. The ADHD and ODD scores are obtained by summing all of the item scores for those item lists. The score for conduct disorder is simply a count of the number of items answered yes. Norms are available only for the ADHD items from the ADHD-IV Rating Scale by DuPaul and colleagues (DuPaul, Power, Anastopoulos, & Reid, 1998). Parents completed this scale for all of their children who were 3 years of age and older.

Behavior Assessment System for Children (BASC) (Reynolds & Kamphaus, 1994)

This scale consists of 131 items each requiring a response using a 4-point Likert scale. The items deal with various symptoms of child psychopathology. Broad-band scores can be obtained for total externalizing and internalizing problems, total behavior problems, and adaptive skills. More narrow-band scales can also be computed for dimensions reflecting hyperactivity, aggression, conduct problems, anxiety, depression, somatization, atypicality, withdrawal, attention problems, adaptability, social skills, and leadership. Raw scores are converted to *T*-scores (*M* of 50, *SD* 10) based on norms provided by the publisher. Parents completed this scale for all of their children who were 3 years of age and older.

Parenting Stress Index (PSI) (Abidin, 1986)

The PSI is a multiple-choice parent self-report form. We used the PSI Short Form, which consists of 36 items derived from the PSI and comprises three scales: Parental Distress, Difficult Child Characteristics, and Dysfunctional Parent-Child Interaction. Reitman, Currior, and Stickle (2002) examined the psychometric characteristics of the 36-item Parenting Stress Index—Short Form (PSI-SF) in a low-income, predominantly minority population. Internal consistencies for the PSI-SF were very good to excellent. However, confirmatory factor analysis (CFA) indicated that a three-factor model comprising of Parental Distress, Difficult Child, and Parent–Child Dysfunctional Interaction subscales was only marginally superior to a single-factor model. The PSI-SF Difficult Child subscale was most strongly associated with a measure of child oppositionality, and the Parental Distress subscale was most highly associated with self-reported psychological symptoms and low income. Parent–Child Dysfunctional Interaction was associated with parent reports of psychological symptoms as well as low income and education. Parents completed this scale based on their relationship with just one of their children 3 years of age or older.

Before proceeding to the results, we need to examine the sex of the parent completing these scales across the groups. There was a significant difference among the groups in the proportion of mothers versus fathers who completed these scales. For the ADHD group, it was 55% mothers and 45% fathers. For the Clinical controls, it was 35% mothers and 65% fathers. And for the Community controls, it was the reverse, 83% mothers and 17% fathers. Pairwise comparisons of the groups showed that the ADHD and Clinical control groups did not differ significantly in these proportions. But these two clinical groups differed significantly from the Community control group in this respect. As a consequence, in all analyses of dimensional measures, the sex of parent completing the scale was used as a separate factor to examine its potential contribution to the results.

Another issue to consider is whether or not the parents' ADHD may bias the reports of their children's ADHD. Two previous studies have not found this to be a problem. Minde et al. (2003) found that teachers of the offspring of adults with ADHD reported as many symptoms of inattention and externalizing problems as did parents. Attention problems scores correlated .83 ($p < .001$) between these sources using the Child Behavior Checklist. Faraone and colleagues also studied this issue specifically and found no evidence for parental bias in reporting (Faraone, Monuteaux, Biederman, Cohen, & Mick, 2003). In view of no evidence of such bias, we believe we can place some faith in the reports of the parents having ADHD concerning their children's ADHD and psychological adjustment.

Our results indicated that the offspring of the ADHD group were rated significantly higher on all scales from the DBDRS than were the offspring in both

TABLE 12.3. Age of Parent and Offspring and Offspring Behavioral Ratings for Each Group in the UMASS Study

Measure	ADHD Mean	SD	Clinical Mean	SD	Community Mean	SD	F	p	Pairwise contrasts
Parent age (years)	39.9	7.5	42.9	4.8	40.7	5.9	2.5	NS	
Offspring age (years)	10.2	4.5	10.0	4.3	10.6	3.3	0.2	NS	
DBDRS (raw scores)									
Inattention	11.8	7.2	8.8	7.7	4.4	3.6	14.6	< .001	1 > 2 > 3
Hyperactive–impulsive	9.7	7.3	6.1	6.0	3.1	3.7	14.3	< .001	1 > 2 > 3
Oppositional-defiant	8.3	5.1	4.9	4.2	3.8	3.6	13.7	< .001	1 > 2,3
Conduct disorder	0.9	1.5	0.3	0.5	0.3	0.8	4.5	.013	1 > 2,3
BASC (T-scores)									
Hyperactive	57.9	15.0	47.3	11.8	42.9	9.1	15.9	< .001	1 > 2,3
Aggression	55.8	11.4	47.8	10.7	46.6	9.1	10.8	< .001	1 > 2,3
Conduct problems	53.7	8.7	46.9	8.0	47.3	9.9	6.3	.003	1 > 2,3
Anxiety[S]	52.0	9.6	48.5	11.4	43.5	8.1	9.0	< .001	1,2 > 3
Depression[S]	54.2	13.0	46.8	9.5	42.1	8.1	14.3	< .001	1 > 2 > 3
Somatization[S]	51.1	11.9	43.7	10.2	43.7	7.6	8.6	< .001	1 > 2,3
Atypicality[S, GxS]	53.6	14.1	45.0	8.4	42.1	4.3	13.2	< .001	1 > 2,3
Withdrawal	52.7	13.5	50.8	12.5	47.8	10.1	0.9	NS	
Attention problems	59.4	12.9	53.3	13.4	47.9	9.6	8.3	< .001	1 > 2 > 3
Adaptability	41.2	10.2	45.7	11.1	52.3	9.3	5.9	.004	1,2 < 3
Social skills	43.9	9.6	48.6	11.0	50.0	10.7	2.6	NS	
Leadership	47.2	8.9	50.4	11.5	50.0	9.5	0.8	NS	
Externalizing problems	57.5	11.9	47.0	10.7	44.9	9.6	16.5	< .001	1 > 2,3
Internalizing problems[S]	52.9	11.8	44.8	10.8	41.4	7.5	15.4	< .001	1 > 2,3
Behavioral symptoms[S]	58.2	13.3	48.2	12.1	41.8	7.9	22.4	< .001	1 > 2 > 3
Adaptive skills	43.5	10.2	47.8	12.2	50.1	9.9	2.7	NS	
Parenting stress									
Parent domain	80.5	21.6	73.4	24.6	34.2	27.9	20.7	< .001	1,2 > 3
Parent–child interaction	84.0	15.3	65.7	38.8	45.0	35.7	9.7	< .001	1,2 > 3
Child domain	78.0	23.5	60.7	36.2	40.9	33.3	8.4	.001	1,2 > 3
Total stress	88.6	14.4	68.0	36.3	42.2	35.6	14.2	< .001	1 > 2 > 3

Note. Sample sizes for the DBDRS are ADHD = 56, Clinical control = 33, Community control = 53. For the BASC they are ADHD = 49, Clinical control = 31, Community control = 52. For the Parenting Stress Index they are ADHD = 26, Clinical = 15, Community = 26. Age ranges of the children by group are ADHD = 3–20, Clinical control = 4–17, Community control = 5–17. SD = standard deviation; F = F-test results of the analysis of variance (or covariance); p = probability value for the F-test; NS = not significant; [S] = significant main effect for sex of parent completing the scale (where this was found, mothers reported higher scores than fathers); [GxS] = group × sex of parent interaction was significant for this measure (see text for details); DBDRS = Disruptive Behavior Disorders Rating Scale (raw scores); BASC = Behavior Assessment System for Children.

Statistical analysis: Groups were initially compared using two-way (group × sex of parent completing scale) analysis of variance. Where this analysis was significant (p < .05) for the main effect for group, pairwise comparisons of the groups were conducted, the results of which are shown in the last column.

the Clinical and Community control groups. The results are graphically illustrated in Figure 12.2. Offspring of the ADHD group had more DSM-IV symptoms of inattention, hyperactive–impulsive behavior, ODD, and CD relative to both control groups. And while the offspring of the Clinical control group also had more inattention and hyperactive–impulsive symptoms than those of the Community control group, they fell significantly below the offspring of the ADHD group in those respects. This obviously supports a striking familial transmission of the symptoms of ADHD within the ADHD families.

Findings for the scales from the BASC were much the same. On 12 of the 16 scales, significant group differences were found and, in every instance, the children of the ADHD group were rated significantly higher than those in the Community control group. And in 10 of these scales, the children in the ADHD group were also rated significantly higher than those in the Clinical control group. The two scales on which the ADHD and Clinical control children did not differ were Anxiety and Adaptability. The groups did not differ among themselves on the remaining four BASC scales of social skills, leadership, withdrawal, and adaptive skills. These findings suggest a more pervasive psychological morbidity among the offspring of the ADHD group than simply their expected elevated risk for having ADHD symptoms. Symptoms of aggression, conduct

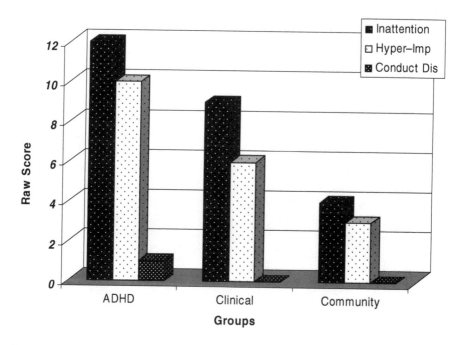

FIGURE 12.2. Raw scores for offspring on the Disruptive Behavior Disorders Rating Scale (DBDRS) subscales for each group in the UMASS Study.

problems, anxiety, depression, somatization, atypicality, and adaptability are also elevated in the children of the adults with ADHD above those in the Community control group.

Some effects due to the sex of the parent completing these scales occurred on 4 of the 16 BASC scales. In all instances, mothers across all groups reported higher scores than fathers; specifically, this occurred on the scales of Anxiety, Depression, Somatization, and Atypicality and, as a consequence, on both the Internalizing and Behavioral Symptoms broad-band scales. There was one significant interaction of the sex of the parent with the grouping factor and that was on the BASC Atypicality scale. Further analyses of this interaction found that, for mothers ratings, the main effect for group was significant and the group pairwise comparisons were such that the ADHD group had higher scores than the Clinical and Community control groups, who also differed from each other (Clinical Community). For fathers, the main effect for group was not significant (.075) but marginally so, which may have been due to the low representation of fathers in the control group ($N = 9$). Within groups, in both the ADHD and Clinical controls, mothers reported significantly higher scores than fathers. The sex difference was not significant in the Community control group. On the remaining 12 BASC scales, the 4 DBDRS scales, and the 4 PSI-SF scales, the sex of the parent had no significant effects on the ratings. Since most of our significant group differences were on those scales, it does not appear that sex of the parent completing the forms can account for our differences among the groups.

We then computed the percentage of the children in each group who could be considered to be clinically disordered on each of the narrow-band scales from the DBDRS and BASC. Our results appear in Table 12.4. The clinical range for the BASC scales was set at a T-score ≥ 65 (+1.5 SD or the 93rd percentile). For the DBDRS, the 93rd percentile score was 16 for boys and 11 for girls on both Inattention and Hyperactive–Impulsive symptom scales using the norms from DuPaul et al. (1998) for these items. The Combined ADHD scale represents children who met the clinical cutoff on both the Inattention and Hyperactive scales. There are no norms for the ODD subscale. We therefore used the results for the Community control group and defined ODD as having a score at or above +1.5 SD above the mean for that group (score = ≥ 9). For the Conduct Disorder scale, a score of 3 was chosen based on the DSM-IV threshold of three symptoms for a diagnosis of CD. We fully understand that these results are not indicative of clinical diagnoses of disorders made by clinicians using full DSM criteria, but they do suggest whether there is a greater risk for such disorders among the children who place in the clinically elevated range.

Our results show that 22 to 43% of the children of the ADHD group received clinically elevated scores on one or both of the ADHD symptom scales from the DBDRS. The results are also depicted in the graph in Figure 12.3. These findings are consistent with earlier reports of a substantially elevated risk of

TABLE 12.4. Proportion of Children in Each Group in the Clinically Elevated Range ≥ 93rd percentile) on the Child Behavior Rating Scales in the UMASS Study

Measure	ADHD		Clinical		Community		χ^2	p	Pairwise contrasts
	N	%	N	%	N	%			
DBDRS (raw scores)									
ADHD inattention	23	43	10	30	1	2	24.9	< .001	1,2 > 3
ADHD hyperactive–impulsive	17	32	4	12	2	4	15.5	< .001	1 > 2,3
Combined ADHD scales	12	22	4	12	1	2	10.4	.006	1,2 > 3
ODD	26	48	6	18	4	7	24.4	< .001	1 > 2,3
Conduct disorder	7	13	0	0	2	4	6.7	.035	1 > 2
BASC (T-scores)									
Hyperactive	16	33	2	6	0	0	24.6	< .001	1 > 2,3
Aggression	11	22	3	10	2	4	8.4	.015	1 > 3
Conduct problems	6	14	0	0	4	8	4.0	NS	
Anxiety[S]	5	10	2	7	0	0	5.3	NS	
Depression[S]	11	22	2	6	1	2	11.9	.003	1 > 3
Somatization[S]	8	16	2	6	0	0	9.7	.008	1 > 3
Atypicality[S, GxS]	8	16	0	0	0	0	14.4	.001	1 > 2,3
Withdrawal	7	14	5	16	3	6	2.7	NS	
Attention problems	18	37	8	26	3	6	14.5	.001	1,2 > 3

Note. Sample sizes for the DBDRS are ADHD = 56, Clinical control = 33, Community control = 53. For the BASC they are ADHD = 49, Clinical control = 31, Community control = 52. N = sample size in the clinical range; % = percent of group endorsing this item; χ^2 = results of the omnibus chi-square test; p = probability value for the chi-square test; pairwise contrasts = results of the chi-square tests involving pairwise comparisons of the three groups; DBDRS = Disruptive Behavior Disorders Rating Scale (raw scores); BASC = Behavior Assessment System for Children.

The clinical range for the BASC scales was a T-score ≥ 65 (93rd percentile). For the DBDRS, the 93rd percentile score was 16 for boys and 11 for girls on both scales on inattention and on hyperactive–impulsive scales. Combined type, above, means that a child met the clinical cutoff on both the inattention and hyperactive scales. For ODD, we used the mean and SD for the Community control group to determine presence of ODD. A score of 9 (+1.5 SD) was the threshold representing the 93rd percentile. For the conduct disorder scale, a score of 3 was chosen, based on the DSM-IV threshold of three symptoms for diagnosis of CD.

ADHD in the offspring of adults with ADHD discussed above (Biederman et al., 1992; Minde et al., 2003). Significantly more of those children fell in the clinical range on both the Inattention and Hyperactive–Impulsive scales than did children in the Community control group. The children in the ADHD group also differed significantly from those in the Clinical control group only on the percentage having elevations on the Hyperactive–Impulsive scale as well as on the Conduct Disorder scale. We also found a significantly elevated risk for ODD among the offspring of adults with ADHD (48%) relative to the two control groups that did not differ from each other in prevalence of ODD. Indeed, ODD was the most common disorder among the offspring of adults with ADHD. Our findings suggest some risk among children of the non-ADHD Clinical control

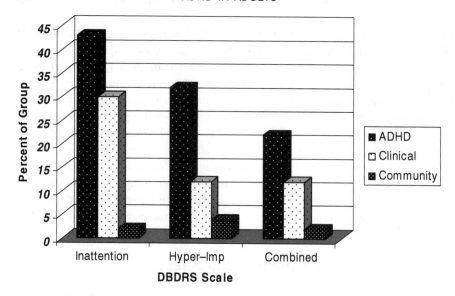

FIGURE 12.3. Percentage of each group falling in the clinically elevated range (≥ 93rd percentile) on the two Disruptive Behavior Disorders Rating Scale (DBDRS) ADHD subscales or their combination in the UMASS Study. Hyper–Imp = Hyperactive–Impulsive Scale. Combined means the case exceeded the clinical cutoff on both the Inattention and Hyperactive–Impulsive scales.

group for clinically elevated symptoms of inattention, which would certainly be in keeping with the same results found for their parents symptoms of inattention (Chapter 4). But they further suggest that being the offspring of an adult with ADHD specifically elevates their risk for hyperactive–impulsive behavior, CD, and especially ODD beyond the risk seen in the children of non-ADHD adults.

For the scales on the BASC, we found that significantly more of the children of the adults with ADHD were in the clinically impaired range on the scales of hyperactive, aggressive, depression, somatization, atypicality, and attention problems than were the children of the Community control adults. Such results are not only consistent with those found on the more DSM-specific scales of the DBDRS for ADHD symptoms but suggest a more pervasive psychological morbidity in the offspring of the ADHD group on scales related to internalizing problems. The children of the ADHD group also differed from those of the Clinical control group in having a higher percentage in the impaired range on the hyperactive and atypicality scales. Interestingly, only on the BASC attention problems scale did the children of the Clinical control adults have a higher proportion in the clinically impaired range relative to children of the Community control adults. In short, the offspring of non-ADHD clinic-referred adults may be at high risk for clinically elevated symptoms of inattention, as are the offspring of adults with ADHD. But the latter offspring also carry a significantly greater risk for a wider array of maladjustments as evident in their clinically elevated symptoms in other areas of ADHD symptoms (hyperactive–impulsive), CD, as well as internalizing disorders (depression, somatization, and atypicality).

These results agree with the only other study of the psychological adjustment of the offspring of adults with ADHD—that by Minde et al. (2003). That study also found higher rates of ADHD specifically and impaired psychological adjustment more generally among the offspring of adults with ADHD compared a normal control group. Our results go further in showing that many of these areas of maladjustment may also distinguish the offspring of adults with ADHD from those of other clinic-referred adults who are not diagnosed with ADHD.

Parenting and Stress

Parenting stress would be expected to be elevated in parents with ADHD by virtue of their own disorder and the comorbid disorders and psychological maladjustment associated with it (see Chapter 8). Add to this the possibility that some of the children have the same disorder as well as ODD and it is clear that parenting could be more distressing in such families than where either the parent or child does not have ADHD. The results for the Parenting Stress Index indicated that parents in both the ADHD and Clinical control groups were significantly higher than in the Community control group in parent, child, and parent–child domain stress scores but did not differ from each other on these domain-specific scales. However, parents in the ADHD group had significantly higher Total Stress scores on this instrument than did parents in either the Clinical or Community control groups. The latter result is certainly in keeping with the elevated levels of psychological maladjustment on both internalizing and externalizing scales from the BASC and DBDRS noted above.

To determine which features of child disruptive behavior contributed significantly to parenting stress, we used linear regression, in which we regressed the four scores from the DBDRS (inattention, hyperactive–impulsive behavior, ODD symptoms, and CD symptoms) onto each PSI-SF stress domain. We did not use all of the BASC scales for this analysis because of the small sample size and the large number of scales from the BASC, which would have created a very small sample size:measure ratio for such an analysis. We used the entire sample of parents completing the scales collapsed across the groups. The sample size was only $N = 63$, so these results should be viewed as purely preliminary findings. While child age may be thought to influence ratings of parent stress, we found no significant correlations between it and any stress domains; therefore we did not include it in the analyses. We made two sets of regression analyses. In the first set, we examined just the child behavior ratings as predictors of parent stress. In the second set, we added parent self-report ratings of ADHD symptoms as well as the parental SCL-90-R Depression and Anxiety scores. We did so in order to see which parent characteristics may be contributing to parenting stress and because past research has shown that such stress is related to these parent characteristics, particularly depression (Johnston & Mash, 2001)

The results are shown in Table 12.5. In considering just child behavior predictors, it can be seen that parenting stress is largely a function of two dimensions of child disruptive behavior, these being inattention and ODD symptoms. Parental domain and total stress are mostly a function of degree of child inattention,

TABLE 12.5. Predicting Parenting Stress Domains from Offspring Disruptive Behavior Scores in the UMASS Study

Stress domain/predictors	Beta	R	R^2	$R^2\Delta$	F	p
Using child behavior predictors only						
Parent domain						
Child inattention score	2.48	.528	.279	.279	23.55	< .001
Parent–child domain						
Child ODD score	3.07	.581	.338	.338	31.09	< .001
Child inattention score	1.31	.618	.382	.044	4.31	.042
Child domain						
Child ODD score	3.94	.694	.482	.482	56.82	< .001
Child inattention score	1.21	.722	.521	.038	4.81	.032
Total stress						
Child inattention score	1.96	.598	.358	.358	34.01	< .001
Child ODD score	2.68	.662	.439	.081	8.65	.005
Using child and parent predictors						
Parent domain						
Parent depression	.664	.757	.574	.574	63.26	< .001
Child inattention	.230	.786	.618	.044	5.31	.026
Child domain						
Parent depression	.437	.647	.418	.418	33.80	< .001
Child ODD score	.424	.744	.554	.136	14.00	.001
Parent–child domain						
Child ODD score	.591	.718	.515	.515	49.96	< .001
Parent depression	.256	.751	.565	.049	5.22	.027
Total stress						
Parent depression	.517	.703	.494	.494	45.86	< .001
Child ODD score	.375	.775	.600	.106	12.23	.001

Note. Beta = standardized coefficient; R = regression coefficient; R^2 = percent of explained variance accounted for by all variables at this step; $R^2\Delta$ = percent of explained variance accounted for by this variable added at this step; F = results of F-test for the equation at this step; p = probability value for the F-test; NS = not significant. Child behavior predictors were parent ratings of ADHD inattention, ADHD hyperactive–impulsive, oppositional defiant disorder, and conduct disorder. Parent predictors were parent self-report ratings of ADHD symptoms and SCL-90-R Depression and Anxiety scores.
Statistical analysis: Multiple linear regression using stepwise conditional method. Sample $N = 63$.

although ODD symptoms make a small additional contribution to the total stress domain. Between 28 and 36% of the variance in these stress domains is accounted for by child inattention symptoms. But the child and parent–child stress domains are mainly predicted from child ODD symptoms (34–48% of variance), while child inattention makes a minor yet significant additional contribution to both (4%). But it is possible that some of these child behavioral problems may have more to do with parental characteristics, such as the link between parental depression and child ODD symptoms, making it possible that some of the child behavior ratings are serving as proxies for parent characteristics that are actually driving the stress ratings found here. We therefore repeated these analyses, entering in three parent characteristics as predictors in addition to the four child behavior predictors studied above. Those results are shown in the lower half of Table 12.4. Our suspicions were correct. Parent depression was significantly predictive of all stress domain scores, replacing some of the significant child behavior predictors found above. However, child inattention continued to have an additional yet much smaller contribution to the parent domain, while child ODD severity made small but significant contributions to the parent–child, child, and total stress domain scores. In summary, it is a mixture of both parental depression and child ODD that contributes to much of the parental stress found here, accounting for 55 to 62% of the variance in stress ratings. Of course, it is possible that parent depression itself is partly a function of the stress induced in raising disruptive children—our results cannot speak to the direction of effects in these relationships.

Our findings agree with a large literature on parenting stress and parent–child interactions in children with ADHD, which has found both parental depression and child ODD symptoms (or social aggression) to be predictors of parenting stress (Johnston & Mash, 2001). Given the numerous findings on the role of parental irritability and depression in disrupting parent–child relationships—not to mention the child symptoms comprising ODD, such as anger, hostility, defiance, temper outbursts—it is not hard to imagine that they would elicit stress during parent–child interactions. But our research extends such findings further by showing that the degree of inattentiveness also makes some contribution to parenting stress. We would have expected hyperactive–impulsive symptoms to be more provocative of parenting stress, given their more disruptive nature, but this is obviously not the case. Inattentiveness in a child appears to be more contributory to parenting stress, probably as a consequence of its adverse impact on compliance, task completion, and remembering and following directions.

Parents with ADHD may have a greater difficulty coping with children and family life more generally than do those without ADHD, as suggested above. Recent studies by Eric Mash and his students have shed further light on this issue, suggesting that these differences may even be evident among women who are expecting their first child. Ninowski, Mash, and Benzies (2007) recently reported a comparison of expectant mothers who had high levels of ADHD symptoms compared to those with lower levels. They found that women with high ADHD severity were less likely to be married, less likely to have gone to college, and less likely to report that they wanted to become pregnant. The level of ADHD symptoms was associated with greater anxiety and depression and less positive expectations about their soon to be born infant and their future maternal role. Such findings are consistent with those reported throughout this book in finding adults with ADHD to be less educated, more likely to have children early, and to have greater levels of anxiety and depression. We also found our adult women with ADHD in the UMASS Study to be less likely to be married.

Watson and Mash (in press) continued this line of research by evaluating women with young infants for their level of ADHD symptoms and their mother–child relations. Again, they found that ADHD severity was associated with higher levels of anxiety and depression but was also contributory to higher levels of maternal hostile–reactive behavior in mothers who had difficult infants. Although the level of maternal ADHD had no effect on perceived parental self-efficacy after controlling for parental anxiety and depression, maternal ADHD severity was associated with a reduced sense of perceived parental impact on child behavior. Perceived social support was unrelated to maternal ADHD symptoms.

The effect of maternal ADHD symptoms was further examined in a study by Banks, Ninowski, Mash, and Semple (in press), who compared women high in levels of ADHD symptoms with those with lower levels. High-ADHD women had more occupational and psychiatric problems, lower parenting self-esteem, and a more external locus of control for their parenting. They also reported less effective disciplinary styles than did women low in ADHD symptoms. While none of these studies used clinically referred women diagnosed with ADHD, they clearly suggest that ADHD in women is likely to have an adverse impact on their parenting roles, parental stress, and parent–child interactions.

Further effects of adult ADHD on parental roles and functioning were found by Murray and Johnston (2006), who recently compared mothers with and without ADHD who all had children with ADHD on various parenting measures and parent–child interaction measures. The mothers with ADHD were found to be poorer at monitoring child behavior and less consistent disciplinarians relative to mothers without the disorder. The mothers with ADHD also appeared to be less effective at problem solving around child behavior issues than control mothers. Results remained the same even after controlling for the severity of child ODD and CD symptoms. Poor parental monitoring of child behavior is a risk factor for accidental injuries and may help to explain the elevated rates of such injuries in children with ADHD (Barkley, 2006), given that parental ADHD may be one source of such lowered levels of child monitoring.

Taken in its entirety, this body of evidence indicates an adverse impact of ADHD in adult women in their roles as mothers. This detrimental impact is over and above that which may be attributable to the comorbid anxiety and depression often seen in conjunction with ADHD in adults. No studies have examined the roles of fathers with ADHD in these domains of parental functioning—a clear void in the literature.

Conclusions and Clinical Implications

This chapter has considered the sexual activity, dating, and marital status and functioning of adults with ADHD as well as their parenting stress and psychological morbidity among the children of these adults in comparison to two control groups.

✓ The Milwaukee Study continued to find higher levels of riskier sexual behavior in the hyperactive than the control groups by age 27, this being most evident in those who were hyperactive as children and had persistent ADHD to that age. Children growing up with ADHD have an earlier start to their sexual careers (intercourse), are more likely to become pregnant (if female) or to impregnate others (if males), are more likely to be parents by ages 21 and 27, and are more likely to contract a sexually transmitted disease by age 21 than are Community control children followed over this same time. These risks deserve greater attention in pediatrics and primary medical care, where efforts to reduce them are, in our opinion, uncommon. Sex and contraception counseling, increased parental supervision, and continued ADHD treatment throughout adolescence should be tested for their utility in reducing these risks.

✓ We did not find differential rates of marriage or higher rates of divorce among the children growing up with ADHD or among the clinic-referred adults with ADHD in keeping with the previous longitudinal studies of hyperactive children and with the inconsistent results of past studies of clinic-referred adults on this issue. But we do find a greater incidence of marital dissatisfaction in both groups of adults with ADHD across these projects as well as poorer quality of dating relationships among those adults with persistent ADHD who were hyperactive as children and are still single and dating.

✓ The spouses of those adults with ADHD were also significantly less satisfied in the marriage than were spouses of the Community control group in the UMASS Study. But such findings may not be specific to adults with ADHD or their spouses because we also found such marital dissatisfaction in our Clinical control adults.

✓ Prior studies found elevated risks for ADHD among the offspring of adults with ADHD, ranging from 43 to 57% of their children. We also found such an elevated risk, with 22 to 43% of the offspring of adults with ADHD falling in the clinically elevated range on either the inattention, hyperactive–impulsive, or combined symptom lists from the DSM-IV. These prevalence figures were certainly higher than those found in our Community control adults, in keeping with prior studies.

✓ But we also used a Clinical control group of adults and found that their off-spring also carried significantly elevated risks for symptoms of inattention as compared with the children of the Community control group, implying that the offsprings' risk for inattention is also found in non–ADHD clinic-referred adults. But risk for hyperactive–impulsive behavior, ODD, and CD appears to be specifically elevated in the offspring of the adults with ADHD.

✓ In fact, ODD would seem to be the most common psychological morbidity to be found in the offspring of adults with ADHD, occurring in nearly half of them (48%).

✓ Our findings are quite consistent with the strong genetic predisposition to ADHD and its high familial transmission, as demonstrated in numerous prior behavior genetic studies of biological family members and twins (Nigg, 2006).

✓ This study also evaluated a wider array of dimensions of children's psycholog-ical maladjustment than prior studies of offspring morbidity had done. Here as well we found that the children of adults with ADHD showed greater symp-toms of both externalizing (ADHD, OD, CD) and internalizing (depression, somatization, atypicality) problems than did children in the Clinical and Community control groups. Our findings suggest a wider range of offspring psychological morbidity associated with ADHD in parents than is the case for parents who do not have ADHD, whether clinically referred or not.

✓ The parents in both the ADHD and Clinical control groups reported higher rates of parenting stress on the specific scales of parent, child, and parent–child domains than did Community control parents, and they did not differ from each other on these scales. But the parents with ADHD reported more total stress in their family lives than did parents in either of the control groups.

✓ Parenting stress, particularly in those domains associated with the child or with parent–child interactions, was primarily predicted by the extent of child ODD symptoms, consistent with prior research in children with ADHD. But degree of child inattentiveness was also a contributor to some domains of par-enting stress, suggesting that it also makes some contribution to the degree of perceived stress reported by parents. However, when parental characteristics of ADHD, depression, and anxiety were considered, our results showed that parental depression may make a large and consistent contribution to all domains of parenting stress. Child ODD symptoms continued to contribute to stress, however, beyond that made by parental depression. The parental level of ADHD did not contribute to levels of parenting stress.

✓ Our findings suggest a wider range of offspring psychological morbidity associated with ADHD in parents than is the case for parents who do not have ADHD, whether clinically referred or not.

✓ Clinicians need to recognize the increased risk of ADHD and related disorders in the offspring of adults with ADHD. Such disorders and psychological problems are likely to require separate evaluation and management from the problems posed by ADHD in the parent. Referral of such cases to child mental health professionals may be needed in some cases.

✓ Parents having ADHD are also likely to do less well in behavioral parent training programs (Sonuga-Barke, Daley, & Thompson, 2002) aimed at management of their child's ADHD and oppositional behavior, suggesting that parent ADHD should be treated before such child behavior management programs are undertaken.

✓ Parents having ADHD are also more likely to experience stress in their roles as parent regardless of the presence or not of ADHD in their children. This may necessitate additional counseling of these adults in stress management and other coping techniques so as to reduce the greater stress and conflict likely to be evident in the families of adults with ADHD.

✓ Marital distress is greater among adults with ADHD but also among non-ADHD clinic-referred adults. Clinicians may need to assess for such disharmony and conflict and make appropriate recommendations for further evaluation and possibly marital intervention as needed.

CHAPTER 13

Neuropsychological Functioning

The domain of neuropsychological functioning is undoubtedly the most studied domain of psychological and adaptive functioning in the literature on adults with ADHD. Studies of children with ADHD followed to adulthood have not explored neuropsychological functioning as much as have studies of clinic-referred adults with ADHD. Given the widespread interest in the potential relationship of ADHD to executive functioning (EF) in children with ADHD, we should also not be surprised to learn that it is this aspect of neuropsychology that has also been the most studied in ADHD in adults.

EF is a very ambiguous term in the field of neuropsychology, and it often means different things to different investigators. The literature on it is typified by descriptions of various activities thought to be involved in EF, while the construct itself goes undefined. For instance, the term has been used to encompass such actions as planning, inhibiting responses, strategy development and use, flexible sequencing of actions, maintenance of behavioral set, and resistance to interference. (Denckla, 1996; Morris, 1996; Spreen, Risser, & Edgell, 1995). Others simply concluded that the EFs are what the frontal lobes do (Stuss & Benson, 1986). Denckla (1994) defined executive functioning by its components: interference control, effortful and flexible organization, and strategic planning or anticipatory, goal-directed preparedness to act. Dennis (1991) did likewise, recognizing the components of regulatory (mental attention), executive (planning), and social discourse (productive verbal interaction with others). And so did Spreen and colleagues in their description of the EFs as inhibition, planning, organized search, self-monitoring, and flexibility of thought and action (Spreen et al., 1995). But nowhere among these lists of component is an opera-

400

tional definition proffered. The most commonly identified EFs are inhibition, working memory (nonverbal and verbal), fluency or generativity, and planning. And even those lists appear to adopt the computer metaphor of the brain, as if it were a passive information processor.

In contrast, Barkley (1997, 2001) has defined EF from a much different perspective. Barkley borrowed from the work of Bronowski (1967/1977) on the evolution of human language and combined it with concepts from Vygotsky's theory of the internalization of speech (see Diaz & Berk, 1992, for a description of this theory and research supporting it) to create a hybrid model of EF. He proposed that the EFs, like the internalization of self-speech, are human self-directed actions (see Chapter 7). These actions are types of self-control. Self-control is any action one uses to alter a subsequent behavior so as to control future consequences. The EFs, according to Barkley's view, are forms of self-control or self-directed action. They have as their function the alteration of one's own subsequent behavior in order to alter the probability of some future consequence. Originally publicly observable actions, like speech, they become progressively more self-directed and private (internalized), being inhibited from public view, until they are finally cognitive or private in form. In the internalization of speech, speech is initially public and directed at others; but around 3 to 5 years of age, it becomes self-directed, though still observable. It then progresses over the next 5 or more years to becoming progressively less observable (quieter, subaudible, then unobservable) while also changing from descriptive to instructive utterances. The individual is using language to guide his or her own behavior, and that language becomes not only more private while being self-directed but also more instructive and controlling of motor behavior. The advantage of this view is that it offers a hypothetical yet testable pathway by which the EFs may have evolved from their more primitive primate counterparts (Barkley, 2001).

The EFs can be thought of as actions to the self aimed at the future, as explained in Chapter 7. Using this perspective, Barkley redefines the list of EFs as (1) inhibition; (2) sensing to the self, especially visual imagery (nonverbal working memory); (3) speech to the self (verbal working memory); (4) the self-regulation of emotion and motivation via emoting to the self; and (5) self-directed play, or analysis and synthesis (generativity, fluency, problem solving, or planning). The latter function refers to the taking apart and recombining and otherwise manipulating of mentally represented information via the two working memory systems. ADHD is argued to disrupt the development of each of these major EFs because of its adverse impact on inhibition—an EF on which the others depend for their own effective execution. Inhibition stops the individual's impulsive responding to the environment, permits a delay in responding during which the other EFs can occur, and protects that delay, the performance of the EFs, and the subsequent chain of goal-directed behavior they will generate from disruption or interference (distractibility).

Whether one adopts this view or not, the fact that ADHD has been shown in neuroimaging research to involve the prefrontal lobes, among other regions (see Nigg, 2006), and that these brain regions are believed to be responsible for the EFs has led ADHD researchers to focus on studying the status of the EFs in patients with ADHD. This has resulted in numerous publications sufficient to warrant separate meta-analyses of child and adult ADHD research (Frazier, Demareem, & Youngstrom, 2004; Hervey, Epstein, & Curry, 2004). The findings for child ADHD have been reviewed elsewhere (Barkley, 1997, 2006) and support the view that inhibition, working memory (especially verbal), and planning and problem solving are adversely affected in this disorder. There is less research on nonverbal working memory and the self-regulation of emotion-motivation, but what does exist suggests some difficulties with this realm as well (Barkley, 2006; Luman, Oosterlaan, & Sergeant, 2005). Generativity or fluency, at least as measured by relatively simple verbal fluency tests, has shown conflicting if not weak evidence for involvement in ADHD (Frazier et al., 2004) while set shifting has received minimal support, at least as reflected in the performance of the Wisconsin Card Sort Test (Frazier et al., 2004).

A Brief Review of EF in Adults with ADHD

As in children with ADHD, research into the neuropsychology of ADHD in adults expanded substantially in the past decade. These studies have used similar or even the same neuropsychological tests employed with children with ADHD and often with comparable results (Hervey et al., 2004). For instance, Matochik et al. (1996) compared 21 ADHD adults against the norms provided with the neuropsychological tests. They found that performance of mental arithmetic and digit span on the Wechsler Adult Intelligence Scale—Revised were significantly below normal, suggesting verbal working memory problems, as are often found in children with ADHD. Barkley et al. (1996) and Kovner et al. (1997) also found adults with ADHD to perform more poorly on this digit span subtest. In contrast, tests of verbal learning, memory, and fluency have shown mixed results with some studies finding no differences from control groups (Barkley et al., 1996; Holdnack, Moberg, Arnold, Gur, & Gur, 1995; Kovner et al., 1997) while others have (Jenkins et al., 1998; Lovejoy et al., 1999), especially when using larger samples (Johnson et al., 2001). This implies that statistical power in the earlier studies may have been limited by smaller sample sizes.

We found performance on the Wisconsin Card Sort Test (WCST) (Barkley et al., 1996) to be within the normal range in young adults with ADHD. Others have also failed to find problems in performance on the WCST in groups of ADHD adults compared to various control groups (see Hervey et al., 2004, for a meta-analysis; Holdnack et al., 1995; Johnson et al., 2001; Seidman, 1997; Rapport, Van Voorhis, Tzelepis, & Friedman, 2001). Only the study by Weyandt, Rice, Linterman, Mitzlaff, and Emert (1998) found differences between their groups on this task. Studies of childhood ADHD also found this task to be quite inconsistent in their results with most finding no group differences (Frazier et al., 2004). This suggests that ADHD does not have an adverse impact on set shifting or whatever neuropsychological function is being tapped by the WCST (Mirsky, 1996).

Barkley et al. (1996) compared a small sample of young adults with ADHD (N = 25) to a control group (N = 23) on several measures of creativity (ideational fluency). No group differences were found as was the case in later studies (Murphy et al., 2001; Rapport et al., 2001). The study by Rapport et al. (2001), however, did find more perseverative and nonperseverative errors on their design fluency task in their ADHD group compared to their control group.

Adults with ADHD were also found in two studies by Barkley et al. (1996; Murphy et al., 2001) to perform significantly worse on a nonverbal working memory task involving the Simon Tone/Color Game, in which increasingly lengthy sequences of tone/color key presses must be imitated to mimic a sample melody. Dowson and colleagues likewise found impaired spatial working memory in their ADHD group compared to those with borderline personality disorder and control adults (Dowson et al., 2004).

In a later study, McClean and colleagues found adults with ADHD (N = 19) to perform more poorly on a computerized cognitive battery assessing spatial working memory, planning, and set shifting and to be slower to respond to targets in a go/no-go task than their matched control group (N = 19) (McClean et al., 2004). A much larger study by Nigg and associates evaluated 105 adults with ADHD and 90 control adults. They reduced their executive function battery by factor analysis to an overall executive factor and a separate speed factor (response output) and found the ADHD group to performed more poorly on both factors (Nigg et al., 2005). The earlier study by Johnson et al. (2001) likewise found adults with ADHD to perform more poorly on tests of response speed as have others using very small samples (Himmelstein & Halperin, 2000; Kovner et al., 1997; Schweiger, Abramovitch, Doniger, & Simon, 2007). These studies are in keeping with similar deficits noted in childhood ADHD (Barkley, 2006; Frazier et al., 2004). Symptoms of inattention in the Nigg et al. study were more closely related to the executive factor, while both inattention and hyperactive–impulsive symptoms were related to the speed factor. The study is significant for demonstrating that these results were not a function of age, IQ, comorbid disorders, sex, or educational level. The relationship of ADHD symptoms to poor adaptive functioning in ADHD adults appears to be mediated by these EF deficits (Stavro, Ettenhoffer, & Nigg, 2007).

Studies of children with ADHD that employ continuous performance tests (CPT) frequently find them to perform these tasks more poorly than do control groups (Barkley, 1996, 2006; Frazier et al., 2004; Nigg, 2001), whether on omission errors and reaction time variability (reflecting inattention) or on commission errors and mean reaction time (reflecting inhibition). Many studies of adults with ADHD have found similar deficits. Barkley et al. (1996) found that their young adults with ADHD also demonstrated more omission and commission errors on a CPT compared to the control group. The same was found by three other studies (Epstein, Conners, Erhardt, March, & Swanson, 1997; Gansler et al., 1998; Seidman, 1997). Yet a few other studies found only commission errors to differentiate their ADHD and control groups (Ossman & Mulligan, 2003; Shaw & Giambra, 1993). Roy-Byrne et al. (1997) compared adults diagnosed with ADHD (probable ADHD) to a group having current adult ADHD symptoms without a persuasive childhood history (possible ADHD) and to a clinical control group using the Conners CPT. They found that those adults who had possible ADHD had a significantly poorer composite CPT score than those in the control group, with the probable ADHD adult group falling between these two groups. Holdnack et al. (1995) also found poorer CPT performance in adults with ADHD, though in this instance it was on the measure of reaction time only and not omission or commission errors. Weyandt, Mitzlaff, and Thomas (2002) found more omission errors in their ADHD group than their control group.

Deficits in inhibition have also been noted on other tests besides CPTs, such as the Stroop task (Hervey et al., 2004; Lovejoy et al., 1999; Rapport et al., 2001), antisaccade tasks (Nigg, Butler, Huang-Pollack, & Henderson, 2002), and negative priming and stopping tasks (Nigg et al., 2002; Ossman & Mulligan, 2003). Prior studies using stop-signal tasks (the participant must withhold quick responding to a cue when signaled by a tone) also find inhibitory deficits for adults with the disorder. Bekker et al. (2005) compared 24 adults with ADHD combined subtype to 24 control adults using this task, along with a stop-change version. In this version, participants had to give an alternative motor response when they heard the tone. Compared to controls, adults with ADHD took a significantly longer time to inhibit and to change their response. Other indices on the stop-change task, including choice error variability, may also reflect impulsivity. Such results indicate that response inhibition is significantly impaired in adults with ADHD, as it is also in childhood ADHD (Nigg, 2001).

Two studies have examined distractibility in adults. One studied college students with a history of hyperactivity in childhood and found greater intrusive task-unrelated thoughts during performance of a CPT (Shaw & Giambra, 1993). Another study found poorer performance of clinically diagnosed adults with ADHD on a test when background noise occurred during the task (Corbett & Stanczak, 1999).

For the most part, neuropsychological studies of adults with ADHD have employed very small sample sizes, often well below those necessary for adequate statistical power to detect small to moderate effect sizes (group differences) in such research. As a consequence, the failure to find group differences on some measures for which differences in the child ADHD literature have been found may simply be a result of low power. In an effort to address this problem, we compared a large sample of adults with ADHD ($N = 105$; ages 17–28 years) to a community control group ($N = 64$) on 14 measures of EFs and olfactory identification using a 2 (groups) × 2 (sex) design (Murphy et al., 2001). The ADHD group performed significantly worse on 11 of these 14 measures. They were significantly worse on the Stroop Color–Word Test, and interference scores (a measure of inhibition and interference control) as well as on measures of verbal working memory (digit span) and fluency. Measures of attention and inhibition from the Conners CPT also revealed deficits in the adults with ADHD similar to those seen in childhood ADHD. Consistent with studies of patients having frontal lobe damage, we found adults with ADHD to make more errors on a smell identification test than did control adults. No sex differences were evident on any measures. No differences were found in the ADHD group as a function of ADHD subtype or comorbid oppositional defiant disorder. These results are in agreement with many studies above, particularly the large study by Nigg et al. (2005), in finding deficits in executive and response speed deficits associated with adult ADHD. We concluded that the EF deficits found in childhood ADHD exist in young adults with ADHD and are largely not influenced by comorbidity.

One neuropsychological study examined expressed emotion and affect recognition in adults with ADHD. It found the adults with ADHD to show a greater intensity of expressed emotion and a greater deficit in affect recognition than in a control group (Rapport, Friedman, Tzelepis, & Van Voorhis, 2002). In the control group, experienced emotion facilitated affect recognition; in the ADHD group, the opposite was the case. The results were in keeping with Barkley's theory of EF deficits in ADHD, noted above, in which affect regulation is hypothesized to be impaired in the disorder. Another study in this same lab also found adults with ADHD to use less emotion-laden words to describe scenes involving emotional interactions (Friedman et al., 2003).

One area related to working memory and executive functioning shown to be deficient in children, teens, and adults with ADHD is the capacity to use one's sense of time to guide motor performance, or more specifically time reproduction. Time reproduction paradigms are typically the most difficult of the timing tasks and place heavy demands on working memory (Zakay, 1990). The individual is shown a sample duration, as by turning a flashlight on and off, but is not told the actual length of the duration. The person must then reproduce the sample duration, typically using the same means by which the sample was presented (in this case, a flashlight). To do this task accurately, the individual must attend to the initial sample interval, hold that duration in mind, and then use it to generate an equivalent duration of response. This test more closely evaluates the capacity of the individual to govern his or her own behavior relative to a mentally represented time interval (the sample duration) than do the other timing paradigms and appears to be more taxing of working memory. For this reason, this task may also be more susceptible to problems with distraction. Supporting this are findings that scores on this task correlate significantly with measures of impulsiveness, apparently more so than other timing tasks (Gerbing, Ahadi, & Patton, 1987). Logically, then, one would expect ADHD to produce impairments on this task, even in the absence of distracting events. All previous studies support this conclusion (see Barkley, 2006, for a review; Barkley, Koplowicz, Anderson, & McMurray, 1997; Barkley, Edwards, et al., 2001; Barkley, Murphy, et al., 2001).

In summary, adults with ADHD appear to show deficits in many of the same EFs as have been found in child ADHD, including inhibition, interference control (resistance to distraction), working memory, emotion regulation, using time to guide behavior, and generativity/fluency, at least on nonverbal measures like design fluency. Tests of planning ability have not been used as extensively in the adult ADHD arena, so its involvement in ADHD is less certain (Hervey et al., 2004). But given the greater frequency of such problems in the verbal reports of those with the disorder (Chapter 4) (De Quiros & Kinsbourne, 2001), it may well turn out to be problematic in adults with ADHD as well. Interestingly, at least one study has found another frontal lobe but non-EF function to be affected by the disorder, and that is smell identification (Murphy et al., 2001)—a finding deserving of replication and consistent with other frontal lobe disorders.

The UMASS Study Results

In Chapter 7, we presented EF-based behavioral symptoms and tested them for their utility in diagnosing ADHD, which they evidently were as all differentiated the ADHD from the Community group and nearly half of them did so from the Clinical control group. But we also selected traditional neuropsychological tests of the major EFs discussed above. In doing so, we used tests of inhibition (Conners CPT), resistance to distraction (Stroop Color–Word Test), nonverbal and verbal working memory (Learning and Memory Battery [LAMB]), and planning or generativity/fluency (LAMB, Five-Point Design Fluency Test). The flexibility or the capacity to shift response patterns has sometimes been considered an EF, while in other models it is a component of attention (Mirsky, 1996). The WCST is typically used to index this component. As noted above, past studies have typically not found performance deficits using it. We included it nonetheless in our battery of neuropsychological tests so as to compare our finding with those of other studies (See the sidebar for a description of these tests).

Our results are presented in Table 13.1. Because of the large number of scores generated for the Conners CPT, WCST, and LAMB, we first analyzed these scores as sets using multivariate analysis of variance for each test. Where

Conners Continuous Performance Test (Conners, 1995)

This is a standardized computer-administered continuous performance test in which single letters are shown on a display screen at three different rates: one every second; one every 2 seconds; or one every 4 seconds. The task lasts 12 minutes. The variation in interstimulus interval allows the examination of this variable on the participant's performance. The task used a response format that is the reverse of most CPTs. The participant presses a button in response to every signal shown but then must cease or inhibit responding when the target signal appears. Norms are available for this CPT from the publisher (Multi-Health Systems, North Tonawanda, N.Y.). The dependent measures employed here were the total number of omissions (missed targets), total commissions (false hits), reaction time (RT), and RT variability. The scores for omissions and RT variability were chosen to assess sustained attention, while the scores for commissions and RT were chosen to assess response inhibition.

Stroop Color–Word Test
(Stroop, 1935; Trenerry, Crosson, Deboe, & Leber, 1989)

This test measures the ability to inhibit competing responses in the presence of salient conflicting information. The version and norms published by Trenerry et al. (1989) were used here. The task comprises three parts. In the first part, the participant reads a repeating list of color names (e.g., red, blue, green) printed in black ink. In the second part, the participant names the colors of a repeated series of X's printed in an ink of those same colors. In the last or Interference condition, the participant must say the color of ink in which a color word is printed. For some words, the color of ink in which it is printed is the same as that of the word, while for others, the color of ink differs from that specified by the word. This portion of the task is believed to reflect problems with the capacity to inhibit habitual or dominant responses (reading the word, in this case). Three scores were derived from this last portion of the test (Interference): the raw scores for the number of items completed and the number of incorrect responses, as well as the percentile score.

Wisconsin Card Sort Test (WCST) (Heaton, 1981)

This test comprises 128 cards each containing sets of geometric designs that vary according to color, shape, and number. The subject is given four cards and then asked to sort the remaining deck using feedback from the examiner. Following 10 correct sorts on a given category (e.g., color), the examiner switches the category unannounced and the subject must now discover the new sorting rule from feedback given by the examiner. While many scores can be derived, we will use the two found by Mirsky (1996) to load on the same factor (Shift), these being percent of correct responses and number of categories successfully identified. Again, we convert the scores from both Trails B and WCST to *T* scores and sum them to create our omnibus Set Shifting score.

Five-Point Test of Design Fluency (Lee et al., 1997)

Originally developed by Regard, Strauss, and Knapp (1982) in an attempt to design a nonverbal version of more commonly used verbal fluency tasks, this test involves a sheet of paper with 40 five-dot matrices on it. Participants are required to produce as many different figures as possible by connecting the dots within each rectangle within a 3-minute time limit. Not all dots have to be used and only straight lines between dots are permitted. No figures are to be repeated. If a violation occurs, participants are given a single warning on the first violation, but the rules are not repeated after any further infractions. Scores are the number of unique designs created, the number of repeated designs (perseveration), the number of rule infractions, and the percentage of designs that are repeated (percent perseveration). Patients with frontal lobe dysfunction have a significantly higher percentage of perseverative errors than do neurological patients without frontal involvement and psychiatric patients (Lee et al., 1997). Using a modified version of this same task, Ruff, Allen, Farrow, Nieman, and Wylie (1994) also found the task to be sensitive to frontal lobe injuries, perhaps more so to right than to left lobe involvement.

Learning and Memory Battery (Schmidt & Tombaugh, 1995)

This battery contains nine separate tests involving verbal learning, verbal memory, and nonverbal memory. Learning is evaluated through the immediate recall of sample information, while retention is evaluated through a delayed retrial on the information presented earlier. We used the delayed recall trials as our index of verbal and nonverbal working memory. The first two tests involve paragraph learning and retention. After a paragraph is read to the participant, he or she tries to recall as much information from the paragraph as possible. There are 31 possible pieces of such information that can be scored. Participants are then given a cued recall trial in which they are prompted with questions about specific items of paragraph content to see if they can now recall that information. The paragraph is then repeated, and once again the participants try to freely recall as much information as they can, after which there is a cued recall trial again involving prompting questions. This is the second task that is scored. After the next test (Word List) is given, the participant is again asked to recall as much as possible concerning the paragraph read to them earlier, which constitutes the delayed retention trial. The next task involves word list learning and retention. Participants are read a list of 15 words and asked to recall as many as they can remember. In the cued recall trial, they are then given a cue as to the semantic category in which the correct specific answer falls (*weapon*, for instance, is the cue for the word *pistol* to be recalled). This task is followed by a word-pair learning task involving 14 word pairs that must be learned. Four trials are given involving four separate word-pair lists. After two other tasks are given, a retention trial is presented for just the first word-pair list. The next task is a digit-span task in which participants are read a string of increasingly longer digit sequences that they must then recall. Each string is presented twice, with recall attempted after each presentation. In the second task, they must recall the digit sequences read to them in backward order. Again each sequence is presented twice. A subsequent task (Supraspan Digit) involves presenting the participant with a digit sequence involving up to 11 digits. The digit sequence given is one greater than the maximum sequence they obtained in the Digit Span forward task. The score is based on the number of trials needed to get the sequence correct in three consecutive trials. Participants are then given two tasks involving a simple and a complex figure which they must reproduce. The complex figure task is similar to the Rey–Osterrieth Complex Figure Task. Each task also involves a retention trial after a delay.

Kaufman Hand Movements Test from the Kaufman Brief Intelligence Test (Kaufman & Kaufman, 1993)

The Hand Movements Test is a well-standardized and normed test for children based on a traditional measure of frontal lobe function in adults. Children are presented with progressively longer sequences of three hand movements, which they must imitate. The test has acceptable reliability and normative data and three studies have shown it to differentiate groups of ADHD from groups of normal children (Grodzinsky & Diamond, 1992; Mariani & Barkley, 1997) and from ADD children who are not hyperactive (Barkley, Grodzinsky, & Dupaul, 1992). Its sensitivity to ADHD may rest in the well-known fine motor coordination difficulties often seen in these children as well as in their inattention to the task itself or deficits in nonverbal working memory, especially as sequences of movements become progressively longer.

Digit Span from the Wechsler Adult Intelligence Scale, Third Edition (WAIS-III) (Wechsler, 1994)

This test involves two subtests. In one, the examinee is given a series of increasingly longer strings of digits by the examiner at a rate of one per second. The examinee must repeat them back in the same numerical sequence. In the second subtest, the examinee must repeat increasingly longer strings of digits in a backward order from that given by the examiner. For both tests, the participant is given two trials at each span length. The test is concluded when the participant fails to repeat both trials correctly at that span length. The score is the longest span length the participant was able to perform correctly on at least one of the two trials. The raw scores from both tests were combined to form a single raw score for this measure. This test was chosen to evaluate verbal working memory.

Simon Game

This is a commercially available game that consists of a circular plastic device housing four large colored keys on its top surface. Each key is a different color. When depressed, each of these keys emits a different tone. When activated, the game automatically presents a sequence of different tones and lights up the key corresponding to each tone as it does so. The subject must then press the keys in their correct sequence to reproduce the melody. With each trial, the sequence of tone/key combinations becomes increasingly longer and thus more complex. The score used here was the longest correctly reproduced sequence. This task was chosen to evaluate nonverbal working memory in a manner equivalent to a digit-span forward task. It is akin to self-ordered pointing tasks (see Lezak, 1995). Our past research with adults with ADHD (Barkley et al., 1996; Murphy, Barkley, et al., 2001) found those adults to be impaired relative to a control group on this measure. It is possible that some adults may be more familiar with this game than others; therefore we inquired about this issue with our participants. The groups did not differ in their familiarity with this game or in the highest level they were able to achieve. They were given two trials at each level of the game (levels I to IV). Most (57–77%) were able to complete level I, but fewer than 10% were able to complete level II.

Tower of London Test (Shallice, 1982)

This test presents the participant with a stand on which there are three spindles of different heights along with three balls of different colors (red, blue, green) arranged on two of these spindles. The participant is then shown a diagram illustrating the goal or final position in which these balls are to be rearranged. In proceeding to rearrange the balls in that final sequence, the participant most do so in the fewest moves. The task requires that participants look ahead to determine the proper order of moves; therefore it is considered a test of planning ability. The test has been used in a number of neuropsychological studies of children with ADHD where planning deficits have been noted (see Barkley, 1997; Grodzinsky & Diamond, 1992; Hervey et al., 2004).

that was significant, subsequent univariate tests were done. Where those were significant, pairwise comparisons were done among the groups to see which group differences were significant. Because there is some controversy over whether or not IQ should be a covariate in such analyses, we repeated the univariate tests a second time controlling for IQ. However, we disagree with doing so for two reasons discussed previously by Barkley (1997). One is that IQ and EF often show a low but significant relationship on many measures of each. Indeed, some of the subtests used in an IQ battery are thought to involve working memory, and recent editions of such tests often permit them to be interpreted as such via a separate score reported for them. Removing IQ through analysis of covariance therefore removes some of the variance in EF tasks with which it is related and would have nothing to do with IQ being a confounding variable due to selection bias. Just as important is the fact that IQ and ADHD often show an inherent negative relationship (see Barkley, 1997), so removing IQ may in fact remove part of the variance in EF tasks that is due to ADHD— the independent variable of interest. For instance, in the UMASS Study the correlation between IQ and number of ADHD symptoms across the entire sample is $r = -.11$ ($p = .04$) while for the Milwaukee Study, the relationship is $r = .22$ ($p = .01$). Although of a low magnitude, the relationships are significant and can be expected to remove some of the variance in the dependent measures that is the result of ADHD. Where this is so, using IQ as a covariate is unacceptable (Miller & Chapman, 2001). For this reason, while we report our results both ways we will interpret the results in the text for when IQ is *not* covaried making comments in footnotes about how results may have changed when IQ was covaried. We review the findings for each test separately below.

Response Inhibition and Inattention (Conners CPT)

The differences among the groups were significant (multivariate test for this set of scores was significant for the main effect for group). No effect of sex or its interaction with the groups was significant. The ADHD group made significantly more errors of omission than either the two control groups. They also had more reaction-time (RT) variability than both control groups. The findings are graphically shown in Figure 13.1 and are consistent with childhood data and other adult studies using CPTs (Frazier et al., 2004; Hervey et al., 2004). Past studies that factor analyzed this test suggested that omission scores and RT error and variability reflect inattentiveness and produce among the most reliable differences from control groups (Murphy et al., 2002). The ADHD group also made more errors of commission than the Community control group, in keeping with prior studies on adults with ADHD (see above); such errors are believed to reflect problems with inhibition (Murphy et al., 2002). But the Clinical control group

TABLE 13.1. Neuropsychological Test Results by Group for the UMASS Study

Measure	ADHD Mean	ADHD SD	Clinical Mean	Clinical SD	Community Mean	Community SD	F	p	Pairwise contrasts	F (–IQ)	p (–IQ)	Pairwise contrasts (–IQ)
Conners CPT							4.34	< .001				
Omission errors[A]	4.1	8.3	2.8	4.5	1.4	2.0	7.7	.001	1 > 2,3	7.1	.001	1 > 3
Commission errors[A]	12.1	6.9	12.6	7.4	7.7	5.9	18.3	.001	1,2 > 3	17.9	< .001	1,2 > 3
Hit RT[A]	385.3	75.9	373.9	73.3	389.9	76.5	1.0	NS				
Hit RT standard error[A]	7.3	3.7	6.4	2.6	5.6	1.8	10.6	< .001	1 > 2 > 3	10.2	< .001	1 > 3
RT variability[A]	11.8	11.4	10.1	7.7	7.0	3.3	10.9	< .001	1 > 2 > 3	10.3	< .001	1 > 3
Attentiveness[A]	3.1	1.0	3.1	1.0	3.8	0.9	20.5	< .001	1,2 < 3	20.1	< .001	1,2 < 3
Risk-taking[A]	.09	.16	.07	.11	.07	.12	1.6	NS				
Wisconsin Cart Sort							.92	NS				
Total errors[A]	95.1	16.1	99.8	13.2	99.2	14.4						
Perseverative responses[A]	98.8	20.0	101.7	14.5	102.6	17.9						
Perseverative errors[A]	98.0	19.9	101.2	13.9	102.0	17.5						
Nonperseverative errors[A]	94.0	14.6	98.9	13.0	97.9	12.9						
Conceptual responses[A]	66.4	14.5	65.7	9.8	64.7	12.7						
Categories completed[A]	5.3	1.4	5.7	1.1	5.5	1.4						
Trials to 1st category[A]	17.8	14.7	14.0	6.7	16.7	12.8						
Failures to maintain set	0.9	1.1	0.5	0.9	0.6	0.9						
Stroop Color–Word Test												
Color–Word Score[A]	100.7	13.6	103.2	13.5	105.1	11.3	3.3	.038	1 < 3	2.9	NS	
Color–Word Net Score[A]	11.1	13.6	7.9	12.9	6.7	11.3	3.6	.028	1 > 3	3.0	.05	1 > 3
Five-Point Design Fluency												
No. of unique designs[A]	26.7	9.3	28.5	9.5	33.2	8.7	14.0	< .001	1,2 < 3	14.7	< .001	1,2 < 3
No. of repeated designs[A]	0.8	1.5	0.6	1.0	0.9	1.2	1.2	NS		1.2	NS	
Perseverative error %[S]	3.2	5.7	2.5	4.0	2.7	3.8	1.8	NS		1.9	NS	
LAMB measures												
Paragraph—Free recall[A]							2.34	.006				
Trial 1 recall[S]	99.8	14.7	99.4	15.6	101.2	14.8	0.7	NS		0.2	NS	
Total recall[S]	95.6	15.5	99.5	15.5	99.4	14.7	2.2	NS		1.1	NS	
Delayed retention[S]	92.6	16.8	98.4	16.2	101.2	14.0	8.4	< .001	1 < 2,3	7.6	< .001	1 < 3

	ADHD M	ADHD SD	Clinical control M	Clinical control SD	Community control M	Community control SD	F	p	Pairwise	F(−IQ)	p(−IQ)	Pairwise (−IQ)
Paragraph—Free and Cued Recall[A]												
Trial 1 recall[S]	97.9	14.3	99.2	14.9	99.6	14.0	0.4	NS		0.2	NS	
Total recall[S]	95.1	17.1	98.8	15.3	99.2	14.4	2.2	NS		1.3	NS	
Delayed retention[S]	105.6	13.4	108.8	12.9	110.0	10.7	3.8	.023	1 < 3	2.8	NS	
Word List—Free Recall												
Trial 1 recall	97.8	13.8	101.6	15.2	98.6	13.8	2.2	NS		1.7	NS	
Total recall	96.5	16.0	100.2	16.8	99.5	15.0	1.4	NS		0.4	NS	
Delayed retention	91.9	17.3	93.1	20.9	98.7	16.3	4.0	.018	1,2 < 3	4.0	.02	1,2 < 3
Word List—Free and Cued Recall							**2.06**	**.018**				
Trial 1 recall	95.9	13.4	100.3	14.9	96.7	13.9	3.1	.044	NS	2.9	NS	
Total recall	93.5	16.6	99.3	15.0	96.9	14.7	3.4	.034	1 < 2	2.3	NS	
Delayed retention	98.0	11.1	99.9	10.2	101.9	8.3	4.7	.010	1 < 3	3.8	.023	1 < 3
Word Pair Learning[A]							**3.44**	**.002**				
Trial 1 recall	99.1	18.2	107.2	17.2	100.3	16.2	5.8	.003	2 > 1,3	4.3	.014	2 > 1,3
Total recall	99.3	18.0	108.8	17.5	100.6	16.2	8.0	< .001	2 > 1,3	6.4	.002	2 > 1,3
Delayed retention	113.1	10.3	114.2	9.0	114.3	7.6	0.6	NS		0.3	NS	
Digit Span							**2.10**	**.023**				
Forward	102.8	12.9	107.6	14.0	108.1	14.4	5.4	.005	1 < 2,3			
Backward	100.8	14.2	105.0	16.4	104.1	15.9	3.0	.05	NS			
Total	102.2	13.9	107.2	15.6	106.6	14.8	4.7	.009	1 < 2,3			
Supraspan												
Learning	96.0	15.4	99.4	15.6	95.3	14.8	1.8	NS				
Retention	96.1	13.7	99.2	13.6	95.9	14.2	1.7	NS				
Simple Figure Task[A]							**5.87**	**.001**				
Trial 1 recall	96.6	16.6	100.0	16.7	95.7	12.8	2.0	NS		1.5	NS	
Total recall	96.6	15.9	100.4	17.2	91.8	13.5	9.6	< .001	3 < 1,2	9.5	< .001	3 < 1,2
Delayed retention	96.2	15.4	99.0	12.9	86.7	14.0	20.5	< .001	3 < 1,2	20.4	< .001	3 < 1,2
Complex Figure Task[A]												
Trial 1 recall	99.3	16.4	105.3	14.9	100.6	15.5	3.6	.029	2 > 1,3	2.3	NS	
Total recall	99.7	17.0	106.6	15.6	99.0	15.4	6.1	.002	2 > 1,3	4.8	.009	2 > 1,3
Delayed retention	102.4	17.0	105.4	17.0	97.4	14.3	6.1	.002	3 < 1,2	6.2	.002	3 < 1,2

Note. Sample sizes are ADHD = 143, Clinical control = 92, Community control = 108. For Nelson–Denny, they are ADHD = 140, Clinical control = 92, Community control = 106. For WCST, they are ADHD = 139, Clinical control = 90, Community control = 104. For the Stroop Color–Word Test, they are ADHD = 135, Clinical control = 90, Community control = 107. For the Five-Point Test, they are ADHD = 119, Clinical control = 77, Community control = 109. For the LAMB, they are ADHD = 135, Clinical control = 89, Community control = 108. SD = standard deviation; F = F-test results of the analysis of variance (or covariance); p = probability value for the F-test; NS = not significant; $F(-IQ)$ = F-test results of the analysis of covariance with IQ covaried; $p(-IQ)$ = probability value for that $F(-IQ)$-test; pairwise contrasts (−IQ) = results of pairwise comparisons using IQ as a covariate; [S] = significant main effect for sex; RT = reaction time; LAMB = Learning and Memory Battery (standard scores).

Statistical analysis: On the CPT, WCST, and LAMB measures, multivariate analyses of variance (MANOVAs) were conducted first on all measures from the CPT and on highly related sets of scores for the LAMB (Paragraph Learning, Word List Learning, Digit Span, and Figure Memory). The results for these MANOVA analyses appear in **bold** next to the name of that set of measures. If the omnibus multivariate F (Wilks lambda), was significant, then univariate analyses of (co)variance were done followed by subsequent pairwise contrasts as necessary. On the remaining tests, groups were initially compared using two way (groups × sex) analysis of variance (or covariance). Where this analysis was significant ($p < .05$) for the main effect for group, pairwise comparisons of the groups were conducted. All analyses were repeated using IQ as a covariate. [A] indicates that age served as a covariate in these analyses.

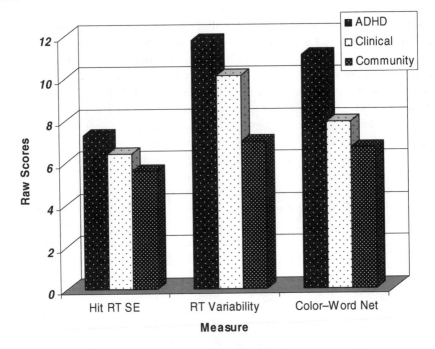

FIGURE 13.1. Raw scores for each group from selected neuropsychological tests on which the ADHD group was significantly different from either the Clinical or Community control group from the UMASS Study. Hit RT SE = hit reaction time standard error score from the Conners CPT; RT variability = reaction time variability from the Conners CPT; Color–Word Net = Stroop Color–Word Test interference score minus the color score. Tests represent inattention and interference control.

also made more such errors, suggesting that these errors may not be specific to ADHD in adults but extend to other disordered populations. Therefore, while the ADHD group shows problems with both inattentiveness and inhibition on the CPT task relative to the Community control group, replicating previous studies with adults with ADHD, our study shows that it is their CPT inattentiveness that distinguishes them from adults having other disorders than ADHD.[1]

We wanted to know which of these various CPT measures was the most useful for discriminating among our groups. We used a discriminant function analysis to determine this issue relative to the Community controls. Two

---

[1] The reanalysis in which we covaried IQ still resulted in a significant multivariate main effect for group. And the same univariate tests were significant. The pairwise contrasts also did not change much except that the Clinical control group no longer differed significantly from the ADHD group on omissions, RT error or RT variability, but those comparisons were marginally significant ($p = .054–.072$) nonetheless. In sum, covarying IQ did not change our findings substantially.

scores were significant at doing so: Hit RT standard error and commission errors (lambda = .821, F = 26.53, df = 2/243, p < .001). They classified 66% of community controls and 75% of ADHD group correctly. We did the same analysis for discriminating the ADHD versus Clinical controls. That showed just one test as being useful: Hit RT standard error again (lambda = .983, F = 4.09, df = 1/230, p = .044). It correctly classified none of the Clinical controls, misclassifying them all as ADHD, but it classified 100% of the ADHD group correctly.

It is again possible that those adults taking medication at study entry may have biased our results. We compared those on medication to those not on medication within each of the ADHD and Clinical control groups and found these two subsets not to differ, implying no obvious bias of our results due to medication status.

Such a result for RT variability is of theoretical or conceptual interest in considering the attention deficit that may be characteristic of ADHD. As many others have noted before us, RT variability appears to be among the most reliable and distinctive differences found in studies using continuous performance and reaction time tasks going back more than 30 years (Douglas, 1972). Many others have reported it since (see Kuntsi, Oosterlaan, & Stevenson, 2001; Rucklidge & Tannock, 2002). In unpublished data, Barkley found RT variability to be associated with higher-density dopamine transport in the striatum in a study using altropane I^{123} to assess dopamine transport activity via SPECT scanning in adults with ADHD and control adults. That was the only CPT score to show such an association after controlling for all other CPT scores. Gilden and Hancock (in press) have recently shown that adults showing such high levels of response variability are also likely to have higher levels of ADHD symptoms and are more likely to be diagnosed as having ADHD. Their application of power spectra analysis to such variability suggests the presence of distinctive noise processes affecting memory and performance in those with high response variability that are not typical of normal cognitive processes or their mere exaggeration. Instead, results for those with high response variability suggest a qualitative difference, what is known as a "random walk contour," to their performance that could serve as a neuropsychological marker or endophenotype for behavioral genetic studies of ADHD. As they have stated:

The reaction time correlation function appears to be under the control of whatever it is that allows people to be vigilant. People that cannot maintain vigilance lose their place at some point in the normal processing chain. Loss of place results in the insertion of an off-task time interval into the reaction time measurement. . . . The off-task intervals are not entirely independent. There is a tendency for people to pause for as long as they have in the recent past and this generates the observed random walk. (p. 6)

To summarize, the CPT reaction time variability and commission error scores may be of some use in distinguishing ADHD cases from normal cases being characteristic of the disorder. But they are not able to distinguish ADHD from other clinical disorders effectively and should not be used as diagnostic tools. And so they are not diagnostic of the disorder. Given that we found that a single interview question involving the symptom of "often being easily distractible by extraneous events" was also able to distinguish normal control adults from those with ADHD with high accuracy, there would be little reason to add a CPT task to that simple interview question if all one wishes to do is determine if a patient is normal or not. If the issue is differential diagnosis of ADHD from other disorders, the CPT will not prove very useful.

Set or Attention Shifting (WCST)

No overall group differences were significant for this set of measures (the multivariate test for the main effect for group was not significant). Our results are certainly in keeping with those of other studies of adults and children with ADHD in showing this test to be of little or no value in documenting EF deficits in those with ADHD (Frazier et al., 2004; Hervey et al., 2004).[2] The sexes were not found to differ on these scores, nor did sex interact with group in any significant way. Comparisons of those on and off medication within the ADHD and Clinical control groups revealed no significant differences, again suggesting no obvious bias of these results due to medication status.

Interference Control or Resistance to Distraction (Stroop Color–Word Test)

The color–word score is a measure of the individual's ability to resist responding to the printed name of a color word while telling the examiner the name of the color of ink in which that word is printed and which may differ from that color named in the word itself. An alternative means of computing this score subtracts out the score for naming colors from the color-word score leaving a net score believed to represent the construct of resistance to distraction that is unbiased by color naming ability. We found our groups to differ significantly on both of these scores. Only the ADHD group differed from the Community controls, consistent with prior studies that made similar comparisons. Neither of these groups differed from the Clinical controls, who placed between the other two groups, although the difference between the ADHD and Clinical controls was marginally significant ($p = .074$). Our results agree with numerous previous studies and also

---

[2] With IQ covaried, the results were unchanged.

show that the problem is one of interference, not just color naming. This suggests that while adults with ADHD may have difficulties with interference control, especially compared to a normal control group, the deficit is not as striking when compared to other clinical control adults.[3] There was no effect of sex of participant on these scores nor did it interact with the group factor in any significant way. Medication status likewise was not found to have any biasing effect on these results.

Noverbal (Design) Fluency (Five-Point Test)

This test is believed to reflect nonverbal fluency or the ability to generate multiple possible responses through the mental manipulation of nonverbal information (see sidebar). We found that both the ADHD and Clinical control groups did more poorly than the Community controls but did not differ from each other on the number of unique designs they created within the time limit. Again we checked our results for a potential medication bias and found that the ADHD adults on medication made more repeated design errors (perseverative errors) and a higher percentage of such errors. We therefore reanalyzed these scores using only those who were not on medication at study entry; we found that the number of unique designs remained significant and the pairwise comparisons showed the same result 1,2 < 3. However, this time the difference between the ADHD and Clinical controls was nearly significant ($p = .052$). For the other two tests, the results were the same (nonsignificant). And so our results suggest that both groups of clinic-referred adults did worse on this test than Community control adults, but the adults with ADHD may be somewhat more impaired than the Clinical control adults, though the difference is hardly clinically impressive.[4]

There was a sex difference on this measure that reached significance. It occurred on Perseverative Errors % and indicated that females had higher scores (3.5) than males (2.3) ($p = .02$).

Verbal and Nonverbal Learning and Working Memory (LAMB)

This is a very complex battery of tests (see sidebar) that was chosen to assess verbal and nonverbal learning and verbal and nonverbal working memory through its use of delayed recall (retention) trials. We discuss the results under each set of conceptually related scores:

---

[3] When controlling for IQ was repeated, the initial group difference on the color-word score became nonsignificant, though only marginally ($p = .057$). The net color word score remained significant.

[4] The results were unchanged when IQ was covaried.

Paragraph Learning and Retention

The groups differed significantly on the set of six scores for Paragraph learning and memory (The multivariate test was significant for the main effect of group).[5] We found that the ADHD group was not impaired on the immediate recall trials of both tasks but were more impaired on the retention trials in comparison to the Community control group on both tests. The adults with ADHD were also more impaired than the Clinical controls on the paragraph task that did not involve cued recall and were marginally so on the free+cued recall task ($p < .06$). This implies that retention of information is more problematic for the ADHD group, perhaps related to a working memory problem. We did find a significant sex difference ($F = 2.69$, $df = 6/320$, $p = .015$) in which females performed better than males on 5 of the 6 scores from these paragraph learning and memory tasks. The interaction of sex with group, however, was not significant. Medication status appeared to have no biasing effects on these measures.

Word List Learning and Memory

For the six scores from the two Word List memory tests, the groups differed significantly from each other on the overall multivariate test (main effect for group was significant). The sex of the participant had no significant effects on these results, nor did it interact with group in any significant way. As with Paragraph memory, once again we see that the problem for the ADHD group is principally with retention. The clinical controls also had some trouble with that on the first free recall test.[6] Again, we find that those with ADHD have the most difficulty with free recall, and cueing makes it less so. Also, a comparison of those on medication to those not on medication in both the ADHD and Clinical control groups revealed no significant differences. Again, this suggests that medication status did not bias these results.

Word Pair List Learning and Memory

For the three tests from the Word Pair memory test, the overall initial (multivariate) analysis found the groups to differ significantly. Of great interest

---

[5] When we repeated the analyses covarying for IQ, these multivariate effects did not change. However, the significant effect on free+cued recall retention test was no longer significant, but only marginally so ($p = .06$). And the pairwise contrast for free recall retention no longer showed a significant difference from the clinical controls—only a marginal one (.079). The clinical controls fall between these two more extreme groups.

[6] The reanalysis covarying for IQ did not change the multivariate results, but one of the measures became nonsignificant (Total Recall for Free and Cued trials).

here is that the Clinical controls outperformed both the ADHD and Community control groups.[7] This is important evidence of a double dissociation between the ADHD and the Clinical control groups, where we find that the Clinical control adults have a selective advantage over the ADHD group, while the inverse was true on the Paragraph and Word List learning tasks above and with Digit Span below. The sex of participant had no effect on these results, nor did medication status.

Digit Span

The groups differed significantly on the overall analysis of the five Digit Span tasks (the multivariate main effect for group was significant). The adults with ADHD had more difficulty than the two control groups mainly in Digit Span forward. But Digit Span backward shows the same trend, and the overall total score was also different, showing a disadvantage for the ADHD group.[8] When we repeated the analyses for the Digit Span tasks comparing just unmedicated subjects, the results remained significant. For Digit Span forward, the pairwise contrasts were the same. For Digit Span backward, the pairwise contrasts were now significant, with the ADHD group worse than the Community control group, whereas they were not previously so. For Digit Span total, the pairwise contrast found the ADHD group to perform worse than both control groups, as before. So, medication status did not change the results other than making the difference between ADHDs and Clinical controls on Digit Span backward more distinct this time. The main effect for sex was also significant. This largely favored males but only for the three Digit Span and not the two supraspan scores. Sex did not interact with the group factor, which again shows no distinctive pattern for females with ADHD than what otherwise would be expected from sex differences in the general population.

Figure (Nonverbal) Learning and Memory

On the Simple and Complex Figures test (six scores), the groups were found to differ significantly (the multivariate main effect for group was significant). The groups differed on five of these six scores. But the individual scores were very surprising in some respects. For instance, the ADHD and Clinical control groups actually performed better on the simple tasks than the Community control group. Also, the Clinical control group outperformed both the ADHD and Community control adults on the complex task. Comparing medicated and

---

[7] The results remained unchanged after covarying IQ.
[8] Controlling for IQ made the multivariate analysis nonsignificant.

unmedicated participants on these scores did show a possible significant biasing effect. We therefore repeated the analyses using just the unmedicated participants, and the results remained the same. The sex of our participants had no significant effect on these scores.

The above findings for the figure tasks were also true above for Word Pair learning. Once again, this implies a possible double dissociation in which the Clinical group not only has no deficits on some tasks but outperforms the adults with ADHD and even normal control adults on those tasks (Word Pair and Complex Figure) on which the ADHD adults are impaired. In contrast, the ADHD group shows selective deficits on other tasks (Paragraph retention) not seen in the Clinical control group. Those tasks on which the ADHD group were most impaired are graphically shown in Figure 13.2.

It is possible that the level of anxiety of participants may be a factor in these results as anxiety may prompt better performance in some ways and may have been more typical of the Clinical control group and ADHD group than the Community control group. We checked this and found partial support for that idea for the simple figure task. Anxiety (SCL-90-R) was significantly though modestly related to simple task performance (rs = .11 and .22 for the simple task scores on which differences were noted, ps = .05 and .001, respectively). But anxiety was negatively related to Word Pair performance for the retention score on which the Clinical controls had done well (r = −.22, p < .001). So we doubt that anxiety alone is the reason for such superior results for the Clinical controls.[9]

Given these group differences on the various LAMB measures, we wished to see which of these tests may have the greatest utility for discriminating our groups. We did a discriminant function analysis comparing the ADHD with the Community control group on just those LAMB measures that were significantly different between these groups. Five measures were found to be useful (significant). They were Paragraph free retention, Word List retention, Digit Span forward, simple figure total recall and simple figure retention. But we found the latter two to be negatively related (inversely) to ADHD because the ADHD group actually performed better on them than the Community control group. These five scores correctly predicted 73% of controls and 77% of ADHD group. When we repeated this analysis comparing the ADHD versus Clinical controls and just one test, Word Pair total recall, it significantly differentiated the groups, but not very well. It classified just 35% of Clinical controls correctly but 81% of ADHDs correctly. These results suggest that while some of the LAMB measures might be modestly useful for distinguishing the ADHD from the Community control

---

[9] We repeated all analyses covarying for IQ. It made no difference here for the results of the multivariate or univariate analyses.

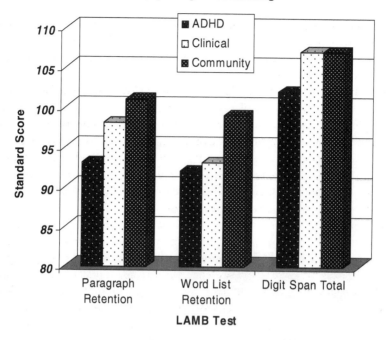

FIGURE 13.2. Standard scores for each group on selected subtests of the Learning and Memory Battery (LAMB) representing verbal working memory deficits in the UMASS Study.

adults, they are less so than the single interview question concerning distractibility noted above (and in Chapter 4). The LAMB measures therefore would not be useful for differential diagnosis of ADHD from other clinical disorders. Once more this illustrates our earlier point that some test score patterns may be characteristic of ADHD yet not be diagnostic of it.

Best Tests for Group Discrimination

We took all the tests which the earlier discriminant functions showed had some utility for the differentiation between the ADHD and Community control groups and used them in a single discriminant function analysis. These tests included those from the CPT and LAMB (and only where ADHDs were worse, not better), the Stroop Color–Word net score, and the five-points unique designs score. Out of these tests, five contributed to differentiating these groups: CPT Hit RT standard error (inattention), CPT Commissions (poor inhibition), unique designs (nonverbal fluency), Paragraph memory free recall retention, and Digit Span forward (verbal working memory). This set of five measures accurately classified 81% of the Community control group and 64% of the ADHD group. We did the same analysis for differentiating the Clinical control group versus the ADHD group. The best test was Paragraph free recall retention, but its accuracy was just 31% for the Clinical control group, though 81% of ADHD group. To summarize, these results indicate that ADHD in adults is associated with selective neuropsychological deficits in attention, inhibition, verbal working memory, and nonverbal fluency relative to the general population (Community group). But any effort to use such tests for classifying cases would yield only moderate results for distinguishing the ADHD and Community control adults and be outperformed by the single interview item having to do with often being easily distractible. These tests would prove of little value in the differential diagnosis of ADHD from other clinical disorders.

The Milwaukee Study Results

The longitudinal Milwaukee Study did not utilize as extensive a battery of neuropsychological tests as did the UMASS Study. Nevertheless, the results for those tests we did employ are in keeping with the results from the UMASS Study and the earlier literature. The results for the measures collected in the Milwaukee Study are displayed in Table 13.2. Once more, we present the findings first without controlling for IQ score and then again with IQ serving as a covariate. Our interest, however, is in the results where IQ is not a covariate for reasons explained above. We chose several measures representing executive functioning, some of which were also used in the UMASS Study. Our measures were the Stroop Color–Word task, again, as our measure of distractibility or interference control, the Simon Game and Kaufman Hand Movements test as our tests of nonverbal working memory (and motor sequencing), the WAIS-III Digit Span subtests as a measure of verbal working memory, the 5-Points Design Fluency test again as our measure of nonverbal fluency, and the Tower of London as a measure of planning ability (see sidebar for test descriptions).

The results for the Stroop Color–Word Test are similar to those found in the UMASS Study in that the H+ADHD group performed significantly worse than the nonpersistent ADHD group (H–ADHD) and the Community control group on the interference portion of this test, believed to reflect resistance to distraction. Yet both hyperactive groups did poorly on the word and color–word scores relative to the Community control group, while the H–ADHD group did worse than the control group on the color score, with the H+ADHD group placing between these two groups. All this suggests that both hyperactive groups may still have difficulty with speed of naming colors and of reading words, consistent with the findings of Nigg et al. (2005) that speed of responding is problematic in ADHD adults. But it is the hyperactive group with current (persistent) ADHD

TABLE 13.2. Neuropsychological Test Results by Group for the Milwaukee Study

Measure	H+ADHD Mean	H+ADHD SD	H-ADHD Mean	H-ADHD SD	Community Mean	Community SD	F	p	Pairwise contrasts	F (-IQ)	p (-IQ)	Pairwise contrasts (-IQ)
Simon Game												
Longest sequence	8.0	2.1	7.9	2.3	9.4	2.4	9.00	< .001	1,2 < 3	3.27	.040	1,2 < 3
Five-Point Design Fluency												
No. of Unique designs	32.4	10.1	30.5	11.7	36.5	9.9	6.15	.003	1,2 < 3	0.93	NS	
No. of Repeated designs	1.3	1.7	1.5	2.5	0.9	1.3	1.71	NS		0.50	NS	
Perseverative error %	3.6	4.7	4.7	8.2	2.5	3.1	2.52	NS		0.80	NS	
No. of Rule infractions	1.2	1.5	1.6	2.5	1.0	1.3	1.55	NS		0.89	NS	
WAIS-III Digit Span	9.6	2.6	9.4	2.7	11.8	2.9	16.68	< .001	1,2 < 3	4.12	.018	1,2 < 3
Stroop Color–Word Test (T-scores)												
Word score	45.3	7.6	44.8	9.5	50.5	8.5	9.51	< .001	1,2 < 3	1.04	NS	
Color score	47.0	6.6	45.6	9.0	49.7	8.9	4.34	.014	2 < 3	0.76	NS	
Color–word score	46.7	8.0	47.9	9.5	54.5	8.2	15.40	< .001	1,2 < 3	2.90	NS	
Interference score	49.5	6.0	51.6	6.0	53.4	6.1	6.10	.003	1 < 2,3	3.25	.041	1 < 2,3
Tower of London												
Total score	30.2	3.2	20.1	4.3	31.1	2.4	2.08	NS		1.38	NS	
No. correct 1st trial	8.1	1.7	8.1	1.6	8.5	1.6	1.39	NS		0.90	NS	
Mean time to first manipulation	4.4	2.9	5.5	3.8	4.5	2.5	2.47	NS		1.69	NS	
Kaufman Hand Movements Test												
No. correct	4.5	2.3	5.2	2.2	6.3	1.9	11.19	< .001	1 < 2 < 3	2.97	.050	1 < 2,3
Longest correct sequence	4.8	1.9	5.4	1.6	5.9	1.2	8.08	< .001	1 < 2 < 3	2.87	NS	

Note. Sample sizes are H+ADHD = 52, H–ADHD = 79, Community control = 73. *SD* = standard deviation; *F* = *F*-test results of the analysis of variance (or covariance); *p* = probability value for the *F*-test; NS = not significant; $F(-IQ)$ = *F*-test results of the analysis of covariance with IQ was covaried; $p(-IQ)$ = probability value for that $F(-IQ)$-test; pairwise contrasts (–IQ) = results of pairwise comparisons using Neuman–Keuls post hoc comparisons when IQ was covaried.

Statistical analysis: Groups were initially compared using one-way (groups) analysis of variance (or covariance). Where this analysis was significant ($p < .05$) for the main effect for group, pairwise comparisons of the groups were conducted. All analyses were repeated using IQ as a covariate.

423

specifically that continues to have problems with resistance to distraction or interference control, a form of inhibition as Barkley noted (1997), consistent with their currently greater levels of ADHD. Thus, as Nigg et al. (2002) earlier discovered, childhood ADHD that persists into adulthood has a specific association with deficits in inhibition.

Both hyperactive groups had difficulties with our two tests of nonverbal working memory, these being the Simon Game and Kaufman Hand Movements Test, relative to the control group. Hyperactive children as adults appear to have deficits in this domain of executive functioning even if their ADHD has not persisted to this age. Yet, the persistently ADHD group had even greater difficulties with the Hand Movements Test than the nonpersistent group, again suggesting somewhat greater executive (working memory) and motor coordination problems in those having more severe ADHD at follow-up. This finding replicates earlier studies of children with ADHD in finding this task to be more impaired in those with ADHD and extends these findings to adults with ADHD with whom this task has not been previously used. Therefore, like clinic-referred adults with ADHD, children with ADHD as adults have difficulties with this domain of executive functioning.

Our sole measure of verbal working memory was the WAIS-III Digit Span Test, which is very similar to though nowhere near as extensive an assessment as the digit span tasks from the LAMB used in the UMASS Study above. As in that study, we found the hyperactive (ADHD) groups to perform this task more poorly than did the Clinical control group but the two hyperactive groups did not differ in this respect. As with nonverbal working memory above, it seems that verbal working memory deficits may persist in hyperactive children as adults regardless of whether or not their ADHD has persisted to this age (27 years). These group differences in nonverbal and verbal working memory deficits are graphically illustrated in Figure 13.3.

Just as in the UMASS Study, we also used the Five-Point Design Fluency Test as a measure of nonverbal fluency, and here again we found ADHD to be associated with difficulties in generating as many unique designs as was our control group. Again, both hyperactive groups performed more poorly on this task yet did not differ from each other. This would seem to suggest that not only do problems with nonverbal working memory exist in children previously diagnosed as ADHD in adults, but nonverbal fluency deficits exist as well whether or not ADHD has persisted to adulthood.

We employed the Tower of London Test here as a measure of planning ability in the belief that this aspect of executive functioning might be associated with ADHD in adulthood. We had not used this task in the UMASS Study, however, precluding comparisons of our findings with that study. We did not find any group differences on this task. Neither did Riccio et al. (2005) in their study of clinic-referred adults with ADHD. Yet studies of children using this or

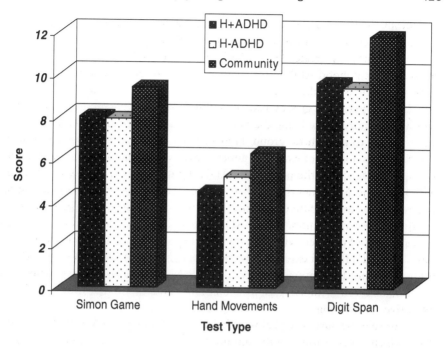

FIGURE 13.3. Tests of working memory from the Milwaukee Study (nonverbal = Simon and Hand Movements tests; verbal = digit span). H+ADHD = hyperactive group that currently has ADHD at age-27 follow-up; H–ADHD = hyperactive group that does not have ADHD at follow-up; Community = Community control group.

similar tower tasks have found ADHD to be associated with problems performing this task (Hervey et al., 2004). Despite adults with ADHD complaining of difficulties with planning ahead (see Chapter 7, also Riccio et al., 2005), those difficulties were not reflected in their performance on this task. All this suggests that either the tower tasks are too simple to detect the planning deficits in adults with ADHD, unlike children with the disorder, or such planning deficits as may be reflected in this sort of task are not a hallmark of the adult stage of the disorder.

The Role of Neuropsychological Tests in the Diagnosis of ADHD

It is our sense that neuropsychological testing has become a rather popular means of evaluating adult patients for ADHD, with some going so far as to claim that specific batteries of neuropsychological tests can serve to confirm the diagnosis of

ADHD in adults, with particular emphasis on tests of inhibition, attention, executive functioning and especially working memory (Biggs, 1995; Epstein, Johnson, Varia, & Conners, 2001). There is a growing body of evidence that adults with ADHD do manifest neuropsychological deficits (Boonstra, Oosterlaan, Sergeant, & Buitelaar, 2005; Hervey et al., 2004; Seidman et al., 2004) similar to those seen in children with ADHD, where the literature is vastly more abundant (Frazier et al., 2004). Our results essentially confirm those seen in earlier studies. Considerable interest therefore exists in the development of tests for adult ADHD, with an implication that these methods are more objective than and hence preferable to the more subjective (and much maligned) but routinely used clinical interviews, rating scales, and DSM diagnostic criteria. Alternative diagnostic strategies for ADHD diagnosis, including use of extensive neuropsychological batteries, are available in many communities and are popular with clinicians and patients. Such popularity, in our opinion, has far outstripped the available evidence supporting the use of these tests for diagnostic purposes, as Barkley and McGough (2004) earlier concluded. The majority of neuropsychological studies of adults with ADHD are limited to small samples sizes and comparisons of ADHD with normal groups as opposed to the more informative comparison of ADHD against non-ADHD clinical groups. As we showed above, such tests are not especially accurate at distinguishing ADHD from other clinical disorders likely to be seen in outpatient clinics.

Furthermore, regardless of the findings that some adults with ADHD demonstrate deficits on neuropsychological testing, clinicians need to guard against overemphasizing an algorithm of test scores, discrepancies, relative weaknesses, or below expected scores as being diagnostic of the disorder. Again, some test patterns can be characteristic of a group with a disorder (ADHD) but not diagnostic of individuals with it. Like McGough and Barkley before us (2004), it is our experience that clinicians sometimes tend to minimize or even ignore the more central features of making the ADHD diagnosis: establishing a childhood or at least adolescent onset of symptoms, showing evidence of chronic and pervasive real world functional impairment in major life activities, and ruling out alternative explanations for the symptoms. Instead, they report a series of test scores as the major rationale for the diagnosis. It may be more appropriate and persuasive to utilize test scores as evidence consistent with a previously made diagnosis that supports the long-standing history of functional impairment established during the nontesting part of the evaluation (interview, reports from collateral informants, and review of historical records ideally). Yet even this concession to neuropsychological testing is questionable when a sizable minority of otherwise well-documented ADHD adult patients achieve scores within the broadly normal range for these tests, as we demonstrated above.

Neuropsychological assessments also involve significantly more expense than rating scales and clinical interviews, further contributing to the need for careful consideration of their incremental value for clinical diagnosis beyond the less costly and more routine interviews and rating scales. Furthermore, testing advocates often fail to acknowledge the likely ceiling effects on many neuropsychological measures for adults, where maximum performance is often attained in early to midadolescent years (Riccio et al., 2005). This makes it highly likely that even adults with ADHD, despite having neuropsychological deficits, may be readily able to perform satisfactorily on such tests. This would make false negatives commonplace, as we saw in reality above in our own studies. Consistent with this view, research to date has shown no proven advantage of such tests in discriminating ADHD from clinical or control groups with reasonable accuracy to warrant widespread clinical use even for children (Barkley & Grodzinsky, 1994; Cohen & Shapiro, 2007; Gordon et al., 2006).

Most problematic in assertions, particularly by test developers and promoters, that one or another neuropsychological measure has clinical diagnostic utility is the frequent failure to provide the proper evidence to support such claims. Findings concerning sensitivity and specificity are the pieces of information most often provided but are not especially relevant for issues of clinical diagnosis despite their use to support the construct or conceptual validity of a particular test. These statistical terms refer to the likelihood that a person will obtain a normal or abnormal test finding *if he or she is already known to have or not have the disorder*. The clinical circumstance is precisely the opposite of this—clinicians must determine whether or not the person has the disorder when given the normal or abnormal score on the test. That requires computation of positive (PPP) and negative predictive power (NPP) or the probability of having the disorder given an abnormal score versus the probability of not having the disorder given a normal score. Their companion statistics are false positives and false negatives. To date, studies examining neuropsychological tests of executive functioning have found relatively high PPP yet unacceptably low NPP for predicting the diagnosis of ADHD. Consequently we, along with other authors, do not recommend use of these tests in clinical settings with children (Barkley & Grodzinsky, 1994) or adults. This suggests that where abnormal scores are found, a disorder may be highly likely, though this does not mean that the disorder is necessarily ADHD. But where normal scores are obtained, the results are not especially helpful in ruling out ADHD given that a substantial minority of these individuals perform normally on these tests.

The few studies of adults with ADHD are even less encouraging than those on children, with reported classification accuracies typically ranging from 44 to 75% (Epstein, Conners, Sitarenios, & Erhardt, 1998; Jenkins et al., 1998; Weyandt et al., 1998). Our results above largely agree with such low to moderate classification levels. The only promising study to date was that of Lovejoy and colleagues (Lovejoy et al., 1999), which reported a PPP of 83 to 100% across a set of six neuropsychological measures, consistent with studies of child ADHD.

But just as consistent were the findings of unsatisfactorily high rates of NPP for most tests. Most studies compare ADHD adults to normal or community control groups. This is not especially informative, as it does not address the issue faced by clinicians—and that is one of differential diagnosis of ADHD from other disorders. The vast majority of clinically referred patients are not normal but have some psychiatric or developmental disorder. The mere fact that someone has asked for an appointment at a psychiatric clinic is often as accurate in predicting that the person will wind up having some disorder on evaluation (being nonnormal). What clinicians require is assistance with differential diagnosis, not determining normalcy, which could probably be done by just using the telephone call to the clinic as a diagnostic tool. Hence demonstrations of ADHD versus normal groups are of little value concerning the utility of tests for diagnosis in clinical practice. For now, as McGough and Barkley concluded earlier (2004), we believe there is insufficient evidence to support the use of neuropsychological tests in confirming the diagnosis of ADHD, although such tests may be helpful in revealing general cognitive delays or specific learning or cognitive processing deficits (Biggs, 1995; Quinlan, 2000). To conclude, clinicians need to appreciate the fact that characteristics of a group with a disorder are not necessarily diagnostic of individuals with that disorder.

Limitations of Our Studies

In any such scientific endeavors as we have reported here, it is important to acknowledge the limitations of the methods and conclusions. Many such limitations were raised and addressed throughout the preceding chapters. Others are worth noting here. We begin with those we believe may have affected follow-up in the Milwaukee Study. One noteworthy methodological limitation was that the examiner was not blind to the original group membership of the participants as being either hyperactive or Community controls at study entry. They were blind, however, to the subgrouping status of the hyperactive participants as currently ADHD by the various diagnostic approaches examined here. This lack of blindness could have introduced some bias into the interview process. Nevertheless, the results of this study for self-reported information are nearly identical to those from the New York and Swedish studies, where examiner blindness was employed, suggesting that any bias that may have occurred here was relatively minimal.

The Community control group used here may also have been problematic for several reasons, not the least of which is its relatively small size and associated problems with limited statistical power for detecting small to moderate effect sizes. The use of volunteer families and a "snowball" recruiting technique combined with rating scale thresholds below which these participants must have placed also may have resulted in an unrepresentative sampling of the general childhood population from this geographical region. This control group therefore may represent a higher-functioning or otherwise skewed sample of individuals than would be typical of a random sampling of the general childhood population. This may have led to some "false-positive" group differences here that might otherwise have not occurred with a more representative sampling technique. However, this would not have affected comparisons between self- and parent-reported information within the hyperactive group. And it would not have affected the comparison of this study to earlier follow-up studies, whose control groups suffered from many of these same limitations. The fact that our Community control group had significant rates of psychiatric disorders, antisocial behavior, drug use, occupational, driving, and money problems, among others, indicates that they were hardly a supernormal group.

The use of this control group to establish the threshold for recovery from ADHD may also have posed a limitation for this study in view of the potentially biased representativeness of that sample. The potential limitations of this control group caution against extending the precise cutoffs we used for symptoms and impairment to other studies and especially to clinical decisions concerning the presence of ADHD in adults.

As for the UMASS Study, it also had several noteworthy limitations. Like the Milwaukee Study, it did not gather information on interjudge agreement concerning the other diagnoses developed from the structured interviews apart from the initial diagnosis of ADHD. Yet the frequency and pattern of these findings are generally consistent with most of those obtained by other investigators, in which reliability of diagnosis from a structured interview was examined; this provides some assurance of the validity of the present results. The examiner in the present study also was not blind to the clinical referral versus control group membership of the individuals that could have introduced some bias into these results. Nevertheless, the examiner was blind to the grouping of clinic-referred participants as either having ADHD or not, so such a bias could not account for the numerous differences found in those crucial comparisons. The consistency of these results with studies of ADHD in children, follow-up studies of ADHD children to adulthood, and other studies of clinically referred adults having ADHD is also somewhat reassuring that such potential for bias does not entirely account for these particular results. Finally, the Clinical control group here could be considered to be better functioning than a general population sample, given the volunteer status and the requirement that they have no history of a serious current psychiatric disorder or current treatment for such disorder. As a consequence, the differences between the ADHD and Community versus Clinical control groups here may have been greater than had a general population sample not screened for current psychiatric disorder been used.

In both studies, each source of information about the participants comes with its own limitations. We tried to correct for these by obtaining information from others who knew the participants and from archival records (such as school transcripts). We also incorporated various psychological tests and standardized self-report instruments in a further effort to present a multimethod, multisource examination of these participant groups. We urge readers to bear these and other limitations of our methods in mind in interpreting the results and conclusions of our studies.

Conclusions and Clinical Implications

In this chapter we have reviewed the previous literature on neuropsychological deficits associated with ADHD in adults with a particular emphasis on the EFs. We used this literature as a background for then discussing the results from both the UMASS Study of clinic-referred adults with ADHD and the Milwaukee Study of children with ADHD grown up.

✓ The executive functions typically include the components of inhibition, resistance to distraction (interference control), verbal and nonverbal working memory, fluency (verbal and nonverbal), and planning, among others. Some investigators have also included the construct of response flexibility or set shifting, typically indexed by the WCST.

✓ Most prior studies compared their adults with ADHD to a normal or community control group. While this helps to distinguish areas of abnormal functioning, such comparisons do not address the specificity of EF deficits for ADHD in adults relative to other psychiatric disorders.

✓ The UMASS study used a relatively comprehensive battery of measures of these EF constructs as well as both a Community and a Clinical control group, which permitted greater identification of any EF deficits that may be more specific to ADHD in adults.

✓ Concerning deficits in attention and inhibition as measured by CPTs, the UMASS Study documented an excess of omission errors and greater reaction-time variability in our adults with ADHD relative to both control groups. The findings are consistent with some prior studies showing such problems with inattention while further identifying them as relatively more impaired and specific in adults with ADHD.

✓ Errors of commission were also greater in the ADHD group than in the Community control group but seemed less specific to the ADHD group given the presence of greater errors in the Clinical control group as well.

✓ Further analyses found that reaction time variability (inattention) and commission errors (inhibition) were the two best CPT measures for distinguishing the ADHD group from the Community control adults, while the former was the only measure of any utility in distinguishing the ADHD group from the Clinical controls. Recent research shows that high levels of response variability may be specifically associated with ADHD in adults and typify an abnormal error pattern associated with impaired vigilance that is not merely an exaggeration of normal variability. Thus, high response variability may be a useful phenotype for behavioral genetic neuroimaging studies of adults with ADHD.

✓ We also studied interference control or resistance to distraction using the Stroop Word–Color Task. Previous studies have found adults with ADHD to have difficulties on this task. Both the UMASS and Milwaukee Studies did as well. But these differences in the UMASS Study were only between the ADHD and Community groups. Such findings suggest that this form of inhibition may not be very specific to ADHD, at least among adults with the disorder. Even so, in the Milwaukee Study, it distinguished the hyperactive children with persistent ADHD to age 27 from those whose ADHD had not persisted.

✓ Prior studies have had little success in identifying problems on the WCST as being reliably associated with ADHD, either in children or adults having the disorder. Our study also found no differences among our groups on any WCST measures. This further supports the conclusion that response flexibility or set shifting is not a problem in adults with ADHD.

✓ Few prior studies have examined fluency or generativity in adults with ADHD. Those that have done so concentrated mainly on verbal fluency measures and have shown mixed results. One study examining design or nonverbal fluency found greater problems with perseverative responses on this task.

✓ Both the UMASS and Milwaukee Studies used a measure of design fluency. The UMASS Study found the adults with ADHD to generate fewer responses on this task than did either the Clinical or Community control group of adults. The Milwaukee Study found that both groups of children who had ADHD in childhood had deficits on this test at adult follow-up regardless of whether their ADHD had persisted to this age or not. Unlike the prior study by Rapport et al. (2001), we did not find more perseverative design responses in either of our studies. Both studies suggest that some problems with nonverbal fluency may be associated with ADHD in adults and that such a deficit persists into adulthood in children with the disorder even if they no longer meet the diagnostic criteria for ADHD.

✓ Among the most reliable findings in past studies have been deficits in verbal working memory as indexed by digit-span tasks, among others. Problems with verbal learning have been mixed, as have past studies using other verbal working memory tasks besides digit span.

✓ Our own studies support the earlier findings of problems with digit-span tasks in adults having ADHD and indicate that they are relatively specific to this disorder compared to our two control groups in the UMASS Study. The Milwaukee Study once again found that clinic-referred children with ADHD followed to adulthood also continue to have deficits in this measure of verbal working memory even if their symptoms no longer meet the criteria for ADHD.

✓ We gave an extensive battery of verbal and nonverbal learning and memory tasks to our participants. In general, we found no evidence of difficulties with immediate verbal learning or recall in such tasks as paragraph, word list, or word-pair learning using the UMASS Study groups.

✓ Our UMASS Study did find deficits associated with ADHD in adults in retention of information over time, such that they were more impaired on delayed recall trials after several intervening tasks had been performed. These retention problems were more evident in free recall and were improved somewhat by cueing of the likely response category. We believe these findings are consistent with a verbal working memory disorder in adults with ADHD similar to that previously shown in children with the disorder and find it to be relatively specific to the disorder relative to both our control groups.

✓ We were surprised to find that our Clinical control group in the UMASS Study actually outperformed both the ADHD and Community control groups on tasks of simple and complex design learning and retention as well as in word-pair learning. This may demonstrate a double dissociation on neuropsychological tasks in which adults with ADHD can be found to be deficient in some areas (verbal working memory, inattention, design fluency) while performing normally in other tasks such as verbal learning, immediate recall, and design learning and recall. In contrast, adults in the Clinical control group excelled at the former tasks and word-pair learning—in fact, they did significantly better than either the ADHD or Community control group.

✓ Although some sex differences were detected on various EF measures, these were routinely main effects for sex in which females were found to typically perform better than males, regardless of group. We found no evidence of any unique profiles that distinguished women from men with ADHD that were not otherwise a part of routine sex differences across the other groups as well.

Our results therefore give no support to the notion that ADHD in women is a qualitatively different neuropsychological disorder from that found in men.

✓ To summarize, ADHD in adults is associated with some relatively specific EF deficits not seen in Community or Clinical control adults. These are most likely to be in measures of inattention, inhibition (interference control), non-verbal and verbal working memory, and design fluency, whereas no deficits in verbal learning, immediate recall, set shifting, or tower planning were evident here.

✓ Clinicians are likely not only to find adults with ADHD complaining more of symptoms of impaired inhibition, attention, and working memory, as reported in Chapter 7, but also to display such deficits on neuropsychological tests that may have been given to these adults.

✓ While such EF deficits characterize adults with ADHD as a group, our results and those of prior studies indicate that such EF deficits are not necessarily diagnostic of ADHD in any given individual. These deficits may also occur in non-ADHD clinical patients with a sufficient frequency to make the level of false positives clinically unacceptable. More likely, however, is that a sizable minority of adults with ADHD can perform these tests sufficiently well to make for an unacceptable level of false negatives for these tests. *We do not recommend the use of any neuropsychological tests at this time to aid in the diagnosis of ADHD in adults.* Such tests may have some utility, however, in illuminating the strengths and weaknesses of an individual, providing additional evidence of weaknesses that may support the need for educational or workplace accommodations, and documenting below average cognitive deficits that may help in meeting the requirements for establishing a disability under the Americans with Disabilities Act.

CHAPTER 14

Summary, Conclusions, and Treatment Implications

In this book we have presented one of the most comprehensive reviews and original research reports published to date on adults with ADHD concerning their symptoms, impairments, and adaptive functioning in many of the important domains of major life activities. We did so while juxtaposing the findings for clinic-referred adults with ADHD against those of clinic-referred children with ADHD followed into adulthood. Our sample sizes in both studies provided sufficient statistical power to detect differences among the groups of at least low-to-moderate effect sizes or greater, ensuring that we were likely to identify those differences that would be robust and also clinically meaningful. By using two control groups in the UMASS Study, we were also able to report not only on the differences between adults with ADHD and general community samples typically reported in previous studies but also on differences that may be most specific to ADHD in adults relative to adults seen at the same clinic who are not diagnosed with ADHD but rather with other disorders. The Milwaukee Study contrasted its adults currently having ADHD against those who, having grown up with ADHD, appeared no longer to have the disorder at age-27 follow-up. Our results relied not only on the self-reports of the adult participants but also on reports from significant others, clinician ratings, employers, official educational and DMV archives, and psychological tests. This extensive battery of measures gave us a multi-informant and multisource perspective on the disorder and its impact on major life activities. It allowed us to conclude that ADHD in adults is a far more impairing disorder across multiple domains of major life activities than are most other disorders likely to be seen in outpatient psychiatric clinics, such as anxiety disorders, or mood disorders.

Across all of our results, one thing seems abundantly clear—ADHD in adults is a significantly impairing disorder. It is associated with numerous difficulties in virtually every domain of major life activity studied here. Whether one studies functioning in education, occupation, social relationships, sexual activities, dating and marriage, parenting and offspring psychological morbidity, crime and drug abuse, health and related lifestyles, financial management, or driving, ADHD can be found to produce diverse and serious impairments. Indeed, its impairments are more substantial than are those seen in other disorders most likely to present to outpatient mental health clinics, such as anxiety disorders, dysthymia, and major depression, among others. This is obvious in the numerous differences we found between adults with ADHD and our Clinical control group. The disorder also deserves its status as one distinct from other forms of psychopathology or developmental disabilities. Its symptoms and impairments are not due simply to general psychopathology. They stand out from other forms of psychopathology in numerous respects. Statements to the effect that ADHD is not a valid disorder, is a myth created by mercenary pharmaceutical companies or mental health professionals for sheer commercial gain, or is indistinct from the other disorders with which it may be associated are not only wrong, they are egregiously so. Numerous differences emerged in the context of these two studies between those with ADHD and general population (Community) controls and between those with ADHD and Clinical control groups that make such assertions moribund. To continue to make such statements in the face of such overwhelming evidence to the contrary is to show either a stunning scientific illiteracy or reflect planned religious or political propaganda intended to deceive the uninformed or unsuspecting general public.

Persistence and Recovery

Along the way, we found some good news for families raising children with ADHD: we were able to examine the percentage of children with ADHD likely to outgrow their disorder by adulthood. For full recovery from both symptoms and impairment (< 84th percentile on both) that figure was 14 to 35%, depending on the source of information and whether agreement between self- and other-reports was required to define full recovery. Not everyone with ADHD in childhood continues to have the disorder in adulthood. We also found that if full DSM criteria are used to define the presence of the disorder, then just 26 to 30% of those who were diagnosed with ADHD in childhood meet the current criteria for the disorder by age 27, depending on whose reports one uses. But we noted that using full DSM criteria for defining ADHD in adults is inappropriate, given that it was designed on children for children. We showed this problem clearly when we examined declines in symptom deviance with age, where we noted that 54% of child cases remain above the 93rd percentile for the control group and 49% remain above the 98th percentile. A sizable percentage of childhood cases of ADHD have clearly remained highly symptomatic into adulthood. Yet in marked contrast to the reports of others, which showed developmental declines in symptoms and disorder, self-reports showed an increase in both between the age-21 and the age-27 follow-ups. This is largely because most childhood cases report themselves to have no disorder at age 21, but apparently they were beginning to realize, in the interim, that they likely do have ADHD symptoms. The reports of others therefore converge on the self-reports over time, whereas they were highly disparate at the age-21 follow-up.

We were curious to know what childhood or adolescent factors may have been associated with full recovery from the disorder (falling below the 84th percentile in symptoms and in impairment, or one or no impairments). This question is somewhat different than that posed in all of our analyses in which we compared those with persistent ADHD to age 27 to those who did not have the disorder (H+ADHD vs. H−ADHD) on the various outcome measures at age 27. We compared those defined as recovered from ADHD based on their self-reports to those who had not recovered on the selection measures used at study entry (Werry–Weiss–Peters Activity Rating Scale, Conners scales, HSQ scale, and childhood IQ) as well as on severity of ADHD, ODD, and CD at adolescent follow-up. We also analyzed the age of onset of ADHD, the duration of stimulant treatment, and years of education. The two groups of hyperactive participants did not differ on any of these measures except that the group that had recovered (by self-report) had more years of education than those who did not (on average, one more year). We repeated these analyses using recovery as defined by other reports. No measures differed significantly. All of this suggests that recovery from ADHD by age 27 is unrelated to severity of disorder, age of onset, childhood IQ, childhood conduct problems at study entry; severity of ADHD, ODD, or CD; or duration of stimulant treatment by adolescence. In short, we cannot distinguish those who will have recovered by age 27 from those who do not. But we have shown that persistent ADHD is associated with a number of adversities in various major life activities by age 27, and that even impersistent ADHD may be associated with some risks.

Best Symptoms for Diagnosis

We examined the utility of DSM symptoms for ADHD when used with adults, demonstrating that a far shorter list of symptoms is required than the 18 presented in the DSM. Surprisingly, the symptom of often being distractible was sufficient to rule out a sizable proportion of our community control groups, while only five to seven more symptoms were needed to then detect those with ADHD among all our clinic-referred adults. Also surprising was that symptoms of hyper-

activity were not especially useful at distinguishing adults with ADHD from those with other disorders, while those of inattention and, to a lesser extent, verbal impulsiveness were more useful at doing so.

One question we sought to address was whether a better set of symptoms designed on and for adults with ADHD could be identified. We succeeded in doing so, finding nine symptoms representing impaired executive functioning (EF) to be useful in this regard and better at identifying the adult stage of the disorder than are most of the symptoms listed in DSM-IV. In view of these findings, we should consider the following nine symptoms that largely reflect EF as a potential item set for ADHD in adulthood:

- Is often easily distracted by extraneous stimuli (DSM-IV-TR) or irrelevant thoughts (EF).
- Often makes decisions impulsively (EF).
- Often has difficulty stopping his or her activities or behavior when he or she should do so (EF).
- Often starts a project or task without reading or listening to directions carefully (EF).
- Often shows poor follow-through on promises or commitments he or she may make to others (EF).
- Often has trouble doing things in their proper order or sequence (EF).
- Often more likely to drive a motor vehicle much faster than others (excessive speeding) (EF).
  - Substitute item for adults without driving experience: Often has difficulty engaging in leisure activities or doing fun things quietly.
- Often has difficulty sustaining attention in tasks or play activities (DSM—optional).
- Often has difficulty organizing tasks and activities (DSM—optional).

A threshold of six of these nine new symptoms appeared to work well at distinguishing the ADHD group from the other two groups, accurately classifying 99% of Community controls, 92% of those with ADHD, and 53% of Clinical controls. These symptoms also map onto the two-dimensional structure of the DSM-IV-TR, aligning either with the dimension of inattention (and working memory) or with that of poor inhibition. Both studies suggested that items emphasizing distractibility, impulsiveness, poor concentration or persistence, and problems with working memory and organization will be the best constructs for identifying adults with ADHD. Items reflecting hyperactivity proved much less useful for doing so.

We further showed that reliance on the age of onset of 7 years for the disorder has no empirical support and should be broadened to ages 14 to 16 or abandoned in favor of a more generically phrased "onset in childhood to adolescence." We found that ADHD has an adverse effect on various domains of major

life activities, the most seriously affected being educational and occupational functioning, money management, and management of daily responsibilities. Our results certainly show that a better set of diagnostic criteria can be developed for the adult stage of ADHD in DSM-V than is currently available in DSM-IV-TR.

General or Global Impairments

As stated earlier (Chapter 6), *the symptoms of ADHD are the behavioral expressions associated with this disorder*—they are the actions demonstrated by those having the disorder that are believed to reflect that disorder (e.g., inattention, distractibility, impulsive responding, hyperactivity, poor executive functioning). In contrast, *impairments are the consequences that ensue for the individual as a result of these cognitive-behavioral expressions.* Symptoms are actions of an individual (cognition/behavior) and impairments are the consequences of those actions (outcomes or social costs). The term "impairment" refers to deficits that are relative to the functioning of the normal population or "average person" and not to an intrapersonal disparity from IQ or comparison to some highly specialized or high-functioning peer group.

In examining the various domains of major life activity specifically in our interviews, we found that with the exception of dating or marriage, the ADHD group in the UMASS Study showed a significantly greater percentage as being impaired in most domains than was the case for either the Clinical or Community control groups. The domain most affected by adult ADHD was education, followed by home responsibilities and occupational functioning and then, to a lesser extent, dating/marriage, and social activities. Community activities such as participating in clubs, sports, or organizations were the least likely to suffer impairment due to ADHD. The Milwaukee Study found a somewhat different pattern of impairment, where current ADHD at age 27 was associated with a somewhat lower likelihood of being impaired in any particular domain. Home and occupational domains were the most likely to be impaired, as was money management and daily responsibilities. Unlike the experience in the UMASS Study, the educational domain was not as likely to be self-reported as impaired in those hyperactive children retaining ADHD at follow-up. This is interesting insofar as the actual evidence for educational impairment was found to be far greater in the hyperactive children grown up than in the clinic-referred adults having ADHD.

We also collected information from retrospective reports on the childhood domains most likely to be impaired. For the ADHD group in the UMASS Study, education or the school setting was far and away the domain most likely to be adversely affected by ADHD (over 90%), followed by daily chores and responsibilities (75%). The same was true for the ratings provided by significant others about the childhood impairments in these groups. While a smaller proportion of each group was rated as being impaired in the reports of others compared to self-

reports, a higher proportion of the ADHD group was rated as impaired in each of the eight domains from childhood than was the case for either control group. And again, the educational setting was the domain in which more of the ADHD group had been affected relative to the other domains surveyed. The Milwaukee Study found that many domains were reported to be impaired, but the domain of social (peer) interactions was the one most likely to be associated with the ADHD group in childhood.

Our findings further indicated that the self-reports of clinic-referred adults in their 30s or older concerning ADHD symptoms or those provided by others who know them well are likely to be impressively correlated with reports within each of these sources about degree of impairment (rs = .70–.80). These relationships are strong, whether they pertain to current functioning or to recall of childhood functioning. Such severity, especially at clinically elevated levels (four or more symptoms), is highly likely to be associated with risk of impairment in one or more major life activities (100% are impaired). The results for children followed to adulthood are somewhat lower but still show significant relationships between severity of ADHD and severity and pervasiveness of impairments.

Comorbidity

There is compelling evidence that ADHD increases the liability for certain other psychiatric disorders. More than 80% of our ADHD groups had at least one other disorder, more than 50% had two other disorders, and more than one-third had at least three other disorders, these being markedly higher than in our control groups in both studies. As in the prior literature on children and adults with ADHD, we found a markedly elevated risk for ODD and, to a lesser extent, for CD in our clinic-referred ADHD group and in our hyperactive children as adults. Current ADHD was especially associated with a childhood history of ODD.

The internalizing disorders of major depressive disorder, dysthymia, and anxiety are more likely to occur in ADHD cases referred to clinics over that risk seen in a Community control group. But MDD and anxiety disorders are also significantly elevated in non-ADHD Clinical control patients seen at the same ADHD clinic and thus may not be as specifically linked to ADHD as to general outpatient psychopathology. Even so, both epidemiological studies in children and adults find some association between ADHD and depression, which makes it unlikely that our findings of a limited association are purely due to referral bias. Nevertheless, the relationships that do exist are not as strong when comparisons to other clinical samples are used than when comparisons to community samples are studied. The Milwaukee Study did not find an elevated risk for MDD specifically in those with persistent ADHD into adulthood but did find an elevated risk for mood disorders more generally and depressive personality disorder, both of which suggest some link between ADHD and level of depressive symptoms, even if not with full syndrome MDD. Neither study found any elevated risk for OCD, bipolar disorder, or schizophrenic spectrum disorders.

Both the ADHD groups in our studies showed a greater risk for alcohol use disorders, while the clinic-referred adults (but not the hyperactive children grown up) also showed a greater risk for cannabis use disorders compared to Community controls. Alcohol use disorders and risk for any drug use disorder may be specifically linked to ADHD, though the level and type of drug use disorder probably has more to do with comorbid CD and antisocial personality disorder as well as local access to specific drugs than with ADHD per se.

We also studied comorbidity dimensionally, using the SCL-90-R and the Young Adult Child Behavior Checklist. Adults with ADHD (whether clinic-referred or children grown up) showed elevations on all scales of the SCL-90-R psychological maladjustment relative to Community controls and on most of the scales relative to the Clinical control group. Our findings are consistent with all but one prior study in the literature on adults with ADHD using this instrument. There is clearly greater maladjustment of all types associated with ADHD than in Clinical or Community comparison groups. Such findings imply that ADHD is a more severe psychological disorder than many outpatient disorders seen in the same clinics.

Concerning the risk of suicidal ideation and attempts, we found that the ADHD group in the UMASS Study had only a slight but not significant increase in risk over the two control groups in both ideation (25% vs. 15–16%) and attempts (6% vs. 2–4%) prior to 18 years of age. But after age 18, both the ADHD and Clinical control groups reported elevated rates of suicidal thinking (27–29%) over that seen in the Community control group (6%). The ADHD group specifically also reported a greater risk of suicide attempts relative to the Community group (8% vs. 1%). The Milwaukee Study also found an elevated risk of suicidal thinking and attempts in the hyperactive groups, particularly before 18 years of age, and an ongoing risk of greater ideation (but not attempts) going forward to follow-ups at ages 21 and 27. But the two hyperactive subgroups did not differ in these risks, indicating that persistent ADHD into adulthood was not the major determinant of such risks. The greater risks of ideation and attempts reported here were largely mediated by the presence of MDD and, to a lesser extent, dysthymia, but they were not especially related to the presence of comorbid CD.

Education

Clinically diagnosed adults with ADHD share some of the same types of academic difficulties in their histories as do children who were hyperactive and followed over development. However, their intellectual levels are higher, their high school graduation rates are higher, they are more likely to have attended college, and their likelihood of having achievement difficulties or learning disabilities is considerably less in most respects than that seen in children with ADHD followed to adulthood. This higher level of intellectual and academic functioning in clinic-referred adults with ADHD makes sense, given that they are self-referred to clinics in comparison to children with ADHD. This fact makes it much more likely that these adults have employment, health insurance, and a sufficient educational level to be so employed and insured. They could also be expected to have a sufficient level of intellect and self-awareness to perceive themselves as being in need of assistance for their psychiatric problems and difficulties in adaptive functioning. Children with ADHD brought to clinics by their parents are less likely to have these attributes by the time they reach adulthood. As adults, they are not as educated, have considerable problems sustaining employment, are more likely to have had a history of aggression and antisocial acts, and are not as self-aware of their symptoms as adults with ADHD who self-refer to clinics. Able, Johnston, Adler, and Swindle (2006) found similar differences between referred and nonreferred adults with ADHD.

The educational careers of the ADHD groups were checkered with adversities. More of the adults with ADHD reported having been retained in grade, received special education, and been diagnosed with learning disabilities or behavioral disorders while in compulsory schooling than adults in either of the two control groups. These risks were even greater in the children with ADHD followed to adulthood. Class rankings and grade-point averages were significantly lower in the ADHD groups than in our control groups. Among those participants who had attended college, more of the ADHD group had unsatisfactory grades and had withdrawn from more classes, as reflected on their college transcripts, than did the two control groups. On tests of educational achievement given in our projects, the ADHD groups were poorer in their arithmetic, spelling, and reading and listening comprehension skills than were adults in the control groups. We also found adults with ADHD to have a higher comorbidity with specific learning disabilities, replicating the substantial literature on children with ADHD. This risk was even higher in the children with ADHD followed to adulthood than in the clinic-referred adults with ADHD. All of this leads us to conclude that of all domains of major life activity adversely affected by ADHD in adults, the domain of education is the most pervasively affected and affects more such adults.

Occupational Functioning

Both clinic-referred adults with ADHD and children growing up with the disorder experienced significant problems in their occupational histories. In the UMASS Study, adults with ADHD were rated by a clinician as functioning at a lower level overall than adults in the other groups. They were also found to have experienced a number of problems in a higher percentage of their previous jobs than adults in the two control groups. These problems were related to getting along with others, demonstrating behavior problems, being fired, quitting out of boredom, and being disciplined by supervisors, all of which were more frequent in the work histories of the adults with ADHD than in either of the control groups. The Milwaukee follow-up study found much the same results except that growing up as a child with ADHD was associated with lower job status and fewer current working hours per week regardless of its persistence into adulthood. Even so, the group with persistent ADHD experienced even more difficulties in their current workplace functioning than did either the H–ADHD or the Community control group. This was also true in comparison to the clinic-referred adults with ADHD; those who had had ADHD as children had been fired from their jobs far more often or experienced disciplinary actions than did clinic-referred adults with the disorder. We corroborated these problems through employer ratings in both studies (UMASS Study currently, Milwaukee Study at age 21). The ADHD groups were rated as having significantly more symptoms of inattention in the workplace and as being more impaired in performing assigned work, pursuing educational activities, being punctual, using good time management, and managing daily responsibilities. Both projects provide direct evidence that ADHD has an adverse impact on workplace functioning not only by self-reports but also by employer blinded corroborative ratings.

Drug Use

Prior research shows that children with ADHD followed to adulthood carry an elevated risk for later substance use and abuse as well as for many antisocial acts and their legal consequences (arrests, jail). In both instances, it is the presence of CD in childhood or adolescence that greatly elevates these risks and accounts for them entirely in some cases. However, ADHD does convey some elevated risk for nonviolent activities—such as drug use, possession, or sale—and may convey an elevated risk for tobacco and alcohol use even in the absence of CD. What little research exists on clinic-referred adults with ADHD likewise suggests a greater likelihood of drug-use disorders and antisocial personality disorder. But prior studies have not examined rates of drug use or specific forms of antisocial activities in as much detail as has the literature on children with ADHD followed to adulthood. We explored these risks further in both of our studies.

The UMASS Study found that adults with ADHD were likely to be past or current smokers; to be users of marijuana, cocaine, LSD, or prescription drugs; and to have been treated for previous alcohol and drug-use disorders than was the case in the Community control group. But the Clinical control group also showed some elevated risks for some drug use problems, primarily past tobacco use and current marijuana use. The ADHD group differed from that clinical group chiefly in having more members who had tried cocaine and LSD. Like past studies of children with ADHD grown up, we found that the presence of CD appears to account for the significantly higher frequency of some drugs used by the ADHD group relative to the control groups. We believe that the presence of childhood CD may not account for whether an adult with ADHD ever tries a particular substance at least once, but it does seem to contribute to the frequency with which they may subsequently continue to use that drug in many instances.

The longitudinal Milwaukee Study largely corroborated the UMASS Study in finding a greater risk for being a smoker, using alcohol, getting drunk, or using illegal prescription drugs among both hyperactive (childhood ADHD) groups at age 27. It also found a greater frequency of caffeine use for those groups than for the control group. However, it is largely being referred and diagnosed as ADHD in childhood that is related to risk for later substance use and abuse than whether or not that ADHD is persistent to age 27. While the ADHD groups in both projects appear to be more likely to abuse both legal and illegal substances, the children with ADHD growing up may carry a greater risk for using alcohol and tobacco, while clinic-referred adults with ADHD seem more likely to use marijuana, cocaine, and LSD.

Worth reiterating are the findings from the Milwaukee Study that found no evidence that treatment with stimulants in childhood was associated with increased drug use or abuse in any category of illegal drugs. In fact, some evidence showed that being treated with stimulants as a child reduced the likelihood of using certain types of drugs, such as speed (amphetamines) or illegally obtained prescription drugs. These findings are consistent with the vast majority of other research on this issue, further solidifying the conclusion that childhood stimulant treatment is *not* associated with risk for later drug use or abuse, no matter how critics, fringe religious zealots, and the popular media wish to portray this issue.

Antisocial Behavior and Its Consequences

Adults who had ADHD as children are routinely found in follow-up studies to be more likely to engage in antisocial acts, to be arrested, and to be jailed than those who did not have ADHD. We found this to be the case in both projects. More clinic-referred adults with ADHD had engaged in shoplifting, stealing without confronting a victim, breaking and entering, assaults with fists, carrying an illegal weapon, being arrested, and being sent to jail. And more adults with ADHD had sold drugs illegally in comparison to the Community control group. The Clinical control group did not differ from either of these two groups on this outcome. The most common forms of antisocial activity for the adults with

ADHD were shoplifting (53%), followed by assaulting someone with their fists (35%) and selling illegal drugs (21%). While much of this risk for antisocial behavior was mediated by the presence of a childhood history of CD (established retrospectively), even the non-CD subset of those having ADHD still committed more antisocial acts than the control groups. Likewise, the Milwaukee Study continued to find markedly higher proportions of the hyperactive group to have committed various antisocial acts than the control group. In most cases, this elevated risk was not related to whether or not the ADHD had persisted to age 27. This suggested to us that while ADHD in both projects is clearly associated with a greater risk of antisocial activity than in control groups, when it occurs in children and leads to early clinic referral and diagnosis, it is associated with an even greater risk for later antisocial acts, arrests, and being jailed than is seen in clinic-referred adults with ADHD.

Both projects found that lifetime criminal diversity and arrest frequency were likely to be predicted by childhood hyperactivity or ADHD as well as the earlier appearance of CD symptoms. The Milwaukee Study also found that diversity of teen drug use also makes an independent contribution to both of these outcomes. This implies a spiraling effect over time between teen antisocial behavior and teen drug use, in which each contributes to the maintenance and increase in the other at later developmental stages. We also found much the same for level of education, such that it makes an independent contribution to crime diversity and arrest frequency beyond that made by the earlier severity of antisocial behavior. Such analyses inform us that it is not so much severity of ADHD that is associated with crime and arrest rates, although childhood hyperactivity makes a small contribution to risk (about 7–8%); rather, additional and greater contributions are made by childhood conduct problems, teen antisocial activity and drug use, and low education, whereas the persistence of ADHD across development did not contribute to these outcomes.

Health and Related Lifestyles

Lifestyle and personality factors, especially conscientiousness, were noted earlier to be significant contributors to human longevity. Half or more of all deaths in the United States are related to drug use, diet, exercise, sexual behavior, driving, and risk taking more generally. Adults with ADHD are more likely to possess these high-risk characteristics, leading us to speculate that they will be in poorer health or at least, going forward, carry significantly higher risks for coronary artery disease, cancer, and accidental death, among others. We found good evidence to support such concerns. The adults with ADHD in the UMASS Study had a higher percentage of individuals reporting problems with sleep, social relationships, family interactions, tobacco use, nonmedical drug use, medical/dental care, motor vehicle safety, work and leisure, and emotional health than did the Community control group. But illicit drug use, driving, and emotional health are areas in which adults with ADHD differed specifically from other clinic-referred adults who do not have ADHD. Similar though not identical elevations in life-style and health risks were also detected in the Milwaukee Study, with eating habits, sleep, social relations, tobacco use, nonmedical drug use, and emotional health also being concerns for a significantly greater percentage of those hyperactive children having persistent ADHD to age 27 (the H+ADHD group) compared to the Community control group. But even those hyperactive children whose ADHD did not persist to adulthood had more members reporting concerns about sleep and tobacco use than did the Community control group.

The Milwaukee Study took a detailed look at current health, medical history, and risk of future coronary heart disease (CHD). It found that the hyperactive group had a significantly greater risk of injury, nonsurgical hospitalizations, and poisonings and experienced more such events than the Community control group in their medical histories. A significantly greater number of current health complaints was evident in the medical histories of those with persistent ADHD relative to those who no longer had ADHD at follow-up. The former also had more such medical complaints than the Community control group. These complaints were associated with elevated levels of somatization, depression, and phobic anxiety, implying that they may be more indicative of psychiatric than of medical problems. We also identified a slight but significantly higher risk lipid profile and a greater risk for CHD over the next 5 and 10 years, mainly for the H+ADHD group compared to the Community control group. That group also reported less regular exercise than the other groups, while both hyperactive groups were more likely to be smokers and consumers of alcohol than the control group. If such trends continue over the next decade, it will become more evident that individuals with ADHD persisting into adulthood carry a higher future risk of heart disease (and possibly cancer) than the general population.

Money Management

Individuals who are more impulsive, have a penchant for immediate gratification, discount future consequences, and are generally poorer at self-regulation can be expected to have problems managing their finances. Given that these characteristics typify adults with ADHD, we hypothesized that those adults would have considerable problems managing money. Our hypotheses were largely borne out. The adults with ADHD in the UMASS Study had a higher proportion of its members reporting problems with managing money, saving money, buying on impulse, nonpayment of utilities resulting in their termination, missing loan payments, exceeding credit card limits, having a poor credit rating, and not saving for retirement. Relative to the normal control group, the adults with ADHD appear to be having relatively pervasive problems with the management of their finances. Four areas of money management were specifically elevated in the ADHD group as compared to both the Clinical and Community control groups, these having to do with deferred gratification (saving and putting money away for retirement), impulse buying, and meeting financial deadlines (nonpayment of utilities resulting in their termination). On all six frequency measures of money management, the adults with ADHD reported more difficulties more often than did the adults in our Community control group. Money difficulties were also more common in the ADHD than in the Clinical control group in at least four of these six areas, those being missing rent payments, missing utility payments, missing loan payments, and having more total money problems. Numerous financial problems were also associated with the hyperactive group in the Milwaukee Study, although these were most frequent in the group whose ADHD had persisted until age 27. Both studies have found a clear, robust, and specific relationship of adult ADHD to a diversity of financial problems, regardless of how adult ADHD patients were ascertained (clinic-referred or children followed to adulthood).

Driving Risks

Driving has probably been the most thoroughly studied major life activity affected by ADHD in the existing adult literature. Our results only add to this burgeoning evidence of significant and pervasive risks. Such risks do not seem to be due to the common comorbid disorders associated with ADHD. Clinic-referred adults with ADHD compared to the Community control group were more likely to have had their licenses suspended or revoked, to have driven without a valid driver's license, to have crashed while driving, to have been at fault in such a crash, and to have been cited for speeding and even reckless driving. Several of these risks were also documented on official DMV records. The ADHD group also had more license suspensions/revocations, more crashes, more speeding citations, and were held to be at fault in more such crashes than either the Clinical or Community control adults. On the DMV record, the adults with ADHD again had more speeding citations and more total citations. Similar though less robust differences were evident between the hyperactive and control groups in Milwaukee, perhaps in part because they are younger and have had less driving experience than adults in the UMASS Study. But as in the UMASS Study, those who were hyperactive as children experienced a higher risk for frequent crashes, a greater risk for reckless driving, more citations for such driving, and a greater risk of license suspensions and revocations. Driving risks were associated with not only ADHD severity but also other factors such as age, more diverse criminal activity, poorer credit ratings, greater hostility (e.g., road rage), and low levels of anxiety (e.g., fearlessness), depending upon the driving outcome being predicted.

Sex, Dating, Marriage, and Offspring

As discussed earlier, two prior studies have documented a riskier sexual lifestyle in teens and adults with ADHD, one of which was the Milwaukee Study at age-21 follow-up. We continued to identify this area as one of concern and greater medical and public health attention for those with ADHD. Childhood ADHD is associated with earlier initiation of sexual activity and intercourse, more sexual partners, more casual sex, and more partner pregnancies or female pregnancies if the woman has ADHD. These risks are further elevated by higher levels of conduct problems, but such problems do not account for the separate contribution made by ADHD. The Milwaukee Study continued to find evidence for concern in this domain of life activity. Those who have grown up with ADHD are more likely to become pregnant (if female) or impregnate others (if males), are more likely to be parents by ages 21 or 27, and are more likely to contract a sexually transmitted disease by age 21 than are Community controls followed over this same time.

We did not find differential rates of marriage or higher rates of divorce among those who had grown up with ADHD or among the clinic-referred adults with ADHD, in keeping with the previous longitudinal studies of hyperactive children and with the inconsistent results of past studies of clinic-referred adults on this issue. We did find some evidence that women with ADHD were less likely to be married at the time of our studies. We also found a greater incidence of marital dissatisfaction in both groups of adults with ADHD across these projects, as well as poorer quality of dating relationships among those with persistent ADHD who were hyperactive as children and are still single and dating. The spouses of those adults with ADHD were also significantly less satisfied in the marriage than were spouses of the Community control group in the UMASS Study. But such findings may not be specific to adults with ADHD or their spouses, because we also found such marital dissatisfaction in our Clinical control adults.

Prior studies discussed earlier have also found elevated risks for ADHD among the offspring of adults with ADHD, ranging from 43 to 57% of their children. We also found such an elevated risk, with 22 to 43% of the offspring of adults with ADHD falling in the clinically elevated range on either the inattention, hyperactive–impulsive, or combined symptom lists from the DSM-IV-TR. These prevalence figures were certainly higher than those found in our Community control adults in keeping with these prior studies. But we also used a Clinical control group of adults and found that their offspring also carried significantly elevated risks for symptoms of inattention than did the children of the Community control group, implying that offspring risk for inattention is also found in non-ADHD clinic-referred adults. In contrast, risk for hyperactive–impulsive behavior, oppositional defiant disorder, and conduct disorder appears to be specifically elevated in the offspring of the adults with ADHD. ODD appeared to be the most common psychological morbidity to be found in the offspring of adults with ADHD, occurring in nearly half of them (48%). Such findings are quite consistent with and supportive of the strong genetic predisposition to ADHD and its high familial transmission, as demonstrated in numerous prior behavioral genetic studies of biological family members and twins. Yet our research also evaluated a wider array of dimensions of children's psychological maladjustment than prior studies of offspring morbidity. Here as well we found that the children of adults with ADHD showed greater symptoms of both externalizing (ADHD, ODD, CD) and internalizing (depression, somatization, atypicality) problems than did children in the Clinical and Community control groups. There is a wider range of offspring psychological morbidity associated with ADHD in parents than is the case for parents who do not have ADHD, whether clinically referred or not.

The parents in both the ADHD and Clinical control groups reported higher rates of parenting stress on the specific scales of parent, child, and parent–child domains than did Community control parents and did not differ from each other on these scales. But the parents with ADHD reported more total stress in their family lives than did parents in either of the control groups. Parenting stress, particularly in those domains associated with the child or with parent–child interactions, was primarily predicted by the extent of child ODD symptoms, consistent with prior research in children with ADHD. But degree of child inattentiveness was also a contributor to some domains of parenting stress, suggesting that it also makes some contribution to the degree of perceived stress reported by parents. However, when parental characteristics of ADHD, depression, and anxiety were considered, our results showed that parental depression may make a large and consistent contribution to all domains of parenting stress. Child ODD symptoms continued to contribute to stress, however, beyond that made by parental depression. Parental level of ADHD did not contribute to levels of parenting stress.

Neuropsychological Functioning

Substantial research exists on the neuropsychological performance of adults with ADHD, especially on measures thought to index the executive functions, which typically include the components of inhibition, resistance to distraction (interference control), verbal and nonverbal working memory, fluency (verbal and nonverbal), sense and use of time, and planning, among others. All of these have been found to be impaired in prior studies, though planning less consistently so. The UMASS study documented an excess of omission errors and greater RT variability on a continuous performance test in our adults with ADHD relative to both control groups. The findings are consistent with some prior studies showing such problems with inattention while further identifying them as relatively more impaired and specific in ADHD in adults. Errors of commission were also greater in the ADHD group than the Community control group but seemed less specific to the ADHD group, given the presence of greater errors in the Clinical control group as well. Further analyses found that RT variability (inattention) and commission errors (inhibition) were the two best CPT measures for distinguishing the ADHD group from the Community control adults, while the former was the only measure of much utility in identifying the ADHD group from the Clinical control adults. Recent research shows that high levels of RT variability may be specifically associated with ADHD in adults and may typify an abnormal error pattern associated with impaired vigilance that is not merely an exaggeration of normal variability. We therefore suggest that high RT variability may be a useful phenotype for behavioral genetic or neuroimaging studies of adults with ADHD.

Interference control or resistance to distraction, assessed using the Stroop Word–Color Task, was found to be impaired in adults with ADHD in both the UMASS and Milwaukee Studies. But these differences in the UMASS Study were found only between the ADHD and Community groups. Such findings suggest that this form of inhibition may not be very specific to ADHD, at least among adults with the disorder. Even so, it distinguished the hyperactive children with persistent ADHD to age 27 from those whose ADHD had not persisted in the Milwaukee Study.

Prior studies have had little success in identifying problems on the Wisconsin Card Sort Task as being reliably associated with ADHD, either in children or adults having the disorder. Our study also found no differences among our groups on any WCST measures. This further supports the conclusion that response flexibility or set shifting is not a problem in adults with ADHD.

Few prior studies have examined fluency or generativity in adults with ADHD. Those that have concentrated mainly on verbal fluency measures have shown mixed results. One study examining design or nonverbal fluency found greater problems with perseverative responses on this task. Both of our studies used a measure of design fluency. The UMASS Study found the adults with ADHD to generate fewer responses on this task than did either control group of adults. The Milwaukee Study found that both groups who had ADHD in childhood had deficits on this test at adult follow-up regardless of whether or not their ADHD had persisted to this age. But we did not find more perseverative design responses in either of our studies. Both studies suggest that some problems with nonverbal fluency may be associated with ADHD in adults and that such a deficit persists into adulthood in children with the disorder even if they no longer meet diagnostic criteria for ADHD.

Among the most reliable findings in past studies have been deficits in verbal working memory as indexed by digit-span tasks, among others. Problems with verbal learning have been mixed, as have past studies using other verbal working memory tasks besides digit span. Our own studies support the earlier findings of problems with digit-span tasks in adults having ADHD—that such problems are relatively specific to this disorder as compared to our two control groups in the UMASS Study. The Milwaukee Study once again found that clinic-referred children with ADHD followed to adulthood also continued to have deficits in this measure of verbal working memory, even if their symptoms no longer met the criteria of ADHD.

The UMASS Study used an extensive battery of verbal and nonverbal learning and memory tasks. In general, we found no evidence of difficulties with immediate verbal learning or recall in such tasks as paragraph, word list, or word pair learning using the UMASS Study groups. Our UMASS Study did find deficits associated with ADHD in adults in retention of information over time, such that they were more impaired on delayed recall trials after several intervening tasks had to be performed. These retention problems were more evident in free recall and were improved somewhat by cueing of the likely response category. We believe that these findings are consistent with a disorder of verbal working memory in adults with ADHD, similar to that previously shown in children with the disorder, and find it to be relatively specific to the disorder relative to both our control groups.

To summarize, ADHD in adults is associated with some relatively specific EF deficits not seen in Community or Clinical control adults. These are most likely to be in measures of inattention, inhibition (interference control), nonverbal and verbal working memory, and design fluency. But no deficits in verbal learning, immediate recall, set shifting, or tower planning were evident here.

Sex Differences

We wish to return here to one of the major aims of the UMASS Study—an examination of possible sex differences between men and women with ADHD. This addresses the issue of whether ADHD in females is different, perhaps qualitatively so, than it is in men. Claims have been made concerning women with ADHD, that the disorder may be uniquely different in them than it is in men with the disorder in ways other than what would be expected from general sex differences in the population (Nadeau & Quinn, 2002; Ratey, Miller, & Nadeau, 1995; Solden, 1995). Yet such assertions are based either on studies of clinic-referred children with ADHD or entirely on clinical experience supported only by anecdotes. This is because there are very few scientific studies of clinic-referred women with ADHD on which to base any such conclusions. We tried to address this lack of information on women with ADHD throughout this text by reporting on the sex differences among our samples whenever they were statistically significant across the myriad domains of symptoms and adaptive functioning studied here. Sex differences were not evident on most measures. The majority of our results indeed undercut any such claims by advocates of anything special to or specific about ADHD as it occurs in women.

For instance, it has been said that "the diagnosis of ADD in women escapes even the best clinicians, because these women often lack the typical symptoms of hyperactivity and impulsivity in childhood or adulthood" (Ratey et al., 1995, p. 260). Our results, in fact, show this claim to be false. We found no differences in the number of hyperactive or impulsive symptoms between men and women with ADHD in this study.

In examining self-reported symptoms (Chapter 3), we found that males self-reported more current symptoms in the interview than females, regardless of group, but men and women did not differ in their recall of childhood ADHD. The same pattern was evident on the rating scales of these symptoms. But we also found that the group × sex interaction was significant on some measures. This would imply that some sex differences might be evident within particular groups that were not evident in the other groups. We found that men and women with ADHD did not differ in their self-ratings of either their current or childhood symptoms. The sex difference of note was found in our Clinical control group, where women reported higher symptom ratings than men. There also were no significant sex differences found in the ratings of ADHD symptoms provided by others. And while a significant group × sex interaction did appear in the employer ratings, it was once again limited to the Clinical control group, where employers rated men as having more ADHD symptoms than women in the workplace. In short, women with ADHD do not differ from men in the severity of their symptoms, the age of onset of those symptoms, the number of domains in which they are impaired (Chapter 5), the total severity of impairment they experience, or the age of onset of specific domains of impairment in any way that can be specifically attributed to their having ADHD. Nor do they differ in the severity of the new EF symptom list we developed as the best list for the diagnosis of ADHD in adults (Chapter 7). In general, men report more total symptoms of ADHD by interview across the groups and rate themselves as having higher impairment scores on rating scales than do females, but such findings are not specific to the ADHD group. All of this suggests that men and women with ADHD have the same disorder and have no qualitative differences in their disorder as a result of their sex. What quantitative differences exist are those found between men and women generally.

It has also been claimed that women with ADHD may be more prone to exhibit symptoms of depression and anxiety and may be less aggressive than males with ADHD (Ratey et al., 1995). In a study by Rucklidge and Kaplan (1997), women with ADHD were in fact found to have more depression and anxiety, mores stress, a more external locus of control, and lower self-esteem compared to women in a control group. But men were not evaluated in this study, so it is highly possible that these findings are not specific to women with ADHD but merely characterize ADHD across both genders. A later study by these authors found this to be so. Again, our results point to just such a conclusion. On the dimensional ratings of depression from the SCL-90-R, no effects of sex were significant. And while women reported higher rates of anxiety, this was typical of women in all three of our groups and was not specific to women with ADHD versus men with the disorder. We did find that women with ADHD actually reported higher rates of attention problems on the Young Adult Behavior Self-Report Form (Chapter 6), *but they were also rated by others as being more aggressive than males with ADHD.* These are among the few differences that were specific to the ADHD group and not evident in our control groups. They run counter to the earlier assertions by clinicians.

In their educational careers, we again did not find much that was specific to women with ADHD that was not typical of women in general in the other two control groups. Women generally were less likely to have been retained in grade in school, to have been suspended from school, to have received special educational services, to have been identified as learning disabled or a behavior problem, or to have perceived themselves as being punished as much as men. All of these findings are consistent with the well-known adversities that boys and men experience in their educational careers relative to girls and women. Such sex differences were found across groups and reflected nothing exceptional about ADHD as it exists in women. The only sex difference evident on educational testing was that women, on average, had higher spelling scores than men, regardless of group. If anything, these results show that women in this study were, on average, less educationally impaired in their school histories than were men.

The results for occupational functioning likewise found little evidence of anything specific to ADHD as it occurs in women. The only such finding was that women with ADHD were more likely to be rated as impaired in relations with clients than were men with ADHD—findings that were not apparent in either control group. Men in general had worked longer at their jobs than had women, worked more hours per week, earned a higher salary, yet had also been fired from more jobs than had women in general. Those findings cut across all groups, reflecting nothing specific about women with ADHD relative to men with the disorder.

On our measures of health and lifestyle concerns, we found that regardless of group, males were more likely than females to have concerns/risks in their eating habits, tobacco and alcohol use, nonmedical drug use, and motor vehicle safety domains. Within the ADHD group, males were more likely to have motor vehicle safety risks, as well as work and leisure concerns. In the Clinical controls, females were more likely to have social, sexual, and work concerns than males, while males were more likely to have concerns about nonmedical drug use. In the Community controls, males were more likely to have risks or concerns about nonmedical drug use, medical/dental, and motor vehicle safety. Such a pattern suggests that the group status did not interact with sex to produce qualitatively different patterns of sex differences within our groups that differed from the overall differences we found between men and women regardless of group. Again, women with ADHD do not differ from men with the disorder other than reflecting the sex differences evident in the general population. The Milwaukee Study did imply that women with ADHD may have larger body mass indexes and may have more of relatively vague medical complaints, which we found to be significantly associated with anxiety, depression, and somatization. It is therefore possible that women with ADHD have somewhat different health concerns than do men. But our prediction of future coronary heart disease suggested that men were at greater risk, particularly those with current ADHD, largely owing to their sex and its differentially greater risks for heart disease than was seen in women in this study. The Milwaukee samples of women, however, were quite small and so may not be reliable. Further study of the health risks associated with ADHD and in women with the disorder specifically is to be recommended.

Not surprisingly, men in general were also more likely to be abusing the various substances that we surveyed in this study and certainly had higher rates of various antisocial acts than did women. Higher rates of CD symptoms were also more likely in the childhood histories of men than women. Much the same thing was reported by Biederman and colleagues (Biederman et al., 1994). In their driving careers, men were also more likely to have experienced various adverse events and did so more often than did women. Women, in contrast, had written more bad checks than men in general. Once again, these are general sex differences applying to males and females across our three groups.

On the neuropsychological measures, only a few sex differences were evident. They showed, not surprisingly, that women performed better on some verbal learning and memory tasks than men. But again, such findings of sex differences were few in number relative to the total number of comparisons in these various domains and, more tellingly, were not specific to the ADHD group. Very similar results were reported by Murphy et al. (2001) on their extensive neuropsychological test battery, which contained large enough samples of each sex to permit an evaluation of sex differences. In another recent study of sex differences in neuropsychological performance in ADHD, Rucklidge (2006) found only one sex difference among the various measures she employed with her adolescent samples. Males with ADHD made more errors of inhibition than females—a difference that became nonsignificant after controlling for reading ability, comorbidity, and IQ. Hence these results provide no support for the notion that the disorder is somehow more uniquely expressed in the neuropsychological deficits of women than of men in a way that is not typical of women in general.

One earlier paper did report some interesting differences between men and women with ADHD on measures of electroencephalographic (EEG) activity and autonomic arousal (skin conductance) (Hermans et al., 2004). They found that the adults with ADHD generally had greater EEG theta (slow-wave) activity and lower skin conductance than their control adults, consistent with earlier research on such measures. But the group differences in EEG activity were attributable entirely to males with ADHD, while those on skin conductance appeared to be due entirely to females with ADHD. The sample sizes of ADHD males ($N = 21$) and females ($N = 14$) were so small, however, as to greatly restrict the statistical power of this study and to call into question just how representative these samples might be of the larger population of men and women with the disorder. While the authors argued that distinctly different mechanisms may underlie the disorder in males than in females, such judgments really ought to be withheld until we can see if the study can be replicated with larger and possibly more representative clinical samples. All of the results of the present study would certainly disagree with such a conclusion.

In summary, where sex differences were evident, the typical pattern of our findings was that few of them reflected specific differences between men and women with ADHD. Instead, they largely represented sex differences in the general populations sampled by our control groups. We largely found little evidence that ADHD in females is different from that in males in any ways that are not typical of sex differences in the general population, and we found no evidence that it is qualitatively different. A few differences in risks emerged for women with ADHD (obesity, somatic complaints, client relations in the workplace) that are worthy of further study but do not rise to the level of advocating a vastly different nature to the disorder in women. Most sex differences cut across all our groups, reflecting general differences between men and women; when such differences were found, they were most often found to be more marked in men than in women.

Treatment Implications

Our numerous findings that were specific to the ADHD groups overwhelmingly support the validity of this disorder in adults, in keeping with prior research and reviews on this issue (Spencer et al., 1994; Wilens et al., 2004). For the most part, adults with ADHD that has persisted from childhood are remarkably similar to clinic-referred adults newly diagnosed with it. Yet some noteworthy differences were evident here. Most of them found the clinic-referred adults with ADHD to be less impaired with one exception, and that was in risk for comorbid psychiatric disorders and especially anxiety and depression. Those who have grown up with ADHD report significantly lower risks for these disorders. Yet those same adults report greater impairment in their educational careers and occupational functioning as do clinic-referred adults with the disorder. Those who have grown up with ADHD also seem to have greater difficulties with antisocial behavior, frank antisocial personality disorder, and possibly drug use than do clinic-referred adults with the disorder. Both groups display significant problems in their health and lifestyle, money management, and driving. The Milwaukee Study also began to document evidence that the disorder may pose risks for future cardiovascular disease and shorter life expectancy if current findings of greater body mass index, smoking, alcohol use, and lower HDL cholesterol, and regular exercise continue over the next decade of their lives.

Our findings have significant implications not only for the design of better diagnostic criteria and for the validity of the disorder itself but also for clinicians who would evaluate and manage this disorder in adults. The myriad impairments we have identified as being associated with ADHD will call for a variety of psychiatric, psychological, educational, and occupational interventions and accommodations to more effectively assist these adults in the management of their disorder and in the reduction of the impairments associated with it. For a detailed discussion of treatments for ADHD in adults, including counseling and medications, see the text by Barkley (2006).

Specifically, clinicians need to be aware of and specifically to assess for the high *comorbidity* of ADHD with other psychiatric disorders, particularly dysthymia, depression, ODD, CD, and alcohol and drug-use disorders more generally. Noteworthy is that the elevated risk for suicidal ideation and attempts associated with the disorder is driven largely by comorbid mood disorders and not so much by ADHD specifically. Such comorbid disorders and psychological problems are highly likely to require separate treatment approaches than those likely to be aimed at the management of ADHD symptoms and their related impairments. Thus, a package of treatments is more likely to be put in place for most adults with ADHD to address this complexity of clinical presentation than is any single drug or psychological therapy.

Our studies lead us to believe that ADHD in adults, particularly when seen in clinic-referred adults, is therefore likely to require polypharmacy more than is the case for childhood ADHD, given these higher risks for comorbid mood and anxiety disorders. While anti-ADHD drugs, such as stimulants and nonstimulant selective norepinephrine reuptake inhibitors, are clearly indicated for such cases, they are unlikely to address the risk for mood disorders evident here, which are likely to require separate medical (i.e., antidepressant) and psychological (i.e. cognitive-behavioral) treatments in their own right. The elevated risk for anxiety disorders in both clinic-referred ADHD adults and those with persistent ADHD in adulthood also suggests (1) that the nonstimulant, atomoxetine, may be of some benefit for these comorbid cases, in view of recent findings that it does not exacerbate anxiety and may reduce it to some extent, and (2) that cognitive-behavioral interventions having utility in management of anxiety disorders generally may be of some benefit for this comorbid population.

Drug detoxification and rehabilitation programs will also be required for that subset of comorbid ADHD cases having drug-use disorders, many of whom are also likely to have antisocial personality disorder or a history of CD. Early and aggressive treatment of the ADHD seen in these comorbid cases at initial entry into rehabilitation programs offers the best chance of assisting these individuals with their rehabilitation efforts. Ignoring ADHD is highly likely to result in recurrent treatment failures due to the significant self-regulation and executive deficits we have identified with this disorder.

Educational and occupational impairments were nearly ubiquitous in the adults with ADHD, whether clinic-referred or children grown up. Clinicians therefore are likely to be asked to involve themselves in the educational impairments of those adults with ADHD still pursuing further education at the time of clinical evaluation. They may be asked to make recommendations concerning the need for and types of accommodations these adults are likely to require in those settings. In so doing, as we noted earlier, clinicians will need to familiarize themselves with the standards of evidence required under the American with Disabilities Act for obtaining such accommodations. They may also be asked to involve themselves in workplace impairments and the types of accommodations that may be needed to deal with these impairments. Where untrained or uncomfortable in doing so, clinicians should refer their patients having such concerns to other professionals specializing in vocational assessment, accommodations, and rehabilitation for the expertise that may be required to address the workplace difficulties of adults with ADHD. Here again, familiarity with the appropriate aspects of the Americans with Disabilities Act will be required to obtain such accommodations.

We noted previously our belief that long-acting ADHD medications will likely prove as useful for assisting adults with ADHD or more so as they have with children with ADHD. We base this on the fact that adults carry responsibilities for themselves and others, their work and ongoing education, and their self-care and family responsibilities across longer periods of the day than do children. In fact, long-acting medications may even need to be further supplemented with immediate-release medications to provide the additional hours of coverage these adults are likely to require beyond that necessary to cover a child's school day. We are fully aware that behavioral interventions have proven very useful in educational settings for ADHD children, but they seem to us to be much less likely to be feasible or be adopted in employment settings. Where they are feasible, then they should be encouraged. But we believe that the nature of adult employment makes medication a more convenient, effective, and private form of intervention for adults with the disorder. Workplace accommodations may offer some additional benefits beyond medication for adults with ADHD, but no research is available to demonstrate the actual efficacy of such accommodations.

Both of our studies documented higher rates of *antisocial behavior and drug use* in both adults with ADHD and those who have grown up with the disorder. Thus, clinicians are advised that a significant minority of adults with ADHD seen in clinical settings are likely to have a past history of substance-use disorders and antisocial activities and that both may be ongoing at the time of clinical presentation. These may require interventions that may be independent of those being implemented for the management of ADHD. We strongly recommend treating the ADHD first in order to determine the extent to which it may be contributing to any ongoing drug use or antisocial activities prior to engaging in rehabilitation efforts aimed directly at these latter problems. This recommendation is based on the fact that medication treatment of ADHD among antisocial individuals who are substance abusers is likely to assist with their rehabilitation, whereas leaving their self-regulation deficits untreated may well contribute to risk for relapse or recidivism, respectively. If the clinician is untrained or uncomfortable in addressing these drug-use and antisocial difficulties, he or she should certainly refer ADHD patients to other professionals who are expert in these domains of rehabilitation for the comanagement of such cases. Practitioners are also likely to find themselves embroiled in criminal or other legal proceedings related to the increased risks of these adults for both drug-use disorders and antisocial acts. They should be prepared to seek expert legal advice concerning such involvement. As noted earlier, there may also be increased issues of personal safety for clinicians in dealing with the antisocial subset of adults with ADHD, thus warranting the taking of preventive measures in the clinical settings where these adults are to be evaluated and treated.

The domain of *health and associated lifestyles* was also an area in which many risks were evident in conjunction with ADHD in adults. Practitioners need to pay more attention to the health and lifestyle risks likely to be present in adults they diagnose with ADHD, apart from their obvious focus on ADHD and comorbid psychiatric disorders. Primary care clinicians in particular need to be better trained to recognize ADHD in adults as a significant risk factor, leading to lifestyles and health behavior choices that place such individuals at greater risk for later CHD. These health and lifestyle risks will likely increase the need for various medical management and health improvement measures beyond just those interventions aimed at the management of ADHD itself. They are also likely to warrant referral to other medical and health professionals who are expert in the management of these health risk and lifestyle problem areas, such as smoking cessation programs, dietary management, and exercise regimens.

Financial management was another domain of major life activity pervasively affected by ADHD in adults. This makes it of paramount importance that clinicians become more aware of community resources—such as banks, credit unions, etc.—that may be of assistance in addressing the money management problems likely to exist in the adaptive functioning of adults with ADHD. Debt reorganization, credit counseling, budgeting advice, bankruptcy assistance, cognitive-behavioral treatments for impulse buying, and so forth, may be needed for some adults with ADHD. Although there is no research on the issue, it is likely that ADHD medications may be as helpful to improving the money management problems of adults with ADHD as they have proven to be in other areas of symptom management and adaptive functioning.

Driving, or the operation of motor vehicles, is an area of impairment for adults with ADHD that is often underappreciated by clinicians. Yet both of our studies and numerous prior ones have consistently documented this domain as a serious and potentially life-threatening arena deserving of clinical attention. Fortunately, recent studies cited earlier have also shown that driving performance can be improved by the use of stimulants and atomoxetine. What also may be needed here is greater attention to the timing of when these adults are likely to drive to ensure that they are receiving adequate levels of medication to address their driving risks at those hours, as in late-night driving, when earlier doses, even of extended-release compounds, may be dissipating. More study is needed to determine the extent to which psychosocial treatments may be useful for this domain of impairment, given that no studies have examined this issue to date. The driving performance problems noted in adults with ADHD may be made differentially worse than in normal adults by the consumption of alcohol; therefore clinicians should encourage their adult ADHD patients to show more restraint in using alcohol if they plan to drive.

As noted above, children growing up with ADHD lead a *riskier sexual lifestyle*. They have an earlier start to their sexual careers (intercourse), are more likely to become pregnant (if female) or to impregnate others (if males), are more likely to be parents by age 21 or 27, and are more likely to contract a sexually transmitted disease by age 21 than are Community controls followed over this same time. These risks deserve greater attention in pediatrics and primary medical care, where efforts to reduce them are uncommon, in our opinion. Sex and contraception counseling, increased parental supervision, and continued ADHD treatment throughout adolescence should be tested for their utility in reducing these risks.

Once adults with ADHD have children, clinicians need to recognize the increased risk of ADHD and related *disorders in the offspring* of these adults. Those disorders and more general psychological problems are likely to require separate evaluation and management from the problems posed by ADHD in the parent. Referral of such cases to child mental health professionals may be needed in some cases. Parents having ADHD are also likely to do less well in behavioral parent training programs, as noted previously, suggesting that parental ADHD be treated prior to undertaking such child behavioral management programs. Parents having ADHD are also more likely to experience stress as parents, regardless of the presence of ADHD in their children. This may necessitate additional counseling of these adults in stress management and other coping techniques to reduce the greater stress and conflict likely to be evident in families where the adults have ADHD. Practitioners should understand that while some of the distress experienced by these parents is due to their offsprings' greater disruptive behavior, some of it is also related to the parents' mental health, and especially depression. This suggests that management of these adults' ADHD may be inadequate in dealing with the distress they experience in child raising if depression is also a comorbidity. Clinical management of the parents' depression may also be necessary. Finally, we noted that marital distress is greater in adults with ADHD than in the general population. Yet it is also elevated in non-ADHD clinic-referred adults and so may not be specific just to ADHD. This implies that clinicians may need to look for such disharmony and conflict and possibly make appropriate recommendations for further evaluation and possibly marital intervention.

Yet in addressing the symptoms and impairments specifically associated with ADHD, we must emphasize that a purely information-based or skill training program aimed at any particular symptom domain or area of impairment is unlikely to correct it. Such programs assume that the basic deficit behind the impairment is a lack of knowledge or skill and that, hence, conveying that information to the client should result in correction of the problem. Barkley (1997) has specified the reasons why such approaches have not proven especially useful in childhood ADHD and may be unlikely to do so for ADHD in adults as well.

Barkley's theory of ADHD argues that the problems those with ADHD experience in major life activities have more to do with not using what they know at critical points of performance in their natural environments than with not knowing what to do. To use the knowledge one has acquired in life, one must stop responding impulsively to immediate events so as to pause the ongoing action and permit the executive system to generate the information necessary to guide a more appropriate response in that situation. This will be done by engaging the retrospective aspects of working memory that lead to hindsight, from which will be gleaned information about similar past experiences and how best to deal with it now. From hindsight will be constructed the prospective aspects of working memory or foresight that prepare the individual to act and guide that ongoing action toward the desired goal. Self-directed speech will further serve these retrospective and prospective aspects of working memory through self-questioning (a means of interrogating one's own history for relevant information) and the generation of verbal rules to further assist in guiding behavior. These activities are likely to foster a sense of the future and a window on time that can determine the temporal foreperiod over which decisions about the future are being made (how long in advance of the event decisions about it are being prepared). The mental imagery and rules that derive from these activities will require the self-generation of motivation in order to support or drive the planned behavior toward its intended goal. And should problems or obstacles to the intended goal or the proposed plan to attain it be encountered, another executive function will provide the analytic (taking apart) and synthetic (recombining) functions that permit mental play with information to discover a means around the obstacle. The problems those with ADHD experience are therefore not ones about which such individuals lack knowledge or skill in what to do; lacking are those executive mechanisms that take what one already knows and the skills one already possesses and apply them, producing more effective behavior toward others and the future.

ADHD is therefore viewed as being a disorder of performance—of doing what one knows rather than knowing what to do. Like patients with injuries to the frontal lobes, those with ADHD find that it has partially cleaved or dissociated intellect from action or knowledge from performance. Thus, the individual with ADHD may know how to act but may not act that way when placed in social settings where such action would be beneficial. The timing and timeliness of behavior in ADHD is disrupted more than is the basic knowledge or skill about that behavior.

From this vantage point, treatments for ADHD will be most helpful when they assist with the performance of a particular behavior at the *point of performance* in the natural environments where and when such behavior should be performed. A corollary of this is that the further away in space and time a treatment is from this point of performance, the less effective it is likely to be in assisting with the management of ADHD. Not only is assistance at the "point of performance" going to prove critical to treatment efficacy, but so is assistance with the time, timing, and timeliness of behavior in those with ADHD, not just in the training of the behavior itself. Nor will there necessarily be any lasting value or maintenance of treatment effects from such assistance if it is removed too soon, once the individual is performing the desired behavior. The value of such treatments lies not only in providing assistance with eliciting behavior that is likely to already be in the individual's repertoire at the point of performance where its display is critical but also in maintaining the performance of that behavior over time in that natural setting.

Disorders of performance in ADHD cause great consternation for the mental health and educational arenas of service. At the core of such problems is the vexing issue of just how one gets people to behave in ways that they know are good for them yet which they seem unlikely, unable, or unwilling to perform. Conveying more knowledge does not prove as helpful as altering the motivational parameters associated with the performance of that behavior at its appropriate point of performance. Coupled with this is the realization that such changes in behavior are maintained only as long as those environmental adjustments or accommodations are as well. To expect otherwise would seem to approach the treatment of ADHD with outdated or misguided assumptions about its essential nature.

The conceptual model of ADHD introduced earlier (Chapter 7) (see also Barkley, 1997, 2006) brings with it many other implications for the management of ADHD in adults. Some of these are briefly mentioned below:

1. If the process of regulating behavior by internally represented forms of information (working memory or the internalization of behavior) is delayed in those with ADHD, then they will be best assisted by "externalizing" those forms of information; the provision of physical representations of that information will be needed in the setting at the point of performance. Since covert or private information is weak as a source of stimulus control, making that information overt and public may assist with strengthening control of behavior by that information.

2. The individual's inability to organize behavior both within and across time is one of the ultimate disabilities due to the disorder. ADHD is to time what nearsightedness is to spatial vision; it creates a temporal myopia in which the individual's behavior is governed even more than normal by events close to or within the temporal now and immediate context rather than by internal information that pertains to longer-term, future events. This helps us to understand why adults with ADHD make the decisions they do, shortsighted as they seem to be to others around them. If one has little regard for future events, then much of one's behavior will be aimed at maximizing immediate rewards and escaping from immediate hardships or aversive circumstances without concern for the delayed consequences of those actions. Those with ADHD may be helped, with the assistance of caregivers and others, by presenting time itself more externally, reducing or eliminating gaps in time among the components of a behavioral contingency (event, response, outcome), and bridging temporal gaps related to future events.

3. Given that the model hypothesizes a deficit in internally generated and represented forms of motivation needed to drive goal-directed behavior, those with ADHD will require the provision of externalized sources of motivation. For instance, the provision of artificial rewards, such as tokens, may be needed throughout the performance of a task or other goal-directed behavior when there are otherwise few or no immediate consequences associated with that performance. Such artificial reward programs become, for the child with ADHD

like prosthetic devices for the physically disabled, allowing them to perform more effectively in some tasks and settings with which they otherwise would have considerable difficulty. The motivational disability created by the disorder makes such motivational prostheses nearly essential for most children with ADHD and probably adults as well.

4. Given the considerations listed above, clinicians should likely reject most approaches to intervention for adults with ADHD that do not involve helping patients with an active intervention at the point of performance.

This theory suggests another implication for the management of ADHD. Only a treatment that can result in improvement or normalization of the underlying neuropsychological (neurogenetic) deficit in behavioral inhibition is likely to result in an improvement or normalization of the executive functions dependent on such inhibition. To date, the only existing treatment that can is medication, such as the use of stimulants or the nonstimulant atomoxetine. These improve or normalize the neural substrates in the prefrontal regions and related networks which likely underlie this disorder. Evidence to date suggests that this improvement or normalization in inhibition and some of the EF may occur as a temporary consequence of active treatment with stimulant medication, yet only during the time course the medication remains within the brain. Research shows that clinical improvement in behavior occurs in as many as 75 to 92% of those with ADHD and results in normalization of behavior in approximately 50 to 60% of these cases on average. The model of ADHD developed here, then, implies that medication is not only a useful treatment approach for the management of ADHD but also the predominant treatment approach among those currently available because it is the only one known to produce such improvement/normalization rates, albeit temporarily.

It can also be reasoned that if ADHD results in an undercontrol of behavior by internally represented forms of information via the EFs, then that information should be "externalized" as much as possible whenever feasible. It should be made physical outside of the individual once again, as it must have been in earlier development. The internal forms of information generated by the executive system, if they have been generated at all, appear to be extraordinarily weak in their ability to control and sustain the behavior of those with ADHD. Self-directed visual imagery, audition, and the other covert resensing activities that form nonverbal working memory as well as covert self-speech, if they are functional at all in certain times and contexts, do not yield up information of sufficient power to control behavior in this disorder. That behavior remains largely under the control of the salient aspects of the immediate context. The solution to this problem is not to nag those with ADHD to simply try harder or to remember what they are supposed to be working on or toward. It is instead to take charge of that immediate context and fill it with physical cues comparable to their internal counterparts, which are proving so ineffective. In a sense, clinicians treating those with ADHD must beat the environment at its own game. Sources of high-appealing distracters that may serve to subvert, pervert, or disrupt task-directed behavior should be minimized whenever possible. In their place should be cues, prompts, and other forms of information that are just as salient and appealing yet are directly associated with or an inherent part of the task to be accomplished. Such externalized information serves to cue the individual to do what he or she knows.

If the rules that are understood to be operative during educational or occupational activities, for instance, do not seem to be controlling the adult's behavior, they should be externalized. The rules can be externalized by posting signs around the school or work environment that are related to these rules and then making sure that the adult frequently refers to them. Having the adult verbally self-state these rules aloud before and during these individual work performances may also be helpful. One can also record these reminders on a cassette tape to which the adult listens through earphones while working. It is not the intention of this chapter to articulate the details of the many treatments that can be designed from this model. That is done in other textbooks. All we wish to do here is simply to show the principle that underlies them—put external information around the person and within their sensory fields so that it may serve to guide their behavior more appropriately. With the knowledge this model provides and a little ingenuity, many of these forms of internally represented information can be externalized for better management of the child or adult with ADHD.

Chief among these internally represented forms of information that either need to be externalized or removed entirely from the tasks are those related to time. As stated earlier, time and the future are the enemies of people with ADHD when it comes to task accomplishment or performance toward a goal. An obvious solution, then, is to reduce or eliminate these problematic elements of a task when feasible. For instance, rather than assign a behavioral contingency that has large temporal gaps among its elements to someone with ADHD, those temporal gaps should be reduced whenever possible. In other words, the elements should be made more contiguous. Rather than tell such a person that a project must be completed over the next month, assist him or her with doing a step a day toward that eventual goal, so that when the deadline arrives, the work will have been done but done in small daily work periods, with immediate feedback and incentives.

Yet there is a major caveat to all these implications for externalizing forms of internally represented information. This caveat stems from the component of the model that deals with self-regulation of emotion, motivation, and arousal: no matter how much clinicians, educators, and caregivers externalize prompts, cues, and other signals of the internalized forms of information by which they desire the person with ADHD to be guided (stimuli, events, rules, images, sounds, etc.), their efforts are likely to prove only partially successful. Even then, they will prove only temporarily so. Internal sources of motivation must be augmented with more powerful external forms as well. It is not only the internally represented information that is weak in those with ADHD but also the internally generated sources of motivation associated with them. In the absence of external motivation in the immediate context, those sources of motivation are critical to driving goal-directed behavior toward tasks, the future, and the intended outcome. Addressing one form of internalized information without addressing the other is a sure recipe for ineffectual treatment. Anyone wishing to treat those with ADHD must understand that sources of motivation must also be externalized in those contexts in which tasks are to be performed, rules followed, and goals accomplished. Complaining to these individuals about their lack of motivation (laziness), drive, will power, or self-discipline will not suffice to correct the problem. Pulling back from assisting them to let the natural consequences occur, as if this would teach them a lesson that could correct their behavior, is likewise a recipe for disaster. Instead, artificial means of creating external sources of motivation must be arranged *at the point of performance* in the context in which the work or behavior is desired.

The methods of behavior modification are particularly well suited to achieving these ends. Many techniques exist within this form of treatment that can be applied to those with ADHD. What first needs to be recognized, as this model of ADHD stipulates, is that (1) internalized, self-generated forms of motivation are weak at initiating and sustaining goal directed behavior; (2) externalized sources of motivation, often artificial, must be arranged within the context at the point of performance; and (3) these compensatory, prosthetic forms of motivation must be sustained for long periods.

The foregoing leads to a much more general implication of this model of ADHD: the approach taken to its management must be the same as that taken in the management of other chronic medical or psychiatric disabilities. We frequently use diabetes as an analogous condition to ADHD in trying to help parents and other professionals to grasp this point. At the time of diagnosis, all involved realize that as yet there is no cure for the condition. Still, multiple means of treatment can provide symptomatic relief from the deleterious effects of ADHD, including taking daily doses of medication and changing settings, tasks, and lifestyles. Immediately following diagnosis, the clinician must educate the patient and family on the nature of the chronic disorder and then designs and implement a treatment package for it. This package must be maintained over long periods to sustain the symptomatic relief that the treatments initially achieve. Ideally, the treatment package, so maintained, will reduce or eliminate the secondary consequences of leaving the condition unmanaged. However, each patient is different, and so is each instance of the chronic condition being treated. As a result, symptom breakthroughs and crises are likely to occur periodically over the course of treatment, which may demand reintervention or the design and implementation of modified or entirely new treatment packages. Changes to the environment that may assist those with the disorder are not viewed as somehow correcting earlier faulty learning or leading to permanent improvements that can permit the treatments to be withdrawn. Instead, the more appropriate view of psychological treatment is one of designing a prosthetic social environment that enables the individual to cope better with and compensate for the disorder. Behavioral and other technologies used to assist adults with ADHD are akin to artificial limbs, hearing aids, wheelchairs, ramps, and other prostheses that reduce the handicapping impact of a disability and give the individual greater access to and better performance of their major life activities.

Throughout all this, the goal of the clinician, family members, and patients themselves is to try to achieve an improvement in the patient's quality of life and overall success, although never totally normal. We can only hope that the science-based findings presented in this text along with the theoretically driven treatment guidelines given above will help researchers, clinicians, and patients to achieve that goal.

References

Abidin, R. R. (1995). *The Parenting Stress Index—Short Form.* Lutz, FL: Psychological Assessment Resources.

Able, S. L., Johnston, J. A., Adler, L. A., & Swindle, R. W. (2006). Functional and psychosocial impairment in adults with undiagnosed ADHD. *Psychological Medicine, 37,* 97–107.

Achenbach, T. M. (1991). *Child Behavior Checklist and Child Behavior Profile—Cross-Informant Version.* Burlington, VT: Author.

Achenbach, T. M. (1991). *Manual for the Child Behavior Checklist/4–18 and 1991 Profile.* Burlington, VT: Author.

Achenbach, T. (2001). *Young Adult Behavior Checklist and Young Adult Self-Report Forms.* Burlington, VT: Author.

Ackerman, P., Dykman, R., & Peters, J. E. (1977). Teenage status of hyperactive and nonhyperactive learning disabled boys. *American Journal of Orthopsychiatry, 47,* 577–596.

Adler, L. (2006). *Scattered minds: Hope and help for adults with attention deficit hyperactivity disorder.* New York: Putnam.

Alberts-Corush, J., Firestone, P., & Goodman, J. T. (1986). Attention and impulsivity characteristics of the biological and adoptive parents of hyperactive and normal control children. *American Journal of Orthopsychiatry, 56,* 413–423.

American Psychiatric Association. (1968). *Diagnostic and statistical manual of mental disorders* (2nd ed.). Washington, DC: American Psychiatric Press.

American Psychiatric Association. (1980). *Diagnostic and statistical manual of mental disorders* (3rd ed.). Washington, DC: American Psychiatric Press.

American Psychiatric Association. (1987). *Diagnostic and statistical manual of mental disorders* (3rd ed., rev.). Washington, DC: American Psychiatric Press.

American Psychiatric Association. (1994). *Diagnostic and statistical manual of mental disorders* (4th ed.). Washington, DC: American Psychiatric Press.

American Psychiatric Association (2000). *Diagnostic and statistical manual of mental disorders* (4th ed., text rev.). Washington, DC: American Psychiatric Press.

Angold, A., Costello, E. J., & Erkanli, A. (1999). Comorbidity. *Journal of Child Psychology and Psychiatry, 40,* 57–88.

Applegate, B., Lahey, B. B., Hart, E. L., Waldman, I., Biederman, J., Hynd, G. W., et al. (1997). Validity of the age of onset criterion for ADHD: A report from the DSM-IV field trials. *Journal of the American Academy of Child and Adolescent Psychiatry, 36,* 1211–1221.

Armstrong, T. D., & Costello, E. J. (2002). Community studies on adolescent substance use, abuse, or dependence and psychiatric comorbidity. *Journal of Consulting and Clinical Psychology, 70,* 1224–1239.

Arthur, W., Tubre, T., Day, E. A., Sheehan, M. K., Sanchez-Cu, M. L., Paul, D., et al. (2001). Motor vehicle crash involvement and moving violations: Convergence of self-report and archival data. *Human Factors, 45,* 1–11.

August, G. J., & Stewart, M. A. (1983). Family subtype of childhood hyperactivity. *Journal of Nervous and Mental Disease, 171,* 362–368.

August, G. J., Stewart, M. A., & Holmes, C. S. (1983). A four-year follow-up of hyperactive boys with and without conduct disorder. *British Journal of Psychiatry, 143,* 192–198.

Babinski, L. M., Hartsough, C. S., & Lambert, N. M. (1999). Childhood conduct problems, hyperactivity-impulsivity, and inattention as predictors of adult criminal activity. *Journal of Child Psychology and Psychiatry, 40,* 347–355.

Banks, T., Ninowski, J. E., Mash, E. J., & Semple, D. L. (in press). Parenting behavior and cognitions in a community sample of mothers with and without symptoms of attention-deficit/hyperactivity disorder. *Journal of Child and Family Studies.*

Barkley, R. A. (1981). *Hyperactive children: A handbook for diagnosis and treatment.* New York: Guilford Press.

Barkley, R. A. (1982). Guidelines for defining hyperactivity in children (attention deficit disorder with hyperactivity). In B. Lahey & A. Kazdin (Eds.), *Advances in clinical child psychology* (Vol. 5, pp. 137–180). New York: Plenum Press.

Barkley, R. A. (1990). *Attention deficit hyperactivity disorder: A handbook for diagnosis and treatment.* New York: Guilford Press.

Barkley, R. A. (1994). *ADHD in adults* [videotape and manual]. New York: Guilford Press.

Barkley, R. A. (1997a). *ADHD and the nature of self-control.* New York: Guilford Press.

Barkley, R. A. (1997b). Inhibition, sustained attention, and executive functions: Constructing a unifying theory of ADHD. *Psychological Bulletin, 121,* 65–94.

Barkley, R. A. (1998). *Attention deficit hyperactivity disorder: A handbook for diagnosis and treatment* (2nd ed.). New York: Guilford Press.

Barkley, R. A. (2001a). Accidents and ADHD. *The Economics of Neuroscience, 3,* 64–68.

Barkley, R. A. (2001b). The executive functions and self-regulation: An evolutionary neuropsychological perspective. *Neuropsychology Review, 11,* 1–29.

Barkley R. A. (2004). Driving impairments in teens and adults with attention-deficit/hyperactivity disorder. *Psychiatric Clinics of North America, 27*(2), 233–260.

Barkley, R. A. (2006). *Attention deficit hyperactivity disorder: A handbook for diagnosis and treatment* (3rd ed.) New York: Guilford Press.

Barkley, R. A., Anastopoulos, A. D., Guevremont, D. G., & Fletcher, K. F. (1991). Adolescents with attention deficit hyperactivity disorder: Patterns of behavioral adjustment, academic functioning, and treatment utilization. *Journal of the American Academy of Child and Adolescent Psychiatry, 30,* 752–761.

Barkley, R. A., Anderson, D., & Kruesi, M. (2007). A pilot study of the effects of atomoxetine on the driving performance of adults with attention deficit hyperactivity disorder, *Journal of Attention Disorders, 10*, 306–316.

Barkley, R. A., & Biederman, J. (1997). Toward a broader definition of the age-of-onset criterion for attention deficit hyperactivity disorder. *Journal of the American Academy of Child and Adolescent Psychiatry, 36*, 1204–1210.

Barkley, R. A., & Cox, D. (2007). A review of driving risks and impairments associated with attention-deficit/hyperactivity disorder and the effects of stimulant medication on driving performance. *Journal of Safety Research, 38*, 113–138.

Barkley, R. A., DuPaul, G. J., & McMurray, M. B. (1990). A comprehensive evaluation of attention deficit disorder with and without hyperactivity. *Journal of Consulting and Clinical Psychology, 58*, 775–789.

Barkley, R. A., Edwards, G., Laneri, M., Fletcher, K., & Metevia, L. (2001). Executive functioning, temporal discounting, and sense of time in adolescents with attention-deficit/hyperactivity disorder and oppositional defiant disorder. *Journal of Abnormal Child Psychology, 29*, 541–556.

Barkley, R. A., & Fischer, M. (2005). Suicidality in children with ADHD, grown up. *The ADHD Report, 13(6)*, 1–6. New York: Guilford Press.

Barkley, R. A., Fischer, M., Edelbrock, C. S., & Smallish, L. (1990). The adolescent outcome of hyperactive children diagnosed by research criteria: I. An 8-year prospective follow-up study. *Journal of the American Academy of Child and Adolescent Psychiatry, 29*, 546–557.

Barkley, R. A., Fischer, M., Edelbrock, C. S., & Smallish, L. (1991). The adolescent outcome of hyperactive children diagnosed by research criteria: III. Mother–child interactions, family conflicts, and maternal psychopathology. *Journal of Child Psychology and Psychiatry, 32*, 233–256.

Barkley, R. A., Fischer, M., Smallish, L., & Fletcher, K. (2002). The persistence of attention-deficit/hyperactivity disorder into young adulthood as a function of reporting source and definition of disorder. *Journal of Abnormal Psychology, 111*, 279–289.

Barkley, R. A., Fischer, M., Smallish, L., & Fletcher, K. (2003). Does the treatment of ADHD with stimulant medication contribute to illicit drug use and abuse in adulthood? Results from a 15-year prospective study. *Pediatrics, 111*, 109–121.

Barkley, R. A., Fischer, M., Smallish, L., & Fletcher, K. (2004). Young adult follow-up of hyperactive children: Antisocial activities and drug use. *Journal of Child Psychology and Psychiatry, 45*, 195–211.

Barkley, R. A., Fischer, M., Smallish, L., & Fletcher, K. (2006). Young adult follow-up of hyperactive children: Adaptive functioning in major life activities. *Journal of the American Academy of Child and Adolescent Psychiatry, 45*, 192–202.

Barkley, R. A., & Grodzinsky, G. (1994). Are tests of frontal lobe functions useful in the diagnosis of attention deficit disorders? *Clinical Neuropsychologist, 8*, 121–139.

Barkley, R. A., Grodzinsky, G., & DuPaul, G. J. (1992). Frontal lobe functions in attention-deficit disorder with and without hyperactivity: A review and research report. *Journal of Abnormal Child Psychology, 20*, 163–188.

Barkley, R. A., Karlsson, J., & Pollard, S. (1985). Effects of age on the mother-child interactions of hyperactive boys. *Journal of Abnormal Child Psychology, 13*, 631–637.

Barkley, R. A., Karlsson, J., Pollard, S., & Murphy, J. (1985). Developmental changes in the mother-child interactions of hyperactive boys: Effects of two dose levels of Ritalin. *Journal of Child Psychology and Psychiatry, 26*, 705–715.

Barkley, R. A., Karlsson, J., Strzelecki, E., & Murphy, J. (1984). The effects of age and Ritalin dosage on the mother–child interactions of hyperactive children. *Journal of Consulting and Clinical Psychology, 52,* 750–758.

Barkley, R. A., Koplowicz, S., Anderson, T., & McMurray, M. B. (1997). Sense of time in children with ADHD: Effects of duration, distraction, and stimulant medication. *Journal of the International Neuropsychological Society, 3,* 359–369.

Barkley, R. A., & Murphy, K. (1998). *Attention deficit hyperactivity disorder: A clinical workbook* (2nd ed.). New York: Guilford Press.

Barkley, R. A., & Murphy, K. (2006). *Attention deficit hyperactivity disorder: A clinical workbook* (3rd ed.). New York: Guilford Press.

Barkley, R. A., Murphy, K. R., & Bush, T. (2001). Time estimation and reproduction in young adults with attention deficit hyperactivity disorder (ADHD). *Neuropsychology, 15,* 351–360.

Barkley, R. A., Murphy, K. R., DuPaul, G. I., & Bush, T. (2002). Driving in young adults with attention deficit hyperactivity disorder: Knowledge, performance, adverse outcomes, and the role of executive functioning. *Journal of the International Neuropsychological Society, 8,* 655–672.

Barkley, R. A., Murphy, K. R., & Kwasnik, D. (1996). Psychological adjustment and adaptive impairments in young adults with ADHD. *Journal of Attention Disorders, 1,* 41–54.

Barkley, R. A., Murphy, K. R., O'Connell, T., Anderson, D., & Connor, D. F. (2006). Effects of two doses of alcohol on simulator driving performance in adults with attention deficit hyperactivity disorder. *Neuropsychology, 20,* 77–87.

Barkley, R. A., Shelton, T. L., Crosswait, C., Moorehouse, M., Fletcher, K., Barrett, S., et al. (2002). Preschool children with disruptive behavior: Three-year outcome as a function of adaptive disability. *Development and Psychopathology, 14,* 45–67.

Barkley, R. A., Smith, K., Fischer, M., & Navia, B. (2006). An examination of the behavioral and neuropsychological correlates of three ADHD candidate gene polymorphisms (DRD4 7+, DBH TaqI A2, and DAT1 40bp VNTR) in hyperactive and normal children followed to adulthood. *American Journal of Medical Genetics: Neuropsychiatric Genetics, 141B* (5), 487–498.

Batalla, A., Hevia, S., Reguero, J. R., Cubero, G. L., & Cortina, A. (2000). Is the number of coronary risk factors a predictor of the severity of early coronary disease? *Cardiology, 94,* 130.

Bekker, E. M., Overtoom, C. C. E., Kooij, S., Buitelaar, J. K., Verbatem, M. N., & Kenemans, L. (2005a). Disentangling deficits in adults with attention-deficit/hyperactivity disorder. *Archives of General Psychiatry, 62,* 1129–1136.

Bekker, E. M., Overtoon, C. C. E., Kooij, S., Buitelaar, J. K., Verbaten, N. M., & Kenemans, J. L. (2005b). Stopping and changing in adults with ADHD. *Psychological Medicine, 35,* 807–816.

Belendiuk, K. A., Clarke, T. L., Chronis, A. M., & Raggi, V. L. (2007). Assessing concordance of measures used to diagnose adult ADHD. *Journal of Attention Disorders, 10,* 276–287.

Berenson, G. S., Srinivasan, S. R., Bao, W., Newman, W. P. III, Tracy, R. E., & Wattigney, W. A. (1998). Association between multiple cardiovascular risk factors and atherosclerosis in children and young adults. The Bogalusa Heart Study. *The New England Journal of Medicine, 338,* 1650–1656.

Biederman, J. (2004). Impact of comorbidity in adults with attention-deficit/hyperactivity disorder. *Journal of Clinical Psychiatry, 65 (Supplement 3),* 3–7.

Biederman, J., Faraone, S. V., Keenan, K., Benjamin, J., Krifcher, B., Moore, C., et al. (1992).

Further evidence for family-genetic risk factors in attention deficit hyperactivity disorder. Patterns of comorbidity in probands and relatives in psychiatrically and pediatrically referred samples. *Archives of General Psychiatry, 49,* 728–738.

Biederman, J., Faraone, S. V., Knee, D., & Munir, K. (1990). Retrospective assessment of DSM-III attention deficit disorder in nonreferred individuals. *Journal of Clinical Psychiatry, 51,* 102–106.

Biederman, J., Faraone, S. V., Mick, E., Spencer, T., Wilens, T., Kiely, K., et al. (1995). High risk for attention deficit hyperactivity disorder among children of parents with childhood onset of the disorder: A pilot study. *American Journal of Psychiatry, 152,* 431–435.

Biederman, J., Faraone, S. V., Spencer, T., Wilens, T., Mick, E., & Lapey, K. (1994). Gender differences in adults with attention-deficit/hyperactivity disorder. *Psychiatry Research, 53,* 13–29.

Biederman, J., Faraone, S., Spencer, T., Wilens, T., Norman, D., Lapey, K. A., et al. (1993). Patterns of psychiatric comorbidity, cognition, and psychosocial functioning in adults with attention deficit hyperactivity disorder. *American Journal of Psychiatry, 150,* 1792–1798.

Biederman, J., Mick, E., & Faraone, S. V. (2000). Age-dependent decline of symptoms of attention deficit hyperactivity disorder: Impact of remission definition and symptom type. *American Journal of Psychiatry, 157,* 816–818.

Biederman, J., Wilens, T., Mick, E., Faraone, S. V., Weber, W., Curtis, S., et al. (1997). Is ADHD a risk factor for psychoactive substance use disorders? Findings from a four-year prospective follow-up study. *Journal of the American Academy of Child and Adolescent Psychiatry, 36,* 21–29.

Biederman, J., Wilens, T., Mick, E., Milberger, S., Spencer, T. J., & Faraone, S. V. (1995). Psychoactive substance use disorders in adults with attention deficit hyperactivity disorder 9ADHD): Effects of ADHD and psychiatric comorbidity. *American Journal of Psychiatry, 152,* 1652–1658.

Biggs, S. H. (1995). Neuropsychological and psychoeducational testing in the evaluation of the ADD adult. In K. G. Nadeau (Ed.), *A comprehensive guide to attention deficit disorder in adults* (pp. 109–134). New York: Brunner/Mazel.

Blouin, A. G., Bornstein, M. A., & Trites, R. L. (1978). Teenage alcohol abuse among hyperactive children: A five year follow-up study. *Journal of Pediatric Psychology, 3,* 188–194.

Boonstra, A. M., Oosterlaan, J., Sergeant, J. A., & Buitelaar, J. K. (2005). Executive functioning in adult ADHD: A meta-analytic review. *Psychological Medicine, 35,* 1097–1108.

Borland, H. L., & Heckman, H. K. (1976). Hyperactive boys and their brothers: A 25-year follow-up study. *Archives of General Psychiatry, 33,* 669–675.

Bronowski, J. (1967/1977). Human and animal languages. *A sense of the future* (pp. 104–131). Cambridge, MA: MIT Press.

Brook, J. S., Whiteman, M., Finch, S. J., & Cohen, P. (1996). Young adult drug use and delinquency: Childhood antecedents and adolescent mediators. *Journal of the American Academy of Child and Adolescent Psychiatry, 35,* 1584–1592.

Brown, T. E. (1996). *Brown Attention-Deficit Disorder Scales.* San Antonio, TX: Psychological Corporation.

Burke, J. D., Loeber, R., & Lahey, B. B. (2001). Which aspects of ADHD are associated with tobacco use in early adolescence? *Journal of Child Psychology and Psychiatry, 42,* 493–502.

Cantwell, D. P. (1972). Psychiatric illness in the families of hyperactive children. *Archives of General Psychiatry, 27,* 414–417.

Cantwell, D. P. (1975). *The hyperactive child.* New York: Spectrum.

Castellanos, F. X., Giedd, J. N., Marsh, W. L., Hamburger, S. D., Vaituzis, A. C., Dickstein, D. P., et al. (1996). Quantitative brain magnetic resonance imaging in attention-deficit hyperactivity disorder. *Archives of General Psychiatry, 53*, 607–616.

Chilcoat, H. D., & Breslau, N. (1999). Pathways from ADHD to early drug use. *Journal of the American Academy of Child and Adolescent Psychiatry, 38*, 1347–1354.

Claude, D., & Firestone, P. (1995). The development of ADHD boys: A 12-year follow-up. *Canadian Journal of Behavioral Science, 27*, 226–249.

Cohen, A. J., & Shapiro, S. K. (2007). Exploring the performance differences on the Flicker Task and the Conners Continuous Performance Test in adults with ADHD. *Journal of Attention Disorders, 10*, 49–63.

Conners, C. K. (1995). *The Conners Continuous Performance Test.* North Tonawanda, NY: Multi-Health Systems.

Conners, C. K., Erhardt, D., & Sparrow, E. (1998). *Conners Adult ADHD Rating Scales (CAARS).* North Tonawanda, NY: Multi-Health Systems, Inc.

Conners, C. K., Erhardt, D., Epstein, J. N., Parker, J. D. A., & Sitarenios, G. (2006). *Self-ratings of ADHD symptoms in adults: Normatiev data, factor structure, reliability, and diagnostic sensitivity.* Unpublished manuscript, Duke University Medical Center, Durham, NC.

Connor, D. F. (2006). Stimulants. In R. A. Barkley (Ed.), *Attention-deficit/hyperactivity disorder: A handbook for diagnosis and treatment* (pp. 608–647). New York: Guilford Press.

Corbett, B., & Stanczak, D. E., (1999). Neuropsychological performance of adults evidencing attention-deficit/hyperactivity disorder. *Archives of Clinical Neuropsychology, 14*, 373–387.

De Quiros, G. B., & Kinsbourne, M. (2001). Adult ADHD: Analysis of self-ratings on a behavior questionnaire. In J. Wasserstein, L. Wolf, & F. Lefever (Eds.), Adult attention deficit disorder: Brain mechanisms and life outcomes. *Annals of the New York Academy of Sciences, 931*, 140–147.

Denckla, M. B. (1994). Measurement of executive function. In G. R. Lyon (Ed.), *Frames of reference for the assessment of learning disabilities: New views on measurement issues* (pp. 117–142). Baltimore: Brookes.

Denckla, M. B. (1996). A theory and model of executive function: A neuropsychological perspective. In G. R. Lyon & N. A. Krasnegor (Eds.), *Attention, memory, and executive function* (pp. 263–277). Baltimore: Brookes.

Dennis, M. (1991). Frontal lobe function in childhood and adolescence: A heuristic for assessing attention regulation, executive control, and the intentional states important for social discourse. *Developmental Neuropsychology, 7*, 327–358.

Derogatis, L. (1986). *Manual for the Symptom Checklist 90 Revised (SCL-90-R).* Baltimore, MD: Author.

Deutscher, B., & Fewell, R. R. (2005). Early predictors of attention deficit hyperactivity disorder and school difficulties in low birth weight premature children. *Topics in Early Childhood Special Education, 25*, 71–79.

Devroey, D., Vantomme, K., Betz, W., Vandevoorde, J., & Kartounian, J. (2004). A review of the treatment guidelines on the management of low levels of high-density lipoprotein cholesterol. *Cardiology, 102*, 61–66.

Diaz, R. M., & Berk, L. E. (1992). *Private speech: From social interaction to self-regulation.* Mahwah, NJ: Lawrence Erlbaum.

Dougherty, D. D., Bonab, A. A., Spencer, T. J., Rauch, S. L., Madras, B. K., & Fischman, A. J. (1999). Dopamine transporter density in patients with attention deficit hyperactivity disorder. *Lancet, 354*, 2132–2133.

Douglas, V. I. (1972). Stop, look, and listen: The problem of sustained attention and impulse control in hyperactive and normal children. *Canadian Journal of Behavioural Science, 4,* 259–282.

Dowson, J. H., McClean, A., Bazanis, E., Toone, B., Young, S., Robbins, T. W., et al. (2003). Impaired spatial working memory in adults with attention-deficit/hyperactivity disorder: comparisons with performance in adults with borderline personality disorder and in controls. *Acta Psychiatrica Scandinavica, 110,* 45–54.

Dunn, L. M., & Dunn, L. M. (1981). *Peabody Picture Vocabulary Test—Revised.* Circle Pines, MN: American Guidance Service.

DuPaul, G. J., Power, T. J., Anastopoulos, A. D., & Reid, R. (1998). *The ADHD Rating Scale–IV: Checklists, norms, and clinical interpretation.* New York: Guilford Press.

DuPaul, J. G., Schaughency, El. A., Weyandt, L. L., Tripp, G., Kiesner, J., Ota, K., et al. (2001). Self-report of ADHD symptoms in university studies: Cross-gender and cross-national prevalence. *Journal of Learning Disabilities, 34,* 370–379.

Dykman, R. A., & Ackerman, P. T. (1992). Attention deficit disorder and specific reading disability: Separate but often overlapping disorders. In. S. Shaywitz & B. A. Shaywitz (Eds.), *Attention deficit disorder comes of age: Toward the twenty-first century* (pp. 165–184). Austin, TX: PRO-ED.

Edelbrock, C. S., & Costello, A. (1988). Convergence between statistically derived behavior problem syndromes and child psychiatric diagnoses. *Journal of Abnormal Child Psychology, 16,* 219–231.

Eisenberg, L. (1973). The overactive child. *Hospital Practice, 8,* 151–160.

Epstein, J. N., Conners, C. K., Erhardt, D., March, J. S., & Swanson, J. M. (1997). Asymmetrical hemispheric control of visual–spatial attention in adults with attention deficit hyperactivity disorder. *Neuropsychology, 11,* 467–473.

Epstein, J. N., Conners, C. K., Sitarenios, G., & Erhardt, D. (1998). Continuous performance test results of adults with attention deficit hyperactivity disorder. *Clinical Neuropsychologist, 12,* 155–168.

Epstein, J. N., Johnson, D. E., Varia, I. M., & Conners, C. K. (2001). Neuropsychological assessment of response inhibition in adults with ADHD. *Journal of Clinical and Experimental Neuropsychology, 23,* 362–371.

Eyestone, L. L., & Howell, R. J. (1994). An epidemiological study of attention-deficit hyperactivity disorders and major depression in a male prison population. *Bulletin of the American Academy of Psychiatry and Law, 22,* 181–193.

Faraone, S. V., & Biederman, J. (1997). Do attention deficit hyperactivity disorder and major depression share familial risk factors? *Journal of Nervous and Mental Disease, 185,* 533–541.

Faraone, S. V., Biederman, J., & Friedman, D. (2000). Validity of DSM-IV subtypes of attention-deficit/hyperactivity disorder: A family study perspective. *Journal of the American Academy of Child and Adolescent Psychiatry, 39,* 300–307.

Faraone, S. V., Biederman, J., Lehman, B., Keenan, K., Norman, D., Seidman, L. J., et al. (1993). Evidence for the independent familial transmission of attention deficit hyperactivity disorder and learning disabilities: Results from a family genetic study. *American Journal of Psychiatry, 150,* 891–895.

Faraone, S. V., Biederman, J., Mennin, D., Wozniak, J., & Spencer, J. T. (1997). Attention deficit hyperactivity disorder with bipolar disorder: A familial subtype? *Journal of the American Academy of Child and Adolescent Psychiatry, 36,* 1387–1390.

Faraone, S. V., Biederman, J., Spencer, T., Mick, E., Murray, K., Petty, C., et al. (2006). Diagnosing adult attention-deficit hyperactivity disorder: Are late onset and subthreshold diagnoses vaild? *American Journal of Psychiatry, 163,* 1720–1729.

Faraone, S. V., Biederman, J., Weiffenbach, B., Keith, T., Chu, M. P., Weaver, A., et al. (1999). Dopamine D4 gene 7-repeat allele and attention deficit hyperactivity disorder. *American Journal of Psychiatry, 156*, 768–770.

Faraone, S. V., & Doyle, A. E. (2001). The nature and heritability of attention-deficit/hyperactivity disorder. *Child and Adolescent Psychiatric Clinics of North America, 10*, 299–316.

Faraone, S. V., Monuteaux, M. C., Biederman, J., Cohan, S. L., & Mick, E. (2003). Does parental ADHD bias maternal reports of ADHD symptoms in children? *Journal of Consulting and Clinical Psychology, 71*, 168–175.

Fayyad, J., DeGraaf, R., Kessler, R., Alonso, J., Angeermeyer, M., Demyttenaere, K., et al. (2007). Cross-national prevalence and correlates of adult attention-deficit hyperactivity disorder. *British Journal of Psychiatry, 190*, 402–409.

Fergusson, D. M., & Horwood, L. J. (1995). Early disruptive behavior, IQ, and later school achievement and delinquent behavior. *Journal of Abnormal Child Psychology, 23*, 183–199.

Filipek, P. A., Semrud-Clikeman, M., Steingard, R. J., Renshaw, P. F., Kennedy, D. N., & Biederman, J. (1997). Volumetric MRI analysis comparing subjects having attention-deficit hyperactivity disorder with normal controls. *Neurology, 48*, 589–601.

Fischer, M. (1990). Parenting stress and the child with attention deficit hyperactivity disorder. *Journal of Clinical Child Psychology, 19*, 337–346.

Fischer, M., & Barkley, R. A. (2006). Young adult outcome of hyperactive children: Leisure, financial and social activities. *International Journal of Disability, Development, and Education, 53*, 229–245.

Fischer, M., Barkley, R. A., Edelbrock, C. S., & Smallish, L. (1990). The adolescent outcome of hyperactive children diagnosed by research criteria: II. Academic, attentional, and neuropsychological status. *Journal of Consulting and Clinical Psychology, 58*, 580–588.

Fischer, M., Barkley, R. A., Fletcher, K., & Smallish, L. (1993a). The adolescent outcome of hyperactive children diagnosed by research criteria: V. Predictors of outcome. *Journal of the American Academy of Child and Adolescent Psychiatry, 32*, 324–332.

Fischer, M., Barkley, R. A., Fletcher, K., & Smallish, L. (1993b). The stability of dimensions of behavior in ADHD and normal children over an 8 year period. *Journal of Abnormal Child Psychology, 21*, 315–337.

Fischer, M., Barkley, R. A., Smallish, L., & Fletcher, K. (2002). Young adult follow-up of hyperactive children: Self-reported psychiatric disorders, comorbidity, and the role of childhood conduct problems. *Journal of Abnormal Child Psychology. 30*, 463–475.

Fischer, M., Barkley, R. A., Smallish, L., & Fletcher, K. (2004). Hyperactive children as young adults: Deficits in inhibition, attention, and response perseveration and their relationship to severity of childhood and current ADHD and conduct disorder. *Developmental Neuropsychology, 27*, 107–133.

Fischer, M., Barkley, R. A., Smallish, L., & Fletcher, K. (2007). Hyperactive children as young adults: Driving ability, safe driving behavior, and adverse driving outcomes. *Accident Analysis and Prevention, 39*, 94–105.

Fletcher, K., Fischer, M., Barkley, R. A., & Smallish, L. (1996). A sequential analysis of the mother–adolescent interactions of ADHD, ADHD/ODD, and normal teenagers' neutral and conflict discussions. *Journal of Abnormal Child Psychology, 24*, 271–298.

Flory, K., Lynam, D., Milich, R., Leukefeld, C., & Clayton, R. (2001, August). *Attention-deficit/hyperactivity disorder as a moderator of the relation between conduct disorder and drug abuse.* Poster presented at the annual meeting of the American Psychological Association, San Francisco, CA.

Flory, K., Molina, B. S. G., Pelham, W. E., Jr., Gnagy, E., & Smith, D. (2006). Childhood

ADHD predicts risky sexual behavior in young adulthood. *Journal of Clinical Child and Adolescent Psychology, 35*, 571–577.

Frazier, T. W., Demareem H. A., & Youngstrom, E. A. (2004). Meta-analysis of intellectual and neuropsychological test performance in attention-deficit/hyperactivity disorder. *Neuropsychology, 18*, 543–555.

Frick, P. J., Kamphaus, R. W., Lahey, B. B., Loeber, R., Christ, M. A. G., Hart, E. L., et al. (1991). Academic underachievement and the disruptive behavior disorders. *Journal of Consulting and Clinical Psychology, 59*, 289–294.

Fried, R., Petty, C. R., Surman, C. B., Reimer, B., Aleardi, M., Martin, J. M., et al. (2006). Characterizing impaired driving in adults with attention-deficit/hyperactivity disorder: a controlled study. *Journal of Clinical Psychiatry, 6*, 567–574.

Friedman, H. S., Tucker, J. S., Schwartz, J. E., Tomlinson-Keasey, C., Martin, L. R., Wingard, D. L., et al. (1995). Psychosocial and behavioral predictors of longevity: The aging and death of the "Termites." *American Psychologist, 50*, 69–78.

Friedman, S. R., Rapport, L. J., Lumley, M., Tzelepis, A., Van Voorhis, A., Stettner, L., et al. (2003). Aspects of social and emotional competence in adult attention-deficit/hyperactivity disorder. *Neuropsychology, 17*, 50–58.

Gansler, D. A., Fucetola, R., Krengel, M., Stetson, S., Zimering, R., & Makary, C. (1998). Are there cognitive subtypes in adult attention-deficit/hyperactivity disorder? *Journal of Nervous and Mental Disease, 186*, 776–781.

Gerbing, D. W., Ahadi, S. A., & Patton, J. H. (1987). Toward a conceptualization of impulsivity: Components across the behavioral and self-report domains. *Multivariate Behavioral Research, 22*, 357–379.

Gilden, D. L., & Hancock, H. (in press). Response variability in attention deficit disorders. *Psychological Science.*

Gittelman, R., Mannuzza, S., Shenker, R., & Bonagura, N. (1985). Hyperactive boys almost grown up: I. Psychiatric status. *Archives of General Psychiatry, 42*, 937–947.

Goldbouart, U., Yaari, S., & Medalie, J. H. (1993). Factors predictive of long-term coronary heart disease mortality among 10,059 male Israeli civil servants and municipal employees: A 23-year mortality follow-up in the Israeli ischemic heart disease study. *Cardiology, 82*, 100–121.

Goldstein, S., & Ellison, A. T. (2002). *Clinician's guide to adult ADHD: Assessment and intervention.* Boston: Academic Press.

Gomez, R. L., Janowsky, D., Zetin, M., Huey, L., & Clopton, P. L. (1981). Adult psychiatric diagnosis and symptoms compatible with the hyperactive syndrome: A retrospective study. *Journal of Clinical Psychiatry, 42*, 389–394.

Gordon, M., & Keiser, S. (Eds.). (1998). *Accommodations in higher education under the Americans with Disabilities Act (ADA): A no-nonsense guide for clinicians, educators, administrators, and lawyers.* New York: Guilford Press.

Gordon, M., & McClure, D. (1996). *The down and dirty guide to adult ADD.* DeWitt, NY: GSI.

Gordon, M., Antshel, K., Faraone, S., Barkley, R., Lewandowski, L., Hudziak, J., et al. (2006). Symptoms versus impairment: The case for respecting DSM-IV's Criterion D. *Journal of Attention Disorders, 9*, 465–475.

Gordon, M., Barkley, R. A., & Lovett, B. J. (2006). Tests and observational measures. In R. A. Barkley (Ed.), *Attention-deficit/hyperactivity disorder: A handbook for diagnosis and treatment* (3rd ed., pp. 369–389). New York: Guilford Press.

Goyette, C. H., Conners, C. K., & Ulrich, R. F. (1978). Normative data for Revised Conners Parent and Teacher Rating Scales. *Journal of Abnormal Child Psychology, 6*, 221–236.

Greene, R. W., Biederman, J., Faraone, S. V., Sienna, M., & Garcia-Jetton, J. (1997). Adolescent outcome of boys with attention-deficit/hyperactivity disorder and social disability: Results from a 4-year longitudinal follow-up study. *Journal of Consulting and Clinical Psychology*, *65*, 758–767.

Grodzinsky, G. M., & Diamond, R. (1992). Frontal lobe functioning in boys with attention-deficit hyperactivity disorder. *Developmental Neuropsychology*, *8*, 427–445.

Gunstad, J., Paul, R. H., Cohen, R. A., Tate, D. F., Spitznagel, M. B., & Gordon, E. (2007). Elevated body mass index is associated with executive dysfunction in otherwise healthy adults. *Comprehensive Psychiatry*, *48*, 57–61.

Hallowell, E. M., & Ratey, J. J. (1994). *Driven to distraction*. New York: Pantheon.

Hallowell, E. M., & Ratey, J. J. (2005). *Delivered from distraction*. New York: Ballantine.

Harrison, A. G., Edwards, M. J., & Parker, K. C. H. (2007). Identifying students faking ADHD: Preliminary findings and strategies for detection. *Archives of Clinical Neuropsychology*, *22*, 577–588.

Hart, E. L., Lahey, B. B., Loeber, R., Applegate, B., & Frick, P. J. (1995). Developmental changes in attention-deficit hyperactivity disorder in boys: A four-year longitudinal study. *Journal of Abnormal Child Psychology*, *23*, 729–750.

Harticollis, P. (1968). The syndrome of minimal brain dysfunction in young adult patients. *Bulletin of the Menninger Clinic*, *32*, 102–114.

Hartmann, T. (1993). *Attention deficit disorder: A different perception*. Lancaster, PA: Underwood-Miller.

Hartsough, C. S., & Lambert, N. M. (1985). Medical factors in hyperactive and normal children: Prenatal, developmental, and health history findings. *American Journal of Orthopsychiatry*, *55*, 190–210.

Harvey, E. (1998). Parental employment and conduct problems among children with attention-deficit/hyperactivity disorder: An examination of child care workload and parenting well-being as mediating variables. *Journal of Social and Clinical Psychology*, *17*, 476–490.

Heaton, R. K. (1981). *A manual for the Wisconsin Card Sorting Test*. Odessa, TX: Psychological Assessment Resources.

Heilengenstein, E., Conyers, L. M., Berns, A. R., Miller, M. A., & Smith, M. A. (1998). Preliminary normative data on DSM-IV attention deficit hyperactivity disorder in college students. *Journal of American College Health*, *46*, 185–188.

Henry, B., Moffitt, T. E., Caspi A., Langley, J., & Silva, P. A. (1994). On the "remembrance of things past": A longitudinal evaluation of the retrospective method. *Psychological Assessment*, *6*, 92–101.

Hermans, D. F., Williams, L. M., Lazzaro, I., Whitmont, S., Melkonian, D., & Gordon, E. (2004). Sex differences in adult ADHD: A double dissociation in brain activity and autonomic arousal. *Biological Psychology*, *66*, 221–233.

Hervey, A. S., Epstein, J. N., & Curry, J. F. (2004). Neuropsychology of adults with attention-deficit/hyperactivity disorder: A meta-analytic review. *Neuropsychology*, *18*, 495–503.

Hill, J. C., & Schoener, E. P. (1996). Age-dependent decline of attention deficit hyperactivity disorder. *American Journal of Psychiatry*, *153*, 1143–1146.

Himmelstein, J., & Halperin, J. M. (2000). Neurocognitive functioning in adults with attention-deficit/hyperactivity disorder. *CNS Spectrums*, *5*, 58–64.

Hinshaw, S. P. (1987). On the distinction between attentional deficits/hyperactivity and conduct problems/aggression in child psychopathology. *Psychological Bulletin*, *101*, 443–447.

Holdnack, J. A., Moberg, P. J., Arnold, S. E., Gur, R. C., & Gur, R. E. (1995). Speed of processing and verbal learning deficits in adults diagnosed with attention deficit disorder. *Neuropsychiatry, Neuropsychology, and Behavioral Neurology, 8*, 282–292.

Hollingshead, J. (1975). *A four-factor index of social position.* New Haven, CT: Author.

Hudziak, J., Heath, A., Madden, P., Reich, W., Bucholz, K., Slutske, W., et al. (1998). Latent class and factor analysis of DSM-IV ADHD: A twin study of female adolescents. *Journal of the American Academy of Child and Adolescent Psychiatry, 37*, 848–850.

Huessy, H. J. (1974). The adult hyperkinetic. *American Journal of Psychiatry, 131*, 724–725.

Jastak, J. F. & Jastak, S. (1993). *The Wide Range Achievement Test 3.* Wilmington, DE: Jastak Associates.

Jenkins, M., Cohen, R., Malloy, P., Salloway, S., Johnson, E. G., Penn, J., et al.(1998). Neuropsychological measures which discriminate among adults with residual symptoms of attention deficit disorder and other attentional complaints. *Clinical Neuropsychologist, 12*, 74–83.

Johnston, C., & Mash, E. J. (2001). Families of children with attention-deficit/hyperactivity disorder: Review and recommendations for future research. *Clinical Child and Family Psychology Review, 4*, 183–207.

Johnson, D. E., Epstein, J. N., Waid, L. R., Latham, P. K., Voronin, K. E., & Anton, R. F. (2001). Neuropsychological performance deficits in adults with attention-deficit/hyperactivity disorder. *Archives of Clinical Neuropsychology, 16*, 587–604.

Kalbag, A. S., & Levin, F. R. (2005). Adult ADHD and substance abuse: Diagnostic and treatment issues. *Substance Use & Misuse, 40*, 1955–1981.

Kannel, W. B., & Larson, M. (1993). Long-term epidemiologic prediction of coronary disease: The Framingham experience. *Cardiology, 82*, 137–152.

Kaufman, A. S., & Kaufman, N. L. (1993). *Kaufman Assessment Battery for Children.* Circle Pines, MN: American Guidance Services.

Kelly, K., & Ramundo, P. (1992). *You mean I'm not lazy, stupid, or crazy?* Cincinnati: Tyrell & Jerem.

Kessler, R. C., Adler, L., Barkley, R. A., Biederman, J., Conners, C. K., Demler, O., et al. (2006). The prevalence and correlates of adult ADHD in the United States: Results from the National Comorbidity Survey replication. *American Journal of Psychiatry, 163*, 716–723.

Kessler, R. C., Berglund, P., Demler, O., Jin, R., & Walters, E. E. (2005). Lifetime prevalence and age-of-onset distribution of DSM-IV disorders in the National Comorbidity Survey replication. *Archives of General Psychiatry, 62*, 593–602.

Klein, R. G., & Mannuzza, S. (1991). Long-term outcome of hyperactive children: A review. *Journal of the American Academy of Child and Adolescent Psychiatry, 30*, 383–387.

Knouse, L. E., Bagwell, C. L., Barkley, R. A., & Murphy, K. R. (2005). Accuracy of self-evaluation in adults with attention-deficit hyperactivity disorder. *Journal of Attention Disorders, 8*, 221–234.

Kollins, S. H., McClerman, J., & Fuemmeler, B. F. (2005). Association between smoking and attention-deficit/hyperactivity disorder symptoms in a population-based sample of young adults. *Archives of General Psychiatry, 62*, 1142–1147.

Kooij, J. J. S., Buitellar, J. K., van den Oord, E. J., Furer, J. W., Rijnders, C. A. T., & Hodiamont, P. P. G. (2004). Internal and external validity of attention-deficit hyperactivity disorder in a population-based sample of adults. *Psychological Medicine, 35*, 817–827.

Kovner, R., Budman, C., Frank, Y., Sison, C., Lesser, M., & Halperin, J. M. (1997). *Neuro-*

psychological testing in adult attention deficit hyperactivity disorder: A pilot study. Unpublished Manuscript.

Krause, K. H., Dresel, S. H., Krause, J., Kung, H. F., Tatsch, K., & Ackenheil, M. (2002). Stimulant-like action of nicotine on striatatl dopamine transporter in the brain of adults with attention deficit hyperactivity disorder. *International Journal of Neuropsychopharmacology, 5,* 111–113.

Kuntsi, J., Oosterlaan, J., & Stevenson, J. (2001). Psychological mechanisms in hyperactivity: I. response inhibition deficit, working memory impairment, delay aversion, or something else? *Journal of Child Psychology and Psychiatry, 42,* 199–210.

Kuperman, S., Schlosser, S. S., Kramer, J. R., Bucholz, K., Hesselbrock, V., Reich, T., et al. (2001). Developmental sequence from disruptive behavior diagnosis to adolescent alcohol dependence. *American Journal of Psychiatry, 158,* 2022–2026.

Lahey, B. B., Applegate, B., McBurnett, K., Biederman, J., Greenhill, L., Hynd, G. W., et al. (1994). DSM-IV field trials for attention deficit/hyperactivity disorder in children and adolescents. *Journal of the American Academy of Child and Adolescent Psychiatry, 151,* 1673–1685.

Lambert, N. M. (2002). Stimulant treatment as a risk factor for nicotine use and substance abuse. In P. S. Jensen, J. R. Cooper, (Eds.), *Diagnosis and treatment of attention deficit hyperactivity disorder: An evidence-based approach.* New York: American Medical Association Press.

Lambert, N. M., & Hartsough, C. S. (1998). Prospective study of tobacco smoking and substance dependencies among samples of ADHD and non-ADHD participants. *Journal of Learning Disabilities, 31,* 533–544.

Lambert, N. M., & Sandoval, J. (1980). The prevalence of learning disabilities in a sample of children considered hyperactive. *Journal of Abnormal Child Psychology, 8,* 33–50.

Lee, G. P., Strauss, E., Loring, D. W., McCloskey, L., Haworth, J. M., & Lehman, R. A. W. (1997). Sensitivity of figural fluency on the Five-Points Test to focal neurological dysfunction. *Clinical Neuropsychologist, 11,* 59–68.

Levy, F., Hay, D. A., McStephen, M., Wood, C., & Waldman, I. (1997). Attention-deficit hyperactivity disorder: A category or a continuum? Genetic analysis of a large-scale twin study. *Journal of the American Academy of Child and Adolescent Psychiatry, 36,* 737–744.

Lezak, M. D. (1995). *Neuropsychological assessment* (3rd Ed.). New York: Oxford University Press.

Locke, H. J., & Wallace, K. M. (1959). Short marital adjustment and prediction tests: Their reliability and validity. *Journal of Marriage and Family Living, 21,* 251–255.

Loeber, R., Burke, J. D., Lahey, B. B., Winters, A., & Zera, M. (2000). Oppositional defiant and conduct disorder: A review of the past 10 years, Part I. *Journal of the American Academy of Child and Adolescent Psychiatry, 39,* 1468–1484.

Loeber, R., Green, S. M., Lahey, B. B., Christ, M. A. G., & Frick, P. J. (1992). Developmental sequences in the age of onset of disruptive child behaviors. *Journal of Child and Family Studies, 1,* 21–41.

Lorch, E. P., Milich, R., Sanchcez, R. P., van den Broek, P., Baer, S., Hooks, K., et al.(2000). Comprehension of televised stories in boys with attention deficit/hyperactivity disorder and nonreferred boys. *Journal of Abnormal Psychology, 109,* 321–330.

Lorch, E. P., O'Neill, K., Berthiaume, K. S., Milich, R., Eastham, D., Brooks, T. (2004). Story comprehension and the impact of studying on recall in children with attention deficit hyperactivity disorder. *Journal of Clinical Child and Adolescent Psychology, 33,* 506–515.

Lorch, E. P., Sanchez, R. P., van den Broek, P., Milich, R., Murphy, E. L., Lorch, R. F. Jr., et al. (1999). The relation of story structure properties to recall of television stories in young children with attention-deficit/hyperactivity disorder and nonreferred peers. *Journal of Abnormal Child Psychology, 27,* 293–309.

Lovejoy, D. W., Ball, J. D., Keats, M., Stutts, M. L., Spain, E. H., Janda, L., et al. (1999). Neuropsychological performance of adults with attention deficit hyperactivity disorder (ADHD): Diagnostic classification estimates for measures of frontal lobe/executive functioning. *Journal of the International Neuropsychological Society, 5,* 222–233.

Luman, M., Oosterlaan, J., & Sergeant, J. A. (2005). The impact of reinforcement contingencies on AD/HD: A review and theoretical appraisal. *Clinical Psychology Review, 25,* 183–213.

Lynskey, M. T., & Fergusson, D. M. (1995). Childhood conduct problems, attention deficit behaviors, and adolescent alcohol, tobacco, and illicit drug use. *Journal of Abnormal Child Psychology, 23,* 281–302.

Mann, H. B., & Greenspan, S. I. (1976). The identification and treatment of adult brain dysfunction. *American Journal of Psychiatry, 133,* 1013–1017.

Mannuzza, S., & Gittelman, R. (1986). Informant variance in the diagnostic assessment of hyperactive children as young adults. In J. E. Barrett & R. M. Rose (Eds.), *Mental disorders in the community* (pp. 243–254). New York: Guilford Press.

Mannuzza, S., Gittelman-Klein, R., Bessler, A., Malloy, P., & LaPadula, M. (1993). Adult outcome of hyperactive boys: Educational achievement, occupational rank, and psychiatric status. *Archives of General Psychiatry, 50,* 565–576.

Mannuzza, S., Klein, R. G., Bonagura, N., Malloy, P., Giampino, H., & Addalli, K. A. (1991). Hyperactive boys almost grown up: Replication of psychiatric status. *Archives of General Psychiatry, 48,* 77–83.

Mannuzza, S., Klein, R., Bessler, A., Malloy, P., & LaPadula, M. (1998). Adult psychiatric status of hyperactive boys grown up. *American Journal of Psychiatry, 155,* 493–498.

Mannuzza, S., Klein, R. G., Klein, D. F., Bessler, A., & Shrout, P. (2002). Accuracy of adult recall of childhood attention deficit hyperactivity disorder. *American Journal of Psychiatry, 159,* 1882–1888.

Manshadi, M., Lippman, S., O'Daniel, R. G., & Blackman, A. (1992). Alcohol abuse and attention deficit disorder. *Journal of Clinical Psychiatry, 44,* 379–380.

Mariani, M., & Barkley, R. A. (1997). Neuropsychological and academic functioning in preschool children with attention deficit hyperactivity disorder. *Developmental Neuropsychology, 13,* 111–129.

Marks, D. J., Newcorn, J. H., & Halperin, J. M. (2001). Comorbidity in adults with attention-deficit/hyperactivity disorder. In J. Wasserstein, L. E. Wolf., & F. F. Lefever (Eds.) Adult attention deficit disorder: Brain mechanisms and life outcomes. *Annals of the New York Academy of Sciences, 931,* 216–238.

Matochik, J. A., Rumsey, J. M., Zametkin, A. J., Hamburger, S. D., & Cohen, R. M. (1996). Neuropsychological correlates of familial attention-deficit/hyperactivity disorder in adults. *Neuropsychiatry, Neuropsychology, and Behavioral Neurology, 9,* 186–191.

McClean, A., Dowson, J., Toone, B., Young, S., Bazanis, E., Robbins, T. W., et al. (2004). Characteristic neurocognitive profile associated with adult attention-deficit/hyperactivity disorder. *Psychological Medicine, 34,* 681–692.

McGinnis, J. M., & Foege, W. H. (1993). Actual causes of death in the United States. *Journal of the American Medical Association, 270,* 2207–2212.

McGough, J. J., & Barkley, R. A. (2004). Diagnostic controversies in adult ADHD. *American Journal of Psychiatry, 161,* 1948–1956.

McGough, J. J., Smalley, S. L., McCracken, J. T., Yang, M., Del'Homme, M., Lynn, D. E., et al. (2005). Psychiatric comorbidity in adult attention deficit hyperactivity disorder: Findings from multiplex families. *American Journal of Psychiatry, 162,* 1621–1627.

McInnes, A., Humphries, T., Hogg-Jonson, S., & Tannock, R. (2003). Listening comprehension and working memory are impaired in attention-deficit hyperactivity disorder irrespective of language impairment. *Journal of Abnormal Child Psychology, 31,* 427–443.

Mendelson, W., Johnson, N., & Stewart, M. A. (1971). Hyperactive children as teenagers: A follow-up study. *Journal of Nervous and Mental Disease, 153,* 273–279.

Menkes, M., Rowe, J., & Menkes, J. (1967). A five-year follow-up study on the hyperactive child with minimal brain dysfunction. *Pediatrics, 39,* 393–399.

Michelson, D., Adler, L., Spencer, T., Reimherr, F., West, S., Allen, A., et al. (2003). Atomoxetine in adults with ADHD: Two randomized, placebo-controlled studies. *Biological Psychiatry, 53,* 112–120.

Mick, E., Faraone, S. V., & Biederman, J. (2004). Age-dependent expression of attention-deficit/hyperactivity disorder symptoms. In T. J. Spencer (Ed.), *Psychiatric Clinics of North America, 27,* 215–224.

Milberger, S., Biederman, J., Faraone, S. V., Chen, L., & Jones, J. (1997). ADHD is associated with early initiation of cigarette smoking in children and adolescents. *Journal of the American Academy of Child and Adolescent Psychiatry, 36,* 37–44.

Milich, R., Widiger, T. A., & Landau, S. (1987). Differential diagnosis of attention deficit and conduct disorders using conditional probabilities. *Journal of Consulting & Clinical Psychology, 55,* 762-767.

Miller, G. A., & Chapman, J. P. (2001). Misunderstanding analysis of covariance. *Journal of Abnormal Psychology, 110,* 40–48.

Milstein, R. B., Wilens, T. W., Biederman, J., & Spencer, T. J. (1997). Presenting ADHD symptoms and subtypes in clinically referred adults with ADHD. *Journal of Attention Disorders, 2,* 159–166.

Minde, K., Eakin, L., Hechtman, L., Ochs, E., Bouffard, R., Greenfield, B., et al. (2003). The psychosocial functioning of children and spouses of adults with ADHD. *Journal of Child Psychology and Psychiatry, 44,* 637–646.

Mirsky, A. F. (1996). Disorders of attention. In R. G. Lyon & N. A. Krasnegor (Eds.), *Attention, memory, and executive function* (pp. 71–96). Baltimore: Brookes.

Molina, B. S. G., Smith, B. H., & Pelham, W. E. (1999). Interactive effects of attention deficit hyperactivity disorder and conduct disorder on early adolescent substance use. *Psychology of Addictive Behaviors, 13,* 348–358.

Morris, R. D. (1996). Relationships and distinctions among the concepts of attention, memory, and executive function: A developmental perspective. In G. R. Lyon & N. A. Krasnegor (Eds.), *Attention, memory, and executive function* (pp. 11–16). Baltimore: Brookes.

Morrison, J. R. (1980). Adult psychiatric disorders in parents of hyperactive children. *American Journal of Psychiatry, 137,* 825–827.

Morrison, J. R., & Minkoff, K. (1975). Explosive personality as a sequel to the hyperactive child syndrome. *Comprehensive Psychiatry, 16,* 343–348.

Morrison, J. R., & Stewart, M. (1973). The psychiatric status of the legal families of adopted hyperactive children. *Archives of General Psychiatry, 28,* 888–891.

Mota, V. L., & Schachar, R. J. (2000). Reformulating attention-deficit/hyperactivity disorder according to signal detection theory. *Journal of the American Academy of Child and Adolescent Psychiatry, 39,* 1144–1151.

Murphy, K. R., & Barkley, R. A. (1996a). Attention deficit hyperactivity disorder adults: Comorbidities and adaptive impairments. *Comprehensive Psychiatry, 37*, 393–401.

Murphy, K. R., & Barkley, R. A. (1996b). Prevalence of DSM-IV ADHD symptoms in adult licensed drivers. *Journal of Attention Disorders, 1*, 147–161.

Murphy, K. R., Barkley, R. A., & Bush, T. (2001). Executive functioning and olfactory identification in young adults with attention deficit hyperactivity disorder, *Neuropsychology, 15*, 211–220.

Murphy, K. R., Barkley, R. A., & Bush, T. (2002). Young adults with ADHD: Subtype differences in comorbidity, educational, and clinical history. *Journal of Nervous and Mental Disease, 190*, 147–157.

Murphy, K. R., & Gordon, M. (2006). Assessment of adults with ADHD. In R. A. Barkley (Ed.), *Attention deficit hyperactivity disorder: A handbook for diagnosis and treatment* (3rd ed., pp. 425–452). New York: Guilford Press.

Murphy, K. R., & LeVert, S. (1995). *Out of the fog.* New York: Hyperion.

Murphy, P., & Schachar, R. (2000). Use of self-ratings in the assessment of symptoms of attention deficit hyperactivity disorder in adults. *American Journal of Psychiatry, 157*, 1156–1159.

Murray, C., & Johnston, C. (2006). Parenting in mothers with and without attention-deficit/hyperactivity disorder. *Journal of Abnormal Psychology, 115*, 51–61.

Nadeau, K. (1995). *A comprehensive guide to adults with attention deficit hyperactivity disorder.* New York: Brunner/Mazel.

Nadeau, K. G., & Quinn, P. (2002). *Understanding women with AD/HD.* Silver Spring, MD: Advantage.

Nigg, J. T. (2001). Is ADHD an inhibitory disorder? *Psychological Bulletin, 125*, 571–596.

Nigg, J. T. (2006). *What causes ADHD?* New York: Guilford Press.

Nigg, J. T., Butler, K., Huang-Pollack, C., & Henderson, J. M. (2002). Inhibitory processes in adults with persistent childhood-onset ADHD. *Journal of Consulting and Clinical Psychology, 70*, 153–157.

Nigg, J. T., Stavro, G., Ettenhofer, M., Hambrick, D., Miller, T., & Henderson, J. M. (in press). Executive functions and ADHD in adults: Evidence for selective effects on ADHD symptom domains. *Journal of Abnormal Psychology, 114*, 706–717.

Ninowski, J. E., Marh, E. J., & Benzies, K. M. (2007). Symptoms of attention-deficit/hyperactivity disorder in first-time expectant women: Relations with parenting cognitions and behaviors. *Infant Mental Health Journal, 28*, 54–75.

O'Donnell, J. P., McCann, K. K., & Pluth, S. (2001). Assessing adult ADHD using a self-report symptom checklist. *Psychological Reports, 88*, 871–881.

O'Leary, K. D., & Arias, I. (1988). Assessing agreement of reports of spouse abuse. In G. T. Hotaling, D. Finkelhor, J. T. Kilpatrick, & M. A. Straus (Eds.), *New directions in family violence research* (pp. 218–227). Newbury Park, CA: Sage.

Ossman, J. M., & Mulligan, N. W. (2003). Inhibition and attention-deficit/hyperactivity disorder in adults. *American Journal of Psychology, 116*, 35–50.

Packer, S. (1978). Treatment of minimal brain dysfunction in a young adult. *Canadian Psychiatric Association Journal, 23*, 501–502.

Patterson, D. A., & Lee, M.-S. (1995). Field trial of the Global Assessment of Functioning Scale–Modified. *American Journal of Psychiatry, 152*, 1386–1388.

Pontius, A. A. (1973). Dysfunction patterns analogous to frontal lobe system and caudate nucleus syndromes in some groups of minimal brain dysfunction. *Journal of the American Medical Women's Association, 26*, 285–292.

Quay, H. C. (1988). Attention deficit disorder and the behavioral inhibition system: The relevance of the neuropsychological theory of Jeffrey A. Gray. In L. M. Bloomingdale & J. Sergeant (Eds.), *Attention deficit disorder: Criteria, cognition, intervention* (pp. 117–126). New York: Pergamon Press.

Quinlan, D. M. (2000). Assessment of attention-deficit/hyperactivity disorder and comorbidities. In T. E. Brown (Ed.), *Attention-deficit disorders and comorbidities in children, adolescents, and adults.* (pp. 455–508). Washington, DC: American Psychiatric Press.

Quitkin, F., & Klein, D. F. (1969). Two behavioral syndromes in young adults related to possible minimal brain dysfunction. *Journal of Psychiatric Research, 7*, 131–142.

Ramirez, C. A., Rosen, L. A., Deffenbacher, J. L., Hurst, H., Nicolette, C., Rosencranz, T., et al. (1997). Anger and anger expression in adults with high ADHD symptoms. *Journal of Attention Disorders, 2*, 115–128.

Ramsay, J. R., & Rothstein, A. L. (2007). *Cognitive-behavioral therapy for adult ADHD: An integrative psychosocial and medical approach.* New York: Routledge.

Rapport, L. J., Friedman, S. L., Tzelepis, A., & Van Voorhis, A. (2002). Experienced emotion and affect recognition in adult attention-deficit/hyperactivity disorder. *Neuropsychology, 16*, 102–110.

Rapport, L. J., Van Voorhis, A., Tzelepis, A., & Friedman, S. R. (2001). Executive functioning in adult attention-deficit/hyperactivity disorder. *Clinical Neuropsychologist, 15*, 479–491.

Rapport, M. D., Scanlan, S. W., & Denney, C. B. (1999). Attention-deficit/hyperactivity disorder and scholastic achievement: A model of dual developmental pathways. *Journal of Child Psychology and Psychiatry, 40*, 1169–1183.

Rasmussen, K., Almvik, R., & Levander, S. (2001). Attention-deficit/hyperactivity disorder, reading disability, and personality disorders in a prison population. *Journal of the American Academy of Psychiatry and the Law, 29*, 186–193.

Rasmussen, P., & Gillberg, C. (2001). Natural outcome of ADHD with developmental coordination disorder at age 22 years: A controlled, longitudinal, community-based study. *Journal of the American Academy of Child and Adolescent Psychiatry, 39*, 1424–1431.

Ratey, J., Miller, A. C., & Nadeau, K. G. (1995). Special diagnostic and treatment considerations in women with attention deficit disorder. In. K. G. Nadeau (Ed.), *A comprehensive guide to attention deficit disorder in adults: Research, diagnosis, treatment* (pp. 260–283). New York: Brunner/Mazel.

Raylu, N., & Oei, T. P. S. (2002). Pathological gambling: A comprehensive review. *Clinical Psychology Review, 22*, 1009–1061.

Regard, M., Strauss, E., & Knapp, P. (1982). Children's production on verbal and non-verbal fluency tasks. *Perceptual and Motor Skills, 123*, 17–22.

Reitman, D., Currier, R. O., & Stickle, T. R. (2002). A critical evaluation of the Parenting Stress Index-Short Form (PSI-SF) in a Head Start population. *Journal of Clinical Child and Adolescent Psychology, 31*, 384–392.

Reynolds, C., & Kamphaus, R. (1994). *Behavioral Assessment System for Children.* Circle Pines, MN: American Guidance Service.

Riccio, C. A., Wolfe, M., Davis, B., Romine, C. R., George, C., & Lee, D. (2005). Attention deficit hyperactivity disorder: manifestation in adulthood. *Archives of Clinical Neuropsychology, 20*, 249–269.

Richards, T. L., Deffenbacher, J. L., Rosen, L. A., Barkley, R. A., & Rodricks, T. (2006). Driving anger and driving behavior in adults with ADHD. *Journal of Attention Disorders, 10*, 54–64.

Ridenour, T. A., Cottler, L. B., Robins, L. N., Compton, W. M., Spitznagel, E. L., & Cunningham-Williams, R. M. (2002). Test of the plausibility of adolescent substance use playing a causal role in developing adulthood antisocial behavior. *Journal of Abnormal Psychology, 111,* 144–155.

Riverside Publishing Company (1993). *The Nelson–Denny Reading Test.* Itasca, IL: Author.

Rosolova, H., Simon, J., & Sefrna, F. (1993). Impact of cardiovascular risk factors on morbidity and mortality in Czech middle-aged men: Pilsen longitudinal study. *Cardiology, 82,* 61–68.

Routh, D. K., Schroeder, C. S., & O'Tuama, L. (1974). The development of activity level in children. *Developmental Psychology, 10,* 163–168.

Roy-Byrne, P., Scheele, L., Brinkley, J., Ward, N., Wiatrak, C., Russo, J., et al. (1997). Adult attention-deficit hyperactivity disorder: Assessment guidelines based on clinical presentation to a specialty clinic. *Comprehensive Psychiatry, 38,* 133–140.

Rucklidge, J. J. (2006). Gender differences in neuropsychological functioning of New Zealand adolescents with and without attention-deficit/hyperactivity disorder. *International Journal of Disability, Development, and Education, 53,* 47–66.

Rucklidge, J. J., & Kaplan, B. J. (1997). Psychological functioning of women identified in adulthood with attention-deficit/hyperactivity disorder. *Journal of Attention Disorders, 2,* 167–176.

Rucklidge, J. J., & Tannock, R. (2002). Neuropsychological profiles of adolescents with ADHD: Effects of reading difficulties and gender. *Journal of Child Psychology and Psychiatry, 43,* 988–1003.

Rucklidge, K., Brown, D., Crawford, S., & Kaplan, B. (2007). Attributional styles and psychosocial functioning of adults with ADHD: Practice issues and gender differences. *Journal of Attention Disorders, 10,* 288–298.

Ruff, R. M., Allen, C. C., Farrow, C. E., Nieman, H., & Wylie, T. (1994). Figural fluency: Differential impairment in patients with left versus right frontal lesions. *Archives of Clinical Neuropsychology, 9,* 41–55.

Rybak, W. S. (1977). More adult minimal brain dysfunction. *American Journal of Psychiatry, 134,* 96–97.

Safren, S. A., Otto, M., Sprich, S., Winett, C., Wilens, T., & Biederman, J. (2005). Cognitive-behavioral therapy for ADHD in medication-treated adults with continued symptoms. *Behaviour Research and Therapy, 43,* 831–842.

Safren, S., Perlman, C., Sprich, S., & Otto, M. W. (2005). *Therapist guide to The Mastery of Your Adult ADHD: A cognitive behavioral treatment program.* New York: Oxford University Press.

Sanchez, R. P., Lorch, E. P., Milich, R., & Welsh, R. (1999). Comprehension of televised stories by preschool children with ADHD. *Journal of Clinical Child Psychology, 28,* 376–385.

Sarkis, S. M. (2005). *10 simple solutions to adult ADD.* Oakland, CA: New Harbinger.

Satterfield, J. H., Faller, K. F., Crinella, F. M., Scjell, A. M., Swanson, J. M., & Homer, L. D. (2007). A 30-year prospective follow-up study of hyperactive boys with conduct problems: Adult criminality. *Journal of the American Academy of Child and Adolescent Psychiatry, 46,* 601–610.

Satterfield, J. H., & Schell, A. (1997). A prospective study of hyperactive boys with conduct problems and normal boys: Adolescent and adult criminality. *Journal of the American Academy of Child and Adolescent Psychiatry, 36,* 1726–1735.

Schmidt, J. P., & Tombaugh, T. N. (1995). *Learning and Memory Battery.* North Tonawanda, NY: Multi-Health Systems.

Schweiger, A., Abramovitch, A., Doniger, G. M., & Simon, E. S. (2007). A clinical construct validity study of a novel computerized battery for the diagnosis of ADHD in young adults. *Journal of Clinical and Experimental Neuropsychology, 29,* 100–111.

Secnik, K., Swensen, A., & Lage, M. J. (2005). Comorbidities and costs of adult patients diagnosed with attention-deficit hyperactivity disorder. *Pharmacoeconomics, 23,* 93–102.

Seidman, L. J. (1997, October). *Neuropsychological findings in ADHD children: Findings from a sample of high-risk siblings.* Paper presented at the annual meeting of the American Academy of Child and Adolescent Psychiatry, Toronto, Canada.

Seidman, L. J., Doyle, A., Fried, R., Valera, E., Crum, K., & Matthews, L. (2004). Neuropsychological function in adults with attention-deficit/hyperactivity disorder. *Psychiatric Clinics of North America, 27,* 261–282.

Semrud-Clikeman, M., Biederman, J., Sprich-Buckminster, S., Lehman, B. K., Faraone, S. V., & Norman, D. (1992). Comorbidity between ADDH and learning disability: A review and report in a clinically referred sample. *Journal of the American Academy of Child and Adolescent Psychiatry, 31,* 439–448.

Shaffer, D. (1994). Attention deficit hyperactivity disorder in adults. *American Journal of Psychiatry, 151,* 633–638.

Shallice, T. (1982). Specific impairments of planning. *Philosophical Transactions of the Royalty Society of London, 298,* 199–209.

Shaw, G. A., & Giambra, L. (1993). Task-unrelated thoughts of college students diagnosed as hyperactive in childhood. *Developmental Neuropsychology, 9,* 17–30.

Shekim, W., Asarnow, R. F., Hess, E., Zaucha, K., & Wheeler, N. (1990). An evaluation of attention deficit disorder-residual type. *Comprehensive Psychiatry, 31*(5), 416–425.

Shelley, E. M., & Riester, A. (1972). Syndrome of minimal brain damage in young adults. *Diseases of the Nervous System, 33,* 335–339.

Shipley, W. C. (1946). *The Shipley Institute of Living Scale.* Los Angeles: Western Psychological Services, Inc.

Skinner, H. A. (1994). *Computerized Lifestyle Assessment.* North Tonawanda, NY: Multi-Health Systems.

Smalley, S. L., McGough, J. J., Del'Homme, M., Newelman, J., Gordon, E., Kim, T., et al. (2000). Familial clustering of symptoms and disruptive behaviors in multiplex families with attention-deficit/hyperactivity disorder. *Journal of the American Academy of Child and Adolescent Psychiatry, 39,* 1135–1143.

Solden, S. (1995). *Women with attention deficit disorder.* Grass Valley, CA: Underwood.

Sonuga-Barke, E. J. S., Daley, D., & Thompson, M. (2002). Does maternal ADHD reduce the effectiveness of parent training for preschool children's ADHD? *Journal of the American Academy of Child and Adolescent Psychiatry, 41,* 696–702.

Span, S. A., Earleywine, M., & Strybel, T. Z. (2002). Confirming the factor structure of attention deficit hyperactivity disorder symptoms in adult, nonclinical samples. *Journal of Psychopathology and Behavioral Assessment, 24,* 129–136.

Spencer, T. (1997, October). *Chronic tics in adults with ADHD.* Paper presented at the annual meeting of the American Academy of Child and Adolescent Psychiatry, Toronto, Canada.

Spencer, T. (2006). Antidepressant and specific norepinephrine reuptake inhibitor treatments. In R. A. Barkley, *Attention deficit hyperactivity disorder: A handbook for diagnosis and treatment* (3rd ed., pp. 648–657). New York: Guilford Press.

Spencer, T. (Ed.). (2004). Adult attention-deficit/hyperactivity disorder. *Psychiatric Clinics of North America, 27*(2), 187–390.

Spencer, T., Biederman, J., Wilens, T., Doyle, R., Surman, C., Prince, J., et al. (2005). A large double blind randomized clinical trial of methylphenidate in the treatment of adults with ADHD. *Biological Psychiatry, 57,* 456–463.

Spencer, T., Biederman, J., Wilens, T., & Faraone, S. V. (1994). Is attention-deficit hyperactivity disorder in adults a valid disorder? *Harvard Review of Psychiatry, 1,* 326–335.

Spencer, T., Biederman, J., Wilens, T., Faraone, S. V., Prince, J., Geerard, K., et al. (2001). Efficacy of a mixed amphetamine salts compound in adults with attention- deficit/hyperactivity disorder. *Archives of General Psychiatry, 58,* 775–782.

Spencer, T., Biederman, J., Wilens, T., Prince, J., Hatch, M., Jones, J., et al. (1998). Effectiveness and tolerability of tomoxetine in adults with attention deficit hyperactivity disorder. *American Journal of Psychiatry, 155,* 693–695.

Spencer, T., Wilens, T., Biederman, J., Faraone, S. V., Ablon, S., & Lapey, K. (1995). A double-blind, crossover comparison of methylphenidate and placebo in adults with childhood onset attention-deficit hyperactivity disorder. *Archives of General Psychiatry, 52,* 434–443.

Spencer, T., Wilens, T., Biederman, J., Wozniak, J., & Harding-Crawford, M. (2000). Attention-deficit/hyperactivity disorder with mood disorders. In T. E. Brown (Ed.), *Subtypes of attention deficit disorders in children, adolescents, and adults* (pp. 79–124). Washington, DC: American Psychiatric Press.

Spitzer, R. L., Davies, M., & Barkley, R. A. (1990). The DSM-III-R field trial for the disruptive behavior disorders. *Journal of the American Academy of Child and Adolescent Psychiatry, 29,* 690–697.

Spitzer, R. L., Williams, J., Gibbon, M., & First, M. B. (1995). *The Structured Clinical Interview for DSM-IV (SCID).* New York: biometric Research Department, New York State Psychiatric Institute.

Spreen, O., Risse, A. H., & Edgell, D. (1995*). Developmental neuropsychology.* New York: Oxford University Press.

Stamler, J., Dyer, A. R., Shekelle, R. B., Neaton, J., & Stamler, R. (1993). Relationship of baseline major risk factors to coronary and all-cause mortality, and to longevity: Findings from long-term follow-up of Chicago cohorts. *Cardiology, 82,* 191–222.

Stavro, G. M., Ettenhoffer, M. L., & Nigg, J. T. (2007). Executive functions and adaptive functioning in young adult attention-deficit/hyperactivity disorder. *Journal of the International Neuropsychological Society, 13,* 324–334.

Stewart, M. A., Mendelson, W. B., & Johnson, N. E. (1973). Hyperactive children as adolescents: How they describe themselves. *Child Psychiatry and Human Development, 4,* 3–11.

Still, G. F. (1902). Some abnormal psychical conditions in children. *Lancet, 1,* 1008–1012, 1077–1082, 1163–1168.

Stroop, J. P. (1935). Studies of interference in serial verbal reactions. *Journal of Experimental Psychology, 18,* 643–662.

Stuss, D. T., & Benson, D. F. (1986). *The frontal lobes.* New York: Raven.

Swensen, A. R., Allen, A. J., Kruesi, M. P., Buesching, D. P., & Goldberg, G. (2004). *Risk of premature death from misadventure in patients with attention-deficit/hyperactivity disorder.* Unpublished manuscript, Eli Lilly Co., Indianapolis, IN.

Szatmari, P., Offord, D. R., & Boyle, M. H. (1989). Correlates, associated impairments, and patterns of service utilization of children with attention deficit disorders: Findings from the Ontario Child Health Study. *Journal of Child Psychology and Psychiatry, 30,* 205–217.

Tannock, R. (2000). Attention deficit disorders with anxiety disorders. In T. E. Brown (Ed.),

Subtypes of attention deficit disorders in children, adolescents, and adults (pp. 125–170). Washington, DC: American Psychiatric Press.

Tannock, R., & Brown, T. (2000). Attention-deficit disorders with learning disorders in children and adolescents. In T. Brown (Ed.), *Attention-deficit disorders and comorbidities in children, adolescents, and adults* (pp. 231–296). Washington, DC: American Psychiatric Press.

Tapert, S. F., Baratta, M. V., Abrantes, A. M., & Brown, S. A. (2002). Attention dysfunction predicts substance involvement in community youths. *Journal of the American Academy of Child and Adolescent Psychiatry, 41,* 680–686.

Tapert, S. F., Granholm, E., Leedy, N. G., & Brown, S. A. (2002). Substance use and withdrawal: Neuropsychological functioning over 8 years in youth. *Journal of the International Neuropyschological Society, 8,* 873–883.

Tercyak, K. P., Lerman, C., & Audrain, J. (2002). Association of attention-deficit/hyperactivity disorder symptoms with levels of cigarette smoking in a community sample of adolescents. *Journal of the American Academy of Child and Adolescent Psychiatry, 41,* 799–805.

Tercyak, K. P., Peshkin, B. N., Walker, L. R., & Stein, M. A. (2002). Cigarette smoking among youth with attention-deficit/hyperactivity disorder: Clinical phenomenology, comorbidity, and genetics. *Journal of Clinical Psychology in Medical Settings, 9,* 35–50.

Torgersen, T., Gjervan, B., & Rasmussen, K. (2006). ADHD in adults: a study of clinical characteristics, impairment, and comorbidity. *Nordic Journal of Psychiatry, 60,* 38–43.

Trenerry, M., Crosson, B., Deboe, J., & Leber, W. (1989). *Stroop Neuropsychological Screening Test.* Odessa, FL: Psychological Assessment Resources.

Triolo, S. J. (1999). *Attention deficit hyperactivity disorder in adulthood: A practitioner's handbook.* New York: Brunner/Mazel.

Tzelepis, A., Schubiner, H., & Warbasse, L. H. III. (1995). Differential diagnosis and psychiatric comorbidity patterns in adult attention deficit disorder. In K. Nadeau (Ed.), *A comprehensive guide to attention deficit disorder in adults: Research, diagnosis, treatment* (pp. 35–57). New York: Brunner/Mazel.

Volk, H. E., Henderson, C., Neuman, R. J., & Todd, R. D. (2006). Validation of population-based ADHD subtypes and identification of three clinically impaired subtypes. *American Journal of Medical Genetics Part B (Neuropsychiatric Genetics), 141B,* 312–318.

Wakefield, J. C. (1992). Disorder as harmful dysfunction: A conceptual critique of DSM-III-R's definition of mental disorder. *Psychological Review, 99,* 232–247.

Wakefield, J. C. (1999). Evolutionary versus prototype analyses of the concept of disorder. *Journal of Abnormal Psychology, 108,* 374–399.

Ward, M. F., Wender, P. H., & Reimherr, F. W. (1993). The Wender Utah Rating Scale: An aid in the retrospective diagnosis of childhood attention deficit hyperactivity disorder. *American Journal of Psychiatry, 150,* 885–890; see correction, *150,* 1280.

Watson, S. J., & Mash, E. J. (in press). The relationship between subclinical levels of symptoms of attention-deficit/hyperactivity disorder and self-reported parental cognitions and behaviors in mothers of young infants. *Journal of Reproductive and Infant Psychology.*

Wechsler, D. (1994). *Wechsler Adult Intelligence Scale—III* (3rd ed.). San Antonio, TX: The Psychological Corporation.

Wechsler, D. (1997). *Manual for the Wechsler Adult Intelligence Test 3rd Ed. (WAIS-III).* San Antonio, TX: Psychological Corp.

Weiss, G., & Hechtman, L. (1993). *Hyperactive children grown up* (2nd ed.). New York: Guilford Press.

Weiss, G., Hechtman, L., Milroy, T., Perlman, T. (1985). Psychiatric status of hyperactives as adults: A controlled prospective 15-year follow-up of 63 hyperactive children. *Journal of the American Academy of Child Psychiatry, 23*, 211–220.

Weiss, G., Minde, K., Werry, J., Douglas, V., & Nemeth, E. (1971). Studies on the hyperactive child: VIII. Five year follow-up. *Archives of General Psychiatry, 24*, 409–414.

Weiss, L. (1992). *ADD in adults.* Dallas: Taylor.

Weiss, M., Hechtman, L. T., & Weiss, G. (1999). *ADHD in adulthood: A guide to current theory, diagnosis, and treatment.* Baltimore: Johns Hopkins University Press.

Wender, P. (1995). *Attention-deficit hyperactivity disorder in adults.* New York: Oxford University Press.

Wenwei, Y. (1996). An investigation of adult outcome of hyperactive children in Shanghai. *Chinese Medical Journal, 109*, 877–880.

Werry, J., & Sprague, R. (1970). Hyperactivity. In C. G. Costello (Ed.), *Symptoms of psychopathology* (pp. 397–417). New York: Wiley.

Weyandt, L. L., Linterman, I., & Rice, J. A. (1995). Reported prevalence of attentional difficulties in a general sample of college students. *Journal of Psychopathology and Behavioral Assessment, 17*, 293–304.

Weyandt, L. L., Mitzlaff, L., & Thomas, L. (2002). The relationship between intelligence and performance on the Test of Variables of Attention (TOVA). *Journal of Learning Disabilities, 35*, 114–120.

Weyandt, L. L., Rice, J. A., Linterman, I., Mitzlaff, L., & Emert, E. (1998). Neuropsychological performance of a sample of adults with ADHD, developmental reading disorder, and controls. *Developmental Neuropsychology, 14*, 643–656.

Whalen, C. K., Jamner, L. D., Henker, B., Delfino, R. J., & Lozano, J. M. (2002). The ADHD spectrum and everyday life: Experience sampling of adolescent moods, activities, smoking, and drinking. *Child Development, 73*, 209–227.

Wigle, D. T., Semenciw, M. R., McCann, C., & Davies, J. W. (1990). Premature deaths in Canada: Impact, trends, and opportunities for prevention. *Canadian Journal of Public Health, 81*, 376–381.

Wilens, T. (2004). Attention-deficit/hyperactivity disorder and the substance use disorders: The nature of the relationship, subtypes at risk, and treatment issues. In T. Spencer (Ed.), Adult attention-deficit/hyperactivity disorder. *Psychiatric Clinics of North America, 27*(2), 283–302.

Wilens, T. E., Faraone, S. V., & Biederman, J. (2004). Attention-deficit/hyperactivity disorder in adults. *Journal of the American Medical Association, 292*, 619–623.

Wilens, T. E., Faraone, S. V., Biederman, J., & Gunawardene, S. (2003). Does stimulant therapy of attention deficit/hyperactivity disorder beget later substance abuse? A meta-analytic review of the literature. *Pediatrics, 11*(1), 179–185.

Willcutt, E. G., Pennington, B. F., & DeFries, J. C. (2000). Etiology of inattention and hyperactivity/impulsivity in a community sample of twins with learning difficulties. *Journal of Abnormal Child Psychology, 28*, 149–159.

Wilson, J. M., & Marcotte, A. C. (1996). Psychosocial adjustment and educational outcome in adolescents with a childhood diagnosis of attention deficit disorder. *Journal of the American Academy of Child and Adolescent Psychiatry, 35*, 579–587.

Wood, D. R., Reimherr, F. W., Wender, P. W., & Johnson, G. E. (1976). Diagnosis and treatment of minimal brain dysfunction in adults: A preliminary report. *Archives of General Psychiatry, 33*, 1453–1460.

Zachary, R. A. (1988). *Institute of Living Scale—Revised Manual*. Los Angeles: Western Psychological Services.

Zakay, D. (1990). The evasive art of subjective time measurement: Some methodological dilemmas. In R. A. Block (Ed.), *Cognitive models of psychological time* (pp. 59–84). Hillsdale, NJ: Lawrence Erlbaum Associates.

Zametkin, A. J., Nordahl, T. E., Gross, M., King, A. C., Semple, W. E., Rumsey, J., et al., (1990). Cerebral glucose metabolism in adults with hyperactivity of childhood onset. *New England Journal of Medicine, 323*, 1361–1366.

Index

t indicates a table; f indicates a figure

489

Psychiatric disorders. *See also* Comorbid
  psychiatric disorders
  health and lifestyle domains and, 343
  overview, 205–209
  symptoms for adults and, 36–37
Psychoanalytic theory, history of ADHD and,
  10–11
Psychological maladjustment. *See also* Comorbid
  psychiatric disorders
  clinical implications of, 243–244
  Milwaukee Study and, 232–234, 234*t*
  in the offspring of adults with ADHD, 384–
    393, 388*t*, 389*f*, 391*t*, 392*f*
  overview, 205–209, 228–229, 228*t*, 241–244
  parenting stress and, 393
  UMASS Study and, 229–232, 229*t*, 231*t*, 232*f*,
    233*f*
Psychological treatments, history of ADHD and,
  16–17

R

Reading comprehension problems. *See* Learning
  disabilities
Reading disorders. *See* Learning disabilities
Recovery from ADHD, 435–436
Relational functioning. *See also* Dating
  functioning; Marital adjustment
  Milwaukee Study and, 145*t*, 146*f*, 147*t*, 379*t*
  overview, 380–384, 382*t*, 397–399, 447–448
  treatment implications and, 458–459
  UMASS Study, 140*f*, 142*t*
Retrospective childhood symptom ratings
  global impairments and, 438–439
  Milwaukee Study and, 90–91
  UMASS Study and, 96*t*, 97–98
  validation of severity of, 91–94
Rewards programs, 461–462

S

Schizophrenic spectrum disorders, 440
School environment. *See also* Educational
  functioning
  behavioral interventions and, 456–457
  educational functioning and, 245–246
  impaired educational settings and, 250–251, 251*t*
Screening adults for ADHD, with an DSM-IV
  based scale, 113–116, 114*t*
Self-appraisals, driving ability impairment and,
  362

Self-directed play, executive functioning and, 401
Self-esteem, sex differences and, 452
Self-monitoring, 115
Self-questioning, 460
Self-regulation. *See also* Symptoms of ADHD,
  new
  executive functioning and, 401
  money management functioning and, 353–354
  overview, 171–175
Self-report assessments
  comorbid psychiatric disorders and, 224–225,
    227
  diagnosis and, 48–49
  global impairments and, 439
  Milwaukee Study and, 62–64, 66–67, 71
  sex differences and, 451
  UMASS Study and, 45–47
Self-reported symptoms, validation of severity of,
  91–94
Separation, marital, 381, 397. *See also* Marital
  adjustment
Set shifting
  neuropsychological functioning and, 431
  Wisconsin Card Sort Test (WCST) and, 416
Sex differences
  achievement test scores, 261*f*
  adverse educational outcomes, 252
  antisocial activities and, 310, 312*f*, 314
  comorbid psychiatric disorders and, 216
  driving ability impairment and, 364–365, 366,
    368*f*
  educational performance, 258–259, 259*f*
  executive functioning and, 433
  extent of impairment and, 136–137, 137*f*
  health and lifestyle domains and, 348–349, 374
  issue of age of onset criteria and, 119–120
  learning disabilities and, 267–268
  Milwaukee Study and, 5, 56, 72–73
  occupational functioning and, 280–281
  offspring of adults with ADHD and, 385, 390
  other-reported symptoms and, 89–90, 89*f*
  overview, 450–454
  parenting stress and, 396
  psychological maladjustment and, 230–231,
    232*f*, 233*f*
  relationship functioning and, 382–383
  sexual behavior and, 379–380
  substance dependence and abuse and, 296–
    297, 300
  suicidality and, 237
  symptom severity and, 82–83, 82*f*, 83*f*
  UMASS Study and, 50–52, 50*t*, 51*f*, 52*t*, 72–
    73, 89–90, 89*f*